WOUND HEALING - NEW INSIGHTS INTO ANCIENT CHALLENGES

Edited by **Vlad Adrian Alexandrescu**

Wound Healing - New insights into Ancient Challenges
http://dx.doi.org/10.5772/61906
Edited by Vlad Adrian Alexandrescu

Contributors

Allison Cowin, Anuradha Majumdar, Ilknur Altunay, Aslı Aksu Cerman, Christian Agyare, Yaw Duah Boakye, Susanna Oteng Dapaah, Theresa Appiah, Samuel Oppong Bekoe, Emelia Oppong Bekoe, Shiu-Nan Chen, Fan-Hua Nan, Yu-Sheng Wu, Sherwin Chen, Junna Ye, Vlad Alexandrescu, Maggie Hodges, Carlos Zgheib, Kenneth Liechty, Junwang Xu, Craig Mandato, Tatsuya Kato, Eric Boucher, Francisco Jose Nicolas, Carmen Insausti, Ángel Bernabé-García, José María Moraleda, Antonio Piñero, Gregorio Castellanos, Joshua Boateng, Omar Sarheed, Asif Ahmed, Douha Shouqair, Edel P Kavanagh, Sherif Sultan, Niamh Hynes, Wael Tawfick, Moyassar Basil Hadi Al-Shaibani, Anne Dickinson, Penny Lovat, Xiao Wang, Shailesh Chaturvedi, Peter Mekhail, Kazuhito Satomura, Reiko Tokuyama-Toda, Jill Monfre, Mayland Chang, Shahriar Mobashery, Trung Nguyen, Lina Fu, Michele Colonna, Flavia Lupo, Francesco Stagno D'Alcontres, Gabriele Delia, Amir Feily, Luigi Ambrosio, Federica Paladini, Mauro Pollini, Alessandro Sannino, Mohammad Bayat

Published by InTech

Janeza Trdine 9, 51000 Rijeka, Croatia

Publishing Process Manager Andrea Koric

Technical Editor SPi Global

Cover InTech Design team

First published October, 2016

Printed in Croatia

Additional hard copies can be obtained from orders@intechopen.com

Wound Healing - New insights into Ancient Challenges, Edited by Vlad Adrian Alexandrescu

p. cm.

Print ISBN 978-953-51-2678-2
Online ISBN 978-953-51-2679-9

For EU product safety concerns:
IN TECH d.o.o., Prolaz Marije Krucifikse Kozulić 3, 51000 Rijeka, Croatia,
info@intechopen.com or visit our website at intechopen.com.

Meet the editor

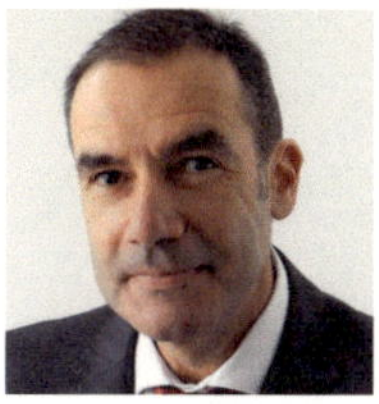

Born in 1958, Dr. Alexandrescu graduated at the Leuven Medical University (UCL, Saint-Luc University) in Brussels in 1994 (with honorary distinction).Adding further to postgraduate stages, he acquired complementary endovascular skills (particularly in carotid, aortic, and below-the-knee peripheral revascularizations) in Saint Joseph Hospital in Marseille (Pr. P. Bergeron and Pr. J. Jausseran), France, and earned particular experience in lower limb CTO recanalization techniques in Leicester Royal Infirmary (Professors P. R. Bell and N. J. London, Vascular Dept. University of Leicester), UK. Currently Dr. Alexandrescu assumes the Chief Department function of the General, Thoracic, and Vascular Surgery Department of the "Princess Paola" Hospital and also Senior Vascular Consultant in the Cardiovascular and Thoracic Surgery Department, CHU Sart Tilman Hospital, University of Medicine, Liège, Belgium. He equally affects institutional "coordination for surgical trainees" in general and vascular surgery, affiliated to the Liège University of Medicine in Belgium. Since 2001, he established and currently participates at the "Multidisciplinary Diabetes Foot Clinic" activities in "Princess Paola" Hospital. Owning more than 53 publications dedicated to endovascular peripheral treatment, diabetic limb-salvage techniques, and tissue regeneration in different surgical and medical journals, Dr. Alexandrescu promotes specific inferior limb reperfusion techniques such as targeted below-the-knee angioplasties following the "angiosome" model of vascularization.

Contents

Preface

I decided to bring up a multidisciplinary volume concerning wound healing, since in my everyday activity, as a surgeon, I am constantly confronted to impressive complexity of tissue regeneration process, singular yet multifaceted for each given patient. Wound regeneration unceasingly staggers scientists and clinicians in revealing its intricacy and constant unfolding, as life's movement itself. Tissue repair seems to bear thousands of overlapping molecular and macroscopic processes, all capable to target specific dysfunctions also parallel remedies, only partially revealed to our knowledge.

My main goal in building this work is to try to uplift the reader's awareness on the latest genetic, molecular, pharmaceutical, medical, surgical, and physiotherapeutic approaches for tissue regeneration, at this moment of soaring technologies and bursting medical information. Many of yesterday's "hopeless foot wounds" reveal nowadays unanticipated limb preservation longings and new expectation for survival. The chapters of this book are conventionally gathered in four main groups of interest, although largely overlapping by indisputable entangled content. As technology evolves, parallel new challenges in cell and tissue engineering, gene, or nanotechnologies (part I), clinical diagnostic, drugs, surgical or endovascular novel approaches (part II), pharmacological research, serviceable dressings (part III), or traditional medications (part IV) become highly indispensable in daily medical practice. Therefore, it is with particular admiration that I greet all participant authors for kindly sharing their erudition and compiling each dedicated chapter at highest scientific level, although influential building blocks of this volume.

I long for that this book may enable the eager clinician or researcher to overcome part of undeniable challenges in his or her current practice and partake with their teams and patients a greater diligence in wound treatment and tissue healing. I would like to express my real gratitude to all remarkable scientists, medical colleagues, specialized nurses, physiotherapists, and statisticians and all those who contributed in fulfilling this work and for every step forward that they eventually enhanced throughout this publication.

Vlad-Adrian Alexandrescu, MD

Department of Vascular, Endovascular and Thoracic Surgery

Princess Paola Hospital, Marche-en-Famenne, IFAC/Vivalia

CHU Sart Tilman Hospital, University of Medicine, Liège, Belgium

Section 1

Molecular and Cellular Aspects for Tissue Regeneration

Chapter 1

The Role of MicroRNAs in Impaired Diabetic Wound Healing

Maggie M. Hodges, Carlos Zgheib, Junwang Xu and Kenneth W. Liechty

Additional information is available at the end of the chapter

http://dx.doi.org/10.5772/63637

Abstract

Diabetes mellitus is a worldwide pandemic, affecting 29 million Americans, resulting in substantial morbidity and mortality, and accounting for an annual healthcare expenditure exceeding $176 billion in the US alone. This burden of disease is the result of a progressive disease associated with numerous complications and the development of chronic wounds, which remain the leading cause of hospital admissions and nontraumatic lower extremity amputations in diabetic patients. Despite clinical strategies aimed at prevention and early detection, patients with diabetes continue to remain at risk of developing chronic diabetic wounds due to poor patient compliance and progression of the diabetic phenotype. Development of the diabetic phenotype and wound healing impairment is associated with dysregulation of microRNAs that regulate inflammation, extracellular matrix composition, and angiogenesis; here we present evidence from the studies that demonstrate correction of microRNA dysregulation expedites wound healing and reverses the diabetic skin phenotype.

Keywords: microRNA, diabetic wound healing, inflammation, angiogenesis, extracellular matrix

1. Introduction

Diabetes mellitus is a worldwide pandemic, affecting 29 million Americans and over 171 million peoples worldwide, resulting in substantial morbidity and mortality, and accounting for an annual healthcare expenditure exceeding $176 billion in the US alone (Data from the 2014 National diabetes fact sheet; available at http://www.cdc.gov/diabetes/pdfs/data/2014-report-estimates-of-diabetes-and-its-burden-in-the-united-states.pdf). This burden of disease is the result of a progressive disease process associated with numerous complications, such as retinopathy, neuropathy, and nephropathy, as well as the development of chronic wounds. Chronic wounds remain the leading cause of hospital admissions and nontraumatic lower extremity amputations in patients with diabetes, with nearly 80% of all amputations performed in patients with diabetes preceded by a diabetic wound [1]. Risk factors for the development of diabetic wounds include the presence of the "pathogenic triad" of neuropathy, ischemia, and trauma [2–4]. In addition, foot deformities, lower extremity edema, and use of inappropriate footwear also contribute to the development of diabetic wounds [2–4].

Despite clinical strategies aimed at prevention and early detection of diabetic neuropathy and diabetic wounds, patients with diabetes continue to have a 12–25% lifetime risk of developing a chronic diabetic wound due to poor patient compliance and progression of the diabetic phenotype [5, 6]. Projections indicate that by 2025 diabetes will affect over 300 million people worldwide, with a rising proportion of the burden borne by patients in developing countries [7, 8]. Given this anticipated rise in the burden of disease attributable to diabetes, and the potential concomitant rise in development of chronic wounds, the impetus for developing more effective wound care strategies cannot be understated.

After injury, patients with diabetes suffer from an impaired wound healing response; the standard wound healing response, in which the tissue passes through consecutive, but overlapping phases of coagulation, inflammation, proliferation, and remodeling, is disrupted [2]. Notably, patients with diabetes demonstrate a phenotype characterized by decreased angiogenesis, impaired leukocyte migration, decreased growth factor production, sustained inflammation, impaired fibroblast function, and imbalance of extracellular matrix deposition and remodeling, and delayed wound healing [9]. A longer duration of diabetes has been associated with a greater risk of impaired wound healing; consistent with this observation, duration of diabetes has been correlated with more profound diabetic neuropathy, increasingly compromised biomechanical properties of diabetic skin, and an increasingly delayed rate of endothelial progenitor cell proliferation. While the cytokines, chemokines, and cellular components of the wound healing response have been extensively studied, recent attention has focused upon the role that microRNAs (miRNAs) play in the impaired healing of diabetic wounds [3].

MiRNAs are a class of small, noncoding RNA molecules, 20-22 nucleotides long, that regulate gene expression at the posttranscriptional level [10]. Complementary binding of miRNAs to the 3′-untranslated region (UTR) of their target messenger RNA (mRNA) results in posttranscriptional repression and/or mRNA degradation, thereby regulating the expression of downstream targets [11]. MiRNA are thought to regulate over one-third of all physiologic processes, including regulation of cell cycle progression, apoptosis, cytokine transcription, cellular metabolic function, signal transduction, proliferation, and determination of cell fate [12, 13]. MicroRNAs are being investigated for their role as biomarkers, diagnostic tools, and therapies in a variety of disease states, including diabetes and numerous types of cancer [14, 15]. Key to the development of the diabetic phenotype is the dysregulation of the expression of miRNA that regulate inflammation, extracellular matrix composition, and angiogenesis.

Here we discuss data that demonstrate correction of microRNA dysregulation expedites wound healing and reverses the diabetic phenotype in skin [16–18].

2. Methods

2.1. Murine model of diabetic wound healing

We utilized a murine model of diabetes, using genetically diabetic female mice homozygous for the leptin receptor mutation (db/db, C57BKS.Cg-m-/-*Leprdb*/J) and age-matched, nondiabetic, heterozygous controls (db/-), obtained from the Jackson Laboratory (Bar Harbor, ME). Leptin is a centrally acting hormone that modulates both satiety and body fat content [19, 20]. Mice homozygous for the leptin receptor mutation develop hyperphagia, obesity, hyperglycemia, insulin resistance, and hyperlipidemia, leading to their extensive use as a murine model of diabetes [19, 20]. Between 4 and 6 weeks of age, the diabetic mice are significantly more obese and hyperglycemic than their nondiabetic counterparts (**Figure 1**), and by 10–14 weeks of age, diabetic mice weigh greater than 45 g, with serum glucose levels in excess of 400 mg/dL, whereas nondiabetic mice weighed less than 25 g, with serum blood glucose levels less than 250 mg/dL [21]. Most noteworthy for our analysis, diabetic mice also demonstrate significantly delayed wound healing when compared with nondiabetic mice, requiring up to 5 days longer to close cutaneous wounds (**Figure 2**) [21, 22].

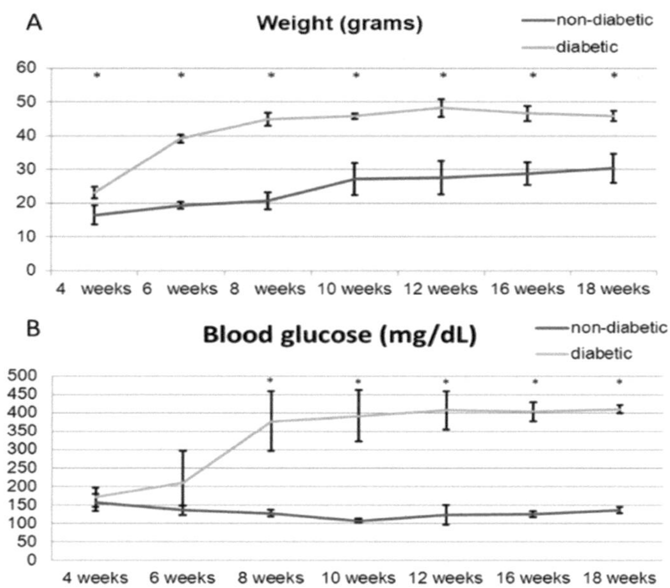

Figure 1. Weight (A) and serum blood glucose (B) of diabetic and nondiabetic mice. (A) Weight of diabetic (C57BKS.Cg-m-/-*Leprdb*/J) and nondiabetic (C57BKS.Cg-m-/+*Leprdb*/J) mice at different ages. **(B)** Serum blood glucose levels in diabetic and nondiabetic mice at different ages. Asterisk (*) indicates $p < 0.05$ for any given time point (Image reproduced from Zgheib *et al.* [21] with permission of the authors.)

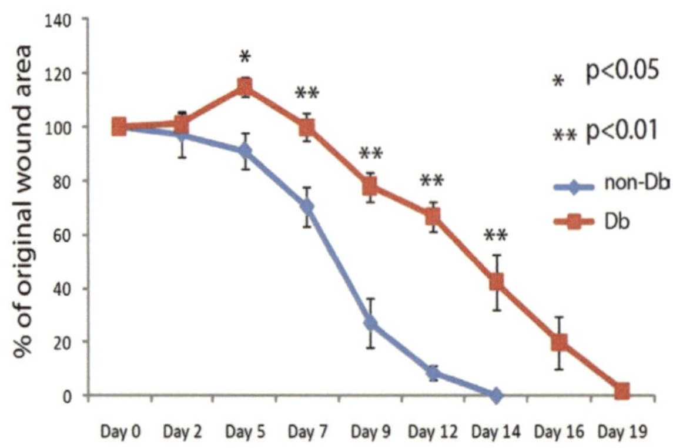

Figure 2. Wound closure in diabetic and nondiabetic mice. The percent (%) of original wound area remaining at various time points during the wound healing process in diabetic and nondiabetic mice. Asterisk (*) indicates $p < 0.05$ and (**) indicates $p < 0.001$.

To obtain a baseline, unwounded skin from the dorsum of diabetic and nondiabetic mice was harvested, and the cranial-caudal orientation was preserved for the purposes of biomechanical testing. Diabetic and nondiabetic mice between 10 and 14 weeks of age had full thickness, excisional dermal wounds created using an 8 mm dermal punch biopsy (Miltex, Inc., York, PA) through the panniculus carnosus, as previously described [17, 21]. Following the initial wounding, mice were treated with either phosphate buffered saline (PBS), 10^6 mesenchymal stem cells (MSCs),and 1×10^6 plaque forming units (PFU) of either an empty lentiviral vector or a lentiviral construct containing a mutated stromal cell derived factor (SDF-1α) transgene, or 10 μL of 100 ng/mL of recombinant human SDF-1α protein. The wounded skin was harvested at 1, 3, 7, 14, and 21 days after initial wounding and animals were euthanized by inhalation of carbon dioxide followed by cervical dislocation.

2.2. Isolation of MSCs

MSCs were isolated from the femurs and tibia of adult C57BL/6TbN (act-GFP) OsbY01 transgenic (GFP) mice, as described previously [17]. Mononuclear cells were then separated by density gradient separation using Ficoll before being suspended at a density of 2.5×10^4 cells/μL in PBS [23].

2.3. Human skin analysis

Human skin samples were obtained via the National Disease Research Interchange (NDRI). Human skin samples measuring 5 × 5 cm were obtained from the anterior portion of the lower extremities within 8 h postmortem. The samples were obtained from patients who were between 45 and 75 years old, without significant comorbidity, malignancy, or a history of radiation or chemotherapy. While it was known whether or not the patients carried an existing diagnosis of diabetes, as well as what medications the individual was currently taking, data regarding the duration of diabetes, degree of blood glucose control, or intensity of sun exposure was not available. Following receipt of the sample, subcutaneous tissues were sharply excised from the dermis and the skin samples intended for biomechanical analysis were immediately flash frozen in liquid nitrogen.

2.4. Culture of dermal fibroblasts

Human skin samples and murine skin samples were processed in order to enable the culture of dermal fibroblasts for further *in vitro* analysis. Skin samples were washed in 70% ethanol for 2 min, followed by 3 washes in PBS. Subcutaneous tissues were sharply excised from overlying dermis, and the remaining dermis was minced before being digested in 2 mL of 1000 u/mL Collagenase for 1 h at 37°C. The sample was then centrifuged at 1000 rpm for 5 min, the supernatant was removed, and the sample was then digested in 5 mL of dispase (1.9 u/mL) for 30 min at 37°C. The sample was again centrifuged at 1000 rpm for 5 min, the supernatant was removed, and the remaining pieces of dermis were mixed with 10 mL of DMEM with 10% fetal bovine serum (FBS, Life Technologies, Calrsbad, CA) and 1% antibiotic-antimycotic (Life Technologies, Calrsbad, CA) and plated in a 100 mm tissue culture plate (Corning Incorporate, Corning, NY). When fibroblasts were observed to proliferate and adhere to the tissue culture plate independent of the pieces of dermis, the dermis was removed, the plate was washed twice with 10 mL PBS, and the culture media was replaced. Cells between passage 1 and 4 were used for these experiments.

2.5. Lentiviral construction

The SDF-1α mutant that was utilized binds the CXCR4 receptor without activating it [24, 25]. According to the manufacturer's instruction, a complementary DNA (cDNA) library was prepared from mouse tissues using TRIzol and Superscript (Invitrogen, Carlsbad, CA). After sequence analysis confirmed the SDF1α cDNA and the SDF1α inhibitor (SDFαi), the CS-CG HIV-1 transfer plasmid was used to generate a self-inactivating lentiviral vector designed to convey expression of either the green fluorescent protein reporter gene (GFP, Clontech Laboratories, Mountain View, CA) or the mutant SDF1αi with the GFP reporter gene under the control of a cytomegalovirus promoter [25–27]. The ability of the plasmid to effectively transfect cells was tested on murine dermal fibroblasts *in vitro* prior to *in vivo* use.

2.6. Biomechanical testing

In order to assess the biomechanical properties of murine and human diabetic and nondiabetic skin, all samples immediately underwent biomechanical testing after harvesting. Biomechanical testing was performed on the diabetic and nondiabetic murine samples at baseline, 4 weeks, and 7 weeks after wounding. Prior to testing, the subcutaneous tissues were removed, and a uniform dumbbell-shaped testing unit was stamped out from the sampled skin [28, 29]. The cranial–caudal orientation of each sample was maintained, and the healed wound, if present, was centrally located within the testing unit. Two lines of Verhoeff stain were placed on either end of the sample, thereby identifying the length of the testing area. The mean cross-sectional area of each sample was then measured using a custom laser band [30]. Each sample underwent testing to calculate the modulus of elasticity and the maximum stress until failure, as previously described [29].

2.7. Immunohistochemistry

Endogenous peroxidase activity was blocked with 0.3% hydrogen peroxide in methanol. GFP was detected with application of rabbit anti-GFP primary antiserum (1:100; Invitrogen, Carlsbad, CA) followed by biotinylated antirabbit secondary antibody (1:200), and the slides were developed using avidin–biotin complex (Vector Laboratories, Burlingame, CA). Slides were counterstained with hematoxylin. For double-immunofluorescent staining, sections were blocked with 1% sodium borohydrate (Sigma–Aldrich, St. Louis, MO) in PBS. Platelet endothelial cell adhesion molecule-1 (CD31) was used an endothelial marker. CD31 was detected by using rat anti-mouse CD31 antibody (1:20 dilution; Invitrogen, Carlsbad, CA and AbCam, Cambridge, MA) followed by biotinylated rabbit anti-rat secondary antibody and detection with the alkaline phosphatase detection system (Vector Laboratories, Burlingame, CA). GFP was detected by using the same rabbit anti-GFP primary antiserum followed by Alexa-Fluor-488-conjugated F (ab') 2 secondary antibodies (1:100; Invitrogen). Slides were counterstained with 4,6-diamidino-2-phenylindole (Vector Laboratories, Burlingame, CA).

Sections were stained for cluster of differentiation (CD) 45, which was used as a cellular marker for inflammatory cells, and antigen retrieval was performed using 13 Antigen Retrieval Citra (BioGenex HK086-9k, Fremont, CA) in a decloaking chamber using the factory default settings (Biocare Medical, Concard, CA). Slides were rinsed three times in 0.1% PBST (0.1% Triton100 in PBS), blocked in 20% goat serum in 0.4% PBST for 60 min at room temperature, and incubated overnight at room temperature with primary antibodies against CD 45 (rabbit polyclonal ab10558, 1:100; Abcam, Cambridge, MA) in 5% goat serum and 0.1% PBST. The following day, slides were washed three times in 0.1% PBST and incubated with the appropriate anti-rabbit biotinylated secondary antibodies for 1 h at room temperature. Slides were washed three times in 0.1% PBST and mounted in Vectashield (Vector Laboratories, Burlingame, CA). The slides were then incubated with avidin–biotin–peroxidase complex (Vector Laboratory) and developed, as described by the manufacturer. The mean number of either CD45 or CD31 positive cells per high power field (hpf) was calculated as the average of 5 hpf per slide.

2.8. Enzyme-linked immunosorbent assay and Western Blot

Skin samples had their subcutaneous tissues removed before being flash frozen in liquid nitrogen immediately after harvest. Collagen content was quantified by Western Blot. Skin samples were cut into 1-mm pieces and homogenized in a 0.5 M acetic acid solution containing 1× protease inhibitor cocktail and 5 mmol/L EDTA, in order to solubilize total collagen. The solution was then centrifuged for 4 h at 4°C at 16.1×10^3 G, the lipid layer was aspirated, and this process was repeated. Bicinchoninic acid protein assay was used to quantify the total protein concentration of the supernatant, and Western blot was performed using standard techniques, and final protein concentrations were standardized to 1 μg/2 μL using a sample buffer before being boiled at 95°C for 5 min. Tris–acetate gels (3–8%) were run at 150 V for 1 h, transferred to 30 V overnight at 4°C, rinsed with Tris-buffered saline, and were subsequently blocked with 5% milk in Tris-buffered saline with 0.1% Tween for 1 h. Collagen I antibody (Abcam Inc., Cambridge, MA) was diluted to 1:2000 (collagen III to 1:1000) and blots were incubated for 1 h at room temperature, washed with Tris-buffered saline with 0.1% Tween, and incubated with secondary antibody (anti-rabbit IgG horseradish peroxidase; GE Healthcare, Marlborough, MA) at 1:10,000 for 1 h at room temperature. Western blots were washed with Tris-buffered saline with 0.1% Tween and then Tris-buffered saline. The blots were then developed using a standard chemiluminescence solution (ECL solution A and B; GE Healthcare, Marlborough, MA) and incubated for 1 min.

2.9. Real-time polymerase chain reaction

Total RNA was extracted and purified from skin samples after homogenization in TRIzol (Invitrogen and Life Technologies, Carlsbad, CA), following the manufacturer's instructions. RNA was converted into cDNA using the SuperScript First-Strand Synthesis System (Invitrogen and Life Technologies, Carlsbad, CA). Random primers were used for the reverse transcription reaction and real-time quantitative polymerase chain reaction (PCR) was performed with either the CFX96 real-time PCR thermal cycler (Bio-Rad, Hercules, CA) or the ABI 7900 realtime PCR thermal cycler (Applied Biosystems, Foster City, CA). These samples were amplified in triplicate using primers for NFkB, IRAK1, TRAF6, IL-6, MIP-2 (IL-8), col1a2, col3a1, VEGF, BCL-2, HIF-1α, miR-146a, miR-15b, and miR-29a (TaqMan gene expression assay, Applied Biosystems, Foster City, CA). Internal normalization was achieved by using the 18 s housekeeping gene as an internal control for mRNA and the U6 housekeeping gene as an internal control for miRNA.

3. Impaired wound healing observed in diabetes is associated with impaired microRNA expression

3.1. Sustained inflammation: the role of mir-146a

While inflammation plays an integral role in normal wound healing, the presence of pathologically sustained inflammation is a chief component of the dysregulated wound healing observed in patients with diabetes [15, 31]. The inflammatory phase of wound healing is characterized by increased infiltration of inflammatory cells (neutrophils and macrophages) and release of inflammatory mediators, such as cytokines [32]. Both the cellular and cytokine response to injury are mediated by microRNA. Specifically, miR-146a has been identified as a key regulator of the nuclear factor kappa-B (NFkB) pathway, which is known to regulate numerous inflammatory processes, as well as the transcription of several inflammatory cytokines [33, 34]. Following activation of the NFkB pathway by toll-like receptors (TLRs), NFkB expression is positively regulated by interleukin-1 receptor-associated kinase 1 (IRAK1) and TNF receptor associated factor 6 (TRAF6) [35]. Increased activity of IRAK1 and TRAF6 result in increased NFkB activity, which then upregulates the expression of genes coding for the key proinflammatory cytokines interleukin-6 (IL-6) and IL-8 [17]. However, NFkB activity can also induce the expression of miR-146a, which inhibits IRAK1 and TRAF6, thereby acting as a brake on the NFkB dependent innate immune response [36].

Analysis of skin samples obtained from wounded diabetic and nondiabetic mice demonstrates significant downregulation of the anti-inflammatory miR-146a in diabetic mice during the course of wound healing (**Figure 3**) [17]. In addition to down regulation of miR-146a, wounded diabetic skin demonstrates significantly elevated expression of mRNA coding for IRAK1, TRAF6, NFkB, and the proinflammatory cytokines IL-6 and IL-8 (with MIP2 being the murine equivalent of IL-8) (**Figure 3**) [17].

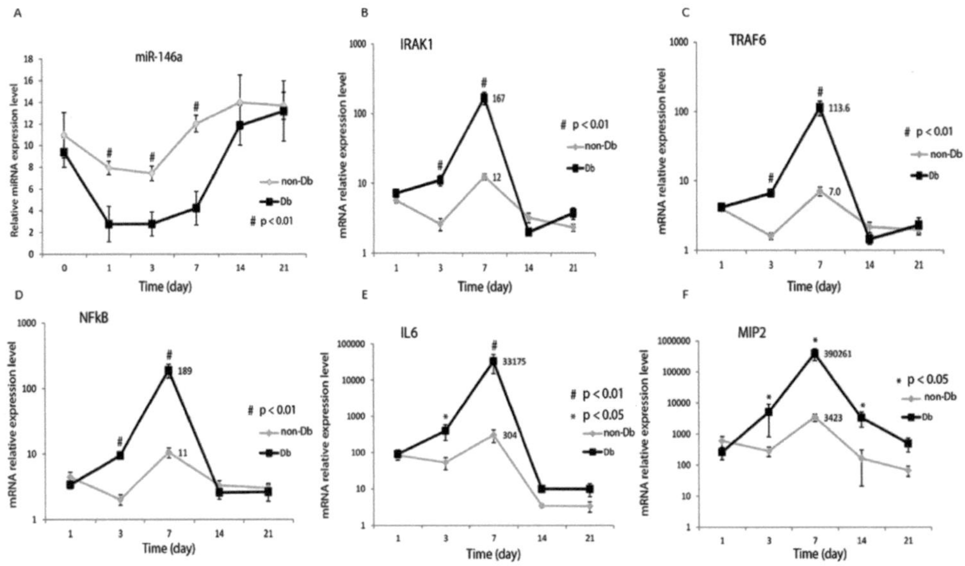

Figure 3. Quantification of miRNA-146a and components of the NFkB pathway in diabetic and nondiabetic wounds. Real-time PCR quantification of miR-146a **(A)**, IRAK1 **(B)**, TRAF6 **(C)**, NFkB **(D)**, and the downstream end products IL-6 **(E)** and MIP2 **(F)** (the murine equivalent of IL-8) days 0–21 after wounding in diabetic and nondiabetic mice. Results are presented as a mean + SEM for each cohort at each time point. Asterisk (*) indicates $p < 0.05$ and # indicates $p < 0.01$. (Image reproduced from Xu *et al.* [17] with permission of the authors.)

3.2. Impaired biomechanical properties and deposition of extracellular matrix: the role of miR-29a

In addition to dysregulation of the maturation phase of wound healing, diabetic skin has been shown to be biomechanically impaired at baseline, with decreased maximum load, maximum stress prior to failure, and decreased elasticity, as seen in **Figure 4** [21, 29]. It is thought this baseline impairment is one of the many factors that place even intact diabetic skin at a higher risk of injury than nondiabetic skin, with continued dysregulation of extracellular matrix remodeling contributing to impaired healing after injury [15, 29]. In addition, the balance of matrix metalloproteinases (MMPs) and tissue inhibitors of matrix metalloproteinases (TIMPs) in diabetic wounds is weighted toward increased breakdown of extracellular matrix components, contributing to poor wound healing [2, 31, 37].

MiR-29a contributes to this impaired extracellular matrix remodeling by posttranscriptional regulation of collagen content, leading to an inverse relationship between miR-29a levels and collagen content [38, 39]. **Figure 5** details the significant upregulation of miR-29a gene expression that has been detected in both diabetic murine (**Figure 5A**) and diabetic human skin (**Figure 5B**). This miR-29a dysregulation corresponded to elevated gene expression of collagen 1α2 (col1α2) and collagen 3α1 (col3α1) in murine diabetic skin when compared with nondiabetic skin (**Figure 6**); however, Western blot confirmed decreased levels of both col1α2 and col3α1 protein in diabetic murine skin, versus nondiabetic murine skin (**Figure 6**). During the maturation phase of wound healing, the extracellular matrix undergoes remodeling

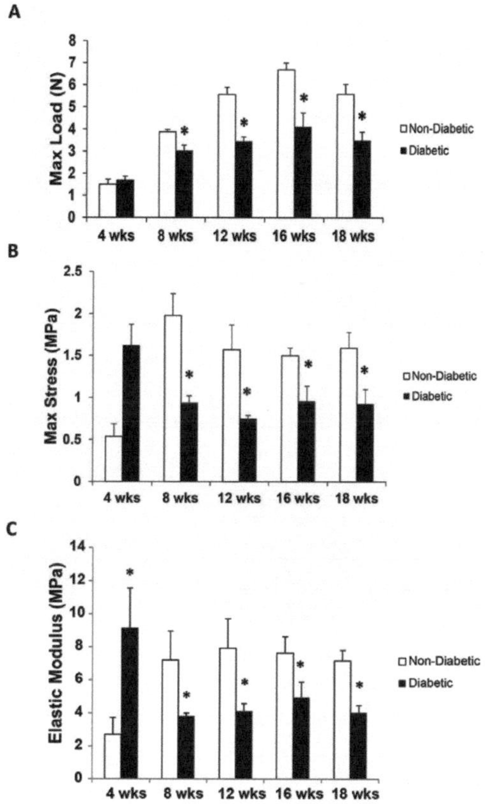

Figure 4. Baseline biomechanical properties of diabetic and non-diabetic skin. (A) The maximum load sustained **(N)** prior to failure in diabetic versus nondiabetic skin samples over 4–18 weeks of age. **(B)** The maximum stress to failure (MPa) in diabetic versus nondiabetic skin samples over 4–18 weeks of age. **(C)**: The elastic modulus (MPa) measured in diabetic versus non-diabetic skin samples over 4–18 weeks of age. Data is presented as a mean + standard error of the mean (SEM) for each cohort. Student's *t*-test was used to compare nondiabetic skin vs. diabetic skin at each time point. Asterisk (*) indicates $p < 0.05$. Abbreviation: Max = Maximum. (Image reproduced from Zgheib *et al.* [21] with permission of the authors.)

characterized by type III collagen being replaced by type I collagen, and this process is thought to be impaired in diabetic skin [15].

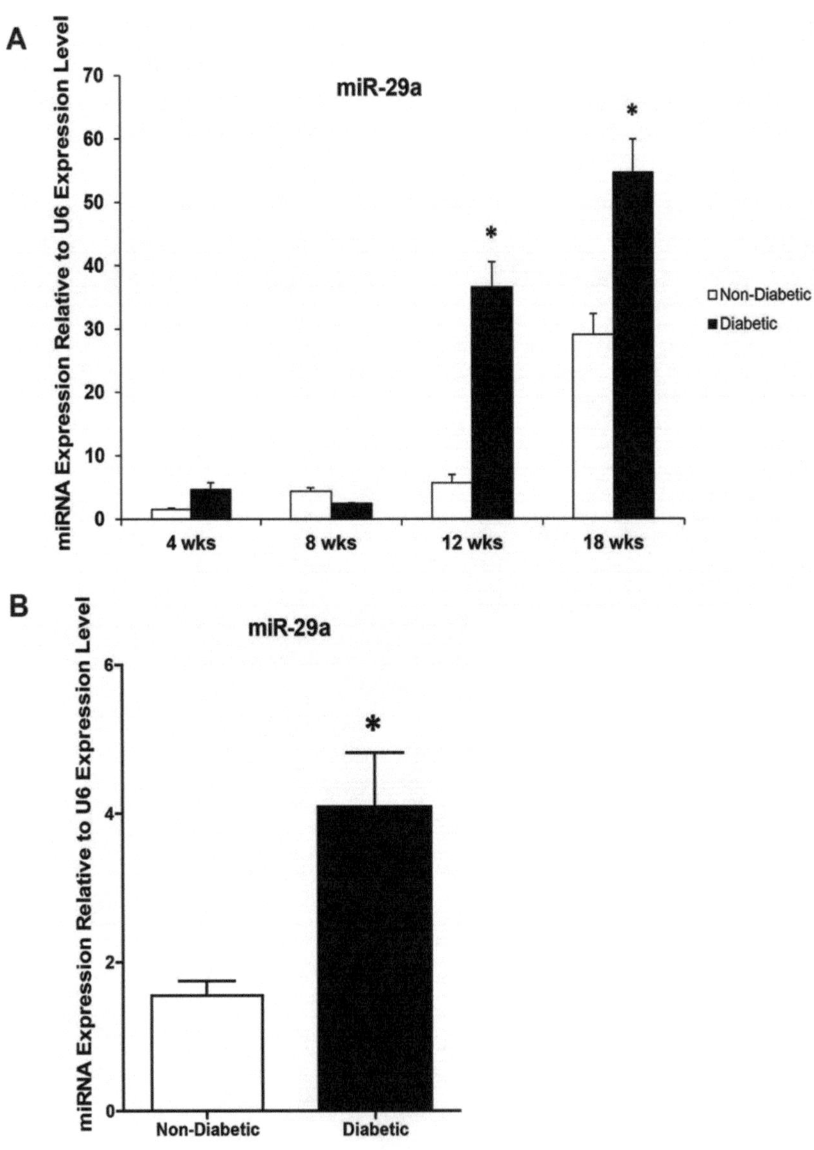

Figure 5. MiRNA-29a gene expression in diabetic and nondiabetic murine (A) and human **(B)** skin. **(A)** Real-time quantitative PCR analysis of miRNA-29a levels in murine diabetic and nondiabetic skin at different age-points. **(B)** Real-time quantitative PCR analysis of miRNA-29a levels in human diabetic and nondiabetic skin. MiR-29a gene expression was calculated after normalizing with U6. Results are presented as a mean + SEM for each cohort. Student's *t*-test was used to compare nondiabetic skin to diabetic skin at each time point. Asterisk (*) indicates $p < 0.05$. (Image reproduced from Zgheib *et al.* [21] with permission of the authors.)

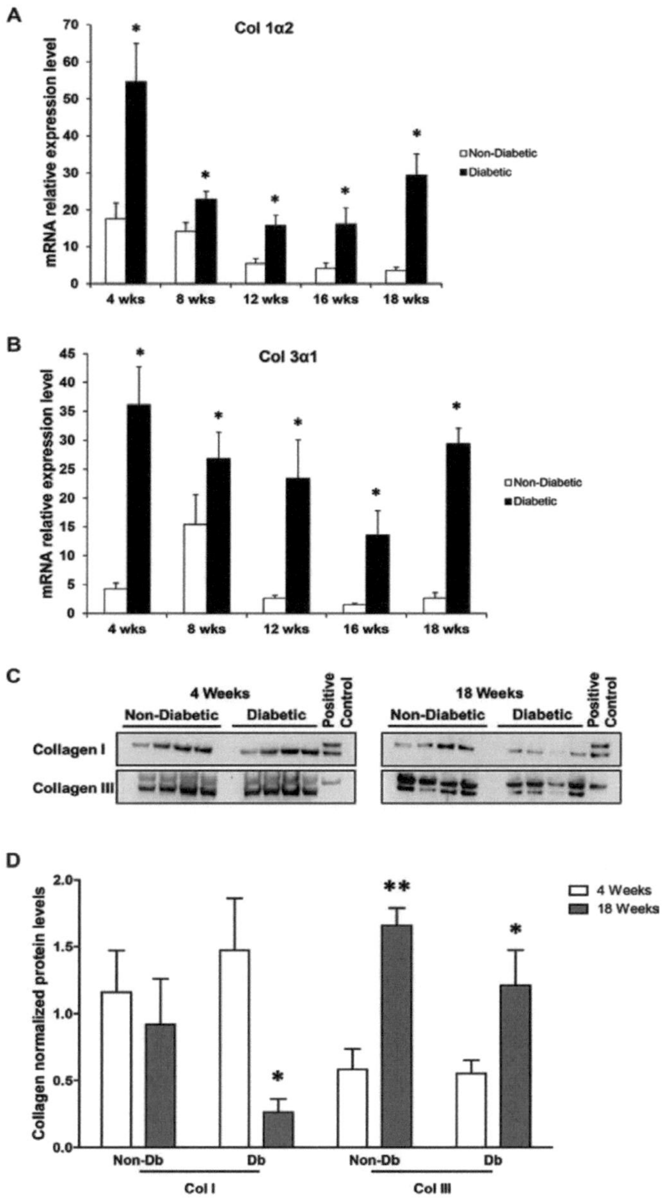

Figure 6. Collagen gene and protein expression in diabetic and non-diabetic murine skin. (A) Relative gene expression for collagen 1α2 in skin samples from diabetic (n = 5) and non-diabetic (n = 5) mice from 4 to 18 weeks of age. **(B)** Relative gene expression for collagen 3α1 in skin samples from diabetic (n = 5) and non-diabetic (n = 5) mice from 4 to 18 weeks of age. **(C)** Collagen I and III protein levels (upper band; black arrows) as demonstrated by western blots, obtained from skin samples from age-matched, non-diabetic and diabetic mice at 4 and 18 weeks of age. **(D)** Collagen I and III protein levels as quantified by western blot. These findings are representative of five independent experiments. Data is presented as a mean + SEM for each cohort. Student's *t*-test was used to compare non-diabetic skin to diabetic skin at each time point. Asterisk (*) indicates $p < 0.05$; ** indicates $p < 0.001$. (Image reproduced from Zgheib *et al.* [21] with permission of the authors.)

3.3. Decreased angiogenesis: the role of miR-15b

Successful angiogenesis requires coordinated extracellular matrix production in order to provide an adequate architecture for formation of new blood vessels [31]. However, angiogenesis within a wound bed is further regulated by numerous angiogenic factors, with vascular endothelial growth factor (VEGF) considered one of the most prominent [40]. Following injury, hypoxia in the wound bed leads to increased expression of hypoxia inducible factor-1 (HIF-1), a transcription factor that increases the expression of numerous proangiogenic proteins, including VEGF [31, 41]. In turn, VEGF attracts endothelial cells to the site of injury, in addition to inducing proliferation and angiogenesis via upregulation of proteins, such as the anti-apoptotic B-cell lymphoma-2 (BCL-2) [16, 40]. BCL-2 is also thought to improve wound healing by stabilizing the alpha subunit of HIF-1 (HIF-1α), mediated by heat shock protein 90 (HSP90), thereby increasing HIF-1 mediated VEGF expression [16]. When compared to nondiabetic murine wounds, diabetic murine wounds have been detailed to have decreased levels of HIF-1a activity, VEGF gene expression, and BCL-2 gene expression, as well as significantly decreased number of cells that stain for the presence of platelet endothelial cell adhesion molecule 31 (CD31), a marker of endothelial cells [42].

MiR-15b negatively regulates angiogenesis by decreasing VEGF expression; this decrease in VEGF expression is associated with decreased cell migration and vascular tubule formation

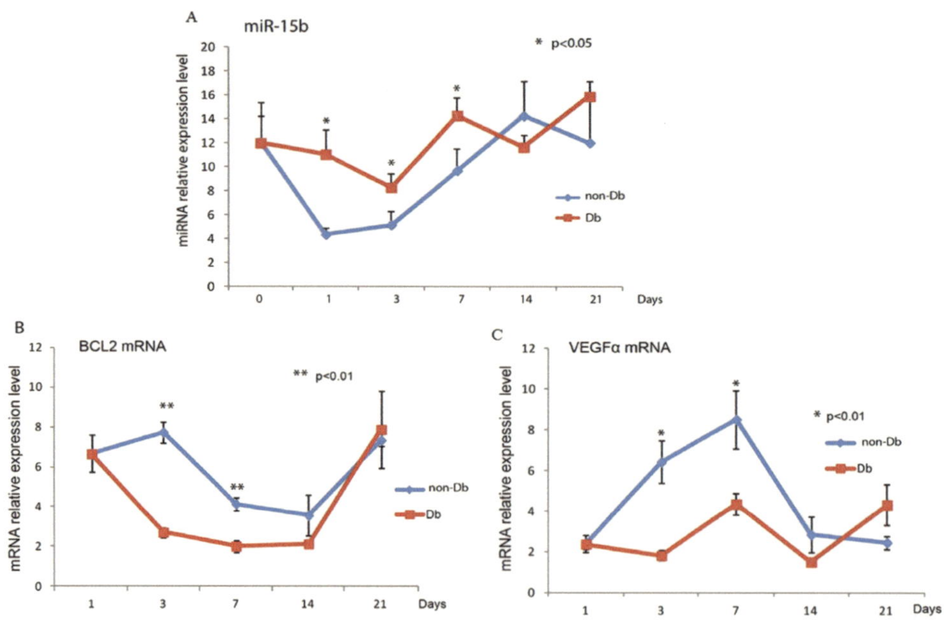

Figure 7. Quantification of miRNA-15b, BCL2, and VEGFα gene expression in diabetic and non-diabetic wounds. Quantification by real-time PCR of miRNA-15b (miR-15b) **(A)**, BCL2 **(B)**, and VEGFα **(C)** gene expression in murine diabetic wounds versus murine non-diabetic wounds, 3–7 days after wounding. Results are presented as a mean + SEM for each cohort at each time point. Asterisk (*) indicates $p < 0.05$ and ** indicates $p < 0.001$. (Image reproduced from Xu *et al.* [16] with permission of the authors.)

in vitro [43]. In nondiabetic humans and mice, the hypoxic conditions following wounding decrease the expression of miR-15b, leading to increased levels of HIF-1α, VEGF, and BCL-2. However, in our murine model of diabetic wound healing, miR-15b expression was significantly upregulated in diabetic mice compared to nondiabetic mice 1, 3, and 7 days after wounding (**Figure 7**). Furthermore, the upregulation in miR-15b expression observed in diabetic mice was associated with a significant downregulation in VEGF and BCL-2 gene expression 3 and 7 days after wounding (**Figure 7**).

4. Therapeutic targets

4.1. The impact of cellular therapies on diabetic wound healing

In the setting of the tremendous clinical and fiscal burden of chronic diabetic wounds, efforts to develop effective wound care strategies are ongoing. The dysregulation of wound healing in patients with diabetes occurs at every stage of healing—whether it be the inflammatory phase, the proliferative phase, or the remodeling phase. Given this widespread dysregulation, therapies directed at individual targets of the wound healing response are unlikely to be completely successful in addressing the diabetic wound healing impairment. As such,

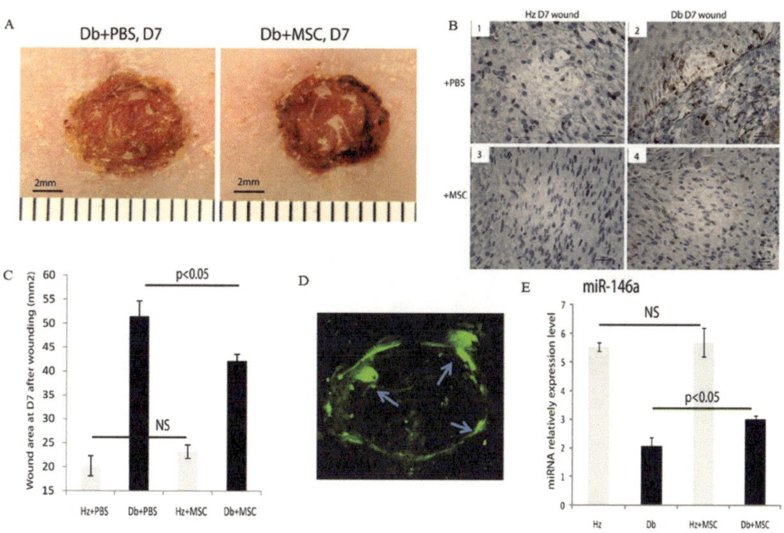

Figure 8. Treatment of diabetic wounds with MSCs expedites wound closure and upregulates miRNA-146a, 7 days after wounding. (A) Diabetic wounds treated with PBS (left) or MSCs (right). **(B)** CD45 immunostaining of diabetic (Db) and nondiabetic (Hz) wounds, following treatment with either PBS or MSCs. **(C)** Quantitative assessment of diabetic (Db) and nondiabetic (Hz) wound closure, following treatment with either PBS or MSCs. **(D)** Flourescent image demonstrating GFP positive cells (MSCs), confirming the persistence of MSCs after injection. Blue arrows indicate injection sites. **(E)** Real-time PCR confirms the upregulation of miRNA-146a gene expression in Db treated with MSCs, compared with Db wounds treated with PBS. Results are presented as a mean + SEM for each cohort at each time point. Asterisk (*) indicates $p < 0.05$ and ** indicates $p < 0.001$. (Image reproduced from Xu *et al.* [17] with permission of the authors.)

attention has been drawn to the use of cell-based therapies for the treatment of chronic diabetic wounds, with the hopes that multipotent cell therapy will address impaired diabetic wound healing at multiple levels of dysregulation [41]. Specifically, MSCs have been a focus due to their capacity for self-renewal, multipotency, and their ease of retrieval from autologous bone marrow [44].

4.1.1. Impact of mesenchymal stem cell treatment on miR-146a

Treatment of diabetic and nondiabetic murine wounds with either MSCs or PBS revealed that treatment of diabetic wounds with MSCs corrected the dysregulated inflammation present in diabetic wounds. Seven days after treatment with MSCs, diabetic murine skin demonstrated more rapid wound healing, a decreased concentration of CD45 positive cells in the periwound tissues, increased expression of miR-146a, and decreased gene expression of IRAK1, TRAF6, NFkB, and the proinflammatory cytokines IL-6 and IL-8/MIP-2 (**Figure 8** and **Figure 9**).

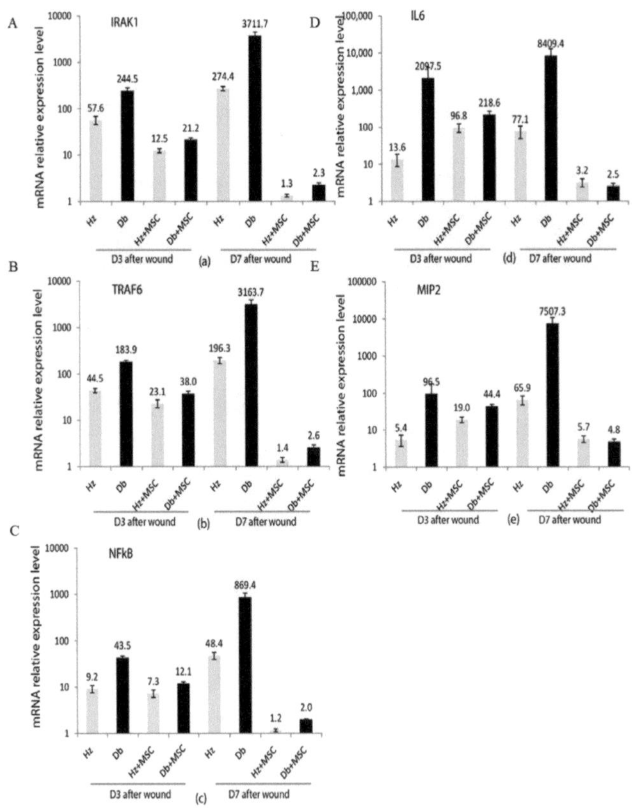

Figure 9. Impact of MSC treatment on IRAK1, TRAF6, NFkB, IL-6, and MIP2 gene expression. Real-time PCR demonstrating the impact of treatment with either MSCs or PBS on gene expression of IRAK1 **(A)**, TRAF6 **(B)**, NFkB **(C)**, IL-6 **(D)**, and MIP2 **(E)** 3 and 7 days after wounding in diabetic and non-diabetic mice Results are presented as a mean + SEM for each cohort at each time point. Asterisk (*) indicates $p < 0.05$ and ** indicates $p < 0.001$. (Image reproduced from Xu *et al.* [17] with permission of the authors.)

4.1.2. *Impact of mesenchymal stem cell treatment on miR-29a*

The expedited diabetic wound healing observed after treatment of diabetic skin with MSCs is not solely associated with decreased inflammation. In addition to upregulating gene expression of miR-146a, treatment with MSCs downregulates miR-29a expression in diabetic murine wounds when compared with nondiabetic murine wounds. The downregulation in miR-29a 4 weeks after treatment with MSCs is accompanied by an upregulation in collagen I and collagen III protein content (**Figure 10**).

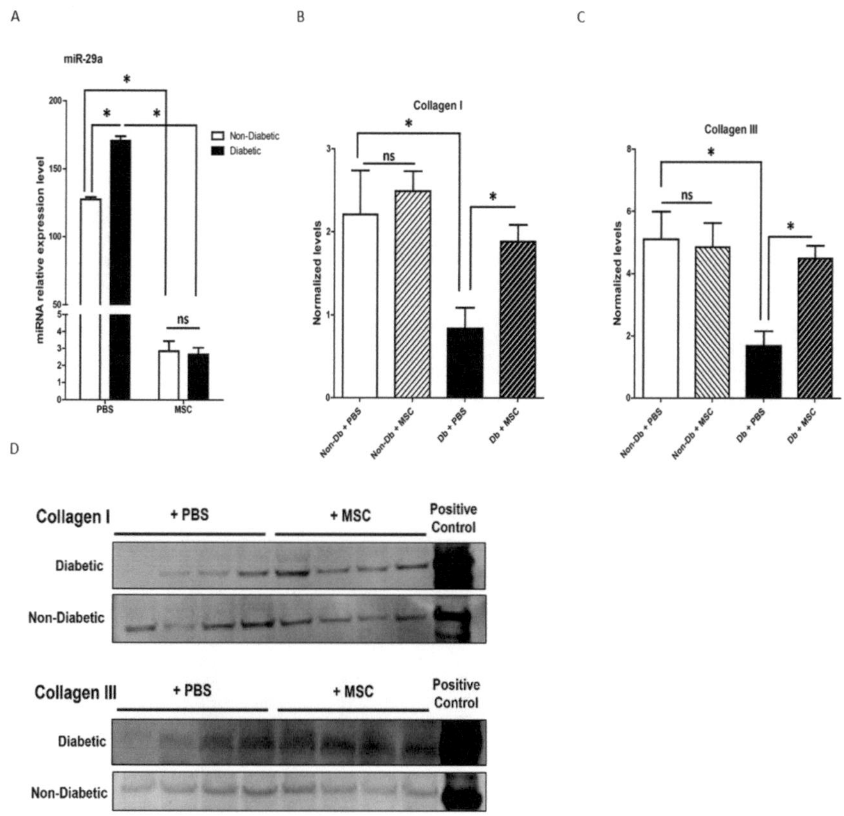

Figure 10. Impact of MSC treatment on collagen protein and gene expression. (A) Real-time PCR quantification of miRNA-29a gene expression in diabetic and non-diabetic murine skin 28 days after treatment with MSCs or PBS. Quantification of **(B)** Collagen I and **(C)** Collagen III protein levels in diabetic skin and non-diabetic skin 28 days after treatment with either MSCs or PBS. **(D)** Western blot depicting the Collagen I and Collagen III protein content in diabetic and non-diabetic wounds 28 days after treatment with either MSCs or PBS. Results are presented as a mean + SEM for each cohort at each time point. Asterisk (*) indicates $p < 0.05$ and ** indicates $p < 0.001$. (Image reproduced from Zgheib *et al.* [21] with permission of the authors.)

4.1.3. *Impact of mesenchymal stem cell treatment on miR-15b*

Treatment with MSCs was also successful at correcting the dysregulated miR-15b expression, further contributing to the improved healing of diabetic wounds observed following treatment with MSCs. Both 3 and 7 days after wounding and treatment with MSCs, diabetic wounds treated with MSCs demonstrated a significant downregulation in miR-15b gene expression when compares to untreated diabetic wounds (**Figure 11**). Additionally, three days after wounding, diabetic wounds treated with MSCs demonstrated significant upregulation in CD31 positive cell sin the wound bed, as well as significant upregulation in HIF-1α, BCL-2, and VEGF gene expression [16].

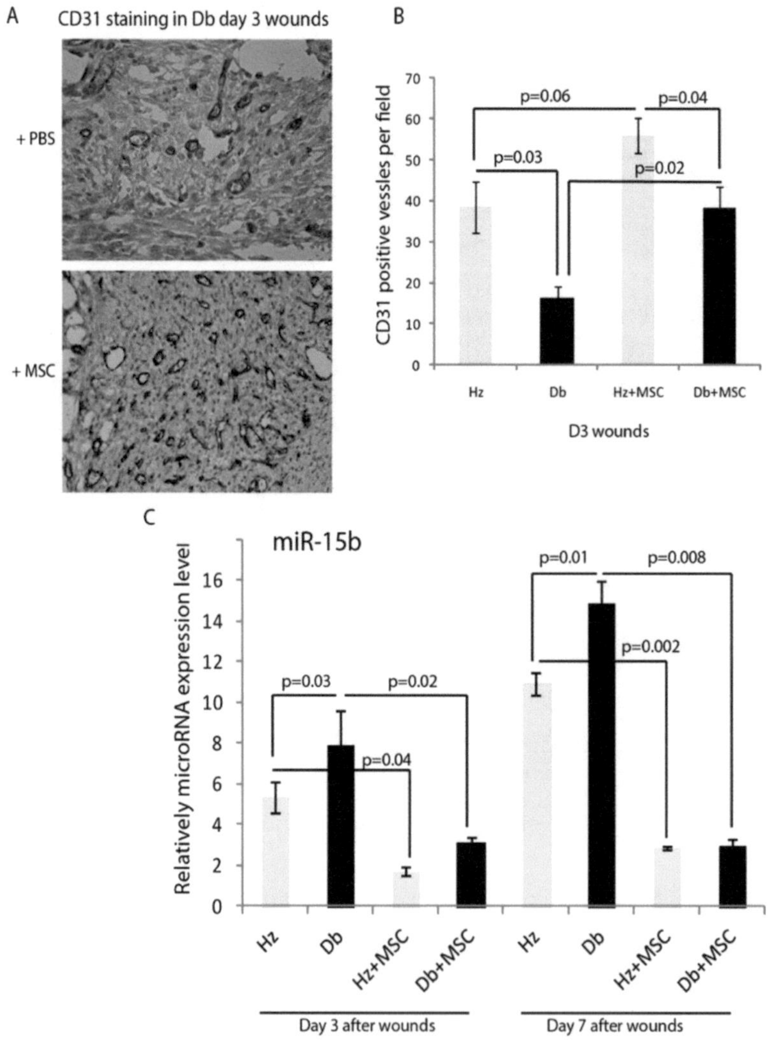

Figure 11. Impact of MSC treatment on angiogenesis and miRNA-15b expression. (A) CD31 immunostaining in diabetic wounds 3 days after wounding and treatment with either PBS or MSCs. **(B)** Quantification of CD31 positive cells in diabetic (Db) and non-diabetic (Hz) wounds 3 days after wounding. **(C)** Real-time PCR quantification of miRNA-15b gene expression 3 and 7 days after wounding in diabetic (Db) and non-diabetic (Hz) skin treated with either PBS or MSCs. Results are presented as a mean + SEM for each cohort at each time point. P-values are included. (Image reproduced from Xu *et al.* [16] with permission of the authors.)

4.2. Adverse effects of MSC treatment

Despite the continued emergence of evidence cataloging the benefits of MSCs in the treatment of diabetic wounds, results are also emerging that detail adverse effects regarding the therapeutic use of MSCs [45]. Specifically, Jeong *et al* (2001) describes the development of soft tissue sarcomas at the site of injection during evaluation of the impact of MSC treatment on both diabetic neuropathy and myocardial regeneration after MI [46]. Similarly, after bone marrow transplant that included systemic administration of 3×10^6 MSCs, Tolar *et al.* reported 12 out of 17 (70.5%) mice developed soft tissue sarcomas, including ectopic ossicles and extremity sarcomas [47]. In addition to the risk of malignant transformation following administration of MSCs, the immunosuppressive impact of MSCs therapy may place patients at risk of infection; although this has not been observed *in vivo* [48].

4.3. The impact of SDF-1α on diabetic wound healing

The time and resources required to harvest and prepare an adequate number of MSCs for autologous transplant has led to investigation in to additional means of simulating the robust improvement in wound healing seen after treatment with MSCs. In attempting to define the mechanism by which MSCs and stromal progenitor cells improve wound healing in diabetic mice, it was noticed that the improved wound healing was associated with upregulation of stromal cell-derived factor-1α (SDF-1α). SDF-1α has long been known as a potent chemokine crucial in the migration and localization of stem cells to wounded tissues [7]. Following injury, SDF-1α expression is upregulated by HIF-1α via VEGF in response to hypoxia in the injured tissues [49]. However, SDF-1α is downregulated in diabetic wounds [7, 22]. We have previously shown that overexpression of SDF-1α in the wound bed is capable of improving the diabetic wound healing impairment [22]. Furthermore, inhibition of SDF-1α via transfection with a mutant SDF-1α that binds the CXCR4 receptor without activation further impairs wound closure, increases inflammatory cytokine production and infiltration of inflammatory cells, and further retards angiogenesis [25]. While these studies support SDF-1α as a key element in mediating the numerous impairments associated with the diabetic wound healing response, there has been no published evaluation of the impact of SDF-1α treatment on miRNA dysregulation in diabetic skin or wounds.

5. Future directions

While we have presented data on the correction of miRNA dysregulation in a diabetic murine model, future directions include extending these explorations to *in vitro* and *in vivo* human models in order to examine the clinical applicability of treating diabetic wounds with either MSCs or SDF-1α, while also investigating how the duration of diabetes impacts miRNA dysregulation in human skin. Furthermore, in no way is the miRNA dysregulation documented in diabetes limited to miR-146a, miR-29a, and miR-15b [14, 15, 39]. Numerous families of miRNA are known to be integral to the wound healing process, and we have only touched on a few of the key regulators. In addition to further evaluating the role these additional miRNA play in regulating the diabetic wound healing response, future directions in this field will likely delve into efforts to make autologous MSC treatment safe and economically feasible, the viability of gene therapy, nanoparticle technology, and improved biomaterials [41, 50, 51]. In addition to regulating protein gene expression, gene therapy could be utilized to upregulate beneficial miRNA expression or downregulate detrimental miRNA expression [39].

The burden of disease attributable to diabetic wounds is projected to intensify as the prevalence of diabetes increases worldwide. As detailed here, patients with diabetes suffer from impaired wound healing, with significant dysregulation at nearly every stage of the wound healing response [2]. This diabetic wound healing phenotype is characterized by decreased angiogenesis, impaired leukocyte migration, decreased growth factor production, sustained inflammation, impaired fibroblast function, imbalance of extracellular matrix deposition and remodeling, and delayed wound healing [9]. Central to the development of this diabetic phenotype is the dysregulation of miRNA that regulate inflammation (miR-146a), extracellular matrix composition (miR-29a), and angiogenesis (miR-15b). We have demonstrated that correction of this microRNA dysregulation through treatment with MSCs expedites wound healing and reverses the diabetic phenotype in skin [16–18], and preliminary results suggest a similar effect following treatment with SDF-1α. Understanding the role that miRNA play in the regulation of wound healing, as well as the numerous ways miRNA are dysregulated in the diabetic state, will be imperative as we strive to develop more effective wound care technologies in the future.

Author details

Maggie M. Hodges*, Carlos Zgheib, Junwang Xu and Kenneth W. Liechty

*Address all correspondence to: maggie.hodges@ucdenver.edu

Laboratory for Fetal and Regenerative Biology, Department of Surgery, University of Colorado Denver, Anschutz Medical Campus and Children's Hospital Colorado, Aurora, CO, USA

References

[1] Reiber GE, Vileikyte L, Boyko EJ, del Aguila M, Smith DG, Lavery LA, et al. Causal pathways for incident lower-extremity ulcers in patients with diabetes from two settings. Diabetes Care. 1999;22(1):157–62.

[2] Falanga V. Wound healing and its impairment in the diabetic foot. Lancet Lond Engl. 2005;366(9498):1736–43.

[3] Leung PC. Diabetic foot ulcers—a comprehensive review. Surg J R Coll Surg Edinb Irel. 2007;5(4):219–31.

[4] Boulton AJM, Kirsner RS, Vileikyte L. Clinical practice. Neuropathic diabetic foot ulcers. N Engl J Med. 2004;351(1):48–55.

[5] Stokes J, Kannel WB, Wolf PA, Cupples LA, D'Agostino RB. The relative importance of selected risk factors for various manifestations of cardiovascular disease among men and women from 35 to 64 years old: 30 years of follow-up in the Framingham Study. Circulation. 1987;75(6 Pt 2):V65–73.

[6] Löndahl M, Katzman P, Nilsson A, Hammarlund C. Hyperbaric oxygen therapy facilitates healing of chronic foot ulcers in patients with diabetes. Diabetes Care. 2010;33(5):998–1003.

[7] Velazquez OC. Angiogenesis and vasculogenesis: inducing the growth of new blood vessels and wound healing by stimulation of bone marrow-derived progenitor cell mobilization and homing. J Vasc Surg. 2007;45(Suppl A):A39–47.

[8] King H, Aubert RE, Herman WH. Global burden of diabetes, 1995–2025: prevalence, numerical estimates, and projections. Diabetes Care. 1998;21(9):1414–31.

[9] Brem H, Tomic-Canic M. Cellular and molecular basis of wound healing in diabetes. J Clin Invest. 2007;117(5):1219–22.

[10] Bartel DP. MicroRNAs: target recognition and regulatory functions. Cell. 2009;136(2): 215–33.

[11] Natarajan R, Putta S, Kato M. MicroRNAs and diabetic complications. J Cardiovasc Transl Res. 2012;5(4):413–22.

[12] Miranda KC, Huynh T, Tay Y, Ang Y-S, Tam W-L, Thomson AM, et al. A pattern-based method for the identification of MicroRNA binding sites and their corresponding heteroduplexes. Cell. 2006;126(6):1203–17.

[13] Banerjee J, Chan YC, Sen CK. MicroRNAs in skin and wound healing. Physiol Genomics. 2011;43(10):543–56.

[14] Zampetaki A, Kiechl S, Drozdov I, Willeit P, Mayr U, Prokopi M, et al. Plasma microRNA profiling reveals loss of endothelial miR-126 and other microRNAs in type 2 diabetes. Circ Res. 2010;107(6):810–7.

[15] Moura J, Børsheim E, Carvalho E. The role of MicroRNAs in diabetic complications-special emphasis on wound healing. Genes. 2014;5(4):926–56.

[16] Xu J, Zgheib C, Hu J, Wu W, Zhang L, Liechty KW. The role of microRNA-15b in the impaired angiogenesis in diabetic wounds. Wound Repair Regen Off Publ Wound Heal Soc Eur Tissue Repair Soc. 2014;22(5):671–7.

[17] Xu J, Wu W, Zhang L, Dorset-Martin W, Morris MW, Mitchell ME, et al. The role of microRNA-146a in the pathogenesis of the diabetic wound-healing impairment: correction with mesenchymal stem cell treatment. Diabetes. 2012;61(11):2906–12.

[18] Caskey RC, Zgheib C, Morris M, Allukian M, Dorsett-Martin W, Xu J, et al. Dysregulation of collagen production in diabetes following recurrent skin injury: contribution to the development of a chronic wound. Wound Repair Regen Off Publ Wound Heal Soc Eur Tissue Repair Soc. 2014;22(4):515–20.

[19] Srinivasan K, Ramarao P. Animal models in type 2 diabetes research: an overview. Indian J Med Res. 2007;125(3):451–72.

[20] Rees DA, Alcolado JC. Animal models of diabetes mellitus. Diabet Med J Br Diabet Assoc. 2005;22(4):359–70.

[21] Zgheib C, Hodges M, Hu J, Beason DP, Soslowsky LJ, Liechty KW, et al. Mechanisms of mesenchymal stem cell correction of the impaired biomechanical properties of diabetic skin: the role of miR-29a. Wound Repair Regen . 2016; 24(2):237-246.

[22] Badillo AT, Chung S, Zhang L, Zoltick P, Liechty KW. Lentiviral gene transfer of SDF-1alpha to wounds improves diabetic wound healing. J Surg Res. 2007;143(1):35–42.

[23] Javazon EH, Keswani SG, Badillo AT, Crombleholme TM, Zoltick PW, Radu AP, et al. Enhanced epithelial gap closure and increased angiogenesis in wounds of diabetic mice treated with adult murine bone marrow stromal progenitor cells. Wound Repair Regen Off Publ Wound Heal Soc Eur Tissue Repair Soc. 2007;15(3):350–9.

[24] Choi W-T, Tian S, Dong C-Z, Kumar S, Liu D, Madani N, et al. Unique ligand binding sites on CXCR4 probed by a chemical biology approach: implications for the design of selective human immunodeficiency virus type 1 inhibitors. J Virol. 2005;79(24):15398–404.

[25] Bermudez DM, Xu J, Herdrich BJ, Radu A, Mitchell ME, Liechty KW. Inhibition of stromal cell-derived factor-1α further impairs diabetic wound healing. J Vasc Surg. 2011;53(3):774–84.

[26] Zennou V, Serguera C, Sarkis C, Colin P, Perret E, Mallet J, et al. The HIV-1 DNA flap stimulates HIV vector-mediated cell transduction in the brain. Nat Biotechnol. 2001;19(5):446–50.

[27] Donello JE, Loeb JE, Hope TJ. Woodchuck hepatitis virus contains a tripartite posttranscriptional regulatory element. J Virol. 1998;72(6):5085–92.

[28] Soslowsky LJ, Thomopoulos S, Tun S, Flanagan CL, Keefer CC, Mastaw J, et al. Neer Award 1999. Overuse activity injures the supraspinatus tendon in an animal model: a histologic and biomechanical study. J Shoulder Elb Surg Am Shoulder Elb Surg Al. 2000;9(2):79–84.

[29] Bermudez DM, Herdrich BJ, Xu J, Lind R, Beason DP, Mitchell ME, et al. Impaired biomechanical properties of diabetic skin implications in pathogenesis of diabetic wound complications. Am J Pathol. 2011;178(5):2215–23.

[30] Favata M. Scarless Healing in the Fetus: Implications and Strategies for Postnatal Tendon Repair (dissertation). University of Pennsylvania; 2006.

[31] Rafehi H, El-Osta A, Karagiannis TC. Epigenetic mechanisms in the pathogenesis of diabetic foot ulcers. J Diabetes Complications. 2012;26(6):554–61.

[32] Mirza RE, Koh TJ. Contributions of cell subsets to cytokine production during normal and impaired wound healing. Cytokine. 2015;71(2):409–12.

[33] Wang X, Ha T, Liu L, Zou J, Zhang X, Kalbfleisch J, et al. Increased expression of microRNA-146a decreases myocardial ischaemia/reperfusion injury. Cardiovasc Res. 2013;97(3):432–42.

[34] Boldin MP, Taganov KD, Rao DS, Yang L, Zhao JL, Kalwani M, et al. miR-146a is a significant brake on autoimmunity, myeloproliferation, and cancer in mice. J Exp Med. 2011;208(6):1189–201.

[35] Taganov KD, Boldin MP, Chang K-J, Baltimore D. NF-kappaB-dependent induction of microRNA miR-146, an inhibitor targeted to signaling proteins of innate immune responses. Proc Natl Acad Sci U S A. 2006;103(33):12481–6.

[36] Hou J, Wang P, Lin L, Liu X, Ma F, An H, et al. MicroRNA-146a feedback inhibits RIG-I-dependent Type I IFN production in macrophages by targeting TRAF6, IRAK1, and IRAK2. J Immunol Baltim Md 2009;183 (3):2150–8.

[37] Blakytny R, Jude E. The molecular biology of chronic wounds and delayed healing in diabetes. Diabet Med J Br Diabet Assoc. 2006;23(6):594–608.

[38] Maurer B, Stanczyk J, Jüngel A, Akhmetshina A, Trenkmann M, Brock M, et al. MicroRNA-29, a key regulator of collagen expression in systemic sclerosis. Arthritis Rheum. 2010;62(6):1733–43.

[39] Banerjee J, Sen CK. MicroRNAs in skin and wound healing. Methods Mol Biol Clifton NJ. 2013;936:343–56.

[40] Ferrara N, Gerber H-P, LeCouter J. The biology of VEGF and its receptors. Nat Med. 2003;9(6):669–76.

[41] Falanga V. Wound healing and its impairment in the diabetic foot. Lancet Lond Engl. 2005;366(9498):1736–43.

[42] Mace KA, Yu DH, Paydar KZ, Boudreau N, Young DM. Sustained expression of Hif-1alpha in the diabetic environment promotes angiogenesis and cutaneous wound repair. Wound Repair Regen Off Publ Wound Heal Soc Eur Tissue Repair Soc. 2007;15(5):636–45.

[43] Chan LS, Yue PYK, Wong YY, Wong RNS. MicroRNA-15b contributes to ginsenoside-Rg1-induced angiogenesis through increased expression of VEGFR-2. Biochem Pharmacol. 2013;86(3):392–400.

[44] Branski LK, Gauglitz GG, Herndon DN, Jeschke MG. A review of gene and stem cell therapy in cutaneous wound healing. Burns J Int Soc Burn Inj. 2009;35(2):171–80.

[45] Jackson WM, Nesti LJ, Tuan RS. Concise review: clinical translation of wound healing therapies based on mesenchymal stem cells. Stem Cells Transl Med. 2012;1(1):44–50.

[46] Jeong J-O, Han JW, Kim J-M, Cho H-J, Park C, Lee N, et al. Malignant tumor formation after transplantation of short-term cultured bone marrow mesenchymal stem cells in experimental myocardial infarction and diabetic neuropathy. Circ Res. 2011;108(11): 1340–7.

[47] Tolar J, Nauta AJ, Osborn MJ, Panoskaltsis Mortari A, McElmurry RT, Bell S, et al. Sarcoma derived from cultured mesenchymal stem cells. Stem Cells Dayt Ohio. 2007;25(2):371–9.

[48] Uccelli A, Moretta L, Pistoia V. Mesenchymal stem cells in health and disease. Nat Rev Immunol. 2008;8(9):726–36.

[49] Ceradini DJ, Kulkarni AR, Callaghan MJ, Tepper OM, Bastidas N, Kleinman ME, et al. Progenitor cell trafficking is regulated by hypoxic gradients through HIF-1 induction of SDF-1. Nat Med. 2004;10(8):858–64.

[50] Chigurupati S, Mughal MR, Okun E, Das S, Kumar A, McCaffery M, et al. Effects of cerium oxide nanoparticles on the growth of keratinocytes, fibroblasts and vascular endothelial cells in cutaneous wound healing. Biomaterials. 2013;34(9):2194–201.

[51] Wu SC, Marston W, Armstrong DG. Wound care: the role of advanced wound-healing technologies. J Am Podiatr Med Assoc. 2010;100(5):385–94.

Chapter 2

The Physiological Roles of Leptin in Skin Wound Healing

Reiko Tokuyama-Toda and Kazuhito Satomura

Additional information is available at the end of the chapter

http://dx.doi.org/10.5772/63368

Abstract

Leptin, a 16 kDa circulating anti-obesity hormone, has many physiological properties such as body weight homeostasis, lipid metabolism, hematopoiesis, thermogenesis, ovarian function, bone formation, and angiogenesis. Interestingly, a certain study showed that skin wound healing delayed in leptin deficient *ob/ob* mice. However, little has been known about the physiological role of leptin in skin wound healing. In this chapter, we introduce whether local and single-dose administration of leptin exerted a promotive influence on the skin wound healing. Immunohistochemical analysis revealed that leptin receptor was expressed in mouse epidermal cells. In addition, topical administration of leptin promoted the healing of chemical burn wounds created on the back skin of mice without any side effects. Then, the mechanisms of the promotive effect of leptin on the wound healing of the skin were demonstrated immunohistochemical and biological analysis; namely, leptin stimulated angiogenesis in the connective tissue beneath the wounded area and the cell proliferation, differentiation/function, and migration of human epidermal keratinocytes. These findings revealed the possible and promising usefulness of leptin as a new wound-healing promoting agent.

Keywords: leptin, skin, wound healing, new promoting agent, local administration

1. Introduction

Leptin, the product of *ob* (*obese*) gene, is a 16 kDa non-glycosylated polypeptide anti-obesity hormone mainly produced and secreted by adipose tissues [1]. Recent studies have demonstrated that leptin is also produced by placenta [2], stomach [3], skeletal muscles [4], brain, and pituitary gland [5, 6]. Leptin influences body weight homeostasis through its effects on food intake and energy expenditure by negative feedback at the hypothalamic nuclei [7]. Leptin is also known to exhibit a variety of physiological actions on lipid metabolism [8], hematopoiesis [9], thermogenesis [10], ovarian function [11], bone formation [12, 13], and angiogenesis [14, 15]. The leptin receptor (Ob-R) is expressed in various tissues including the hypothalamus [16, 17], adipose tissue [18], skeletal muscle [19], and hepatocytes [18, 20]. The multifunctionality of leptin and the wide distribution of its receptor suggest that leptin plays a variety of physiological roles not only as a systemic hormone but also as a local growth factor.

The surface of the body is covered by skin to communicate with the external environment and to protect deeper tissues and organs by separating them from the external environment such as chemical, mechanical, and thermal stresses, infections, and dehydration [21, 22]. Normal dermal wound repair processes, such as inflammation, angiogenesis, contraction, deposition of extracellular matrix, granulation tissue formation, epithelialization, and remodeling, require various cellular and molecular signals [23]. In this biological process, skin fibroblasts interact with surrounding cells such as keratinocytes, inflammatory cells, and endothelial cells [21, 24]. Fibroblasts produce extracellular matrix, glycoproteins, adhesive molecules, and various cytokines [25, 26]. The lack of these signals may result in poor healing of wounds such as diabetic ulcers [27, 28].

A certain study showed that skin wound healing delayed in leptin deficient *ob/ob* mice and that exogenously administered leptin restored this delayed wound healing by enhancing re-epithelialization of the wound in these mice in diabetic condition [29]. Another some studies unveiled the effect of leptin on wound healing by demonstrating that leptin acted as an autocrine/paracrine regulator in the wounded site [30, 31]. These findings strongly suggest the possibility that leptin could be a potential medicine for promoting wound healing in skin. However, all previous studies refer to whole-body dosage administered intraperitoneally, and even when administered locally, the leptin must have been administered every day. So, we investigated whether local and single-dose administration of leptin exerted a promotive influence on the skin wound healing. Because, we thought that local and single administration of leptin could avoid the influence of its adverse effect such as metabolic disorders, hyper/hypoglycemia caused by the fact that leptin is a multifunctional and potent systemic hormone, and could be advantageous for the lowering of patients' distress in some cases in its clinical application.

2. Localization of leptin receptor in mouse skin

An immunohistochemical analysis of mouse skin using anti-leptin receptor antibody revealed that leptin receptor was expressed in prickle and granular cells of epidermis (**Figure 1**). These findings showed that epidermal cells are target of leptin.

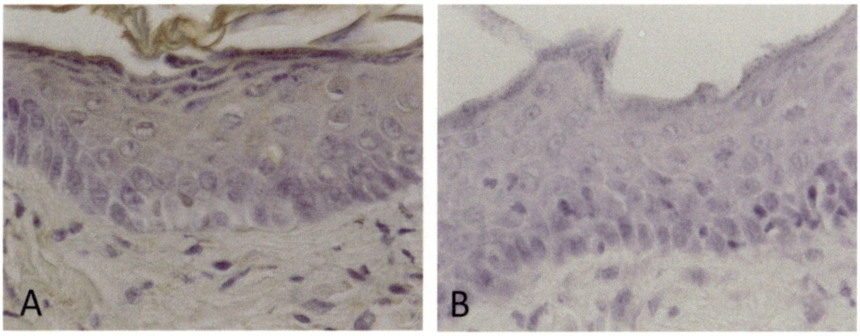

Figure 1. Immunohistochemical localization of leptin receptor in normal mouse skin. (A) Leptin, (B) negative control. Leptin receptor was expressed in prickle and granular cells of epidermis of mouse skin.

3. Effect of leptin on the wound healing of the skin

To elucidate the effect of leptin on the wound healing of the skin, mouse skin chemical burn model was used. Eighteen 6-week-old male ICR mice were fed a normal diet and maintained under a 12-h light/12-h dark cycle. Chemical wounds were created on the back skin by applying two pieces (12 × 12 mm) of filter paper soaked with 20% sodium hypochlorite for 5 min. Wound formation was verified next day, and the wounds were covered with 15 g (12 × 12 × 1 mm) of MedGel (Med GEL Corp., Tokyo, Japan) containing 10 μL of 100 ng/mL leptin (R&D Systems, Minneapolis, USA) or phosphate-buffered saline (PBS) as a control. This hydrogel-contained leptin or PBS was attached to the chemical burn site and dressed. The size of the ulcer was measured on day 4 and 8 after burn formation, and the skin tissue around the wound was obtained for histological analysis. In consequence, at day 4, slightly enhanced re-epithelialization was observed in leptin-treated group, but no significant difference was noted between leptin-treated and control group. In contrast, at day 8, significantly enhanced re-epithelialization was observed in leptin-treated group (**Figure 2**). These experiments showed that the wound area decreased much faster in the leptin-treated group compared with the control group. These findings demonstrated that single and local administration of leptin using bioabsorbable hydrogel promoted the wound healing of skin.

Meanwhile, body weight (BW), and levels of aspartate aminotransferase (AST), alanine aminotransferase (ALT) or blood sugar (BS) were not affected through experiment period, showing that topically administered leptin had no systemic adverse effects (**Figure 3**). These findings certify that topically administered leptin is capable of promoting wound healing of the skin without any systemic adverse effects in this period. However, unfortunately, we could not elucidate whether local and single administration of leptin could avoid or not the influence of its side effect over a long period. This issue should be elucidated in the future investigation.

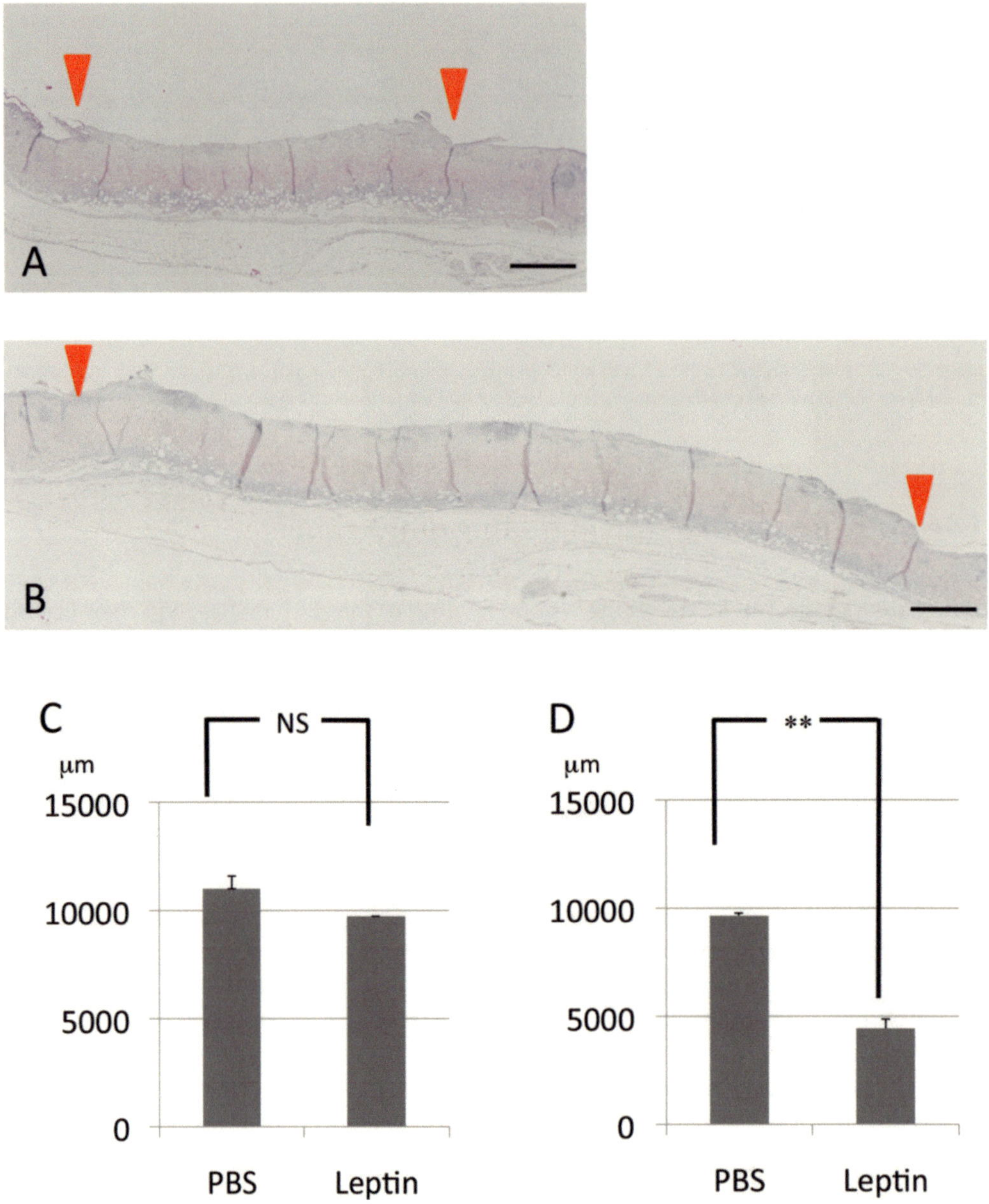

Figure 2. Effect of leptin on the wound healing of the mouse skin. (A) Histological findings of wound repair of skin at day 8 after initial wounding in leptin-treated group. (B) Histological findings of wound repair of skin at day 8 after initial wounding in control group. Spaces between arrow heads show ulcerative area without epithelium. Wound heal is significantly enhanced in leptin-treated group. (C) Skin wound healing at day 4 after wound creation. No significant difference in wound healing was noted between leptin-treated and control group. (D) Skin wound healing at day 8 after wound creation. Significantly enhanced re-epithelialization was observed in leptin-treated group. **$P < 0.01$. H-E staining. Bars: 500 µm.

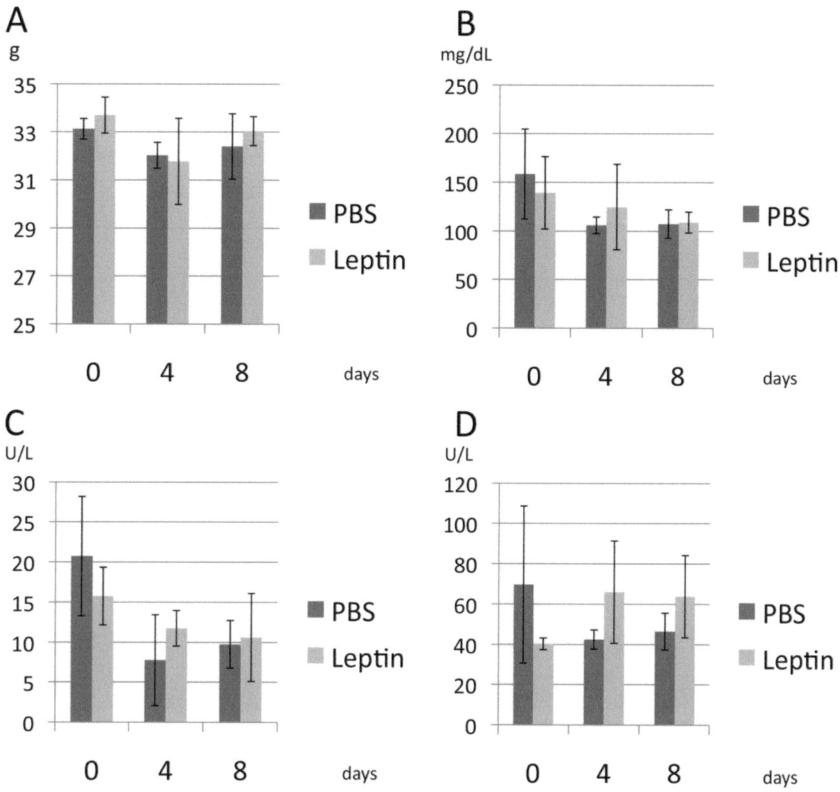

Figure 3. Changes in BW, AST, ALT, and BS. (A) BW, (B) BS, (C) AST, (D) ALT. None of these laboratory parameters were significantly affected by leptin application.

4. Mechanism of the promotive effect of leptin on the wound healing of the skin

4.1. Effect of leptin for angiogenesis on the wound healing of the skin

To elucidate the mechanism of the promotive effect of leptin on the wound healing of the skin, first, the influence of leptin on the angiogenesis in the connective tissues beneath the wound in the skin was revealed by histological analysis. The localization of blood vessels was analyzed by immunohistochemistry by using anti-CD31 antibody. Then, at day 4, after initial wounding, no significant difference on the number of CD31-positive cells was detected between leptin-treated and control group. However, at day 8, after initial wounding, the number of CD31-positive cells significantly increased in leptin-treated group (**Figure 4**). These findings demonstrated that leptin stimulates angiogenesis in the connective tissue beneath the ulcer, and promotes wound healing in the skin by accelerating the supply of nutritions, oxygen, and even some bioactive substances.

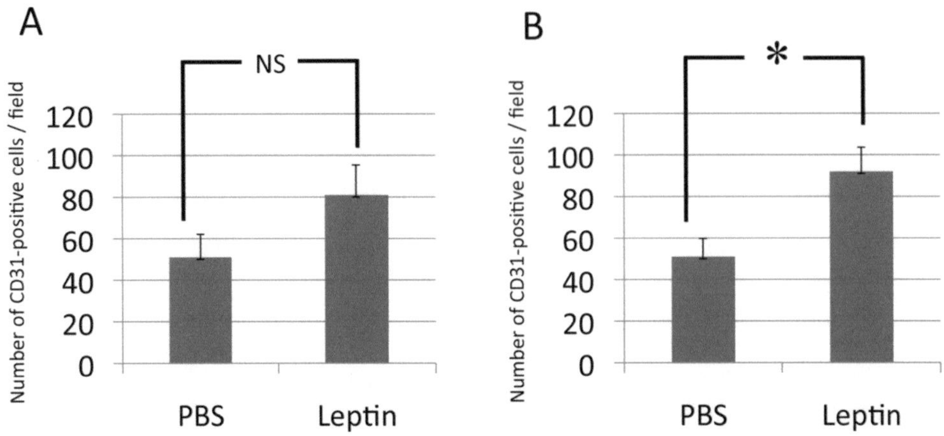

Figure 4. Number of vascular endothelial cells in the dermal connective tissue beneath the ulcerated area. (A) At day 4, after initial wounding, no significant difference in the number of CD31-positive cells between leptin-treated group and control group. (B) At day 8, after initial wounding, more vascular endothelial cells distributed in the connective tissue beneath the ulcer in leptin-treated group compared with control group. *P < 0.05.

4.2. Effect of leptin on the proliferation of human epidermal keratinocytes

To reveal another possible mechanism underlying the promotive effect of leptin on the skin wound healing, cell biological analyses were performed using human epidermal keratinocytes on the premise that the cells were proven to express the mRNA and protein of leptin receptor (*Ob-R*) (data not shown). To elucidate the effect of leptin on the proliferation of human epidermal keratinocytes, the cells were cultured in the absence or presence of various concentrations of leptin. The results indicated that the proliferation of human keratinocytes was significantly enhanced by leptin at a concentration equal to and more than 10 ng/mL

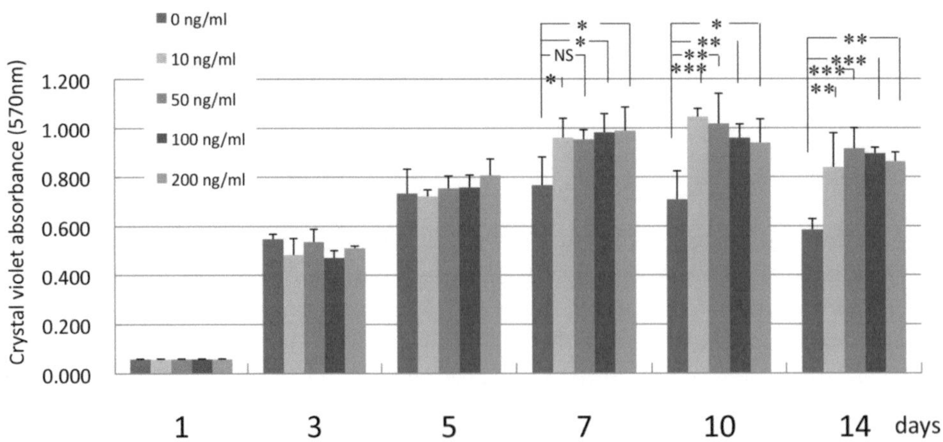

Figure 5. Effect of leptin on the proliferation of human epidermal keratinocytes. Leptin-enhanced cell proliferation at a concentration equal to and more than 10 ng/mL. *P < 0.05, **P < 0.01, ***P < 0.001.

(**Figure 5**). These findings showed the modest stimulatory effect of leptin on the proliferation of human epidermal keratinocytes.

4.3. Effect of leptin on the differentiation/function of human epidermal keratinocytes

Next, the effect of leptin on the differentiation/function of human keratinocytes was demonstrated using quantitative RT-PCR analysis of the expression of mRNA encoding keratinocyte-related genes, that is, *Cytokeratin 13, Cytokeratin 14,* and *Transglutaminase I.* Accordingly, this analysis detected an elevation in expression levels of these gene expressions in the presence of 100 ng/mL leptin (**Figure 6**). These findings showed that leptin has a stimulatory effect on the differentiation/function of human epidermal keratinocytes.

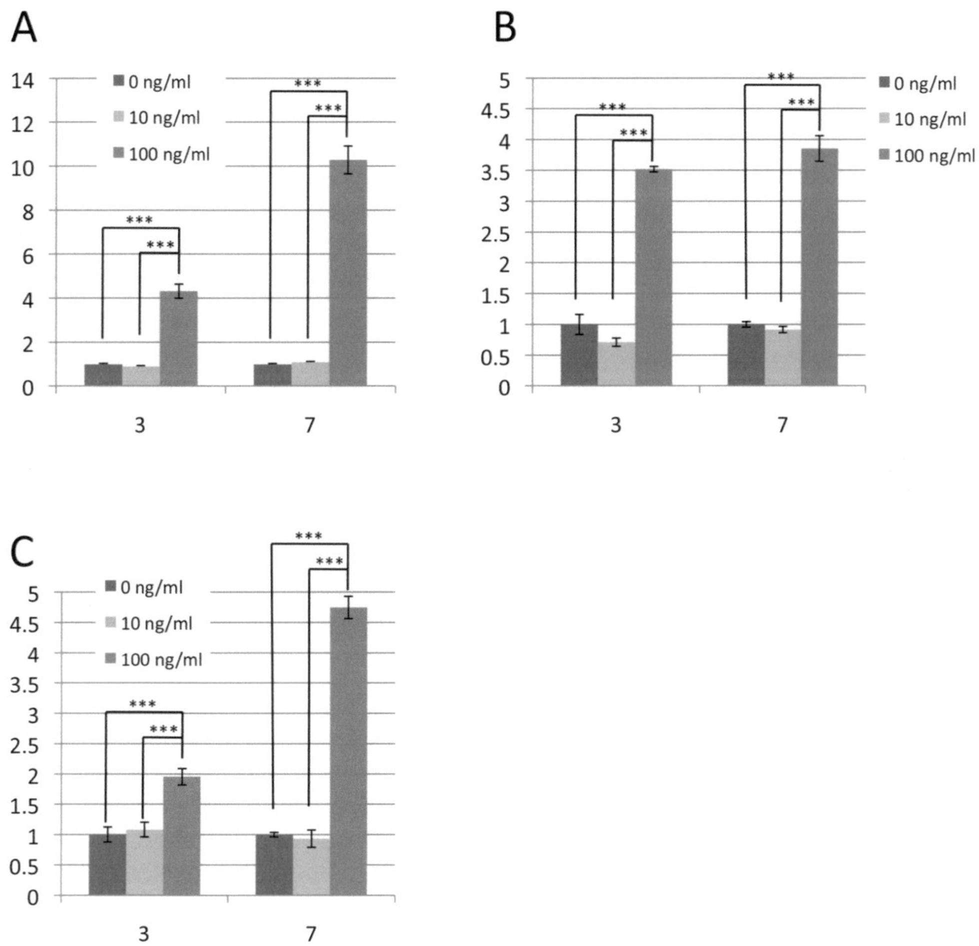

Figure 6. Effect of leptin on the expression of mRNA encoding *Cytokeratin 13, Cytokeratin 14,* and *Transglutaminase I* in human epidermal keratinocytes analyzed by quantitative RT-PCR analysis. (A) *Cytokeratin 13,* (B) *Cytokeratin 14,* (C) *Transglutaminase I.* Leptin exerted stimulatory effect on the gene expression of *Cytokeratin 13, Cytokeratin 14,* and *Transglutaminase I* at the concentration of 100 ng/mL. ***P < 0.001.

4.4. Effect of leptin on the migration of human epidermal keratinocytes

Moreover, to elucidate the effect of leptin on cell migration around the skin wounded area, scratch assay using human epidermal keratinocytes was performed. The assay was performed using CytoSelect Wound Healing Assay kit (Cell Biolabs Inc., San Diego, USA) according to the manufacturer's instructions. After preparation, the cells were treated with or without 100 ng/mL of leptin. Images of wound healing were captured using a phase-contrast microscope at 0, 3, 6, 9, 12, 18, and 24 h after the preparation. The area of open wound field was calculated by using ImageJ software [32]. Consequently, the significant effect was not observed during initial 12 h. However, the area without cells decreased significantly in leptin-treated group compared with control group from 18 to 24 h (**Figure 7**). This assay revealed that leptin significantly accelerated the migration of human epidermal keratinocytes.

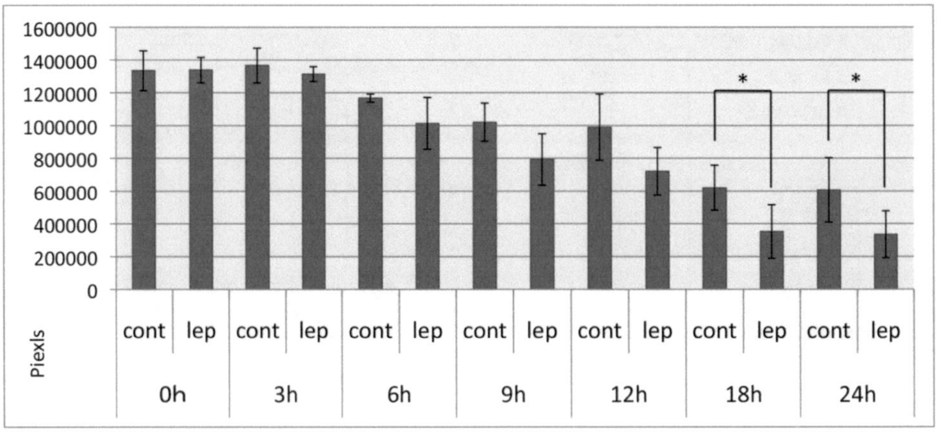

Figure 7. Effect of leptin on the migration of human epidermal keratinocytes. Leptin accelerated the migration of human epidermal keratinocytes, significantly. *$P < 0.05$.

5. Conclusion

Leptin is capable of promoting wound healing of skin by influencing epidermal keratinocytes proliferation, differentiation/function and migration, and angiogenesis in the connective tissue beneath the wounded area. Moreover, we showed that single dose and topically administration of leptin could promote wound healing in the skin without any side effects by using an adequate drug delivery system [33]. In addition to these findings, our previous study demonstrated that local administration of leptin could promote wound healing in the oral mucosa by enhancing epithelial cell migration and angiogenesis in the connective tissue beneath the wound [34]. Taken together, leptin is proven to play physiological roles in wounded area not only as a systemic hormone but also as a local growth factor. Importantly, these findings presented in this chapter declared the possible and promising usefulness of leptin as a new wound-healing promoting agent.

Author details

Reiko Tokuyama-Toda and Kazuhito Satomura*

*Address all correspondence to: satomura-k@tsurumi-u.ac.jp

Department of Oral Medicine and Stomatology, Second Department of Oral and Maxillofacial Surgery, School of Dental Medicine, Tsurumi University, Yokohama, Kanagawa, Japan

References

[1] Zhang Y, Proenca R, Maffei M, Barone M, Leopold L, Friedman JM: Positional cloning of the mouse obese gene and its human homologue. Nature. 1994;372:425–432.

[2] Masuzaki H, Ogawa Y, Sagawa N, Hosoda K, Matsumoto T, Mise H, Nishimura H, Yoshimasa Y, Tanaka I, Mori T, Nakao K: Nonadipose tissue production of leptin: leptin as a novel placenta-derived hormone in humans. Nat Med. 1997;3:1029–1033.

[3] Bado A, Levasseur S, Attuoub A, Kermorgant S, Laigneau JP, Boutoluzzi MN, Moizol L, Lehy T, Guerre-Millo M, Le Marchand-Brustel Y, Lewin MJ: The stomach is a source of leptin. Nature. 1998;394:790–793.

[4] Wang J, Liu R, Hawkins M, Barzilai N, Rossetti L: A nutrient-sensing pathway regulates leptin gene expression in muscle and fat. Nature. 1998;393:684–688.

[5] Jin L, Burguera BG, Couse ME, Scheithauer BW, Lamsan J, Eberhardt NL, Kulig E, Lloyd RV: Leptin and leptin receptor expression in normal and neoplastic human pituitary: evidence of a regulatory role for leptin on pituitary cell proliferation. J Clin Endocrinol Metab. 1999;84:2903–2911.

[6] Morash B, Li A, Murphy PR, Wilkinson M, Ur E: Leptin gene expression in the brain and pituitary gland. Endocrinology. 1999;140:5995–5998.

[7] Friedman JM, Halaas JL: Leptin and the regulation of body weight in mammals. Nature. 1998;395:763–770.

[8] Bryson JM, Phuyal JL, Swan V, Caterson ID: Leptin has acute effects on glucose and lipid metabolism in both lean and gold thioglucose-obese mice. Am J Physiol. 1999;277:E417–E422.

[9] Gainford T, Willson TA, Metcalf D, Handman E, McFarlane C, Ng A, Nicola NA, Alexander WS, Hilton DJ: Leptin can induce proliferation, differentiation, and functional activation of hematopoietic cells. Proc Natl Acad Sci USA. 1996;93:14564–14568.

[10] Hwa JJ, Ghibaudi L, Compton D, Fawzi AB, Strader CD: Intracerebroventricular injection of leptin increases thermogenesis and mobilizes fat metabolism in ob/ob mice. Horm Metab Res. 1996;8:659–663.

[11] Spicer LJ, Francisco CC: The adipose obese gene product, leptin evidence of a direct inhibitory role in ovarian function. Endocrinology. 1997;138:3374–3379.

[12] Ducy P, Amling M, Takeda S, Priemel M, Schilling AF, Beli FT, Shen J, Vinson C, Rueger JM, Karsenty G: Leptin inhibits bone formation through a hypothalamic relay: a central control of bone mass. Cell. 2000;100:197–207.

[13] Kume K, Satomura K, Nishisho S, Kitaoka E, Yamanouchi K, Tobiume S, Nagayama M: Potential role of leptin in endochondral ossification. J Histochem Cytochem. 2002;50:150–169.

[14] Bouloumie A, Drexler HCA, Lafontan M, Busse R: Leptin, the product of ob gene, promotes angiogenesis. Circ Res. 1998;83:1059–1066.

[15] Sierra-Honigmann MR, Nath AK, Murakami C, Garcia-Cardena G, Papapetropoulos A, Sessa WC, Madge LA, Schechner JS, Schwabb MB, Polverini PJ, Flores-Riveros JR: Biological action of leptin as an angiogenic factor. Science. 1998;281:1683–1686.

[16] Fei H, Okano HJ, Li C, Lee G, Zhao C, Darnell R, Friedman JM: Anatomic localization of alternatively spliced leptin receptors (Ob-R) in mouse brain and other tissues. Proc Natl Acad Sci USA. 1997;94:7001–7005.

[17] Mercer JG, Hoggard N, Williams LM, Lawrence CB, Hannah LT, Trayhurn P: Localization of leptin receptor mRNA and the long form splice variant (Ob-Rb) in mouse hypothalamus and adjacent brain regions by in situ hybridization. FEBS Lett. 1996;387:113–116.

[18] De Matteis R, Dashtipour K, Ognibene A, Cinti S: Localization of leptin receptor splice variants in mouse peripheral tissues by immunohistochemistry. Proc Nutr Soc. 1998;57:441–448.

[19] Guerra B, Santana A, Fuentes T, Delgado-Guerra S, Cabrera-Socorro A, Dorado C, Calbet JA: Leptin receptors in human skeletal muscle. J Appl Physiol. 2007;102:1786–1792.

[20] Gohen P, Yang G, Yu X, Soukas AA, Wolfish CS, Friedman JM, Li C: Induction of leptin receptor expression in the liver by leptin and food deprivation. J Biol Chem. 2005;280:10034–10039.

[21] Martin P: Wound healing—aiming for perfect skin regeneration. Science. 1997;276:75–81. doi:10.1126/science.276.5309.75

[22] Tartarini D, Mele E: Adult stem cell therapies for wound healing: biomaterials and computational models. Front Bioeng Biotechnol. 2016;3:206. doi:10.3389/fbioe.2015.00206

[23] Bellavia G, Fasanaro P, Melchionna R, Capogrossi MC, Napolitano M: Transcriptional control of skin reepithelialization. J Dermatol Sci. 2014;73:3–9. doi:10.1016/j.jdermsci.2013.08.007

[24] Chen D, Hao H, Fu X, Han W: Insight into reepithelialization: how do mesenchymal stem cells perform? Stem Cells Int. 2016;2016:6120173. doi:10.1155/2016/6120173

[25] Gosain A, Dipietro LA: Aging and wound healing. World J Surg. 2004;28:321–326.

[26] Kim WS, Park BS, Sung JH, Yang JM, Park SB, Kwak SJ, Park JS: Wound healing effect of adipose-derived stem cells: a critical role of secretory factors on human dermal fibroblasts. J Dermatol Sci. 2007;48:15–24.

[27] Robson MG, Hill DP, Smith PD, Wang X, Meyer-Siegler K, Ko F, VandeBerg JS, Payne WG, Ochs D, Robson LE: Sequential cytokine therapy for pressure ulcer: clinical and mechanistic response. Ann Surg. 2000;231:600–611.

[28] Nambu M, Kishimoto S, Nakamura S, Mizuno H, Yanagibayashi S, Yamamoto N, Azuma R, Nakamura S, Kiyosawa T, Ishihara M, Kanatani Y: Accelerated wound healing in healing-impaired db/db mice by autologous adipose tissue-derived stromal cells combined with atelocollagen matrix. Ann Plast Surg. 2009;63:317–321.

[29] Frank S, Stallmeyer B, Kampfer H, Kolb N, Pfeilscifter J: Leptin enhances wound re-epithelialization and constitutes a direct function of leptin in skin repair. J Clin Investig. 2000;106:501–509.

[30] Murad A, Nath AK, Cha ST, Demir E, Flores-Riveros J, Sierra-Honigmann MR: Leptin is an autocrine/paracrine regulator of wound healing. FASEB J. 2003;17:1895–1897.

[31] Stallmeyer B, Kampfer H, Podda M, Kaufman R, Pfeilschifter J, Frank S: A novel keratinocyte mitogen: regulation of leptin and its functional receptor in skin repair. J Investig Dermatol. 2001;117:98–105.

[32] Schneider CA, Rasband WS, Eliceiri KW: NIH Image to ImageJ: 25 years of image analysis. Nat Methods. 2012;9:671–675.

[33] Tadokoro S, Ide S, Tokuyama R, Umeki H, Tatehara S, Kataoka S, Satomura K: Leptin promotes wound healing in the skin. PLos One. 2015;10:e0121242. doi:10.1371/journal.pone.0121242

[34] Umeki H, Tokuyama R, Ide S, Okubo M, Tadokoro S, Tezuka M, Tatehara S, Satomura K: Leptin promotes wound healing in the oral mucosa. PLos One. 2014;7:e101984. doi:10.1371/journal.pone.0101984

Chapter 3

Roles of Matrix Metalloproteinases in Cutaneous Wound Healing

Trung T. Nguyen, Shahriar Mobashery and
Mayland Chang

Additional information is available at the end of the chapter

http://dx.doi.org/10.5772/64611

Abstract

Wound healing is a complex process that consists of hemostasis and inflammation, angiogenesis, re-epithelialization, and tissue remodeling. Matrix metalloproteinases (MMPs) play important roles in wound healing, and their dysregulation leads to prolonged inflammation and delayed wound healing. There are 24 MMPs in humans, and each MMP exists in three forms, of which only the active MMPs play a role in the pathology or repair of wounds. The current methodology does not distinguish between the three forms of MMPs, making it challenging to investigate the roles of MMPs in pathology and wound repair. We used a novel MMP-inhibitor-tethered affinity resin that binds only the active form of MMPs, from which we identified and quantified active MMP-8 and active MMP-9 in a murine diabetic model with delayed wound healing. We showed that up-regulation of active MMP-9 plays a detrimental role whereas active MMP-8 is involved in repairing the wound in diabetic mice. These studies identified MMP-9 as a novel target for therapeutic intervention in the treatment of chronic wounds. A selective inhibitor of MMP-9 that leaves MMP-8 unaffected would provide the most effective therapy and represents a promising strategy for therapeutic intervention in the treatment of diabetic foot ulcers.

Keywords: MMPs, chronic wounds, wound healing, selective MMP-9 inhibitor, MMP profiling

1. Introduction

Skin is one of the largest organs in humans. Its three main functions are protection against environmental damage, regulation of body temperature, and perception of environmental change. The skin consists of two distinct layers of tissue, the epidermis and dermis. The epidermis is the outermost layer. The inner layer, dermis, provides cushioning and tensile strength for the skin through the support of the extracellular matrix (ECM) [1]. The ECM—a three-dimensional structure, where cutaneous cells and tissues are embedded—comprises approximately 300 proteins, including collagen, proteoglycans, and glycoproteins [2]. Injury to the skin would account for breaks in these protective layers, which become a cutaneous wound. The wound has to be repaired because of its critical role in prevention of infection, and the well-being of the tissue and the organism. Wounds that undergo a well-coordinated cascade of biochemical events in healing are called acute wounds. On the other hand, wounds that are recalcitrant to healing due to prolonged residency in one of the healing stages are called chronic wounds. For wound healing to progress, the ECM has to be remodeled properly, and endopeptidases such as matrix metalloproteinases (MMPs) contribute to this remodeling process. Whereas these subjects have been reviewed in excellent recent articles [3–6], the emphasis in this chapter focuses on the roles of the family of MMPs that are involved in the wound-healing process.

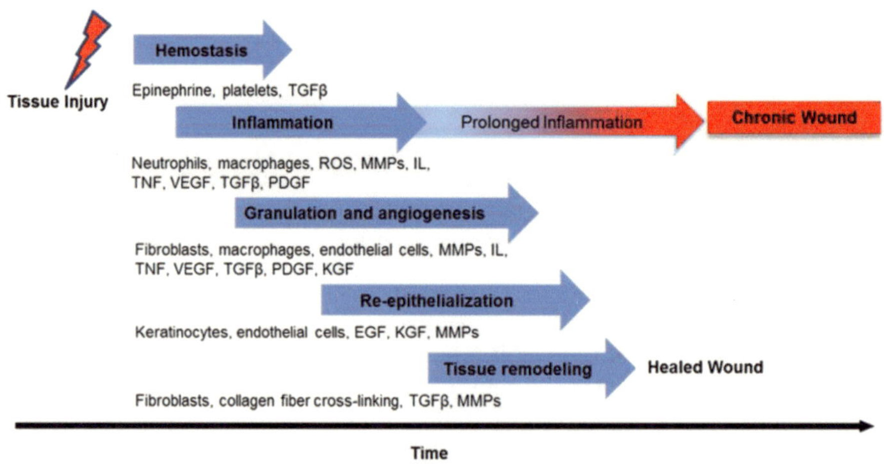

Figure 1. The phases of wound healing. After tissue injury, hemostasis and inflammation start immediately, in which cytokines, growth factors, and ROS are produced to recruit cells to the wound site. The next proliferative phases of wound healing include angiogenesis and re-epithelialization, where new tissue is formed by endothelial cells, fibroblasts, and keratinocytes. In diabetic wound healing, inflammation can be prolonged, causing the wounds to be chronic. The final phase is tissue remodeling. EGF (epidermal growth factor), IL (interleukin), KGF (keratinocyte growth factor), MMPs (matrix metalloproteinases), PDGF (platelet-derived growth factor), ROS (reactive oxygen species), TGF-β (transforming growth factor-beta), TNF (tumour necrosis factor), VEGF (vascular endothelial growth factor). Adapted from Schreml [22].

There are currently at least 24 known MMPs in humans [7]. Not all functions that these enzymes play in humans have been elucidated and concepts in their mechanistic roles in wound healing are emerging only recently. Yet, it is generally appreciated that MMPs play roles in each stage of wound healing, in large measure because of the need for restructuring of the ECM in the process of wound healing. The phases of wound healing consist of (1) hemostasis and inflammation, (2) granulation and angiogenesis, (3) re-epithelialization, and (4) tissue remodeling and are depicted in **Figure 1**. All four phases of wound healing have to be coordinated and integrated properly in a timely and sequential manner for successful healing. The repair processes require the coordination of events involving various cells, the ECM components, growth factors, cytokines, and enzymes. Furthermore, it is increasingly evident that MMPs display a duality of functions in the physiology of the tissue and processes of pathology, as evidenced for chronic wounds, cancers, Parkinson's and Alzheimer's diseases [8–10]. As such, certain MMPs might have a beneficial effect in healing, yet others might exhibit detrimental effect as aberrations in the functions of these enzymes in disease development and progression. The differentiation of these functions—detrimental versus beneficial—has been a challenge. Yet, new tools and capabilities are becoming available to address exactly these issues in various diseases.

1.1. Stages of wound healing

Once injury to the skin takes place, the cutaneous wound immediately enters the first phase of hemostasis (**Figure 1**). The onset of blood vessel constriction prevents excessive bleeding, which is followed by the aggregation of platelets along the damaged endothelium to form a plug. A cascade of events ensues, which leads to the formation of a blood clot. The serine-proteinase thrombin cleaves fibrinogen into insoluble fibrin threads that are aggregated with platelets to create the clot. In addition to stopping the bleeding, the blood clot serves as a provisional matrix for cell migration [11]. The surrounding cells of a blood clot also release inflammatory cytokines and growth factors as signaling molecules to attract a variety of cells

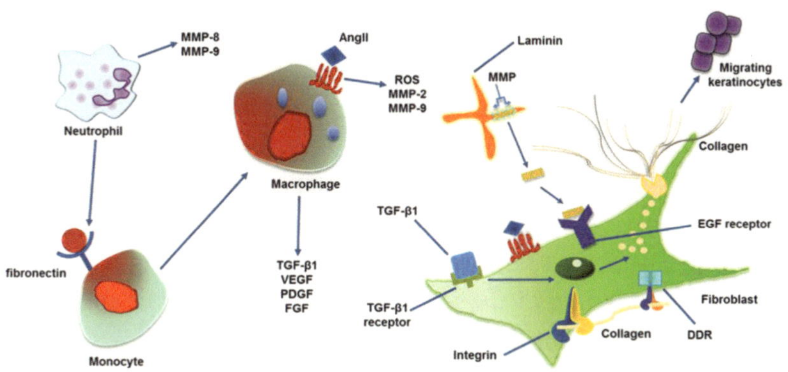

Figure 2. ECM–growth factor interactions and production of MMPs in wound healing. Monocytes migrate to the wound site and bind to fibronectin released by neutrophils. This interaction causes monocytes to differentiate into macrophages that secrete multiple growth factors. TGF-β1 binds to its receptor on fibroblasts and stimulates the cells to produce ECM components such as collagen, fibronectin, and hyaluronic acid. Neutrophils also produce MMP-8 and -9 in the wound. Binding of AngII to macrophages stimulates the cells to produce ROS and MMPs. MMPs can cleave laminin to release a fragment that binds EGF receptor on fibroblasts and stimulates migration and proliferation of keratinocytes. AngII (angiotensin II), ECM (extracellular matrix), DDR (discoidin domain receptor), EGF (epidermal growth factor), FGF (fibroblast growth factor), MMPs (matrix metalloproteinases), PDGF (platelet-derived growth factor), ROS (reactive oxygen species), TGF-β1 (transforming growth factor-beta 1), VEGF (vascular endothelial growth factor).

to the wound site to initiate the inflammatory phase. These cells include neutrophils, macrophages, and lymphocytes, which defend the site from infectious agents [12]. The earliest arrival of neutrophils takes place only a few hours after injury [13]. Neutrophils are responsible for releasing fibronectin, which has multifunctional roles, including a structural function due to its fibrillary composition, mediating interactions between ECM components and other cells, or serving as a bridge between cells [14, 15]. Fibronectin and fibrin act to provide provisional matrix that promotes cellular migration and adhesion, depending on the wound status. Also, during inflammation, fibronectin and other ECM protein fragments can attract monocytes, a type of white blood cells, to the wound site from the bloodstream. The interactions at the wound site cause monocytes to undergo differentiation into additional macrophages (**Figure 2**) [14]. Macrophages are stimulated by growth factors to produce reactive-oxygen species (ROS), MMPs, and multiple growth factors such as platelet-derived growth factor (PDGF), transforming growth factor-β (TGF-β), vascular endothelial growth factor (VEGF), and fibroblast growth factor (FGF) (**Figure 2**) [16]. One factor that can stimulate macrophages is angiotensin II (AngII). The renin–angiotensin system (RAS) is a pathway to regulate angiotensin, a hormone peptide, to eventually produce the primary effector-AngII [17]. This effector is present in macrophages, neutrophils, fibroblasts, and endothelial cells of human skin [18]. With binding and stimulation of AngII, inflammatory cells such as macrophages generate ROS and MMPs that subsequently promote migration and proliferation of keratinocytes. This will be discussed in a later section of this chapter.

Among many growth factors and cytokines, TGF-βs play critical roles in regulating the development of the ECM. There are three isoforms (TGF-β1–3) in humans, with each playing distinct roles in regulating synthesis of the ECM components, and even cellular proliferation or cellular death [19, 20]. TGF-βs are produced in latent forms that need to be activated by cleavage of their pro-peptides, before exerting their activities on the ECM, which include stimulation of cellular production of ECM components [20]. The most well known is TGF-β1, which can control production and degradation of many constituents involved in wound healing [14]. Once TGF-β1 binds to its receptor, this interaction stimulates the synthesis of ECM components such as collagen, fibronectin, and hyaluronic acid in many types of cells, including fibroblasts [21]. Fibroblasts are cells that synthesize collagen and other constituents deposited on the ECM [14]. Besides monocytes/macrophages, fibroblasts also generate ROS, including peroxide anion, hydroxyl ion, and superoxide anion, which are important in defense against pathogenic microorganisms [22]. ROS, in turn, has the effect of stimulating the production of more cytokines that lead to increased production of proteinases such as MMPs to modify components of the ECM [22]. Dualities of functions reveal themselves in ROS as well. The function against the pathogens is beneficial, but high-level ROS can cause damage to the ECM components [22]. This fine balance for ROS could stimulate complex signal pathways that would lead to up-regulation of MMPs in the wounds. The enhanced presence of ROS and the attendant stimulated turnover of ECM components could cause tissue destruction and hinder the repair processes [23]. This duality of roles for ROS was observed in a murine wound model that documented severe damage to the endothelium in a background that lacked ROS-detoxifying enzymes [24]. In diabetic patients with chronic wounds, the production of ROS has been found to exceed the antioxidant capacity, adding more oxidative stress to the wounds that subsequently increases MMP levels by 60-fold over those in acute wounds [12].

Granulation and angiogenesis take place in the next phase of wound repair, which is also known as the proliferative phase (**Figure 1**). Granulation tissue is defined as a matrix of collagen, with microscopic blood vessels that are newly formed from preexisting blood vessels in a process called angiogenesis. New blood capillaries supply oxygen to the wound tissue, which is critical for the healing process. Granulation, in the form of a red or pink soft tissue, forms on the surface of the wound. Macrophages are tasked with initiating this phase by degrading the blood clots and by producing a variety of cytokines and chemokines to attract fibroblasts to enter the wound site [22]. The population of fibroblasts at the wound site will expand by both migration and proliferation through dynamic interaction with growth factors and the ECM. This is mediated by integrins, a set of receptors for fibroblast, which consist of an extracellular domain that binds to the ECM, and an intracellular portion that associates with the cytoskeleton for biochemical signaling [25]. Integrins and discoidin domain receptor 2 (DDR2), another receptor for fibroblasts, bind to type I collagen within the ECM. This interaction stimulates the production of MMP-2 to promote migration of fibroblasts to the wound site through the basement membrane during ECM remodeling [26], as indicated in **Figure 2**. In addition, as mentioned earlier, TGF-β1 can stimulate proliferation of fibroblasts. The wound tissue is hypoxic and would require a supply of oxygen for the demands of the biochemical processes of wound healing [22]. Hypoxia stimulates macrophages, keratinocytes, fibroblasts, and endothelial cells to produce more VEGF, which is a cytokine associated with angiogenesis [22]. The enhanced expression of VEGF causes endothelial cells at the wound bed to migrate, proliferate, and form new blood vessels into the wounds to supply oxygen during angiogenesis [27]. In addition, VEGF has been shown to increase expression of the collagen-binding integrin in the dermal microvasculature [28]. These bindings with integrin help cells adhere to the ECM and promote additional growth factor expression. Rossiter et al. have reported that deletion of keratinocyte-specific VEGF impaired angiogenesis and delayed wound healing in a murine model [29]. Other researchers have shown that overexpression of VEGF can lead to enhanced wound healing in murine excisional wounds [30]. Another receptor that plays an important role in cellular migration during angiogenesis is epidermal growth factor (EGF) receptors, which can bind to EGF and laminin to enhance fibroblast migration [31, 32]. Laminin, which is a fibrous constituent of the basement membrane, plays important roles in cell adhesion, migration, and proliferation [33]. At the wound site, cleavage of laminin-332 (also referred to as laminin-5) by MMPs would generate a fragmented laminin peptide that binds to the EGF receptor and enhances the cellular motility of proliferating keratinocytes [34], demonstrated in **Figure 2**. In addition to its role in angiogenesis, fibroblasts are responsible for the production and deposition of immature collagen (type III collagen), which is essential in providing more strength for the wound ECM [22].

The formation of granulation tissue in the last phase provides a support matrix for epithelial cells to migrate across and to cover the wound surface in a process known as re-epithelialization (**Figure 1**). This stage of wound healing mainly involves keratinocytes, which are a predominant cell type in the epidermis of the skin [35]. In fact, to cover the wound surface with a new layer of epithelium, the keratinocytes at the wound edge need to undergo migration, differentiation, and proliferation. In the basal layer of epidermis, keratinocytes have differentiating characteristics, in which they are able to change into a longer and flatter shape before they begin migration [35]. The migrating keratinocytes need to loosen their adhesion to each other before moving away from the wound edge toward the wound's central point to close the open area [35]. It is interesting to note that these cells need to establish adhesion to the new ECM around them via integrins, but at the same time they develop actin filaments to support cellular migration through a wound matrix of necrotic material, clots, and even bacteria [36, 37]. During this process, the continued enhanced expression of MMPs, released by a variety of cells (macrophages, keratinocytes, endothelial cells, and fibroblasts) plays crucial roles in degrading substrates of the provisional wound matrix [38]. After the first layer of cells that cover the wound area, keratinocytes need to proliferate to have adequate depth of cells in the wound. The onset of proliferation is brought about by a variety of factors such as EGF, TGF-α, TGF-β, keratinocyte growth factor (KGF), and hepatocyte growth factor (HGF) [39]. The migration and proliferation of these cells require increased supply of oxygen in the wound bed [22]. It is important to note that in chronic wounds, the epidermis fails to re-epithelialize due to non-migratory keratinocytes, compared to acute wounds [35]. Following the robust proliferation and epithelial migration, wound healing enters its last phase of tissue remodeling that could potentially last in the order of years. Type III collagen prevalent during this last phase is gradually replaced by the more stable type I collagen [22]. The collagen fibers at the wound site are rearranged, cross-linked, and aligned to increase the wound's tensile strength [40]. The participation of proteinases is necessary to ensure ECM remodeling, which will bring back normality to the tissue.

In the repair of acute wounds, interactions between growth factors and the ECM occur in an orchestrated manner, where each phase is allowed to transition properly to the next, resulting in a healed wound. There are numerous factors that contribute to the impairment of wound healing in patients. Some are local factors that directly affect wound closure such as supply of oxygen, infection, venous sufficiency, and imbalance between proteinases or growth factors [12]. Others are underlying conditions that influence the overall health of a patient, including age, diseases, obesity, medications, and an immunocompromised system [12]. For instance, septic conditions have been shown to delay wound healing in mice [41]. In the case of patients affected by hypoproteinemia, their protein deficiency can impair wound healing by affecting capillary formation, cellular proliferation, collagen deposition, and wound remodeling [12]. The most detrimental disease is diabetes, where patients are more prone to develop non-healing ulcers or chronic wounds. In these wounds, the interactions between growth factors and the ECM are disrupted because of biochemical abnormalities of the ECM and aberrantly elevated activities of MMPs [14]. The imbalance between MMPs and their endogenous regulators can cause excessive degradative activities and critical loss of the newly reformed ECM in wound healing.

1.2. Matrix metalloproteinases (MMPs): structures and regulation

Matrix metalloproteinases are a group of 24 enzymes in humans—there are a total of 28 MMPs known to date, including enzymes from other organisms—which are expressed as zymogenic inactive proteins [7]. These enzymes are highly regulated and one level of regulation is exerted in their proteolytic activation by other proteinases, including by other MMPs [42, 43]. As the pro-domain of the zymogens are removed, the active sites become available for catalysis. Tissue inhibitors of matrix metalloproteinases (TIMPs) are protein inhibitors of these enzymes that form non-covalent complexes with the catalytic domain. The activation events and the inhibition by TIMPs account for various steps in the regulation process, which we will expand on in the following sections. These events are graphically depicted in **Figure 3** for MMP-2.

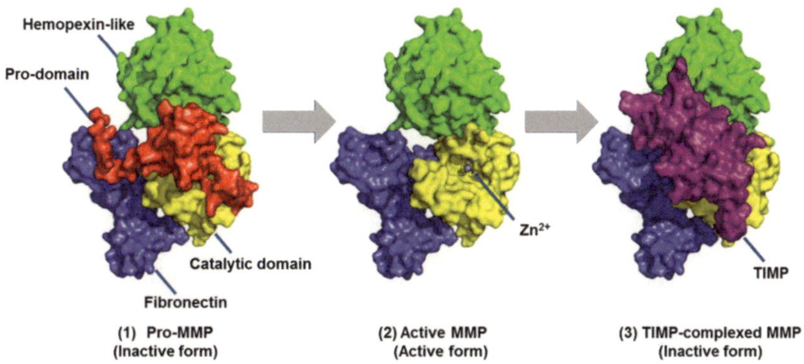

Figure 3. MMPs, as exemplified in this figure by MMP-2, exist in three forms: pro-MMPs (inactive), active MMPs, and TIMP-complexed MMPs (inactive). MMPs are first produced as latent pro-MMPs (1) with a pro-domain (shown in red) blocking the active site (shown in yellow). The removal of the pro-domain is required to activate MMPs by revealing the zinc ion in the catalytic site (2). Active MMPs are then able to cleave substrates. The activity of MMPs is regulated by interaction with TIMPs (shown in purple), which inactivate the MMPs (3).

MMPs are zinc-dependent endopeptidases. They are either secreted into the ECM or are membrane-anchored on the surface of the cell [9, 44, 45]. The most basic components of all MMPs consist of three domains: a signal sequence at the N-terminus, a pro-domain that caps the active site, and a catalytic domain, as depicted in **Figure 4**. This minimal domain organization is present in MMP-7 and MMP-26, also known as the matrilysins. The catalytic domain is characterized by the zinc-binding HExxHxxGxxH motif, containing three conserved histidines [46]. Several MMPs have an additional domain referred to as the hemopexin-like domain, which is linked at the C-terminus of the aforementioned basic sequence. The hemopexin-like domain is believed to play a role in substrate recognition. This organization of domains for MMPs is seen in MMP-3 and -10 (also known as stromelysin-1 and-2), MMP-1, -8, and -13 (also known as collagenases), MMP-12 (metalloelastase), MMP-20 (enamelysin), and MMP-22 and -27 [47] (**Figure 4**). MMP-2 and MMP-9 (or gelatinases) have more complicated structures by having fibronectin repeats inserted into the side of the catalytic sites [47]

(**Figure 4**). The membrane-bound MMPs have two types of membrane anchors. One is a transmembrane peptide domain and another is the GPI anchor (**Figure 4**). There are a few other variations, which are summarized in **Figure 4** graphically. The structural similarities among these MMPs are high. Certainly, individual domains are highly similar in both sequence and three-dimensional structures. As a consequence, these enzymes share significant overlap in their substrate preferences, which is likely a reflection of the fact that the functions of disparate MMPs in the physiology of the organism are critical and they exhibit some redundancy in their turnover of the substrates as a consequence. As it pertains to wound healing, important MMPs and their known substrates are listed in **Table 1**.

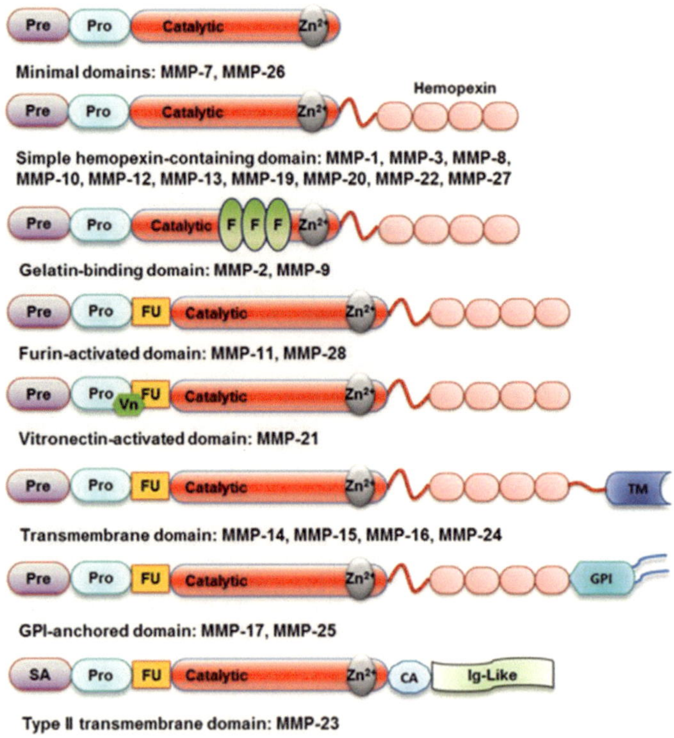

Figure 4. Structures of the MMP family. MMPs are divided into eight subgroups based on structural similarities. Pre: signal sequence, Pro: pro-peptide, Zn^{2+}: zinc-binding site, Catalytic: catalytic domain, F: repeats of fibronectin, Fu: furin-like serine proteinases, Vn: vitronectin-like insert, TM: transmembrane domain, GPI: glycosylphosphatidylinositol, SA: N-terminal signal anchor, CA: cysteine array, Ig-Like: immunoglobulin-like.

As indicated earlier, the functions of these enzymes are highly regulated. This regulation manifests itself at the transcriptional level as well as at the proteome level. Production of MMPs is stimulated in a variety of cells such as keratinocytes, fibroblasts, endothelial cells, and inflammatory cells during wound healing. These cells can be transcriptionally activated by a wide range of cytokines and growth factors including EGF, HGF, FGF, TGF-β, VEGF, PDGF, and KGF, as well as by interleukins and interferons [74]. Since there are many cytokines with

http://dx.doi.org/10.5772/64611

the ability to activate transcription to produce the zymogens, there are numerous signaling pathways implicated in the control of proteinase expression. These pathways include, for instance, mitogen-activated protein kinase (MAPK), or growth factor-dependent pathways of Smad, NF-kB, activation of focal adhesion kinase (FAK) by integrin activation, or Wnt cascade [11]. The highly regulated process is critical for the physiological roles. When the regulation goes awry, these enzymes cause pathological consequences. The pathological outcomes of MMP dysregulation have been the subject of many review articles [8, 10, 75, 76].

MMP	Preferred Substrates	Roles in Wound Healing	Cell culture	Human (H) or Mouse (M) wounds	Detection Method
MMP-1 (collagenase-1)	Collagen I, II, III, VII and X; aggrecan, serpins; alpha2-macroglobulin	• Promotes human keratinocyte migration on fibrillar collagen [38]	X		^{35}S-labeled antisense RNA probes [38]
		• Overexpression in keratinocytes delays re-epithelialization [38]	X		
		• Expressed by keratinocytes at their trailing membrane edge during wound healing [48]	X	H	Competitive ELISA [48]
		• Found to be elevated in diabetic foot ulcer patients [49]		H	
MMP-2 (gelatinase A)	Gelatin; collagen I, IV, V, VII, and X; laminin; aggrecan; fibronectin; tenascin	• Expressed by fibroblasts and endothelial cells in both mouse [50] and human acute wounds [51]		M H	ELISA and gelatin zymography [51]
		• Accelerates cell migration [34]	X		
		• Expressed in platelets, mediates platelet adhesion and aggregation [52]	X		
		• Keratinocyte migration [34]	X		
		• Activates MMP-9 [53]	X		
MMP-3 (stromelysin-1)	Collagen IV, V, IX, and X; fibronectin; elastin; gelatin;	• Expressed by basal keratinocytes in both human acute and chronic wounds [54]		H	^{35}S-labeled antisense RNA probes [54, 57]

MMP	Preferred Substrates	Roles in Wound Healing	Cell culture	Human (H) or Mouse (M) wounds	Detection Method
	aggrecan; nidogen; fibrillin; E-cadherin				
		• Affects wound contraction and delayed healing [55]		M	
		• Activates MMP-9 [56]	X		
MMP-7 (matrilysin)	Elastin; fibronectin; laminin; nidogen; collagen IV; tenascin: versican; α1-proteinase inhibitor; E-cadherin; tumour necrosis factor	• Required for re-epithelialization of mucosal wounds [58]		M	Immunohistochemistry [59]
		• Re-epithelialization of mucosal tissue is impaired in MMP-7 knockout mice [58]		M	
MMP-8 (collagenase-2)	Collagen I, II, and III; aggrecan, serpins; 2-MG	• Mainly expressed by neutrophils [3]			Western blot [62]
		• Promotes cutaneous diabetic wound healing [60]		M	MMP-inhibitor-tethered affinity resin [60]
		• Most prevalent collagenase in wounds [61]		H	
		• MMP-8 knockout mice show delayed wound closure [62]		M	
		• Found to be elevated in diabetic foot ulcer patients [49]		H	
		• Selective inhibition of MMP-8 delays murine diabetic wound healing [60]		M	*In-situ* zymography [63]
		• Topical application of active MMP-8 accelerates murine diabetic wound healing [63]		M	

MMP	Preferred Substrates	Roles in Wound Healing	Cell culture	Human (H) or Mouse (M) wounds	Detection Method
MMP-9 (gelatinase B)	Gelatin; collagen I,III,IV, V and VII; aggrecan; elastin; fibrillin	• Hypoxia induces cell migration through increased expression of MMP-9 [64]		M	Immunohistochemistry and gelatin zymography [51]
		• Upregulation causes detrimental effects in murine diabetic wounds [60]		M	• MMP-inhibitor-tethered affinity resin [60]
		• Keratinocyte migration [65]	X		
		• Increased levels in wound fluid of diabetic foot ulcers, quantified by gelatin zymography [49]		H	
		• MMP-9 knockout diabetic mice have reduced re-epithelialization and delayed wound closure [63]		M	
		• Selective inhibition of MMP-9 accelerates diabetic wound healing [60, 63]		M	*In-situ* zymography [63]
MMP-10 (stromelysin-2)	Collagen IV, V, IX, and X; fibronectin; elastin; gelatin; laminin; aggrecan; nidogen; E-cadherin	• Expressed by epidermal cells three days post-wounding in human wounds [66]		H	^{35}S-labeled antisense RNA probes [57, 66]
		• Overexpression in keratinocytes resulted in normal wound healing but disorganized epithelium [67]		M	• RNA probes [67]
MMP-12 (metalloelastase)	Collagen IV; gelatin; fibronectin; laminin; vitronectin; elastin; fibrillin; apolipoprotein A; α1-proteinase inhibitor	• Expressed specifically in macrophages, but not expressed by epithelial cells [50]		M	RNA isolation and RNase protection analysis [50]
		• Potential regulator of angiogenesis due to ability to generate angiostatin [68]	X		Western blot [68]

MMP	Preferred Substrates	Roles in Wound Healing	Cell culture	Human (H) or Mouse (M) wounds	Detection Method
MMP-13 (collagnase-3)	Collagen I, II, III, IV, IX, X and XIV; gelatin; fibronectin; laminin; tenascin; aggrecan; fibrillin; serpins	• Promotes re-epithelialization indirectly by affecting wound contraction [69]	X		mRNA and immunohistochemistry [70]
		• Keratinocyte migration [70]		M	
		• MMP-13 knockout mice have reduced re-epithelialization and delayed wound closure [70]		M	
MMP-14 (MT1-MMP)	Collagen I,II, and III; gelatin; fibronectin; laminin; vitronectin; aggrecan; tenascin; nidogen; perlecan; fibrillin; α1-proteinase inhibitor, α2-macroglobulin	• Promotes keratinocyte migration and invasion [71]			^{35}S-labeled antisense RNA probes [72]
		• Involved in KGFR expression, and can regulate epithelial cell proliferation [72]		M	
		• Activates MMP-2 [73]	X		

Adapted from Martins and Caley [3].

Table 1. Mammalian MMPs: enzymatic substrates and roles in wound healing.

The complex orchestration of events that we outlined in Section 1.1 on wound healing involves important roles by MMPs. However, since MMPs are highly regulated at the proteome level, the transcriptional regulation is not the full picture. Yet, the transcriptional regulation of MMPs is the most studied, as the tools for it are readily available. For example, the increased transcription leads to higher translation to the inactive MMP zymogens, which have to experience proteolytic activation. This activation may only require disruption of the interaction between the active-site zinc ion and the conserved cysteine residue from the sequence …PRCGVPD… of the pro-domain to give rise to the active MMPs [3]. During physiological processes, pro-MMP activation can be achieved either by serine proteinases or by other MMPs [6]. In particular, membrane-type MMPs have been shown to be capable of activating other pro-MMPs, both directly and indirectly. For instance, MMP-14 (or MT1-MMP) is involved in regulating activation of pro-MMP-9 in osteoclast migration [77]. Activation of MMPs by serine proteinases is regulated by inhibition of plasma proteinase inhibitors, including α1-proteinase and α2-macroglobulin or thrombospondin-1 and thrombospondin-2 [3]. The activity of MMPs is primarily regulated *in vivo* by endogenous tissue inhibitors of metalloproteinases (TIMPs) (**Figure 3**). In mammals, there are four TIMPs (TIMP-1, -2, -3, and -4) that bind specifically to inhibit MMPs [78]. The dysregulation such as imbalance between MMPs and TIMPs ratio leads to up-regulation of proteinase activity and damage to the ECM.

Method	Advantages	Limitations
mRNA and RT-PCR	Quick, simple, and inexpensive	Does not measure amount and activity of the proteinases
Western blot and immunohistochemistry	Simple, sensitive, and specific	Requires specific and expensive antibodies and does not distinguish between zymogen, active, and TIMP-complexed MMPs
Gelatin zymography	Inexpensive materials, semi-quantitative	Unable to distinguish between active and TIMP-complexed MMPs, low sensitivity
In-situ zymography	Identification of MMPs can be done in tissues	Limited to availability of fluorescent substrates, but not quantitative, and hard to discriminate between different MMPs, low sensitivity
Activity-based enzyme profiling	Specificity	Requires library of selective MMP-directed probes
TAPI-2 affinity resin	Identifies active MMPs	Starting materials are very expensive and requires user linking of TAPI to the resin
MMP inhibitor–tethered affinity resin	Identifies and quantifies active MMPs	Requires synthesis of MMP-inhibitor covalently attached to the resin

Adapted from Fisher and Mobashery [76].

Table 2. Profiling methods for MMPs.

Once activated, the only MMP form that is not complexed by TIMPs would have catalytic competence. Hence, tools are needed for analysis at the protein level in the afflicted/diseased tissue. Many current methodologies to profile MMPs are limited because they are unable to detect active MMPs (summarized in **Table 2**). We have applied unique tools to this end in both diabetic and non-diabetic wounds. An MMP-inhibitor-tethered affinity resin that binds exclusively to the active forms of MMPs was used to fish out activated MMPs that exist in wound tissues [60]. Once bound, the active MMPs were digested with trypsin and the peptides were analyzed by liquid chromatography—mass spectrometry/mass spectrometry (LC-MS/MS); the proteinases were identified from the peptides MS/MS data and a protein database search [60] (**Figure 5**). Subsequently, each identified active MMP was quantified using LC-MS/MS methods and custom-synthesized peptides. This analysis led to the discovery of active MMP-8 and MMP-9 in both diabetic and non-diabetic wounds from mice. The quantification revealed that MMP-9 was elevated at statistically significant levels, whereas levels of MMP-8 were slightly up-regulated after seven days from infliction of the wound [60].

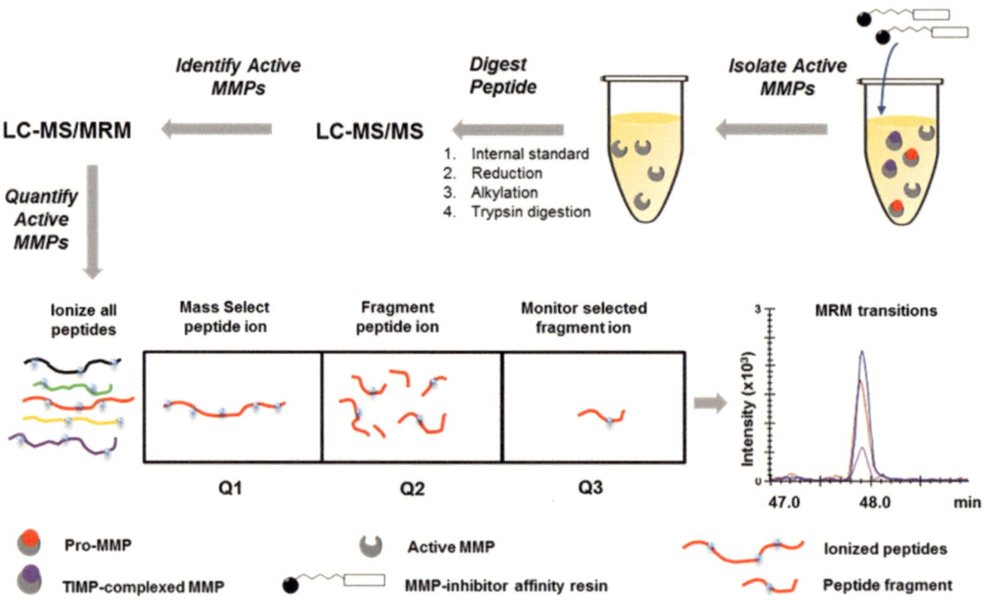

Figure 5. MMP-inhibitor-tethered affinity resin to identify and quantify active MMPs. Wound tissues are homogenized, and the homogenate is incubated with the MMP-inhibitor-tethered affinity resin, which binds only to active MMPs. The isolated active MMPs are reduced (to reduce disulfide bonds between the thiol groups of cysteine in MMPs), alkylated (to prevent reformation of disulfide bonds), and trypsin digested. The resulting peptides are analyzed by liquid chromatography-tandem mass spectrometry (LC-MS/MS) and identified by a protein database. The identified MMPs are quantified using three peptides and three transitions per peptide using LC with multiple-reaction monitoring (MRM). In this highly specific quantitative MS method, the ionized peptide selected in the first quadrupole (Q1) generates to a pool of fragments in the second quadrupole (Q2), where the highest intensity fragment ion is selected for monitoring in the third quadrupole (Q3). This transition from peptide to fragment ion is monitored, and the area under this peak is integrated. Finally, the concentrations of active MMPs in wound samples are quantified by using peak area ratios relative to the internal standard and calibration curve regression parameters.

Whereas these studies were followed up by investigations of knockout mice as well, the knockout mice do not provide a superior opportunity for elucidation of the functions of MMPs in our opinion. Knockout MMP-9 mice, which survive the embryonic stage, were made diabetic to explore the role of the enzyme. We hasten to add that the compensatory activities of other MMPs in light of the overlapping profiles for the substrates create ambiguity in interpretation of the data. These compensatory activities will be present throughout the embryonic development up to the point in which the experiment is conducted with these mice. The more superior approach, in our opinion, in elucidating the roles of the two enzymes (MMP-8 and MMP-9) is the use of selective pharmacological agents that afford total temporal control of abrogation of activity within the wounds in the time course of the experiments. Highly selective or specific inhibitors for the given enzyme are critical for the success of these studies. These investigations indeed revealed the duality of MMP functions, beneficial and detrimental, in diabetic wounds [60, 63]. It was documented that MMP-8 had a beneficial role in wound healing, as it might be the body's response to the healing process. On the other hand, MMP-9 was shown to serve a detrimental role in diabetic wound healing; hence, an aberration in the regulatory events in diabetic animals led to its formation with detrimental consequences. Indeed, pharmacological intervention by selective MMP-9 inhibitors with no activity toward MMP-8 would appear to be a promising approach to speed up healing of diabetic wounds. As the non-healing wounds remain open for a long period of time, they face the fatal threat of infections with methicillin-resistant *Staphylococcus aureus* [79, 80] that lead to amputations like in the case of diabetic foot infections [81]. There is a serious need to develop new approaches to facilitate healing in chronic wounds since current treatments have not been proven effective. The only FDA approved drug Regranex™ (becaplermin), a platelet-derived growth factor, is associated with malignancies and increased risk of death [82]. In addition, the effectiveness of negative-pressure wound therapy is still unclear, stem cell therapies do not clear the infection, or topical antibiotics, and antimicrobial dressings induce antibiotic resistance [81].

2. Detection of matrix metalloproteinases in tissue

As indicated above, MMPs are usually not detectable in normal adult tissues, but are up-regulated in disease. The tools available for assessment of MMP levels are quantification of mRNA, reverse transcription-polymerase chain reaction (RT-PCR), Western blotting and immunohistochemistry, gelatin zymography, *in-situ* gelatin zymography, activity-based enzyme profiling, and TAPI-2 resin [76]. However, these tools generally do not reveal whether the elevated levels of the MMPs that are being monitored are due to the inactive zymogenic forms, the active MMPs, or the MMPs in complex with TIMPs (inactive forms). Quantification of mRNA levels by Northern blot analysis and RT-PCR are limited in that these methods measure mRNA levels and not the amount and activity of the protein. Immunohistochemistry and Western blot require specific antibodies, which usually cannot distinguish between active and TIMP-inhibited MMPs, and might exhibit cross-reactivity. The sensitivity of zymography is not typically high, and this method also detects TIMP-complexed MMPs. *in-situ* zymography is limited by the availability of fluorescent proteinase substrates, which at present can be performed for MMP-1, -2, -3, -7, -8, -9, -12, -13, and -25. This method has limitations for quantitative determinations. Activity-based enzyme profiling of MMPs requires a library of selective MMP-directed probes [76]. A TAPI-2 affinity resin has been reported to identify active MMPs [76]. However, it is very expensive. With the exception of the TAPI-2 resin, the other methods do not identify and quantify the active forms of MMPs. A summary of advantages and limitations of these methods is given in **Table 2**. We add that another complication in these studies is that the active MMPs formed in diseased tissue might be present in minute quantities, such that conventional detection methods at the proteome level might not be able to identify them. We reiterate that of the MMP forms, only the active MMPs in the absence of TIMP complexation would be able to perform its function in manifestation of the disease.

Expression of MMPs in normal uninjured skin is generally low. However, their activities are thought to be up-regulated when cutaneous wounds occur. For instance, low RNA expression levels of MMP-2 and MT1-MMP were reported in uninjured murine skin [50]. Once the cutaneous injury happens, up-regulation and expression of many MMPs have been reported, including collagenases (MMP-1 [83], MMP-8 [60, 61], and MMP-13 [70]), gelatinases (MMP-2 [51] and MMP-9 [51, 60]), stromelysins (MMP-3 and MMP-10 [54]), and other MMPs such as MMP-7 [58], MMP-12 [50], and MMP-14 [51]. However, it should be noted that most of these studies employed methods that do not distinguish between the active or inactive forms of MMPs, except the aforementioned TAPI-2 resin and the recent methodology that couples an MMP-inhibitor-tethered affinity resin with mass spectrometry, as mentioned in the previous section [60]. As such, observation of up-regulation or even the expression of a particular MMP does not necessarily imply a role for that MMP in wound healing. Parallel to MMPs, the expression of TIMPs is often increased in order to regulate the proteinase activities [84]. Hence, the biochemical imbalance that leads to aberrant consequence has to be the focus of research in elucidating the mechanistic basis of disease.

2.1. Beneficial roles of MMPs in wound repair

Collagenases have been implicated in wound healing for many years. As the name implies, these proteinases prefer to turn over various types of collagen (types I, II, and III), which is an important process in wound repair (**Table 1**). MMP-1, expressed by keratinocytes about a week after injury occurs, might facilitate keratinocyte migration when these cells come into contact with type I collagen in the early re-epithelization phase [83]. The interaction between keratinocytes at the wound edge and type I collagen in the matrix via the $\alpha2\beta1$ integrin receptor enhances the expression of MMP-1 [38]. MMP-1 cleaves type I collagen to generate cleaved fragments, which have been suggested to become a less adhesive binding ligand than the native protein and that loosens the matrix environment for cellular movements. Thus, the complex of MMP-1 and $\alpha2\beta1$ promotes migration of keratinocyte on type I collagen in the re-epithelialization phase, as shown in **Figure 6**. However, $\alpha2\beta1$ integrin-deficient mice still retain normal re-epithelialization, collagen deposition, and tensile strength, which indicate a possible compensatory mechanism by another integrin receptor [85]. Once the new basement membrane is established after re-epithelialization, the epidermal expression of MMP-1 is terminated by cellular contacts with proteins from the membrane. Specifically, the contact between keratinocytes with laminin-111 (previously called laminin-1) leads to the repression of MMP-1 in the presence of type I collagen [86]. Expression of MMP-1 has also been observed in fibroblasts during granulation and angiogenesis [83], where the enzyme might act to remodel the ECM of the wound [87]. Interestingly, overexpression of human MMP-1 in the epidermis of transgenic mice resulted in delayed wound closure; however, the genomic modification with human DNA in these animals may have resulted in unwanted phenotypes [88].

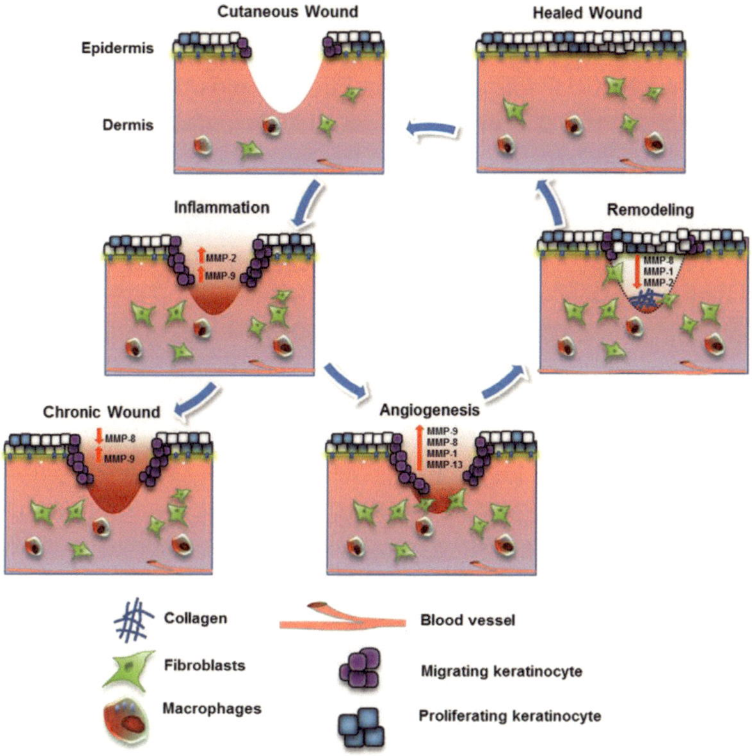

Figure 6. Involvement of MMPs in the wound-healing process. The healed or healthy skin, consisting of ECM and blood vessels, is populated by fibroblasts. Once the skin is damaged by a full-thickness injury, it becomes a cutaneous wound. In the early phase of inflammation, the wound is occupied with fibrin clot to seal the wound, and levels of MMP-2 and MMP-9 are increased. Fibroblasts and macrophages migrate into the wound site, where they are stimulated to release more MMPs to remodel the ECM. The inflammation phase is followed by angiogenesis, in which the up-regulation of a variety of MMPs (including MMP-1, MMP-8, MMP-9, and MMP-13) would stimulate epithelial cells (keratinocytes) to proliferate and migrate to re-epithelialize over the wound area. However, prolonged inflammation could cause the wounds to become chronic, as it has been observed in diabetic foot ulcers. During chronic wounds, the irregular up-regulation of MMP-9 has been associated with reduction of MMP-8 and plays a detrimental role in ECM remodeling. Tissue remodeling and expression of MMPs are attenuated when the epithelial cells proliferate and differentiate in order to reform the new epithelium. During this last phase of wound healing, fibroblasts can continue to remodel the underlying dermis over a period of several months.

Expression of human MMP-1 has shown similar patterns to expression of murine MMP-13 in an excisional wound healing model (**Figure 6**) [50, 89]. Both MMP-1 and MMP-13 may share roles in promoting the survival of fibroblasts while remodeling collagen deposition in the wound ECM [69]. Hattori *et al.* have shown that MMP-13 knockout mice had both delayed re-epithelialization and wound closure (**Table 3**) [70]. However, in another study, MMP-13 knockout mice showed normal efficiency of re-epithelialization, wound closure, inflammatory response, and unaltered remodeling of the wound matrix [90]. The inconclusive evidence on the role of MMP-13 in wound repair could in principle be explained by the redundancy in functions of proteinases that we mentioned earlier. There was up-regulated expression of MMP-8 (or collagenase-2) in these MMP-13-deficient animals [90], for example. The relevance of MMP-8 in wound repair was unclear until this study indicated that there is enzymatic compensation by MMP-8 to facilitate normal wound healing [90]. There is mounting evidence that MMP-8 plays a beneficial role in repairing the wounds. As MMP-8 is expressed and secreted mostly by neutrophils, its expression peaks after four days in non-diabetic wounds, detected by ELISA [61]. In humans, MMP-8 is the most prevalent collagenase in cutaneous wounds, where it is required for debridement of the wound and for the removal of damaged type I collagen [61]. Yet, it is still challenging to conclude whether this is the active form of MMP-8 by the methods that were used. In mice, the exact levels of active MMP-8 were quantitatively determined by the use of an MMP-inhibitor-tethered affinity resin coupled with mass spectrometry [60]. In this study, Gooyit *et al.* also demonstrated that selective inhibition of MMP-8 caused delayed wound healing and incomplete re-epithelialization in diabetic mice [60]. In addition, MMP-8-deficient mice displayed a significant delay in wound healing, caused by a lag in neutrophil infiltration, persistent inflammation and impaired re-epithelialization (**Table 3**) [62]. However, MMP-8 knockout mice show compensation in MMP-9 [62], making it difficult to separate the roles of MMP-8 and MMP-9 in wound healing. Furthermore, topical application of active recombinant MMP-8 on murine diabetic wounds resulted in a significant acceleration in both wound healing and re-epithelialization [63]. These studies reveal the beneficial role of MMP-8 in wound healing, where the neutrophil-derived MMP-8 can facilitate repair processes by providing debridement for damaged proteins and paving a pathway for the formation of the provisional matrix for keratinocyte migration (**Figure 6**).

Gene	Modification	Wound phenotype	Reference
hmmp-1	Overexpression in keratinocytes	Delayed re-epithelialization	[88]
mmp-3	Knockout	Impaired wound contraction	[55]
mmp-8	Knockout	Delayed re-epithelialization, delayed arrival of and prolonged inflammation	[62]
mmp-9	Knockout	Enhanced re-epithelization, accelerated wound closure	[63, 64]
mmp-10	Overexpression in KCs	Unaltered wound closure, scattered epithelialization	[67]
mmp-13	Knockout	Delayed wound closure, and reduced re-epithelialization	[70]
mmp-14	Knockout	Unaltered wound closure over 7 days' but premature morbidity and mortality were observed in these mice	[92, 93]

Table 3. Metalloproteinase gene targeting in mice studies and wound phenotypes.

The underlying cause of diabetic complications leads to up-regulation of MMP-9 compared to MMP-8. For instance, biopsy samples from diabetic patients revealed only two-fold increase in MMP-8, but 14-fold increase in MMP-9 expression when compared to non-diabetic tissues

[49]. Although the application of recombinant MMP-8 accelerated healing of full-thickness wounds in diabetic mice, it might have a similar beneficial mechanism as the marketed drug Santyl®, which is indicated for debridement of chronic dermal ulcers and severely burned areas and contains collagenase derived from *Clostridium histolyticum*. Clinical evidence suggests that collagenase treatment expedites the removal of necrotic tissues and enhances keratinocyte migration [91]. When used after debridement, Santyl® promotes wound healing in patients with pressure ulcers, venous leg ulcers, diabetic ulcers, and severely burnt wounds [91]. However, excessive use of active recombinant MMP-8 may affect the formation of new ECM and may not be beneficial in wound healing. A dose-response study with active recombinant MMP-8 topically administered to wounds of diabetic mice showed that higher levels of this proteinase did not accelerate wound healing [63].

Gelatinases, MMP-2 and MMP-9, are also involved in wound repair. Early expression of both gelatinases is observed in platelets, where MMP-9 is involved in platelet production and MMP-2 mediates platelet adhesion and aggregation [52]. The early expression of gelatinases might contribute to degradation of gelatin matrix in biofilm produced by bacteria [94]. This degradation serves to weaken the attachment of bacterial biofilm to the wound site and might be a strategy in fighting infection [94]. In addition, gelatinases are able to digest various constituents of the wound matrix to initiate angiogenesis in the repair processes. After tissue injury, AngII, which plays roles in inflammation, cell proliferation, and migration, would stimulate macrophages and neutrophils to generate ROS and MMPs to promote cell adhesion and ECM formation [17]. Specifically, AngII has been shown to induce the expression of both gelatinases, MMP-2 [95] and MMP-9 [96, 97]. AngII has been demonstrated to promote angiogenesis via activation of VEGF and endothelial nitric oxide [98], whereas studies with AngII-type 1a receptor knockout mice or with inhibition of AngII receptor have resulted in delayed wound healing with reduced angiogenesis in animals [99]. Given the beneficial role of AngII in angiogenesis of wound healing, it is interesting to note that there is discrepancy in the outcomes of diseases treated with this factor's inhibitors. These inhibitors can either block AngII receptors or inhibit the enzyme that generates factor AngII in the RAS pathway. In cancer, AngII inhibitors have been shown to reduce the tumor-related VEGF expression, angiogenesis, and tumor size [16]. These drugs are also used to treat hypertension, in which dysregulation of RAS causes poor blood flow, inadequate supply of oxygen, and impaired wound healing [12]. When used in anti-hypertensive therapy, drugs such as losartan has been demonstrated to promote wound healing in diabetes-induced mice by improving vascular perfusion, without affecting VEGF expression [100]. To this extent, anti-hypertensive therapy appears to be beneficial for wound healing. Thus, there is a need for further research to elucidate the precise role of these inhibitors in diabetic patients with impaired wound healing.

Expression of MMP-2 is demonstrated to coincide with expression of laminin-332 (also referred to as laminin-5) during enhanced keratinocyte migration in wound healing [101]. Since both MMP-2 and MMP-9 can cleave the gamma-2 chain of laminin-322 [102], they result in a pro-migratory and EGF-like fragment that binds EGF receptor to trigger cell migration of keratinocytes at the wound matrix [34], demonstrated in **Figure 2**. This cleaved fragment has been found in both tumors and tissues that undergo remodeling, except for intact epidermis [34,

103, 104]. Interestingly, MMP-8 also cleaves laminin-332, which indicates the mechanistic redundancy of the roles of MMPs during wound healing [102]. Furthermore, the two gelatinases might contribute to angiogenesis possibly by activating cytokines such as TNF-α (tumor necrosis factor-alpha) [105] and VEGF [106, 107]. However, cleavage of laminin-332 by MMP-2 has only been shown in tumor cells and normal breast epithelial cells, but not in normal keratinocytes in wound repair. Some studies have implicated MMP-2 in cleaving the latency-associated peptide (LAP) of pro-TGF-β and latent TGF-β binding protein (LTBP) to release activated TGF-β to bind the ECM [108–110]. Another study has also indicated that the active form of MMP-2 can activate MMP-9 in cell culture [53]. Pro-MMP-2 itself needs to be activated, and it has been shown that this activation requires the cluster of MMP-14, pro-MMP-2, and $\alpha V\beta 3$ integrin in a model of breast cancer cells [111]. It is important to note that active MMP-2 was not observed in wounds of diabetic and non-diabetic mice in the studies that used the MMP-inhibitor-tethered affinity resin, described earlier [60]. Therefore, the role of MMP-2 during wound healing has remained obscured with no *in vivo* verification to date. In fact, the study that implicated both active MMP-2 and MMP-9 in human wound healing used gelatin zymography as the tool [112]. However, this method lacks the ability to detect exclusively the active MMPs in the wound tissues, because the denaturation of the TIMP-MMP complex during electrophoresis could also result in an active MMP-2 band (**Table 2**). On the other hand, inhibition of MMP-9 activity with an antibody or MMP-9 ablation has delayed keratinocyte migration *in vitro*, which indicates the necessary involvement of MMP-9 during normal wound closure [65]. Others have also demonstrated *in vitro* that MMP-9 appears to promote keratinocyte migration [113]. Indeed, the study with the MMP-inhibitor-tethered affinity resin revealed that active MMP-9 was essentially undetectable in the intact skin, but it was expressed as early as one day after injury and remained up-regulated throughout the two weeks of study in non-diabetic and diabetic mice [60]. In the case of diabetic mice with delayed wound closure, the analysis showed up-regulation of active MMP-9, which could be detrimental to the repair process [60]. Besides promoting angiogenesis, gelatinases and other MMPs interestingly can inhibit angiogenesis by generating anti-angiogenic peptides from other precursor proteins. For instance, distinct proteinases such as MMP-3, -7, -9, -13, and -20 have been shown to generate active endostatin from human collagen XVIII [114] *in vitro*, whereas MMP-2, -3, -7, -9, and -12 are responsible for generating angiostatin from plasminogen [68, 115].

Expression of MMP-3 and MMP-10 (two stromelysins) has been found in epidermal cells during human and murine wound healing using RNA probes (**Table 1**). MMP-3 is expressed by the basal-proliferating keratinocytes, which are in contact with the intact basement membrane and close to the wound edge [54]. Expression of MMP-3 is also detected in fibroblasts during wound healing [11]. Research has shown that wound closure was delayed in non-diabetic MMP-3 knockout mice due to impaired wound contraction (**Table 3**) [55]. The implicated involvement of MMP-3 in normal wound healing may have resulted from demonstration that MMP-3 could activate MMP-9 [56], the gelatinase that plays roles in keratinocyte migration. However, MMP-2 could also trigger activation of MMP-9 [53], which corroborates the possibility of mechanistic compensation by other MMPs in physiology. Thus, the involvement of MMP-3 in the repair processes of wound healing still remains ambiguous. Nonetheless, it has been demonstrated that MMP-3 can activate several pro-MMPs, digest many ECM components, and increase the availability, as well as the activities, of cytokines and growth factors [116]. These findings disclose roles for MMP-3 in cell migration and proliferation during wound repair.

Meanwhile, MMP-10 (stromelysin-2), is expressed with a different pattern even though both MMP-3 and MMP-10 can degrade several collagens and non-collagenous connective tissue substrates, including proteoglycans, gelatin, fibronectin, and laminin [117], as indicated in **Table 1**. Human MMP-10 is expressed by epidermal cells about three days post-wounding, where its regulation seems to depend on EGF, TGF-β, and TNF-α cytokines [66]. The role of MMP-10 in wound repair was investigated by overexpressing a constitutively active MMP-10 mutant in keratinocytes, which resulted in normal wound-healing architecture and normal wound-healing rate in these transgenic mice [67]. However, the epidermal histology was demonstrated to have a disorganized migrating epithelium, composed of degradation in the newly formed matrix via laminin-332, abnormal cell-to-cell contacts of keratinocytes, and finally an increased rate of apoptosis of keratinocytes [67]. These findings indicate that levels of MMP-10 require a tightly regulated expression to facilitate keratinocyte migration during wound healing. Although both stromelysins would appear to be players, more investigations are needed to ascertain the roles of active MMP-3 and MMP-10 in the physiology of wound repair.

In addition to gelatinases and collagenases, other MMPs might have roles in wound healing as well, even though the data are not conclusive. For instance, MMP-7 (matrilysin) has been shown to be expressed in injured epithelia of various mucosal tissues, including lung, kidney, cornea, and gut [58, 118–120], even though MMP-7 is not expressed in epidermal wounds. In the lungs, MMP-7 has been demonstrated to play a role in inducing epithelial migration by facilitating the shedding of syndecan-1, a transmembrane heparin sulfate proteoglycan [58]. In the same study, MMP-7 knockout mice displayed impaired re-epithelialization in the mucosal tissue [58]. Also in the lungs, MMP-7 has been shown to cleave E-cadherin in the process of facilitating cell migration away from the edge of the injured wound [118]. On the other hand, another study has shown that MMP-7 and MMP-13 are expressed at the invasive edge of tumors [121]. Another proteinase that might be important for the wound-repair process is MMP-12 (metalloelastase), which is expressed by macrophages surrounding blood vessels in acute murine excisional wounds [50]. Even though MMP-12 was not detected in either acute- or chronic-wound tissues in the presence of macrophages, this proteinase expression was found to be abundant in different human cutaneous granulomas [122]. In addition to its ability to degrade fibrinogen interfering with blood clotting [123], MMP-12 is a potential regulator of angiogenesis, since it was demonstrated to be most efficient at producing angiostatin [68]. Membrane-type MMPs might also be necessary for wound healing, more specifically MMP-14, which is the most extensively studied to date (**Table 1**). The pivotal role of MMP-14 in angiogenesis of wound healing may be attributed to the enzyme's fibrinolytic and collagenolytic activity that is necessary for cell migration [71]. In addition, MMP-14 is needed for TIMP-2-mediated activation of pro-MMP-2, a process that is coordinated by two MMP-14 molecules and TIMP-2 [73]. Although MMP-14-deficient mice display abnormalities in bone development, impaired angiogenesis, and defective type I collagen [93, 124], wound closure in these animals remains surprisingly unaffected (**Table 3**) [92]. However, MMP-14 has been demonstrated to regulate cell proliferation by altering the expression of the KGF receptor during wound healing in acute airway injury [72]. The overlapping functions of other membrane-type MMPs or other MMPs may compensate for the absence of MMP-14 in these animals, supporting the concept of proteinase redundancy among MMPs.

2.2. Roles of MMPs in the pathology of chronic wounds

Cutaneous injuries that are recalcitrant to healing will become chronic wounds. In addition to delayed wound closure, chronic wounds are characterized by excessive proteolysis, prolonged inflammation, and failure in re-epithelialization [125]. Although MMPs play important roles in restructuring the ECM and repairing the wounds, high levels of MMPs can be blamed for increased proteolysis that leads to excessive degradation of ECM constituents and disruptions of cell migration. These unwarranted events cause the wounds to enter a prolonged inflammation. ELISA was used to document 65-fold higher levels of MMP-1, twofold higher of MMP-8, and twofold lower of TIMP-2, whereas gelatin zymography showed 14-fold higher levels of MMP-9, and sixfold higher of MMP-2 in diabetic foot ulcers than in non-diabetic patients with acute wounds [49]. Up-regulation of MMPs hinders wound repair by degrading ECM components and growth factors excessively [126]. As the wounds stay open too long, the invading bacteria might also release bacterial proteinases to cause rapid degradation of growth factors [94]. In order to defend the wounds against the invading microbes, the body will secrete more ROS and inflammatory factors. High levels of ROS such as hydrogen peroxide cause tissue damage [22], and high levels of inflammatory factors can lead to elevated expression of MMPs, as discussed earlier. The delaying mechanism of this vicious cycle keeps the patient's wound in a chronic stage [127]. Most studies emphasize MMP-9 up-regulation, which is associated with poor wound healing in diabetic foot ulcers and chronic wounds (**Figure 6**). When high levels of exogenous MMP-9, parallel to human chronic wounds, was applied to non-diabetic mice, this treatment delayed wound healing of the animals [128]. In one study, up-regulated levels of MMP-9 were found in wound fluid from patients with unhealed diabetic foot ulcers when compared with healed ulcers, as determined by gelatin zymography [129]. Also, in this same study, the researchers found decreased levels of TGF-β1 and TIMP-1 using ELISA [129]. In another study of patients with diabetic foot ulcer, levels of MMP-9 were measured by Western blot with MMP-9 antibody and were higher in patients with high risk of developing foot ulcers [130]. Expression of this proteinase was detected in migrating epithelial cells by ELISA [50, 51] and in inflammatory cells including T cells and neutrophils by gelatin zymography [131, 132]. Nevertheless, it should be noted that increased levels of MMPs, specifically that of MMP-9, as determined by ELISA, Western blot or gelatin zymography do not necessarily imply that it is active or has any role in the pathology of chronic wounds. ELISA and Western blot depend on the specificity of the antibodies, which likely immunoreact with pro-MMPs, active MMPs, and TIMP-complexed MMPs. Similarly, the active MMP-2 and MMP-9 bands detected by gelatin zymography could be from the TIMP-complexed gelatinases that dissociate during electrophoresis [133]. Therefore, the expression of MMP-9 found in many studies cannot be established conclusively as active MMP-9, the only form of the proteinase that can modify substrates catalytically. Another common research method is the use of MMP knockout animals, which may provide further insights into the roles of MMPs in wound healing (**Table 3**). However, the drawback of knockout animals is the possibility of mechanistic compensation by other MMPs in the absence of the ablated MMP, as discussed earlier. For instance, it has been shown that levels of MMP-9 are increased when MMP-2 or MMP-8 are ablated [62, 134]. Also, many MMPs share the same substrates, indicating the redundancy in the proteinase functions of MMPs [3].

We described earlier the MMP-inhibitor-tethered affinity resin that Gooyit *et al.* used to identify and accurately measure the levels of active MMP-9, which was found to be up-regulated in diabetic mice with delayed wound healing [60]. The dual roles of MMPs are exhibited in this case of MMP-9 up-regulation, which was demonstrated to be detrimental to diabetic wound repair by topical treatment with two distinct selective MMP-9 inhibitors (ND-322 and ND-336) [60, 63]. Inhibition of MMP-9 accelerated wound healing and promoted re-epithelialization. It has been shown that MMP-9 inhibits cell replication during epithelial migration; thus, MMP-9-deficient mice, both diabetic and non-diabetic, display a better rate of wound closure [63, 64]. Similar to MMP-2, MMP-9 can also activate pro-TGF-β and release it from LTBP [108, 109], while TGF-β has been shown to induce pro-MMP-9 in human skin [135]. Since TGF-β1 is a cytokine that elicits recruitment of inflammatory cells during wound healing [136], its up-regulation can regulate wound repair [137]. Interestingly, prolonged elevation in levels of inflammatory cytokines, such as TGF-β, can lead to a prolonged inflammation phase and consequentially delayed wound closure in diabetic mice [138]. However, it has also been shown that non-diabetic MMP-9 knockout mice had delayed wound closure [70]. The apparent conflicting role of MMP-9 may be explained by compensation of other MMPs, such as increased expression of MMP-3 and MMP-13 in MMP-9 knockout animals [139]. In addition, the redundancy of MMP substrates allow other MMP(s) to fulfill the same role, for instance MMP-1, MMP-2, MMP-9, and MMP-13 have a role in keratinocyte migration and can replace MMP-9 during normal wound healing [38, 70, 113, 140]. To date, topical application with a selective MMP-9 inhibitor, by itself or in combination with recombinant MMP-8, has shown therapeutic potential in accelerating murine diabetic wound healing [63]. These treatments improve diabetic wound healing by increasing angiogenesis and restoring levels of inflammatory cytokines, including TGF-β1 [63].

3. Conclusions

MMPs exist in three forms—pro-MMPs, active MMPs, and TIMP-complexed MMPs—of which only the active MMPs play a role in the pathology or repair of acute and chronic wounds. Current methodologies do not distinguish between the three forms of MMPs. Thus, the roles of MMPs in acute and chronic wounds are still not Qualitative and well-characterized quantitative profiling of only the active form of MMPs is necessary for investigating the critical roles of MMPs in remodeling the ECM during wound repair. We used a novel MMP-inhibitor-tethered affinity resin that binds only the active form of MMPs, from which we identified and quantified active MMP-8 and active MMP-9 in a murine diabetic model with delayed wound healing [60]. We showed that up-regulation of active MMP-9 plays a detrimental role whereas active MMP-8 is involved in repairing the wound in diabetic mice [60, 63]. These studies identified MMP-9 as a novel target for therapeutic intervention in the treatment of chronic wounds. A selective inhibitor of MMP-9 that leaves MMP-8 unaffected would provide the most effective therapy and represents a promising strategy for therapeutic intervention in the treatment of diabetic foot ulcers.

Acknowledgements

This work was supported by a grant from the American Diabetes Association Pathway to Stop Diabetes Grant 1-15-ACN-06. Trung T. Nguyen is a Fellow of the Chemistry-Biochemistry-Biology Interface Program supported by training grant T32 GM075762 from the National Institutes of Health.

Author details

Trung T. Nguyen, Shahriar Mobashery and Mayland Chang*

*Address all correspondence to: mchang@nd.edu

Department of Chemistry and Biochemistry, University of Notre Dame, Notre Dame, Indiana, USA

References

[1] Kirby GT, Mills SJ, Cowin AJ, Smith LE. Stem cells for cutaneous wound healing. Biomed Res Int. 2015;2015:285869.

[2] Bonnans C, Chou J, Werb Z. Remodelling the extracellular matrix in development and disease. Nat Rev Mol Cell Biol. 2014;15(12):786–801.

[3] Martins VL, Caley M, O'Toole EA. Matrix metalloproteinases and epidermal wound repair. Cell Tissue Res. 2013;351(2):255–268.

[4] Rohani MG, Parks WC. Matrix remodeling by MMPs during wound repair. Matrix Biol. 2015;44–46:113–121.

[5] Salazar JJ, Ennis WJ, Koh TJ. Diabetes medications: impact on inflammation and wound healing. J Diabetes Complic. 2016;30(4):746–752.

[6] Caley MP, Martins VL, O'Toole EA. Metalloproteinases and wound healing. Adv Wound Care (New Rochelle). 2015;4(4):225–234.

[7] Ugalde AP, Ordonez GR, Quiros PM, Puente XS, Lopez-Otin C. Metalloproteases and the degradome. In: Clark IM, Young DA, Rowan AD, editors. Matrix Metalloproteinase Protocols, vol. 622, 2nd ed. New York: Humana Press 2010. p. 3–29.

[8] Brkic M, Balusu S, Libert C, Vandenbroucke RE. Friends or foes: matrix metalloproteinases and their multifaceted roles in neurodegenerative diseases. Mediat Inflamm. 2015;2015:620581.

[9] Folgueras AR, Pendas AM, Sanchez LM, Lopez-Otin C. Matrix metalloproteinases in cancer: from new functions to improved inhibition strategies. Int J Dev Biol. 2004;48(5–6):411–424.

[10] Chang M. Restructuring of the extracellular matrix in diabetic wounds and healing: a perspective. Pharmacol Res. 2016;107:243–248.

[11] Toriseva M, Kahari VM. Proteinases in cutaneous wound healing. Cell Mol Life Sci. 2009;66(2):203–224.

[12] Guo S, Dipietro LA. Factors affecting wound healing. J Dent Res. 2010;89(3):219–229.

[13] Egozi EI, Ferreira AM, Burns AL, Gamelli RL, Dipietro LA. Mast cells modulate the inflammatory but not the proliferative response in healing wounds. Wound Repair Regen. 2003;11(1):46–54.

[14] Schultz GS, Wysocki A. Interactions between extracellular matrix and growth factors in wound healing. Wound Repair Regen. 2009;17(2):153–162.

[15] Clark RA. Fibronectin matrix deposition and fibronectin receptor expression in healing and normal skin. J Invest Dermatol. 1990;94(Suppl 6):128S–134S.

[16] George AJ, Thomas WG, Hannan RD. The renin-angiotensin system and cancer: old dog, new tricks. Nat Rev Cancer. 2010;10(11):745–759.

[17] Mehta PK, Griendling KK. Angiotensin II cell signaling: physiological and pathological effects in the cardiovascular system. Am J Physiol Cell Physiol. 2007;292(1):C82–C97.

[18] Steckelings UM, Wollschlager T, Peters J, Henz BM, Hermes B, Artuc M. Human skin: source of and target organ for angiotensin II. Exp Dermatol. 2004;13(3):148–154.

[19] Macri L, Silverstein D, Clark RA. Growth factor binding to the pericellular matrix and its importance in tissue engineering. Adv Drug Deliv Rev. 2007;59(13):1366–1381.

[20] Hyytiainen M, Penttinen C, Keski-Oja J. Latent TGF-beta binding proteins: extracellular matrix association and roles in TGF-beta activation. Crit Rev Clin Lab Sci. 2004;41(3): 233–264.

[21] Roberts AB, Heine UI, Flanders KC, Sporn MB. Transforming growth factor-beta. Major role in regulation of extracellular matrix. Ann N Y Acad Sci. 1990;580:225–232.

[22] Schreml S, Szeimies RM, Prantl L, Karrer S, Landthaler M, Babilas P. Oxygen in acute and chronic wound healing. Br J Dermatol. 2010;163(2):257–268.

[23] Gary Sibbald R, Woo KY. The biology of chronic foot ulcers in persons with diabetes. Diabetes Metab Res Rev. 2008;24(Suppl 1):S25–S30.

[24] Kumin A, Schafer M, Epp N, Bugnon P, Born-Berclaz C, Oxenius A, et al. Peroxiredoxin 6 is required for blood vessel integrity in wounded skin. J Cell Biol. 2007;179(4):747–760.

[25] Boudreau NJ, Jones PL. Extracellular matrix and integrin signalling: the shape of things to come. Biochem J. 1999;339(Pt 3):481–488.

[26] Olaso E, Labrador JP, Wang L, Ikeda K, Eng FJ, Klein R, et al. Discoidin domain receptor 2 regulates fibroblast proliferation and migration through the extracellular matrix in association with transcriptional activation of matrix metalloproteinase-2. J Biol Chem. 2002;277(5):3606–3613.

[27] Sen CK, Khanna S, Babior BM, Hunt TK, Ellison EC, Roy S. Oxidant-induced vascular endothelial growth factor expression in human keratinocytes and cutaneous wound healing. J Biol Chem. 2002;277(36):33284–33290.

[28] Senger DR, Claffey KP, Benes JE, Perruzzi CA, Sergiou AP, Detmar M. Angiogenesis promoted by vascular endothelial growth factor: regulation through alpha1beta1 and alpha2beta1 integrins. Proc Natl Acad Sci U S A. 1997;94(25):13612–13617.

[29] Rossiter H, Barresi C, Pammer J, Rendl M, Haigh J, Wagner EF, et al. Loss of vascular endothelial growth factor a activity in murine epidermal keratinocytes delays wound healing and inhibits tumor formation. Cancer Res. 2004;64(10):3508–3516.

[30] Hong YK, Lange-Asschenfeldt B, Velasco P, Hirakawa S, Kunstfeld R, Brown LF, et al. VEGF-A promotes tissue repair-associated lymphatic vessel formation via VEGFR-2 and the alpha1beta1 and alpha2beta1 integrins. FASEB J. 2004;18(10):1111–1113.

[31] Tran KT, Lamb P, Deng JS. Matrikines and matricryptins: Implications for cutaneous cancers and skin repair. J Dermatol Sci. 2005;40(1):11–20.

[32] Panayotou G, End P, Aumailley M, Timpl R, Engel J. Domains of laminin with growth-factor activity. Cell. 1989;56(1):93–101.

[33] Colognato H, Yurchenco PD. Form and function: the laminin family of heterotrimers. Dev Dyn. 2000;218(2):213–234.

[34] Giannelli G, Falk-Marzillier J, Schiraldi O, Stetler-Stevenson WG, Quaranta V. Induction of cell migration by matrix metalloprotease-2 cleavage of laminin-5. Science. 1997;277(5323):225–228.

[35] Pastar I, Stojadinovic O, Yin NC, Ramirez H, Nusbaum AG, Sawaya A, et al. Epithelialization in wound healing: a comprehensive review. Adv Wound Care (New Rochelle). 2014;3(7):445–464.

[36] Golliger JA, Paul DL. Wounding alters epidermal connexin expression and gap junction-mediated intercellular communication. Mol Biol Cell. 1995;6:10.

[37] Paladini RD, Takahashi K, Bravo NS, Coulombe PA. Onset of re-epithelialization after skin injury correlates with a reorganization of keratin filaments in wound edge keratinocytes: defining a potential role for keratin 16. J Cell Biol. 1996;132(3):17.

[38] Pilcher BK, Dumin JA, Sudbeck BD, Krane SM, Welgus HG, Parks CW. The activity of collagenase-1 is required for keratinocyte migration on a type I collagen matrix. J Cell Biol. 1997;137(6):12.

[39] Jacinto A, Martinez-Arias A, Martin P. Mechanisms of epithelial fusion and repair. Nat Cell Biol. 2001;3(5):E117–E123.

[40] Velnar T, Bailey T, Smrkolj V. The wound healing process: an overview of the cellular and molecular mechanisms. J Int Med Res. 2009;37(5):1528–1542.

[41] Sommer K, Sander AL, Albig M, Weber R, Henrich D, Frank J, et al. Delayed wound repair in sepsis is associated with reduced local pro-inflammatory cytokine expression. PLoS One. 2013;8(9):e73992.

[42] Rosenblum G, Meroueh S, Toth M, Fisher JF, Fridman R, Mobashery S, et al. Molecular structures and dynamics of the stepwise activation mechanism of a matrix metalloproteinase zymogen: challenging the cysteine switch dogma. J Am Chem Soc. 2007;129(44): 13566–13574.

[43] Kotra LP, Cross JB, Shimura Y, Fridman R, Schlegel HB, Mobashery S. Insight into the complex and dynamic process of activation of matrix metalloproteinases. J Am Chem Soc. 2001;123(13):3108–3113.

[44] Gomis-Ruth FX. Catalytic domain architecture of metzincin metalloproteases. J Biol Chem. 2009;284(23):15353–15357.

[45] Massova I, Kotra LP, Fridman R, Mobashery S. Matrix metalloproteinases: structures, evolution, and diversification. FASEB J. 1998;12(12):1075–1095.

[46] Lopez-Otin C, Overall CM. Protease degradomics: a new challenge for proteomics. Nat Rev Mol Cell Biol. 2002;3(7):509–519.

[47] Chen P, Parks WC. Role of matrix metalloproteinases in epithelial migration. J Cell Biochem. 2009;108(6):1233–1243.

[48] Saarialho-Kere UK, Kovacs SO, Pentland AP, Olerud JE, Welgus HG, Parks WC. Cell-matrix interactions modulate interstitial collagenase expression by human keratinocytes actively involved in wound-healing. J Clin Invest. 1993;92(6):2858–2866.

[49] Lobmann R, Ambrosch A, Schultz G, Waldmann K, Schiweck S, Lehnert H. Expression of matrix-metalloproteinases and their inhibitors in the wounds of diabetic and non-diabetic patients. Diabetologia. 2002;45(7):1011–1016.

[50] Madlener M, Parks WC, Werner S. Matrix metalloproteinases (MMPs) and their physiological inhibitors (TIMPs) are differentially expressed during excisional skin wound repair. Exp Cell Res. 1998;242(1):201–210.

[51] Mirastschijski U, Impola U, Jahkola T, Karlsmark T, Agren MS, Saarialho-Kere U. Ectopic localization of matrix metalloproteinase-9 in chronic cutaneous wounds. Hum Pathol. 2002;33(3):355–364.

[52] Jurasz P, Chung AW, Radomski A, Radomski MW. Nonremodeling properties of matrix metalloproteinases: the platelet connection. Circ Res. 2002;90(10):1041–1043.

[53] Fridman R, Toth M, Pena D, Mobashery S. Activation of progelatinase B (MMP-9) by gelatinase A (MMP-2). Cancer Res. 1995;55(12):2548–2555.

[54] Vaalamo M, Weckroth M, Puolakkainen P, Kere J, Saarinen P, Lauharanta J, et al. Patterns of matrix metalloproteinase and TIMP-1 expression in chronic and normally healing human cutaneous wounds. Br J Dermatol. 1996;135(1):52–59.

[55] Bullard KM, Lund L, Mudgett JS, Mellin TN, Hunt TK, Murphy B, et al. Impaired wound contraction in stromelysin-1-deficient mice. Ann Surg. 1999;230(2):260–265.

[56] Ogata Y, Enghild JJ, Nagase H. Matrix metalloproteinase 3 (stromelysin) activates the precursor for the human matrix metalloproteinase 9. J Biol Chem. 1992;267(6):3581–3584.

[57] Saarialho-Kere UK, Pentland AP, Birkedal-Hansen H, Parks WC, Welgus HG. Distinct populations of basal keratinocytes express stromelysin-1 and stromelysin-2 in chronic wounds. J Clin Invest. 1994;94(1):79–88.

[58] Chen P, Abacherli LE, Nadler ST, Wang Y, Li Q, Parks WC. MMP7 shedding of syndecan-1 facilitates re-epithelialization by affecting alpha(2)beta(1) integrin activation. PLoS One. 2009;4(8):e6565.

[59] Dunsmore SE, Saarialho-Kere UK, Roby JD, Wilson CL, Matrisian LM, Welgus HG, et al. Matrilysin expression and function in airway epithelium. J Clin Invest. 1998;102(7): 1321–1331.

[60] Gooyit M, Peng Z, Wolter WR, Pi H, Ding D, Hesek D, et al. A chemical biological strategy to facilitate diabetic wound healing. ACS Chem Biol. 2014;9(1):105–110.

[61] Nwomeh BC, Liang HX, Cohen IK, Yager DR. MMP-8 is the predominant collagenase in healing wounds and nonhealing ulcers. J Surg Res. 1999;81(2):189–195.

[62] Gutierrez-Fernandez A, Inada M, Balbin M, Fueyo A, Pitiot AS, Astudillo A, et al. Increased inflammation delays wound healing in mice deficient in collagenase-2 (MMP-8). FASEB J. 2007;21(10):2580–2591.

[63] Gao M, Nguyen TT, Suckow MA, Wolter WR, Gooyit M, Mobashery S, et al. Acceleration of diabetic wound healing using a novel protease-anti-protease combination therapy. Proc Natl Acad Sci U S A. 2015;112(49):15226–15231.

[64] Mohan R, Chintala SK, Jung JC, Villar WV, McCabe F, Russo LA, et al. Matrix metalloproteinase gelatinase B (MMP-9) coordinates and effects epithelial regeneration. J Biol Chem. 2002;277(3):2065–2072.

[65] Kyriakides TR, Wulsin D, Skokos EA, Fleckman P, Pirrone A, Shipley JM, et al. Mice that lack matrix metalloproteinase-9 display delayed wound healing associated with delayed reepithelization and disordered collagen fibrillogenesis. Matrix Biol. 2009;28(2):65–73.

[66] Rechardt O, Elomaa O, Vaalamo M, Paakkonen K, Jahkola T, Hook-Nikanne J, et al. Stromelysin-2 is upregulated during normal wound repair and is induced by cytokines. J Invest Dermatol. 2000;115(5):778–787.

[67] Krampert M, Bloch W, Sasaki T, Bugnon P, Rulicke T, Wolf E, et al. Activities of the matrix metalloproteinase stromelysin-2 (MMP-10) in matrix degradation and keratinocyte organization in wounded skin. Mol Biol Cell. 2004;15(12):5242–5254.

[68] Cornelius LA, Nehring LC, Harding E, Bolanowski M, Welgus HG, Kobayashi DK, et al. Matrix metalloproteinases generate angiostatin: effects on neovascularization. J Immunol. 1998;161(12):6845–6852.

[69] Toriseva MJ, Ala-aho R, Karvinen J, Baker AH, Marjomaki VS, Heino J, et al. Collagenase-3 (MMP-13) enhances remodeling of three-dimensional collagen and promotes survival of human skin fibroblasts. J Invest Dermatol. 2007;127(1): 49–59.

[70] Hattori N, Mochizuki S, Kishi K, Nakajima T, Takaishi H, D'Armiento J, et al. MMP-13 plays a role in keratinocyte migration, angiogenesis, and contraction in mouse skin wound healing. Am J Pathol. 2009;175(2):533–546.

[71] Seiki M. The cell surface: the stage for matrix metalloproteinase regulation of migration. Curr Opin Cell Biol. 2002;14(5):624–632.

[72] Atkinson JJ, Toennies HM, Holmbeck K, Senior RM. Membrane type 1 matrix metalloproteinase is necessary for distal airway epithelial repair and keratinocyte growth factor receptor expression after acute injury. Am J Physiol Lung Cell Mol Physiol. 2007;293(3):L600–L610.

[73] Strongin AY, Collier I, Bannikov G, Marmer BL, Grant GA, Goldberg GI. Mechanism of cell surface activation of 72-kDa type IV collagenase. Isolation of the activated form of the membrane metalloprotease. J Biol Chem. 1995;270(10):5331–5338.

[74] Yan C, Boyd DD. Regulation of matrix metalloproteinase gene expression. J Cell Physiol. 2007;211(1):19–26.

[75] Fisher JF, Mobashery S. Recent advances in MMP inhibitor design. Cancer Metastasis Rev. 2006;25(1):115–136.

[76] Fisher JF, Mobashery S. Mechanism-based profiling of MMPs. In: Clark IM, Young DA, Rowan AD, editors. Matrix Metalloproteinase Protocols, vol 622, 2nd ed. New York: Humana Press; 2010. p. 471–487.

[77] Chellaiah MA, Ma T. Membrane localization of membrane type 1 matrix metalloproteinase by CD44 regulates the activation of pro-matrix metalloproteinase 9 in osteoclasts. Biomed Res Int. 2013;2013:302392.

[78] Baker AH, Edwards DR, Murphy G. Metalloproteinase inhibitors: biological actions and therapeutic opportunities. J Cell Sci. 2002;115(Pt 19):3719–3727.

[79] Esposito S, Noviello S, Leone S. Epidemiology and microbiology of skin and soft tissue infections. Curr Opin Infect Dis. 2016;29(2):109–115.

[80] Bassetti M, Righi E, Carnelutti A. New therapeutic options for skin and soft tissue infections. Curr Opin Infect Dis. 2016;29(2):99–108.

[81] Uckay I, Gariani K, Dubois-Ferriere V, Suva D, Lipsky BA. Diabetic foot infections: recent literature and cornerstones of management. Curr Opin Infect Dis. 2016;29(2): 145–152.

[82] Ziyadeh N, Fife D, Walker AM, Wilkinson GS, Seeger JD. A matched cohort study of the risk of cancer in users of becaplermin. Adv Skin Wound Care. 2011;24(1):31–39.

[83] Inoue M, Kratz G, Haegerstrand A, Stahlebackdahl M. Collagenase expression is rapidly induced in wound-edge keratinocytes after acute injury in human skin, persists during healing, and stops at reepithilialization. J Invest Dermatol. 1995;104(4):479–483.

[84] Vaalamo M, Leivo T, Saarialho-Kere U. Differential expression of tissue inhibitors of metalloproteinases (TIMP-1,-2,-3, and-4) in normal and aberrant wound healing. Hum Pathol. 1999;30(7):795–802.

[85] Grenache DG, Zhang ZH, Wells LE, Santoro SA, Davidson JM, Zutter MM. Wound healing in the alpha 2 beta 1 integrin-deficient mouse: altered keratinocyte biology and dysregulated matrix metalloproteinase expression. J Invest Dermatol. 2007;127(2):455–466.

[86] Sudbeck BD, Pilcher BK, Welgus HG, Parks WC. Induction and repression of collagenase-1 by keratinocytes is controlled by distinct components of different extracellular matrix compartments. J Biol Chem. 1997;272(35):22103–22110.

[87] Pins GD, Collins-Pavao ME, Van De Water L, Yarmush ML, Morgan JR. Plasmin triggers rapid contraction and degradation of fibroblast-populated collagen lattices. J Invest Dermatol. 2000;114(4):647–653.

[88] Di Colandrea T, Wang LS, Wille J, D'Armiento J, Chada KK. Epidermal expression of collagenase delays wound-healing in transgenic mice. J Invest Dermatol. 1998;111(6): 1029–1033.

[89] Ravanti L, Toriseva M, Penttinen R, Crombleholme T, Foschi M, Han J, et al. Expression of human collagenase-3 (MMP-13) by fetal skin fibroblasts is induced by transforming

growth factor beta via p38 mitogen-activated protein kinase. FASEB J. 2001;15(6):1098–1100.

[90] Hartenstein B, Dittrich BT, Stickens D, Heyer B, Vu TH, Teurich S, et al. Epidermal development and wound healing in matrix metalloproteinase 13-deficient mice. J Invest Dermatol. 2006;126(2):486–496.

[91] McCallon SK, Weir D, Lantis JC, 2nd. Optimizing wound bed preparation with collagenase enzymatic debridement. J Am Coll Clin Wound Spec. 2014;6(1–2): 14–23

[92] Mirastschijski U, Zhou ZJ, Rollman O, Tryggvason K, Agren MS. Wound healing in membrane-type-1 matrix metalloproteinase-deficient mice. J Invest Dermatol. 2004;123(3):600–602.

[93] Holmbeck K, Bianco P, Caterina J, Yamada S, Kromer M, Kuznetsov SA, et al. MT1-MMP-deficient mice develop dwarfism, osteopenia, arthritis, and connective tissue disease due to inadequate collagen turnover. Cell. 1999;99(1):81–92.

[94] Gibson D, Cullen B, Legerstee R, Harding KG, Schultz G. MMPs made easy. Int Wound J. 2009;1(1).

[95] Arenas IA, Xu Y, Lopez-Jaramillo P, Davidge ST. Angiotensin II-induced MMP-2 release from endothelial cells is mediated by TNF-alpha. Am J Physiol Cell Physiol. 2004;286(4):C779–C784.

[96] Guo RW, Yang LX, Wang H, Liu B, Wang L. Angiotensin II induces matrix metalloproteinase-9 expression via a nuclear factor-kappaB-dependent pathway in vascular smooth muscle cells. Regul Pept. 2008;147(1–3):37–44.

[97] Kintscher U, Wakino S, Kim S, Fleck E, Hsueh WA, Law RE. Angiotensin II induces migration and Pyk2/paxillin phosphorylation of human monocytes. Hypertension. 2001;37(2 Pt 2):587–593.

[98] Tamarat R, Silvestre JS, Durie M, Levy BI. Angiotensin II angiogenic effect *in vivo* involves vascular endothelial growth factor- and inflammation-related pathways. Lab Invest. 2002;82(6):747–756.

[99] Kurosaka M, Suzuki T, Hosono K, Kamata Y, Fukamizu A, Kitasato H, et al. Reduced angiogenesis and delay in wound healing in angiotensin II type 1a receptor-deficient mice. Biomed Pharmacother. 2009;63(9):627–634.

[100] Kamber M, Papalazarou V, Rouni G, Papageorgopoulou E, Papalois A, Kostourou V. Angiotensin II inhibitor facilitates epidermal wound regeneration in diabetic mice. Front Physiol. 2015;6:170.

[101] Moses MA, Marikovsky M, Harper JW, Vogt P, Eriksson E, Klagsbrun M, et al. Temporal study of the activity of matrix metalloproteinases and their endogenous inhibitors during wound healing. J Cell Biochem. 1996;60(3):379–386.

[102] Mydel P, Shipley JM, Adair-Kirk TL, Kelley DG, Broekelmann TJ, Mecham RP, et al. Neutrophil elastase cleaves laminin-332 (laminin-5) generating peptides that are chemotactic for neutrophils. J Biol Chem. 2008;283(15):9513–9522.

[103] Koshikawa N, Giannelli G, Cirulli V, Miyazaki K, Quaranta V. Role of cell surface metalloprotease MT1-MMP in epithelial cell migration over laminin-5. J Cell Biol. 2000;148(3):615–624.

[104] Gilles C, Polette M, Coraux C, Tournier JM, Meneguzzi G, Munaut C, et al. Contribution of MT1-MMP and of human laminin-5 gamma2 chain degradation to mammary epithelial cell migration. J Cell Sci. 2001;114(Pt 16):2967–2976.

[105] Werner S, Grose R. Regulation of wound healing by growth factors and cytokines. Physiol Rev. 2003;83(3):835–870.

[106] Dean RA, Butler GS, Hamma-Kourbali Y, Delbe J, Brigstock DR, Courty J, et al. Identification of candidate angiogenic inhibitors processed by matrix metalloproteinase 2 (MMP-2) in cell-based proteomic screens: disruption of vascular endothelial growth factor (VEGF)/heparin affin regulatory peptide (pleiotrophin) and VEGF/Connective tissue growth factor angiogenic inhibitory complexes by MMP-2 proteolysis. Mol Cell Biol. 2007;27(24):8454–8465.

[107] Bergers G, Brekken R, McMahon G, Vu TH, Itoh T, Tamaki K, et al. Matrix metalloproteinase-9 triggers the angiogenic switch during carcinogenesis. Nat Cell Biol. 2000;2(10):737–744.

[108] Dallas SL, Rosser JL, Mundy GR, Bonewald LF. Proteolysis of latent transforming growth factor-beta (TGF-beta)-binding protein-1 by osteoclasts. A cellular mechanism for release of TGF-beta from bone matrix. J Biol Chem. 2002;277(24):21352–60.

[109] Yu Q, Stamenkovic I. Cell surface-localized matrix metalloproteinase-9 proteolytically activates TGF-beta and promotes tumor invasion and angiogenesis. Genes Dev. 2000;14(2):163–176.

[110] Imai K, Hiramatsu A, Fukushima D, Pierschbacher MD, Okada Y. Degradation of decorin by matrix metalloproteinases: identification of the cleavage sites, kinetic analyses and transforming growth factor-beta1 release. Biochem J. 1997;322 (Pt 3):809–814.

[111] Deryugina EI, Ratnikov B, Monosov E, Postnova TI, DiScipio R, Smith JW, et al. MT1-MMP initiates activation of pro-MMP-2 and integrin alphavbeta3 promotes maturation of MMP-2 in breast carcinoma cells. Exp Cell Res. 2001;263(2):209–223.

[112] Agren MS, Mirastschijski U, Karlsmark T, Saarialho-Kere UK. Topical synthetic inhibitor of matrix metalloproteinases delays epidermal regeneration of human wounds. Exp Dermatol. 2001;10(5):337–348.

[113] McCawley LJ, O'Brien P, Hudson LG. Epidermal growth factor (EGF)- and scatter factor/hepatocyte growth factor (SF/HGF)- mediated keratinocyte migration is coinci-

dent with induction of matrix metalloproteinase (MMP)-9. J Cell Physiol. 1998;176(2): 255–265.

[114] Heljasvaara R, Nyberg P, Luostarinen J, Parikka M, Heikkila P, Rehn M, et al. Generation of biologically active endostatin fragments from human collagen XVIII by distinct matrix metalloproteases. Exp Cell Res. 2005;307(2):292–304.

[115] O'Reilly MS, Wiederschain D, Stetler-Stevenson WG, Folkman J, Moses MA. Regulation of angiostatin production by matrix metalloproteinase-2 in a model of concomitant resistance. J Biol Chem. 1999;274(41):29568–29571.

[116] Visse R, Nagase H. Matrix metalloproteinases and tissue inhibitors of metalloproteinases: structure, function, and biochemistry. Circ Res. 2003;92(8):827–839.

[117] Murphy G, Cockett MI, Ward RV, Docherty AJ. Matrix metalloproteinase degradation of elastin, type IV collagen and proteoglycan. A quantitative comparison of the activities of 95 kDa and 72 kDa gelatinases, stromelysins-1 and -2 and punctuated metalloproteinase (PUMP). Biochem J. 1991;277 (Pt 1):277–279.

[118] McGuire JK, Li Q, Parks WC. Matrilysin (matrix metalloproteinase-7) mediates E-cadherin ectodomain shedding in injured lung epithelium. Am J Pathol. 2003;162(6): 1831–1843.

[119] Surendran K, Simon TC, Liapis H, McGuire JK. Matrilysin (MMP-7) expression in renal tubular damage: association with Wnt4. Kidney Int. 2004;65(6):2212–2222.

[120] Kure T, Chang JH, Kato T, Hernandez-Quintela E, Ye H, Lu PC, et al. Corneal neovascularization after excimer keratectomy wounds in matrilysin-deficient mice. Invest Ophthalmol Vis Sci. 2003;44(1):137–144.

[121] Kivisaari AK, Kallajoki M, Mirtti T, McGrath JA, Bauer JW, Weber F, et al. Transformation-specific matrix metalloproteinases (MMP)-7 and MMP-13 are expressed by tumour cells in epidermolysis bullosa-associated squamous cell carcinomas. Br J Dermatol. 2008;158(4):778–785.

[122] Vaalamo M, Kariniemi AL, Shapiro SD, Saarialho-Kere U. Enhanced expression of human metalloelastase (MMP-12) in cutaneous granulomas and macrophage migration. J Invest Dermatol. 1999;112(4):499–505.

[123] Hiller O, Lichte A, Oberpichler A, Kocourek A, Tschesche H. Matrix metalloproteinases collagenase-2, macrophage elastase, collagenase-3, and membrane type 1-matrix metalloproteinase impair clotting by degradation of fibrinogen and factor XII. J Biol Chem. 2000;275(42):33008–33013.

[124] Zhou Z, Apte SS, Soininen R, Cao R, Baaklini GY, Rauser RW, et al. Impaired endochondral ossification and angiogenesis in mice deficient in membrane-type matrix metalloproteinase I. Proc Natl Acad Sci U S A. 2000;97(8):4052–4057.

[125] Menke NB, Ward KR, Witten TM, Bonchev DG, Diegelmann RF. Impaired wound healing. Clin Dermatol. 2007;25(1):19–25.

[126] Wlaschek M, Peus D, Achterberg V, Meyer-Ingold W, Scharffetter-Kochanek K. Protease inhibitors protect growth factor activity in chronic wounds. Br J Dermatol. 1997;137(4): 646.

[127] Armstrong DG, Jude EB. The role of matrix metalloproteinases in wound healing. J Am Podiatr Med Assoc. 2002;92(1):12–18.

[128] Reiss MJ, Han YP, Garcia E, Goldberg M, Yu H, Garner WL. Matrix metalloproteinase-9 delays wound healing in a murine wound model. Surgery. 2010;147(2): 295–302.

[129] Liu Y, Min D, Bolton T, Nube V, Twigg SM, Yue DK, et al. Increased matrix metalloproteinase-9 predicts poor wound healing in diabetic foot ulcers. Diabetes Care. 2009;32(1):117–119.

[130] Dinh T, Tecilazich F, Kafanas A, Doupis J, Gnardellis C, Leal E, et al. Mechanisms involved in the development and healing of diabetic foot ulceration. Diabetes. 2012;61(11):2937–2947.

[131] Leppert D, Waubant E, Galardy R, Bunnett NW, Hauser SL. T cell gelatinases mediate basement membrane transmigration *in vitro*. J Immunol. 1995;154(9):4379–4389.

[132] Okada S, Kita H, George TJ, Gleich GJ, Leiferman KM. Migration of eosinophils through basement membrane components *in vitro*: role of matrix metalloproteinase-9. Am J Respir Cell Mol Biol. 1997;17(4):519–528.

[133] Vandooren J, Geurts N, Martens E, Van den Steen PE, Opdenakker G. Zymography methods for visualizing hydrolytic enzymes. Nat Methods. 2013;10(3):211–220.

[134] Hsu JYC, McKeon R, Goussev S, Werb Z, Lee JU, Trivedi A, et al. Matrix metalloproteinase-2 facilitates wound healing events that promote functional recovery after spinal cord injury. J Neurosci. 2006;26(39):9841–9850.

[135] Han YP, Tuan TL, Hughes M, Wu H, Garner WL. Transforming growth factor-beta - and tumor necrosis factor-alpha -mediated induction and proteolytic activation of MMP-9 in human skin. J Biol Chem. 2001;276(25):22341–22350.

[136] Crowe MJ, Doetschman T, Greenhalgh DG. Delayed wound healing in immunodeficient TGF-beta 1 knockout mice. J Invest Dermatol. 2000;115(1):3–11.

[137] Amendt C, Mann A, Schirmacher P, Blessing M. Resistance of keratinocytes to TGFbeta-mediated growth restriction and apoptosis induction accelerates re-epithelialization in skin wounds. J Cell Sci. 2002;115(Pt 10):2189–2198.

[138] Badr G. Camel whey protein enhances diabetic wound healing in a streptozotocin-induced diabetic mouse model: the critical role of beta-Defensin-1, -2 and -3. Lipids Health Dis. 2013;12:46.

[139] Ducharme A, Frantz S, Aikawa M, Rabkin E, Lindsey M, Rohde LE, et al. Targeted deletion of matrix metalloproteinase-9 attenuates left ventricular enlargement and collagen accumulation after experimental myocardial infarction. J Clin Invest. 2000;106(1):55–62.

[140] Makela M, Larjava H, Pirila E, Maisi P, Salo T, Sorsa T, et al. Matrix metalloproteinase 2 (gelatinase A) is related to migration of keratinocytes. Exp Cell Res. 1999;251(1):67–78.

Chapter 4

Delivery Systems in Wound Healing and Nanomedicine

Lina Fu

Additional information is available at the end of the chapter

http://dx.doi.org/10.5772/63763

Abstract

Introduction: Delivery systems in nanomedicine contribute to the improvements in wound healing, tissue regeneration, and anticancer pharmacological fields. Although various wound dressings have been used in wound care treatments, there is a great challenge in the wound management of ulcers, trauma, chronic wounds, and severe injury and burns, especially infected wounds.

Body: To accelerate wound healing, influence tissue repair, reduce scarring, and control infection, various delivery devices have been developed in wound healing. The application of delivery devices has improved early as well as long-term wound care in delayed healing wounds. Main delivery systems are described, including drugs, bioactive proteins/growth factors, genes, and cells, outlining the advantages and limitations of each carrier in wound healing, as well as the mechanisms and release. This chapter reviews biomaterials and scaffolds that provide the carriers of bioactive agents, which include antimicrobial agents, combinations of cells, growth factors and genes, both scaffolds and cell interactions toward regeneration of skin tissues, vascular reconstructions, as well as transdermal carriers. In addition, the regulations, procedures, and clinical trails for delivery systems for wound healing are discussed.

Conclusion: In the past decades, many wound dressings and skin substitutes have been developed to treat skin loss and wounds. Delivery systems can improve wound healing and tissue regeneration. Looking toward the future, the need for delivery wound healing products for chronic and complex wounds will increase. Functionalized delivery systems will probably be the academic interest and industrial focus on wound healing.

Keywords: wound healing, delivery system, wound dressing, skin regeneration, biomaterials

1. Introduction

Nanomedicine has had a significant impact on delivery system development for pharmacological fields that include controlled-release wound dressings and biocompatible nanocarriers for biomedical applications [1]. As the largest organ in the human body, skin gives the body protection, but in so doing sustains a variety of skin wounds that require immediate repair process [2]. Modern wound dressings have been under development for decades. Although there are a wide array of wound dressings, ointments, and medical devices for clinical use, the time-consuming process of wound management is mainly restricted to wound repair rather than regeneration, which are two distinct definitions [3]. The key problem of skin regeneration is how to restore the native structure and function of the injured organ, including blood capillaries. Recently, biomaterial carriers in nanomedicine have shifted the focus from patient survival to quality of skin regeneration in terms of function, scar reduction, and improved aesthetics for reconstruction surgeries and burns [4]. In the formats of wound dressings and transdermal formulations, delivery systems have been applied to accelerate wound healing and to promote tissue regeneration, as well as to treat skin cancers using nanomedicine.

There are different circumstances in which people may need wound care and management. To meet the challenges of wound treatments for acute wounds and chronic wounds, such as large-area skin loss, burns, ulcers (pressure, diabetic, neuropathic, or ischemic), trauma, and especially infected wounds, which are mostly caused by microbes [5], the accurate delivery of antimicrobial agents is attracting much attention from researchers [6–8]. In addition to antimicrobial wound dressing, delivery systems of bioactive proteins, such as peptides and growth factors (platelet-derived growth factor, PDGF; endothelial growth factor, EGF; and fibroblast growth factor 2, FGF2 or bFGF), have demonstrated their promising effects in wound healing [9]. Cell therapy, including stem cell strategy, provides a novel therapeutic approach to wound healing [10]. Interestingly, mesenchymal stem cells (MSCs) and adipose-derived stem cells (ASCs) have emerged as a new approach in skin tissue engineering to accelerate wound closure, which would be of enormous benefit particularly for those wounds experiencing delayed healing in patients with diabetes and elderly [11, 12]. Gene delivery systems for wound healing have been also developed to transfer deoxyribonucleic acid (DNA) and ribonucleic acid (RNA) to wound sites [13, 14]. The regulations of delivery systems in wound healing can be complicated and vary greatly depending on the specific biomaterials and scaffolds, as well as the clinical use in particular [15]. In the commercialization of delivery wound healing systems, developmental and regulatory challenges are greater than in normal wound dressing and wound healing products. The biomaterials and scaffolds used in delivery systems take advantage of different structures, chemical parameters, and sources and so may require more rigorous development and regulation.

This chapter reviews biomaterials and scaffolds used in the design, characterization, and evaluation of delivery systems for wound healing, which include delivering antimicrobial drugs, combinations of proteins (growth factors and peptides), cells, and genes (**Figure 1**). Specific examples of application are summarized. Regenerations of skin tissues and reconstructions of blood capillaries in the wound care process are covered. In addition, the regulatory considerations for delivery systems in the wound healing field are also explored.

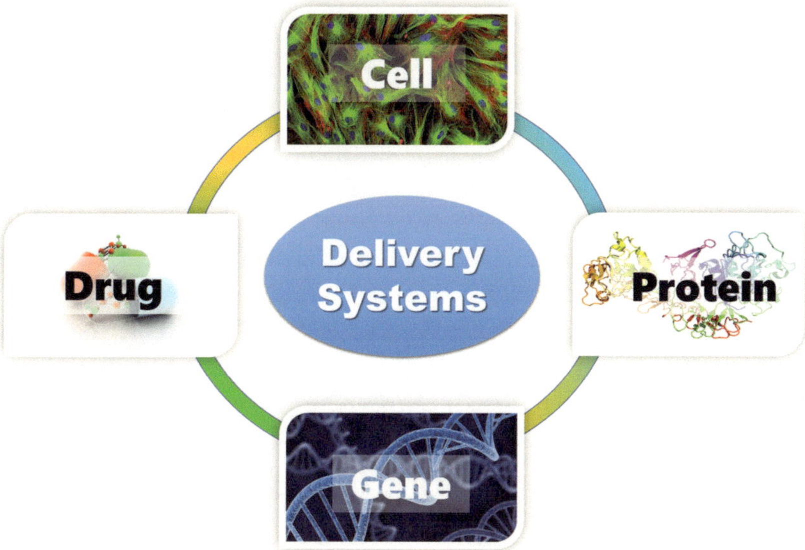

Figure 1. Delivery systems in wound healing.

2. Drug delivery system in wound healing

Chronic wounds and infected wounds currently pose a significant burden worldwide. Drug delivery systems (DDS) in wound healing that release antimicrobial and anti-inflammatory drugs represent a great opportunity to prevent infections or enhance the effectiveness of current commercial drugs. Many biocompatible biomaterials have been extensively investigated to deliver drugs into wound beds and to improve wound healing. Significant efforts have been made to develop DDS using different types of biomaterials, such as polymeric microspheres and nanospheres, lipid nanoparticles, nanofibrous structures, hydrogels, and scaffolds [16].

2.1. Delivery of antibiotics

Wound healing is a complex process that often requires treatment with antibiotics. To optimize and improve the usage of currently available antibiotics, DDS of antibiotics have attracted much attention. Antibiotic drugs used in delivery systems for wound healing are cefazolin [17], gentamicin sulfate [6], ceftazidime pentahydrate [18], ciprofloxacin [19], gentamicin [20], doxycycline hyclate [21], and the anti-inflammatory drug diclofenac [20]. Various biodegradable polymeric scaffolds (electrospun nanofibers, microspheres, composites, and films) were investigated for antibiotic delivery systems, including electrospun nanofibers of poly(lactide-co-glycolide) (PLAGA) [17], composites of a polyglyconate core and a porous poly(DL-lactic-co-glycolic acid) shell [18], chitosan (CS)-gelatin composite films [19], a three-dimensional (3D) polycaprolactone-tricalcium phosphate (PCL-TCP) mesh [6], bacterial cellulose (BC) membranes grafted with RGDC peptides (R for arginine, G for glycine, D for aspartic acid, C for cysteine) [20], poly(vinyl alcohol) (PVA) microspheres sandwiched poly(3-hydroxybutyric acid) (PHB) electrospun fibers [21], and β-cyclodextrin-conjugated hyaluronan hydrogels [22].

Antibiotic agents used in wound healing typically incur adverse effects (e.g., nephrotoxicity for vancomycin, cytotoxicity for ciprofloxacin, and hemolysis for antimicrobial polymers). Loading of antibiotics within polymeric vesicles could attenuate side effects, which has been demonstrated recently [23]. Li et al. reported a general strategy to construct a bacterial strain-selective delivery system for antibiotics based on responsive polymeric vesicles. That was in response to enzymes, including penicillin G amidase (PGA) and β-lactamase (Bla) that are closely associated with drug-resistant bacterial strains. A sustained release of antibiotics enhanced stability and reduced side effects. The results demonstrated that methicillin-resistant *Staphylococcus aureus* (*S. aureus*) (MRSA)-triggered release of antibiotics from Bla-degradable polymeric vesicles *in vitro* inhibited MRSA growth, and enhanced wound healing in an *in vivo* murine model.

2.2. Delivery of silver

To solve the problem of the increased prevalence and growth of multidrug-resistant bacteria, silver is used to reduce and eliminate wound infections using methodologies that limit the ability of bacteria to evolve into further antibiotic-resistant strains. In recent decades, the developments of silver (colloidal silver solution, silver proteins, silver salts, silver sulfadiazine (SSD) and nanosilver)-containing wound dressings for healing promotion and infection reduction have provided promising approaches [24]. The main synthesis approaches of silver monocrystalline silver (nanosilver or silver nanoparticle) include chemical reduction, micro-organism reduction, microwave-assisted photochemical reduction, and laser ablation. Antibacterial wound dressings in the formats of AgNP-embedded poly(vinyl pyrrolidone) (PVP) hydrogels were prepared by γ-irradiation at various doses: 25, 35, and 45 kGy [25]. Antibacterial tests showed that the 1 and 5 mM AgNP-embedded PVP hydrogels were effective, with 99.99% bactericidal activity at 12 and 6 h, respectively. A gamma-irradiated PVA/nanosilver hydrogel was also developed for potential use in burn dressing applications [26]. Interestingly, the wound healing activity of 0.1% w/w AgNPs in Pluronic F127 gels was enhanced to a considerable extent [27]. A new type of high surface area metallic silver in the form of highly porous silver microparticles (AgMPs) was studied [28]. Polylactic acid (PLA) nanofibers were successfully loaded with either highly porous AgMPs or AgNPs. A simulated three-dimensional (3D) coculture system was designed to evaluate human epidermal keratinocytes and *S. aureus* bacteria on the wound dressings. PLA nanofibers containing highly porous AgMPs exhibited steady silver ion release at a greater rate of release than nanofibers containing AgNPs.

Due to its antimicrobial activity, good coagulation and immunostimulating activities, chitosan is one of the native polymers chosen to control infection and enhance wound healing. Chitosan-based wound dressings can be gels, microparticles or nanoparticles, sponges and films [29]. Sacco et al. combined the two antimicrobial agents, silver and chitosan, to develop a silver-containing antimicrobial membrane based on chitosan-tripolyphosphate (TPP) hydrogel for wound treatments. Based on the slow diffusion of TPP, the macroscopic chitosan hydrogels were obtained that included AgNPs stabilized by a lactose-modified chitosan. Besides the good bactericidal properties of the material, the biocompatibility assays on keratinocytes (HaCaT) and fibroblasts (NIH-3T3) cell lines did not prove to have any harmful effects on the viability of cells using the MTT [1-(4,5-dimethylthiazol-2-yl)-3,5-diphenylformazan] method [8]. Chitin was also used to form the composite scaffolds with nanosilver. These chitin/nanosilver composites were found to be bactericidal against *S. aureus* and *Escherichia coli* (*E. coli*) with good blood-clotting ability [30].

Bioelectric wound dressing can also deliver silver to wound beds. *Pseudomonas aeruginosa (P. aeruginosa)* is a common bacterium associated with chronic wound infection. An US Food and Drug Administration (FDA)-approved wireless electroceutical dressing (WED), which in the presence of conductive wound exudate is activated to generate an electric field (0.3–0.9 V), was investigated to test its anti-biofilm properties using a pathogenic *P. aeruginosa* strain PAO1. WED markedly disrupted biofilm integrity in a setting where normal silver dressing was ineffective. Biofilm thickness and number of live bacterial cells were decreased in the presence of WED because WED served a spontaneous source of reactive oxygen species [31].

2.3. Delivery of other drugs

Besides silver, other drugs can be used to improve wound healing, for example, the anti-scar drug astragaloside IV [32]. In a rat full-skin excision model, the**** *in vivo* regulation of 9% astragaloside IV-based solid lipid nanoparticles-gel enhanced the migration and proliferation of keratinocytes, increased drug uptake on fibroblasts *in vitro* ($P < 0.01$) through the caveolae endocytosis pathway, and inhibited scar formation *in vivo* by increasing wound closure rate ($P < 0.05$) and by contributing to angiogenesis and collagen regular organization.

Different from most antibiotics that select for resistant bacteria, curcumin acts using multiple mechanisms. Curcumin (diferuloylmethane) is a bioactive and major phenolic component of turmeric derived from the rhizomes of *Curcuma longa linn.* Owing to its antioxidant and anti-inflammatory properties, curcumin plays a significant beneficial and pleiotropic regulatory role not only in cancers, cardiovascular disease, Alzheimer's disease, inflammatory disorders, and neurological disorders but also in wound healing because of its innate antimicrobial properties. However, the clinical implication of native curcumin is hindered due to low solubility, physicochemical instability, poor bioavailability, rapid metabolism, and poor pharmacokinetics, but these issues can be overcome by efficient delivery systems [33]. A biodegradable sponge, made from chitosan (CS) and sodium alginate (SA) with water uptake ability ranging between 1000 and 4300%, was developed to deliver curcumin as a wound dressing material up to 20 days. The *in vivo* animal test using SD rats showed that this CS/SA sponge had a better effect than cotton gauze, and adding curcumin into the sponge enhanced the therapeutic healing effect and improved collagen arrangement [34]. Curcumin nanoparticles (Curc-np) with an average diameter of 222 ± 14 nm were synthesized [35]. Curc-np represent a significant advance for reducing bacterial load. They can inhibit *in vitro* growth of methicillin-resistant *S. aureus* (MRSA) and *P. aeruginosa* in dose-dependent fashion, and so may represent a novel topical antimicrobial and wound healing adjuvant for infected burn wounds and other cutaneous injuries. Bacterial cellulose (BC) can be used for drug loading and controlled release [36]. The topical or transdermal drug delivery systems of two model drugs (lidocaine hydrochloride and ibuprofen) were developed. Diffusion studies with Franz cells showed that the incorporation of lidocaine hydrochloride in BC membranes provided lower permeation rates than those obtained with the conventional formulations [37].

There is a high mortality in patients with diabetes and severe pressure ulcers, resulting from the reduced neovascularization caused by the impaired activity of the transcription factor hypoxia-inducible factor-1 alpha (HIF-1α). To improve HIF-1α activity, Duscher et al. developed the drug delivery system of an FDA-approved small molecule deferoxamine (DFO), which is an iron chelator that increases HIF-1α transactivation in diabetes by preventing iron-catalyzed reactive oxygen stress [38]. The animal study on a pressure-induced ulcer model in diabetic mice showed a significantly improved wound healing using the transdermal delivery of DFO. DFO-treated wounds demonstrated increased collagen density, improved neovascularization, and reduction of free radical formation, leading to decreased cell death.

3. Bioactive protein delivery systems in wound healing

Wound healing in skin is an evolutionarily conserved, complex, multicellular process, which is executed and regulated by an equally complex signaling network involving numerous growth factors, cytokines, and chemokines [39]. Growth factors are soluble secreted proteins capable of affecting a variety of cellular processes important for tissue regeneration. However, the application of growth factors in clinics remains limited due to lack of good delivery systems and carriers. Recently, biomaterial carriers and sophisticated delivery systems such as nanoparticles and nanofibers for delivery of growth factors and peptides related in wound healing are a main focus in this research area [40].

3.1. Delivery of growth factors

EGF, PDGF, FGF2, keratinocyte growth factor (KGF) [41], transforming growth factor-β (TGF-β), insulin-like growth factor (IGF), vascular endothelial growth factor (VEGF), granulocyte macrophage colony stimulating factor (GM-CSF), and connective tissue growth factor (CTGF) are the main growth factors correlated with the wound healing process of skin [16]. Growth factors usually have short half-life time leading to a rapid deactivation at local wound beds in the body and resulting in a low efficacy. In order to enhance the efficacy of growth factor delivery systems, some bioactive and biodegradable matrixes including extracellular matrixes, have been used as carriers [42].

EGF is one of the most common growth factors used for treating skin wounds. Succinoylated dextrin (~85,000 g/mol; ~19 mol% succinoylation), a clinically well-tolerated polymer, was used to deliver EGF and led to sustained release of free recombinant human EGF over time (52.7% release after 168 h) [43]. Using a layer-by-layer assembly technique, EGF was successfully encapsulated using poly(acrylic acid) (PAA)-modified polyurethane (PU) films [44] or chitosan and alginate films [45]. Johnson and Wang treated the full-thickness wounded mice with a heparin-binding epidermal growth factor coacervate delivery system, and the results exhibited the enhanced migration of keratinocytes with retained proliferative potential, forming a confluent layer for regained barrier function within 7 days [46]. Chitosan-based gel formulations containing egg yolk oil and EGF are better alternatives compared to Silverdin® (1% silver sulfadiazine), given their significant difference ($P < 0.05$) treating wounds in Wistar rats [47]. Since the healing rate of wound is an important factor influencing the outcome of clinical treatments, as well as a crucial step in burn wound treatment, and the quality of wound healing has a direct bearing on the life quality of patients, FGF2 clearly has clinical efficacy in a variety of wound managements [48]. Skin flap survival is a major challenge in reconstructive plastic surgery. A sustained delivery system of FGF2 using heparin-conjugated fibrin was used to improve skin flap survival significantly in a rat animal model [49]. A delivery system composed of fibrin hydrogels doped with bFGF-loaded double emulsion increased the proliferation of endothelial cells compared to sham controls, indicating that the released bFGF was bioactive [50]. An injectable delivery system of PDGF using two-component polyurethane scaffolds was reported to achieve a sustained release for up to 21 days. The *in vitro* bioactivity of the released PDGF was largely preserved by a lyophilized powder. The presence of PDGF attracted both fibroblasts and mononuclear cells, significantly accelerating the degradation of the polymer and enhancing the formation of new granulation tissue as early as day 3 [51]. Hyaluronan-based porous nanoparticles were also investigated for the delivery of PDGF [52]. Recombinant human stromal cell-derived factor-1 (SDF-1), a naturally occurring chemokine that is rapidly overexpressed in response to tissue injury, was delivered in an alginate gel to accelerate wound closure and reduce scar formation [53]. SDF-1 delivery systems were evaluated using an acute surgical Yorkshire pig model. Wounds treated with SDF-1 protein ($n = 10$) and plasmid ($n = 6$)-loaded alginate patches healed faster than the sham ($n = 4$) or control ($n = 4$). At day 9, SDF-1-treated wounds significantly accelerated wound closure (55.0 ± 14.3% healed) compared to nontreated controls (8.2 ± 6.0%, $p < 0.05$).

Recently, it has been increasingly recognized that biodegradable and biocompatible scaffolds incorporated with multiple growth factors might serve as the most promising medical devices for skin tissue regeneration. Beyond drug delivery, BC hydrogel is used to deliver bFGF, EGF, and KGF with modifications of different extracellular matrices (ECMs; collagen, elastin, and hyaluronan) [54]. *In vitro* and *in vivo* evaluation of the applicability of a dextran hydrogel loaded with chitosan microparticles (255 ± 0.9 μm) containing EGF and VEGF were performed, and they accelerated wound healing [55]. Moreover, the histological analysis revealed the absence of reactive or granulomatous inflammatory reaction in skin lesions. Multiple epidermal induction factors (EIF), such as EGF, insulin, hydrocortisone, and retinoic acid (RA), were prepared for blended and core-shell electrospinnings with gelatin (gel) and poly(L-lactic acid)-co-poly-(e-caprolactone) (PLLCL) solutions [56]. An initial 44.9% burst release from EIF blended electrospun nanofibers was observed over a period of 15 days. The epidermal differentiation potential of adipose-derived stem cells (ADSCs) was used to evaluate the scaffolds prepared either by core-shell spinning or by blend spinning. After 15 days of cell culture, the proliferation of ADSCs on EIF-encapsulated core-shell nanofibers was the highest. Moreover, a higher percentage of ADSCs were differentiated to epidermal lineages on EIF-encapsulated core-shell nanofibers compared to the cell differentiation of EIF-blended nanofibers, and this can be attributed to the sustained release of EIF from the core-shell nanofibers. A method for coating commercially available nylon wound dressings using the layer-by-layer process was utilized to control the release of VEGF165 and PDGF-BB [57]. Animal evaluation was performed using a db/db mouse model of chronic wound healing. This combination delivery system promotes significant increases in the formation of granulation tissue and/or cellular proliferation when compared to dressings utilizing single growth factor therapeutics.

3.2. Delivery of peptides

Current therapeutic regiments of wounded patients are static and mostly rely on matrices, gels, and engineered skin tissue. Accordingly, there is a need to design next-generation grafting materials to enable biotherapeutic spatiotemporal targeting from clinically approved matrices. Peptides are good candidates for controlling wound infections. A drug carrier system was designed for delivering an insect metalloproteinase inhibitor (IMPI) drug to enable treatment of chronic wound infections [58]. Poly(lactic-co-glycolic acid) (PLGA) supplies lactate that accelerates neovascularization and promotes wound healing. Delivery systems of LL37 peptide encapsulated in PLGA nanoparticles (PLGA-LL37 NP) were evaluated in full-thickness excisional wounds. A significantly higher collagen deposition, re-epithelialized and neovascularized composition were found in PLGA-LL37 NP-treated group. *In vitro*, PLGA-LL37 NP induced enhanced cell migration but had no effect on the metabolism and proliferation of keratinocytes. Interestingly, it displayed antimicrobial activity on *E. coli* [59]. CM11 peptide (WKLFKKILKVL-NH_2) (128 mg/L), a short cecropin-melittin hybrid peptide, was delivered by an alginate sulfate-based hydrogel as the antimicrobial wound dressing, and its healing effects were tested on skin infections caused by MRSA (200 μL, 3×10^8CFU/mL) in a mouse model [60]. During 8-day period, the 2% mupirocin treatment group and hydrogel containing peptide treatment groups showed similar levels of wound healing.

4. Cell delivery systems in wound healing

Wound healing involves the coordinated efforts of several cell types, including keratinocytes, fibroblasts, endothelial cells, macrophages, and platelets. The migration, infiltration, proliferation, and differentiation of these cells will culminate in an inflammatory response, the formation of new tissue and ultimately wound closure [39]. Cell-based therapies for wound repair are limited by inefficient delivery systems that fail to protect cells from acute inflammatory environments [61]. Wound dressing of cells laden in biomaterials on wound surfaces might not effectively and timely exert functions on deep or chronic wounds, where insufficient blood supply presents. Therefore, cell delivery systems are the main focus in the cell-based therapeutic field. Cell, including stem cells and other cells, delivered wound dressings have recently shown great promise for accelerating wound healing and reducing scar formation.

4.1. Stem cells

Stem cell therapy offers a promising new technique for aiding in wound healing; however, current findings show that stem cells typically die and/or migrate from the wound site, greatly decreasing the efficacy of the treatment. Most stem cells studied in wound healing delivery systems are mesenchymal stem cells (MSCs), endothelial progenitor cells (EPCs), adipose-derived stem cells (ASCs), umbilical cord perivascular cells (UCPCs), and circulating angiogenic cells (CACs). MSCs have been shown to improve tissue regeneration in several preclinical and clinical trials [62]. MSCs from various sources, such as bone marrow and adipose tissue, have been reported in the delivery systems for wound healing [10, 63].

A 3D membrane (FBMSC-CMM) from a freeze-dried bone marrow mesenchymal stem cells-conditioned medium (FBMSC-CM) can hold over 80% of the paracrine factors, which could significantly accelerate wound healing and enhance the neovascularization as well as epithelialization through strengthening the trophic factors in the wound bed [11]. Scaffolds strongly influence key parameters of stem cell delivery, such as seeding efficiency, cellular distribution, attachment, survival, metabolic activity, and paracrine release [64]. Pullulan was used to form a composite with collagen hydrogel for the delivery of MSCs into wounds [65]. Hydrogels induced MSC secretions of angiogenic cytokines and expression of transcription factors associated with the maintenance of pluripotency and self-renewal (Oct4, Sox2, Klf4) when compared to MSCs grown in standard conditions. Engrafted MSCs were found to differentiate into fibroblasts, pericytes, and endothelial cells but did not contribute to the epidermis. Wounds treated with MSC-seeded hydrogels demonstrated significantly enhanced angiogenesis, which was associated with increased levels of VEGF.

There are other kinds of stem cells that have been used in combination with 3D scaffolds as a promising approach in the field of regenerative medicine. For instance, human umbilical cord perivascular cells (HUCPVC) [66], amniotic fluid-derived stem cells (AFSs) [67], EPCs [68], and circulating angiogenic cells (CACs). CACs are known as early EPCs and are isolated from the mononuclear cell fraction of peripheral blood, and provide a potential topical treatment for nonhealing diabetic foot ulcers. A scaffold fabricated from type 1 collagen facilitates topical cell delivery of CACs to a diabetic rabbit ear wound (alloxan-induced ulcer). Increased angiogenesis and increased percentage wound closure were observed with the treatment of collagen and collagen seeded with CSCs [69].

Compared to MSCs and EPCs, adipose-derived mesenchymal stem cells (ASCs) represent an even more appealing source of stem cells because of their abundance and accessibility. ASCs are autologous, non-immunogenic, plentiful, and easily obtained [70]. An acellular dermal matrix (ADM) scaffold made from cadaveric skins of human donors (AlloDerm, LifeCell Corp., Branchburg, NJ, USA) was served as a carrier for the delivery of ASCs [12]. ASCs-ADM grafts secreted various cytokines, including VEGF, HGF, TGFβ, and bFGF. Novel technology and biocompatible biomaterials have been applied for stem cell delivery. A silk fibroin-chitosan (SFCS) scaffold serving as a delivery vehicle for human adipose-derived stem cells (ASCs) was evaluated in a murine soft tissue injury model [71]. Microvessel density at wound bed biopsy sites at 2 weeks postoperative was significantly higher in the ASC-SFCS group vs. SFCS alone (7.5 ± 1.1 vs. 5.1 ± 1.0 blood vessels per high-power field). A newly developed thermoresponsive poly(ethylene) glycol (PEG)-hyaluronic acid (HA) hybrid hydrogel with multiple acrylate functional groups provides an efficient delivery dressing system for human adipose-derived stem cells (hADSCs) [72]. Although cellular proliferation was inhibited, cellular secretion of growth factors, such as VEGF and PDGF production, increased over 7 days, whereas IL-2 and IFNγ release were unaffected. Injectable gelatin microcryogels (GMs) were used to load human ASCs [73]. The results demonstrated the priming effects of GMs on the upregulation of stemness genes and improved secretion of growth factors of hASCs for potential augmented wound healing. In a full-thickness skin wound model in nude mice, multisite injections and dressings of hASC-laden GMs significantly accelerated the healing compared to free stem cell injection.

4.2. Other cells

Endothelial cells (ECs), keratinocytes, and fibroblasts are the most studied cells in terms of accelerated wound healing and improved skin tissue regeneration. A growing number of studies indicate that endothelial cells (ECs) and endothelial progenitor cells (EPCs) may regulate vascular repair in wound healing via paracrine mechanisms [61]. Using dried reagent patches that incorporate dextran (DEX) and a bulk aqueous phase comprising a cell culture medium containing poly(ethylene) glycol (PEG), Bathany et al. made a micro-patterned localized delivery of fluorescent molecules and enzymes for cell detachment [74]. Keratinocytes were delivered to dermal wounds in mice via cell-adhesive peptides attached to chitosan membranes [75]. Two peptides of 12 or 13 amino acids each that bind to cell surface heparin-like receptors (A5G27 and A5G33) were found to promote strong keratinocyte attachment, whereas the one that binds to integrin (A99) was inactive. Recombinant human collagen III (rhCol-III) gel was used as a delivery vehicle for cultured autologous skin cells (keratinocytes only or keratinocyte-fibroblast mixtures) [76]. Its effect on the healing of full-thickness wounds in a porcine wound-healing model was examined. Two Landrace pigs were used for the study. Fourteen deep dermal wounds were created on the back of each pig with an 8-mm biopsy punch. The scaffold enhanced early granulation tissue formation. Interestingly, fibroblast-containing gel was effectively removed from the wound, whereas gels without cells or with keratinocytes only remained intact.

5. Gene delivery systems in wound healing

Gene delivery is an emerging technology in the field of tissue repair and is being used to promote wound healing. Gene delivery is targeted to develop sustained release, to reduce side effects, and to enable both spatial and temporal control of gene silencing afterward. For example, chemical modifications were used to stabilize and reduce nonspecific effects of

http://dx.doi.org/10.5772/63763

siRNA molecules using effective delivery [77]. The controlled delivery of nucleic acids (DNA and RNA) to selected tissues remains an inefficient process are affected by low transfection efficacy, poor scalability because of varying efficiency with cell type and location, and questionable safety as a result of toxicity issues arising from the typical materials (e.g., viral vectors) and procedures employed. Biocompatible materials, in the formats of micro/nanoparticles, scaffolds, hydrogels and electrospun fibers, made from cationic polymers and lipids, have been used as nonviral vectors, which has attracted much attention recently.

5.1. Viral vectors in gene delivery

The TGFβ family plays a critical regulatory role in repair and coordination of remodeling after cutaneous wounding. TGFβ3 has been implicated in an antagonistic role regulating overt wound closure and promoting ordered dermal remodeling. A mutant form of TGFβ3

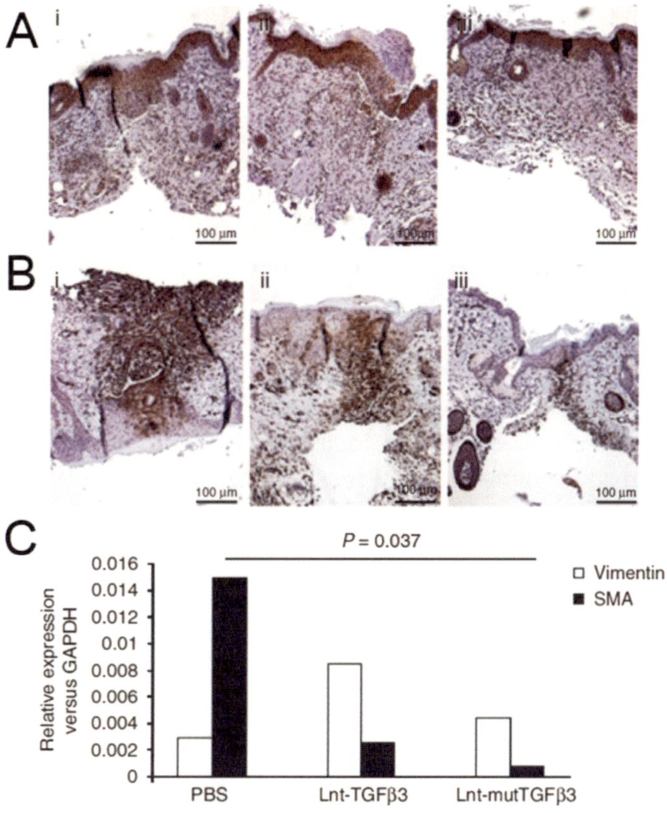

Figure 2. Transgenic overexpression of TGFβ3 decreases fibroblast to myofibroblast differentiation at the site of cutaneous wounding *in vivo*. (A) and (B) wound sections were stained immunohistochemically for fibroblast (a: vimentin) and myofibroblast (b: SMA) markers after treatment with [a and b(i)] PBS, [a and b(ii)] Lnt-TGFβ3, or [a and b(iii)] Lnt-mutTGFβ3. (C) Real-time reverse transcription-PCR showed that both TGFβ3 application groups and the PBS control (n = 4) as well as a significant decrease between the Lnt-mutTGFβ3 and Lnt-TGFβ3 treatment groups. PBS, phosphate-buffered saline; SMA, smooth muscle actin; TGF, transforming growth factor.

(mutTGFβ3) was generated by ablating its binding site for the latency-associated TGFβ-binding protein (LTBP-1) [78]. A localized intradermal transduction using a lentiviral vector expressing the mutTGFβ3 in a mouse skin wounding model was demonstrated to reduce reepithelialization density and fibroblast/myofibroblast trans-differentiation within the wound area. Both of which reduced scar tissue formation (**Figure 2**). Using a noninvasive imaging system, the kinetics of luciferase gene expression was studied when delivered in an adenoviral vector (replication-deficient adenovirus, Ad5). A peak of gene expression occurred at 7 days after delivery [79]. The esophageal cancer-related gene-4 (Ecrg4) delivering a viral-mediated gene was evaluated in a cutaneous wound healing model [80]. Both Ecrg4 mRNA and its protein product were localized to the epidermis, dermis, and hair follicles of healthy mouse skin.

5.2. Nonviral vectors in gene delivery

Gene delivery using adenoviral vectors in tissue regeneration is hindered by a short duration of transgene expression. A fibrin scaffold was used to enhance delivery of the adenovirus to a wound site, precluding the need for high repeated doses [81]. An anti-fibrotic interfering RNA (RNAi) delivery system using exogenous microRNA (miR)-29B was proposed to modulate ECM remodeling following cutaneous injury. A collagen scaffold was used as the carrier of (miR)-29B. The mRNA expressions of collagen type I and collagen type III were reduced up to 2 weeks after fibroblasts culture. *In vivo* evaluation in full-thickness wounds treated with miR-29B delivery revealed that collagen type III/I ratio and matrix metalloproteinase (MMP)-8 to TIMP-1 ratio were improved [82]. Porous (100 and 60 μm) and nonporous (n-pore) hyaluronic acid-MMP hydrogels with encapsulated reporter (pGFPluc) or proangiogenic (pVEGF) plasmids are used as a scaffold-mediated gene delivery [83]. Alginate-DNA gels were used to treat diabetic wounds, which provided sustained release of bioactive factors, such as neuropeptides and VEGF [13]. Silver nanoparticles (AgNPs) can be further augmented for gene delivery applications. The biofunctionalized stable AgNPs with good DNA-binding ability for efficient transfection and minimal toxicity were developed [84]. Polyethylene glycol (PEG)-stabilized chitosan-g-polyacrylamide was used to modify AgNPs. To enhance the efficiency of gene transfection, the Arg-Gly-Asp-Ser (RGDS) peptide was immobilized on the surface of AgNPs. The transfection efficiency of AgNPs increased significantly after immobilization of the RGDS peptide reaching up to $42 \pm 4\%$ and $30 \pm 3\%$ in HeLa and A549 cells, respectively. The transfection efficiency was significantly higher than $34 \pm 3\%$ and $23 \pm 2\%$, respectively, with the use of polyethylenimine (PEI, 25 kDa).

For treating diabetic patients with a threat of limb amputations, genes of various growth factors have been proposed in delivery systems. A simple nonviral gene delivery using minicircle plasmid DNA encoding VEGF was combined with an arginine-grafted cationic dendrimer PAM-RG4 [85]. Mouse ASCs were transfected with DNA plasmid encoding VEGF or green fluorescent protein (GFP) using biodegradable poly (β-amino) esters (PBAE). Cells transfected with Lipofectamine™ 2000, a commercially available transfection reagent, were included as controls. ASCs transfected using PBAEs showed an enhanced transfection efficiency and 12–15-folds higher VEGF production compared with the controls ($^{*}P < 0.05$) [86]. Keratinocyte growth factor-1 (KGF-1) DNA was delivered using NTC8385-VA1 plasmid, a novel minimalized, antibiotic-free DNA expression vector [87].

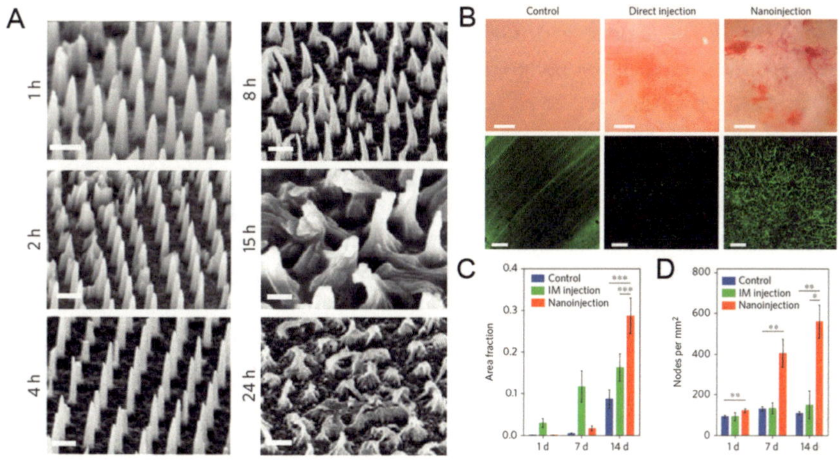

Figure 3. (A) Time course of nanoneedles incubated in cell-culture medium at 37°C. Scale bar = 2 μm. (B) Nanoneedles mediate neovascularization in wound healing. (C) The number of nodes in the vasculature per millimeter square. (D) Within each field of view acquired for untreated control, intramuscular injection (IM), and nanoinjection. $P < 0.05$, $P < 0.01$, $P < 0.001$.

DNA-incorporated electrospun nanofibrous matrix was fabricated to control the release of DNA in response to high concentration of MMPs (matrix metalloproteinases) such as diabetic ulcers [88]. High efficiency and minimal toxicity *in vitro* have been demonstrated that can be used for an intracellular delivery of nucleic acids by using nanoneedles [89]. Biodegradable nanoneedles were fabricated by metal-assisted chemical etching of silicon. These nanoneedles mediated the in situ delivery of an angiogenic gene, VEGF165, and triggered the patterned formation of new blood vessels. The nanoneedles were designed for extremely localized delivery to a few superficial layers of cells (two-dimensional patterning). This gene delivery can access the cytosol to co-deliver DNA and siRNA with an efficiency greater than 90%. *In vivo* studies show that the nanoneedles transfected the VEGF165 gene, improved wound healing and scar-tissue remodeling, and induced sustained neovascularization and a localized sixfold increase in blood perfusion in the target region of the muscle (**Figure 3**). This confined intracellular delivery has the potential to target specific exposed areas within a tissue, further reduce the invasiveness of the injection, and limit the impact on the overall structure of the tissue.

6. Regulatory considerations

The major concerns of commercialization of drug/protein/cell/gene delivery wound dressings are the complicated registration process, specifically regulatory approval, protocol consideration, and clinical trial process. Among all the parameters of delivery wound dressings, the type and source of the materials (e.g., human and animal origin) are critical to the regulatory approval process. A product composed of two or more regulated components, that is, drug/device, biologic/device, drug/biologic, or drug/device/biologic, that are physically, chemically, or otherwise combined or mixed and produced as a single entity is defined as a combination product [90]. The FDA (Food and Drug Administration, United States) regulation of a combination product (e.g., delivery system for wound healing) is mainly determined by the component with the primary mode of action. According to the classification of the product, the clinical trials (for premarket approval, PMA) must provide valid scientific evidence of safety and efficacy to support the indicated use of the wound healing delivery systems. Generally, preclinical studies contain toxicity studies and animal model evaluations. Delivery systems of drugs, bioactive proteins, cells, and genes in wound healing and nanomedicine should test their biocompatibility according to ISO 10993, including dermal irritation, dermal sensitization, cytotoxicity, acute systemic toxicity, hemocompatibility/hemolysis, pyrogenicity, mutagenicity studies, subchronic toxicity, chronic toxicity, and immunogenic potential [91]. Good clinical practices (GCPs) are the standards for designing, conducting, recording, and reporting clinical trials required for Class III medical devices.

For example, autologous stem cells are under clinical trial and are effective in ulcer healing and angiogenesis. However, translating delivery of stem cell application in *in vitro* and *in vivo* experiments from animal models to human clinical trials is still in its infancy. Preclinical studies suggest that cell delivery systems represent an effective and safe therapeutic strategy in the treatment of nonhealing wounds. More clinical studies on human subjects, including better data management of the patients and long-term follow-up of the patients' conditions, are necessary. Improved stem cell delivery vehicles in large-scale human clinical trials may be promising for diabetics with foot ulcers. There are no serious complications or side effects, but its therapeutic mechanisms, effects, and standardization still require further research [92]. While delivery system-based products offer increasingly important strategies for managing complex wounds, potential drawbacks include the risks of infectious agent transfer and immunological rejection. The manufacturing process, transport, and storage of delivery systems in wound healing are major cost implications; thus, their current clinical use remains limited [93]. Many current clinical trials are placing a high emphasis on addressing safety issues in all stem cell therapies, including stem cell delivery in wound healing [94]. The serious adverse effects of stem cell delivery are mainly immune response and tumorigenic potential. Delivery systems used in cell therapy encompass four main approaches, which are systemic administration, injection, topical, and local deliveries. Localized delivery of cells in wound healing is an optimal delivery approach for wound treatments [95]. Nonimmunogenic, nontoxic, biodegradable, and biocompatible biomaterials have been developed as carriers of stem cells that can protect cells and improve wound healing. However, clinical use of stem cells, for example, allogeneic EPCs, is currently inhibited by the risk of immunogenicity and tumorigenicity. To modulate the immune response, mesenchymal stromal cells or umbilical cord blood is already used in clinical trials, but definitive results are still pending. MSCs are known to be hypoimmunogenic [96]. Current challenges are standardized and quality-controlled cell therapy, the differentiation of MSCs to unwanted tissue, and potential tumorigenicity [94]. MSCs have been applied clinically for the treatment of diabetic wounds. Long *in vitro* expansion time and multiple handling procedures are barriers for its clinical application and increase the chances of infection [97]. Autologous induced pluripotent stem cells are nonimmunogenic and can be a promising cell source used in wound healing [98]. By comparison, clinical use of allogeneic cells is more complex and requires additional regulatory, legal, and safety hurdles to be overcome [99]. All things considered, the future prospects for the utilization of both autologous and allogeneic cells in cell delivery systems are bright. In the United States, there are three regulatory processes for the registration of wound healing delivery systems [100]. Only wound dressing with lower complexity and risk that is substantially equivalent to a marketed "predicate" device may be cleared through the 510(k) premarket notification process. In another words, those types of wound dressings are classified as Class I medical device. Clinical data are typically not needed for 510(k) clearance of Class II medical devices. Higher-risk Class III medical devices typically require premarket approval (PMA). In summary, the regulatory processes are depending on multiple factors including the device's classification, the availability of a substantially equivalent predicate, and the level of risk. Before commercialization, investigational devices maybe clinically investigated within the USA through the investigational device exemption (IDE) process, which is a request to conduct clinical research on an investigational device with "significant" risk in the **United States**.

User fees are required with the submissions of 510(k) premarket notifications and PMA application in the **United States**. Recently, Health Canada released a consultation document that discusses the cost recovery (user fee) framework which shows the basis for accountability at Health Canada for the review process [101]. Essentially, the fees "guarantee" a certain level of service from Health Canada—for instance, specifying the target number of days in which Health Canada will process different types of applications. If the targets are not met, that is, if "performance" does not meet the established standard, the entity being charged the user fee will have their future fees reduced by a corresponding amount. Providing a framework for registration approval globally of delivery wound dressings would translate those delivery systems studied from the laboratory investigation stage to clinical use, which will benefit patients' quality of life.

7. Conclusions

In the past few decades, many wound dressings and skin substitutes have been developed to treat skin loss and wounds. Delivery systems have been proven to improve wound healing and skin tissue regeneration. Polymeric microspheres and nanospheres, nanoparticles, nanofibrous structures, hydrogels, and scaffolds have been developed to deliver drugs to wound sites, overcoming the challenges caused by antibiotic-resistant microbial infections. Controlled release of drug delivery systems has been of increasing interest, as well as the applications of nanotechnology and biomaterial scaffolds. Growth factor and peptide delivery systems applied in skin wound healing help in the regeneration of tissue, reduction of scarring, and reconstruction of blood capillaries (neovascularization). Keratinocytes, fibroblasts, endothelial cells, mesenchymal stem cells, adipose-derived stem cells, and endothelial progenitor cells studied in delivery systems have great promise in chronic wounds and diabetic ulcers. Gene therapies now in clinical trials and the discovery of biodegradable polymers, fibrin meshes, and human collagen serving as potential delivery systems may soon be available to clinical wound management. However, regeneration of peripheral nerves is seldom reported. Looking toward the future, these delivery wound healing products may be able to achieve the replacement and regeneration of more normal skin; to gain localized delivery to wound site; to heal severe burns, chronic and complex wounds; to control the release of drugs, growth factors, and cells; and to silence genes.

Author details

Lina Fu

Address all correspondence to: runa0325@gmail.com; lfu28@uwo.ca

Department of Chemical and Biochemical Engineering, Western University, London, Ontario, Canada

Fordham Centre for Biomedical Engineering, London, Ontario, Canada

References

[1] Wan WK, Yang L, Padavan DT. Use of degradable and nondegradable nanomaterials for controlled release. Nanomedicine (Lond). 2007 Aug;2(4):483-509. DOI: 10.2217/17435889.2.4.483

[2] Hurtley S, Hines PJ, Mueller KL, Culotta E. From bench to bedside. Science. 2014 Nov 21; 346(6212):932–3. DOI: 10.1126/science.346.6212.932

[3] Kamolz LP, Griffith M, Finnerty C, Kasper C. Skin regeneration, repair, and reconstruction. BioMed Research International. 2015 Jan 1; 2015. DOI: 10.1155/2015/892031

[4] Orgill DP, Blanco C, editors. Biomaterials for treating skin loss. Cambridge: Woodhead Publishing Limited; 2009 Jan 28.

[5] Gurtner GC, Werner S, Barrandon Y, Longaker MT. Wound repair and regeneration. Nature. 2008 May 15; 453(7193):314–21. DOI:10.1038/nature07039

[6] Teo EY, Ong SY, Chong MS, Zhang Z, Lu J, Moochhala S, Ho B, Teoh SH. Polycaprolactone-based fused deposition modeled mesh for delivery of antibacterial agents to infected wounds. Biomaterials. 2011 Jan 31; 32(1):279–87. DOI:10.1016/j.biomaterials.2010.08.089

[7] Singh B, Sharma S, Dhiman A. Design of antibiotic containing hydrogel wound dressings: biomedical properties and histological study of wound healing. Interna-

tional Journal of Pharmaceutics. 2013 Nov 30; 457(1):82–91. DOI: 10.1016/j.ijpharm.2013.09.028

[8] Sacco P, Travan A, Borgogna M, Paoletti S, Marsich E. Silver-containing antimicrobial membrane based on chitosan-TPP hydrogel for the treatment of wounds. Journal of Materials Science: Materials in Medicine. 2015 Mar 1; 26(3):1–2. DOI: 10.1007/s10856-015-5474-7

[9] Sun BK, Siprashvili Z, Khavari PA. Advances in skin grafting and treatment of cutaneous wounds. Science. 2014 Nov 21; 346(6212):941–5. DOI: 10.1126/science.1253836

[10] Hanson SE, Kleinbeck KR, Cantu D, Kim J, Bentz ML, Faucher LD, Kao WJ, Hematti P. Local delivery of allogeneic bone marrow and adipose tissue-derived mesenchymal stromal cells for cutaneous wound healing in a porcine model. Journal of Tissue Engineering and Regenerative Medicine. 2013 Feb 1. DOI: 10.1002/term.1700.

[11] Peng Y, Xuan M, Zou J, Liu H, Zhuo Z, Wan Y, Cheng B. Freeze-dried rat bone marrow mesenchymal stem cell paracrine factors: a simplified novel material for skin wound therapy. Tissue Engineering Part A. 2014 Dec 9; 21(5–6):1036–46. DOI: 10.1089/ten.TEA.2014.0102

[12] Nie C, Zhang G, Yang D, Liu T, Liu D, Xu J, Zhang J. Targeted delivery of adipose-derived stem cells via acellular dermal matrix enhances wound repair in diabetic rats. Journal of Tissue Engineering and Regenerative Medicine. 2015 Mar 1; 9(3):224–35. DOI: 10.1002/term.1622

[13] Tellechea A, Silva EA, Min J, Leal EC, Auster ME, Pradhan-Nabzdyk L, Shih W, Mooney DJ, Veves A. Alginate and DNA gels are suitable delivery systems for diabetic wound healing. The International Journal of Lower Extremity Wounds. 2015 Jun 1:1534734615580018. DOI: 10.1177/1534734615580018

[14] Kobsa S, Kristofik NJ, Sawyer AJ, Bothwell AL, Kyriakides TR, Saltzman WM. An electrospun scaffold integrating nucleic acid delivery for treatment of full-thickness wounds. Biomaterials. 2013 May 31; 34(15):3891–901. DOI: 10.1016/j.biomaterials.2013.02.016

[15] Narang AS, Chang RK, Hussain MA. Pharmaceutical development and regulatory considerations for nanoparticles and nanoparticulate drug delivery systems. Journal of Pharmaceutical Sciences. 2013 Nov 1; 102(11):3867–82. DOI: 10.1002/jps.23691

[16] Gainza G, Villullas S, Pedraz JL, Hernandez RM, Igartua M. Advances in drug delivery systems (DDSs) to release growth factors for wound healing and skin regeneration. Nanomedicine: Nanotechnology, Biology and Medicine. 2015 Aug 31; 11(6):1551–73. DOI: 10.1016/j.nano.2015.03.002

[17] Katti DS, Robinson KW, Ko FK, Laurencin CT. Bioresorbable nanofiber-based systems for wound healing and drug delivery: optimization of fabrication parameters. Journal

of Biomedical Materials Research Part B: Applied Biomaterials. 2004 Aug 15;70(2):286–96. DOI: 10.1002/jbm.b.30041

[18] Elsner JJ, Zilberman M. Antibiotic-eluting bioresorbable composite fibers for wound healing applications: microstructure, drug delivery and mechanical properties. Acta Biomaterialia. 2009 Oct 31;5(8):2872–83. DOI: 10.1016/j.actbio.2009.04.007

[19] Hima Bindu TV, Vidyavathi M, Kavitha K, Sastry TP, Suresh kumar RV. Preparation and evaluation of ciprofloxacin loaded chitosan–gelatin composite films for wound healing activity. International Journal of Drug Delivery. 2010; 2(2):173–82. DOI: 10.5138/ijdd.2010.0975.0215.02027

[20] Rouabhia M, Asselin J, Tazi N, Messaddeq Y, Levinson D, Zhang Z. Production of biocompatible and antimicrobial bacterial cellulose polymers functionalized by RGDC grafting groups and gentamicin. ACS Applied Materials & Interfaces. 2014 Jan 14;6(3):1439–46. DOI: 10.1021/am4027983

[21] Nagiah N, Ramanathan G, Sobhana L, Sivagnanam UT, Srinivasan NT. Poly (vinyl alcohol) microspheres sandwiched poly (3-hydroxybutyric acid) electrospun fibrous scaffold for tissue engineering and drug delivery. International Journal of Polymeric Materials and Polymeric Biomaterials. 2014 Jul 24;63(11):583–5. DOI: 10.1080/00914037.2013.854230

[22] Li R, Zhang X, Zhang Q, Liu H, Rong J, Tu M, Zeng R, Zhao J. β-Cyclodextrin-conjugated hyaluronan hydrogel as a potential drug sustained delivery carrier for wound healing. Journal of Applied Polymer Science. 2016 Mar 5;133(9):43072(1–8). DOI: 10.1002/app.43072

[23] Li Y, Liu G, Wang X, Hu J, Liu S. Enzyme-responsive polymeric vesicles for bacterial strain-selective delivery of antimicrobial agents. Angewandte Chemie International Edition England. 2016 Jan 26;55(5):1760-4. DOI: 10.1002/anie.201509401

[24] Atiyeh BS, Costagliola M, Hayek SN, Dibo SA. Effect of silver on burn wound infection control and healing: review of the literature. Burns. 2007 Mar 31;33(2):139–48. DOI: 10.1016/j.burns.2006.06.010

[25] Khampieng T, Brikshavana P, Supaphol P. Silver nanoparticle-embedded poly (vinyl pyrrolidone) hydrogel dressing: gamma-ray synthesis and biological evaluation. Journal of Biomaterials Science, Polymer Edition. 2014 May 24;25(8):826–42. DOI: 10.1080/09205063.2014.910154

[26] Oliveira RN, Rouzé R, Quilty B, Alves GG, Soares GD, Thiré RM, McGuinness GB. Mechanical properties and in vitro characterization of polyvinyl alcohol-nano-silver hydrogel wound dressings. Interface Focus. 2014 Feb 6;4(1):20130049. DOI: 10.1098/rsfs.2013.0049

[27] Shankar S, Jaiswal L, Aparna RS, Prasad RG, Kumar GP, Manohara CM. Wound healing potential of green synthesized silver nanoparticles prepared from *Lansium domesticum*

fruit peel extract. Materials Express. 2015 Mar 1;5(2):159–64. DOI: 10.1166/mex.2015.1225

[28] Mohiti-Asli M, Pourdeyhimi B, Loboa EG. Skin tissue engineering for the infected wound site: biodegradable PLA nanofibers and a novel approach for silver ion release evaluated in a 3D coculture system of keratinocytes and *Staphylococcus aureus*. Tissue Engineering Part C: Methods. 2014 Mar 17;20(10):790–7. DOI: 10.1089/ten.tec.2013.0458

[29] Patrulea V, Ostafe V, Borchard G, Jordan O. Chitosan as a starting material for wound healing applications. European Journal of Pharmaceutics and Biopharmaceutics. 2015 Nov 30;97:417–26. DOI: 10.1016/j.ejpb.2015.08.004

[30] Madhumathi K, Kumar PS, Abhilash S, Sreeja V, Tamura H, Manzoor K, Nair SV, Jayakumar R. Development of novel chitin/nanosilver composite scaffolds for wound dressing applications. Journal of Materials Science: Materials in Medicine. 2010 Feb 1;21(2):807–13. DOI: 10.1007/s10856-009-3877-z

[31] Banerjee J, Ghatak PD, Roy S, Khanna S, Hemann C, Deng B, Das A, Zweier JL, Wozniak D, Sen CK. Silver-zinc redox-coupled electroceutical wound dressing disrupts bacterial biofilm. PLoS One. 2015 Mar 24;10(3):e0119531. DOI: 10.1371/journal.pone.0119531

[32] Chen X, Peng LH, Shan YH, Li N, Wei W, Yu L, Li QM, Liang WQ, Gao JQ. Astragaloside IV-loaded nanoparticle-enriched hydrogel induces wound healing and anti-scar activity through topical delivery. International Journal of Pharmaceutics. 2013 Apr 15;447(1):171–81. DOI: 10.1016/j.ijpharm.2013.02.054

[33] Yallapu MM, Nagesh PK, Jaggi M, Chauhan SC. Therapeutic applications of curcumin nanoformulations. The AAPS Journal. 2015 Nov 1;17(6):1341–56. DOI: 10.1208/s12248-015-9811-z

[34] Dai M, Zheng X, Xu X, Kong X, Li X, Guo G, Luo F, Zhao X, Wei YQ, Qian Z. Chitosan-alginate sponge: preparation and application in curcumin delivery for dermal wound healing in rat. BioMed Research International. 2009 Nov 11;2009. DOI: 10.1155/2009/595126

[35] Krausz AE, Adler BL, Cabral V, Navati M, Doerner J, Charafeddine RA, Chandra D, Liang H, Gunther L, Clendaniel A, Harper S. Curcumin-encapsulated nanoparticles as innovative antimicrobial and wound healing agent. Nanomedicine: Nanotechnology, Biology and Medicine. 2015 Jan 31;11(1):195–206. DOI: 10.1016/j.nano.2014.09.004

[36] Huang L, Chen X, Nguyen TX, Tang H, Zhang L, Yang G. Nano-cellulose 3D-networks as controlled-release drug carriers. Journal of Materials Chemistry B. 2013;1(23):2976–84. DOI: 10.1039/c3tb20149j

[37] Trovatti E, Freire CS, Pinto PC, Almeida IF, Costa P, Silvestre AJ, Neto CP, Rosado C. Bacterial cellulose membranes applied in topical and transdermal delivery of lidocaine hydrochloride and ibuprofen: in vitro diffusion studies. International Journal of Pharmaceutics. 2012 Oct 1;435(1):83–7. DOI: 10.1016/j.ijpharm.2012.01.002

[38] Duscher D, Neofytou E, Wong VW, Maan ZN, Rennert RC, Inayathullah M, Januszyk M, Rodrigues M, Malkovskiy AV, Whitmore AJ, Walmsley GG. Transdermal deferoxamine prevents pressure-induced diabetic ulcers. Proceedings of the National Academy of Sciences. 2015 Jan 6;112(1):94–9. DOI: 10.1073/pnas.1413445112

[39] Barrientos S, Stojadinovic O, Golinko MS, Brem H, Tomic-Canic M. Growth factors and cytokines in wound healing. Wound Repair and Regeneration. 2008 Sep 1;16(5):585–601. DOI: 10.1111/j.1524-475X.2008.00410.x

[40] Koria P. Delivery of growth factors for tissue regeneration and wound healing. BioDrugs. 2012 Jun 1;26(3):163–75. DOI: 10.2165/11631850-000000000-0000

[41] Geer DJ, Swartz DD, Andreadis ST. Biomimetic delivery of keratinocyte growth factor upon cellular demand for accelerated wound healing in vitro and in vivo. The American Journal of Pathology. 2005 Dec 31;167(6):1575–86. DOI: 10.1016/S0002-9440(10)61242-4

[42] Yao C, Yao P, Wu H, Zha Z. Acceleration of wound healing in traumatic ulcers by absorbable collagen sponge containing recombinant basic fibroblast growth factor. Biomedical Materials. 2006 Mar 15;1(1):33. DOI:10.1088/1748-6041/1/1/005

[43] Hardwicke J, Ferguson EL, Moseley R, Stephens P, Thomas DW, Duncan R. Dextrin–rhEGF conjugates as bioresponsive nanomedicines for wound repair. Journal of Controlled Release. 2008 Sep 24;130(3):275–83. DOI: 10.1016/j.jconrel.2008.07.023

[44] Kulkarni A, Diehl-Jones W, Ghanbar S, Liu S. Layer-by-layer assembly of epidermal growth factors on polyurethane films for wound closure. Journal of Biomaterials Applications. 2014 Aug 1;29(2):278–90. DOI: 10.1177/0885328214523058

[45] Picheth GF, Sierakowski MR, Woehl MA, Ono L, Cofré AR, Vanin LP, Pontarolo R, De Freitas RA. Lysozyme-triggered epidermal growth factor release from bacterial cellulose membranes controlled by smart nanostructured films. Journal of Pharmaceutical Sciences. 2014 Dec 1;103(12):3958–65. DOI: 10.1002/jps.24205

[46] Johnson NR, Wang Y. Controlled delivery of heparin-binding EGF-like growth factor yields fast and comprehensive wound healing. Journal of Controlled Release. 2013 Mar 10;166(2):124–9. DOI: 10.1016/j.jconrel.2012.11.004

[47] Yenilmez E, Basaran E, Arslan R, Berkman MS, Güven UM, Bayçu C, Yazan Y. Chitosan gel formulations containing egg yolk oil and epidermal growth factor for dermal burn treatment. Die Pharmazie: An International Journal of Pharmaceutical Sciences. 2015 Feb 2;70(2):67–73. DOI: 10.1691/ph.2015.4126

[48] Nunes QM, Li Y, Sun C, Kinnunen TK, Fernig DG. Fibroblast growth factors as tissue repair and regeneration therapeutics. PeerJ. 2016 Jan 12;4:e1535. DOI: 10.7717/peerj.1535

[49] Park HJ, Lee S, Kang KH, Heo CY, Kim JH, Yang HS, Kim BS. Enhanced random skin flap survival by sustained delivery of fibroblast growth factor 2 in rats. ANZ Journal of Surgery. 2013 May 1;83(5):354–8. DOI: 10.1111/j.1445-2197.2012.06194.x

[50] Fabiilli ML, Wilson CG, Padilla F, Martín-Saavedra FM, Fowlkes JB, Franceschi RT. Acoustic droplet–hydrogel composites for spatial and temporal control of growth factor delivery and scaffold stiffness. Acta Biomaterialia. 2013 Jul 31;9(7):7399–409. DOI: 10.1016/j.actbio.2013.03.027

[51] Li B, Davidson JM, Guelcher SA. The effect of the local delivery of platelet-derived growth factor from reactive two-component polyurethane scaffolds on the healing in rat skin excisional wounds. Biomaterials. 2009 Jul 31;30(20):3486–94. DOI: 10.1016/j.biomaterials.2009.03.008

[52] Zavan B, Vindigni V, Vezzù K, Zorzato G, Luni C, Abatangelo G, Elvassore N, Cortivo R. Hyaluronan based porous nano-particles enriched with growth factors for the treatment of ulcers: a placebo-controlled study. Journal of Materials Science: Materials in Medicine. 2009 Jan 1;20(1):235–47. DOI: 10.1007/s10856-008-3566-3

[53] Rabbany SY, Pastore J, Yamamoto M, Miller T, Rafii S, Aras R, Penn M. Continuous delivery of stromal cell-derived factor-1 from alginate scaffolds accelerates wound healing. Cell Transplantation. 2010 Apr 1;19(4):399–408. DOI: 10.3727/096368909X481782

[54] Lin YK, Chen KH, Ou KL, Liu M. Effects of different extracellular matrices and growth factor immobilization on biodegradability and biocompatibility of macroporous bacterial cellulose. Journal of Bioactive and Compatible Polymers. 2011 Sep 1;26(5):508–18. DOI: 10.1177/0883911511415390

[55] Ribeiro MP, Morgado PI, Miguel SP, Coutinho P, Correia IJ. Dextran-based hydrogel containing chitosan microparticles loaded with growth factors to be used in wound healing. Materials Science and Engineering: C. 2013 Jul 1;33(5):2958–66. DOI: 10.1016/j.msec.2013.03.025

[56] Jin G, Prabhakaran MP, Kai D, Ramakrishna S. Controlled release of multiple epidermal induction factors through core–shell nanofibers for skin regeneration. European Journal of Pharmaceutics and Biopharmaceutics. 2013 Nov 30;85(3):689–98. DOI: 10.1016/j.ejpb.2013.06.002

[57] Almquist BD, Castleberry SA, Sun JB, Lu AY, Hammond PT. Combination growth factor therapy via electrostatically assembled wound dressings improves diabetic ulcer healing in vivo. Advanced Healthcare Materials. 2015 Oct 1;4(14):2090–9. DOI: 10.1002/adhm.201500403

[58] Eisenhardt M, Dobler D, Schlupp P, Schmidts T, Salzig M, Vilcinskas A, Salzig D, Czermak P, Keusgen M, Runkel F. Development of an insect metalloproteinase inhibitor drug carrier system for application in chronic wound infections. Journal of Pharmacy and Pharmacology. 2015 Nov 1;67(11):1481–91. DOI: 10.1111/jphp.12452

[59] Chereddy KK, Her CH, Comune M, Moia C, Lopes A, Porporato PE, Vanacker J, Lam MC, Steinstraesser L, Sonveaux P, Zhu H. PLGA nanoparticles loaded with host defense

peptide LL37 promote wound healing. Journal of Controlled Release. 2014 Nov 28;194:138–47. DOI: 10.1016/j.jconrel.2014.08.016

[60] Babavalian H, Latifi AM, Shokrgozar MA, Bonakdar S, Mohammadi S, Moghaddam MM. Analysis of healing effect of alginate sulfate hydrogel dressing containing antimicrobial peptide on wound infection caused by methicillin-resistant *Staphylococcus aureus*. Jundishapur Journal of Microbiology. 2015 Sep;8(9). DOI: 10.5812/jjm.28320

[61] Zhang M, Rehman J, Malik AB. Endothelial progenitor cells and vascular repair. Current Opinion in Hematology. 2014 May;21(3):224. DOI: 10.1097/MOH.0000000000000041.

[62] Xu K, Cantu DA, Fu Y, Kim J, Zheng X, Hematti P, Kao WJ. Thiol-ene Michael-type formation of gelatin/poly (ethylene glycol) biomatrices for three-dimensional mesenchymal stromal/stem cell administration to cutaneous wounds. Acta Biomaterialia. 2013 Nov 30;9(11):8802–14. DOI: 10.1016/j.actbio.2013.06.021

[63] Sánchez-Sánchez R, Brena-Molina A, Martínez-López V, Melgarejo-Ramírez Y, de Dios LT, Gómez-García R, de Lourdes Reyes-Frías M, Rodríguez-Rodríguez L, Garciadiego-Cázares D, Lugo-Martínez H, Ibarra C. Generation of two biological wound dressings as a potential delivery system of human adipose-derived mesenchymal stem cells. Asaio Journal. 2015 Nov;61(6):718. DOI: 10.1097/MAT.0000000000000277

[64] Wahl EA, Fierro FA, Peavy TR, Hopfner U, Dye JF, Machens HG, Egaña JT, Schenck TL. In vitro evaluation of scaffolds for the delivery of mesenchymal stem cells to wounds. BioMed Research International. 2015 Oct 4;2015:1. DOI: 10.1155/2015/108571

[65] Rustad KC, Wong VW, Sorkin M, Glotzbach JP, Major MR, Rajadas J, Longaker MT, Gurtner GC. Enhancement of mesenchymal stem cell angiogenic capacity and stemness by a biomimetic hydrogel scaffold. Biomaterials. 2012 Jan 31;33(1):80–90. DOI: 10.1016/j.biomaterials.2011.09.041

[66] Zebardast N, Lickorish D, Davies JE. Human umbilical cord perivascular cells (HUCPVC) A mesenchymal cell source for dermal wound healing. Organogenesis. 2010 Oct 1;6(4):197–203. DOI: 10.4161/org6.4.12393

[67] Skardal A, Mack D, Kapetanovic E, Atala A, Jackson JD, Yoo J, Soker S. Bioprinted amniotic fluid-derived stem cells accelerate healing of large skin wounds. Stem Cells Translational Medicine. 2012 Nov;1(11):792. DOI: 10.5966/sctm.2012-0088

[68] Kim KL, Han DK, Park K, Song SH, Kim JY, Kim JM, Ki HY, Yie SW, Roh CR, Jeon ES, Kim DK. Enhanced dermal wound neovascularization by targeted delivery of endothelial progenitor cells using an RGD-g-PLLA scaffold. Biomaterials. 2009 Aug 31;30(22):3742–8. DOI: 10.1016/j.biomaterials.2009.03.053

[69] O'Loughlin A, Kulkarni M, Vaughan EE, Creane M, Liew A, Dockery P, Pandit A, O'Brien T. Autologous circulating angiogenic cells treated with osteopontin and delivered via a collagen scaffold enhance wound healing in the alloxan-induced

diabetic rabbit ear ulcer model. Stem cell Research & Therapy. 2013 Dec 1;4(6):1–4. DOI: 10.1186/scrt388

[70] Shingyochi Y, Orbay H, Mizuno H. Adipose-derived stem cells for wound repair and regeneration. Expert Opinion on Biological Therapy. 2015 Sep 2;15(9):1285–92. DOI: 10.1517/14712598.2015.1053867

[71] Altman AM, Yan Y, Matthias N, Bai X, Rios C, Mathur AB, Song YH, Alt EU. IFATS collection: human adipose-derived stem cells seeded on a silk fibroin-chitosan scaffold enhance wound repair in a murine soft tissue injury model. Stem Cells. 2009 Jan 1;27(1): 250–8. DOI: 10.1634/stemcells.2008-0178

[72] Hassan W, Dong Y, Wang W. Encapsulation and 3D culture of human adipose-derived stem cells in an in-situ crosslinked hybrid hydrogel composed of PEG-based hyper-branched copolymer and hyaluronic acid. Stem Cell Research & Therapy. 2013 Mar 21;4(2):32. DOI: 10.1186/scrt182

[73] Zeng Y, Zhu L, Han Q, Liu W, Mao X, Li Y, Yu N, Feng S, Fu Q, Wang X, Du Y. Preformed gelatin microcryogels as injectable cell carriers for enhanced skin wound healing. Acta Biomaterialia. 2015 Oct 1;25:291–303. DOI: 10.1016/j.actbio.2015.07.042

[74] Bathany C, Park J, Cho YK, Takayama S. Dehydrated aqueous two-phase system micro-domains retain their shape upon rehydration to allow patterned reagent delivery to cells. Journal of Materials Chemistry B. 2013;1(44):6020–6. DOI: 10.1039/c3tb21004a

[75] Masuda R, Mochizuki M, Hozumi K, Takeda A, Uchinuma E, Yamashina S, Nomizu M, Kadoya Y. A novel cell-adhesive scaffold material for delivering keratinocytes reduces granulation tissue in dermal wounds. Wound Repair and Regeneration. 2009 Jan 1;17(1):127–35. DOI:10.1111/j.1524-475X.2008.00450.x

[76] Nuutila K, Peura M, Suomela S, Hukkanen M, Siltanen A, Harjula A, Vuola J, Kankuri E. Recombinant human collagen III gel for transplantation of autologous skin cells in porcine full-thickness wounds. Journal of Tissue Engineering and Regenerative Medicine. 2015 Dec 1;9(12):1386–93. DOI: 10.1002/term.1691

[77] Sarett SM, Nelson CE, Duvall CL. Technologies for controlled, local delivery of siRNA. Journal of Controlled Release. 2015 Nov 28;218:94–113. DOI: 10.1016/j.jconrel. 2015.09.066

[78] Waddington SN, Crossley R, Sheard V, Howe SJ, Buckley SM, Coughlan L, Gilham DE, Hawkins RE, McKay TR. Gene delivery of a mutant TGFβ3 reduces markers of scar tissue formation after cutaneous wounding. Molecular Therapy. 2010 Dec 1;18(12): 2104–11. DOI: 10.1038/mt.2010.174

[79] Peterson CY, Shaterian A, Borboa AK, Gonzalez AM, Potenza BM, Coimbra R, Eliceiri BP, Baird A. The noninvasive, quantitative, in vivo assessment of adenoviral-mediated gene delivery in skin wound biomaterials. Biomaterials. 2009 Dec 31;30(35):6788–93. DOI: 10.1016/j.biomaterials.2009.07.069

[80] Shaterian A, Kao S, Chen L, DiPietro LA, Coimbra R, Eliceiri BP, Baird A. The candidate tumor suppressor gene Ecrg4 as a wound terminating factor in cutaneous injury. Archives of Dermatological Research. 2013 Mar 1;305(2):141–9. DOI: 10.1007/s00403-012-1276-7

[81] Breen A, Dockery P, O'Brien T, Pandit A. Fibrin scaffold promotes adenoviral gene transfer and controlled vector delivery. Journal of Biomedical Materials Research Part A. 2009 Jun 15;89(4):876–84. DOI: 10.1002/jbm.a.32039

[82] Monaghan M, Browne S, Schenke-Layland K, Pandit A. A collagen-based scaffold delivering exogenous microRNA-29b to modulate extracellular matrix remodeling. Molecular Therapy. 2014 Apr 1;22(4):786–96. DOI: 10.1038/mt.2013.288

[83] Tokatlian T, Cam C, Segura T. Porous hyaluronic acid hydrogels for localized nonviral DNA delivery in a diabetic wound healing model. Advanced Healthcare Materials. 2015 May 1;4(7):1084–91. DOI: 10.1002/adhm.201400783

[84] Sarkar K, Banerjee SL, Kundu PP, Madras G, Chatterjee K. Biofunctionalized surface-modified silver nanoparticles for gene delivery. Journal of Materials Chemistry B. 2015;3(26):5266–76. DOI: 10.1039/c5tb00614g

[85] Kwon MJ, An S, Choi S, Nam K, Jung HS, Yoon CS, Ko JH, Jun HJ, Kim TK, Jung SJ, Park JH. Effective healing of diabetic skin wounds by using nonviral gene therapy based on minicircle vascular endothelial growth factor DNA and a cationic dendrimer. The Journal of Gene Medicine. 2012 Apr 1;14(4):272–8. DOI: 10.1002/jgm.2618

[86] Nauta A, Seidel C, Deveza L, Montoro D, Grova M, Ko SH, Hyun J, Gurtner GC, Longaker MT, Yang F. Adipose-derived stromal cells overexpressing vascular endothelial growth factor accelerate mouse excisional wound healing. Molecular Therapy. 2013 Feb 1;21(2):445–55. DOI: 10.1038/mt.2012.234

[87] Dou C, Lay F, Ansari AM, Rees DJ, Ahmed AK, Kovbasnjuk O, Matsangos AE, Du J, Hosseini SM, Steenbergen C, Fox-Talbot K. Strengthening the skin with topical delivery of keratinocyte growth factor-1 using a novel DNA plasmid. Molecular Therapy. 2014 Apr;22(4):752. DOI: 10.1038/mt.2014.2

[88] Kim HS, Yoo HS. MMPs-responsive release of DNA from electrospun nanofibrous matrix for local gene therapy: in vitro and in vivo evaluation. Journal of Controlled Release. 2010 Aug 3;145(3):264–71. DOI: 10.1016/j.jconrel.2010.03.006

[89] Chiappini C, De Rosa E, Martinez JO, Liu X, Steele J, Stevens MM, Tasciotti E. Biodegradable silicon nanoneedles delivering nucleic acids intracellularly induce localized in vivo neovascularization. Nature Materials. 2015 May 1;14(5):532–9. DOI: 10.1038/NMAT4249

[90] United States Government Code of Federal Regulations, Title 21 (21CFR), Part 3, Food and Drugs, Office of the Federal Register National Archives and Records Administration, US Government Printing Office, Washington, DC, 2015 April 1.

[91] ISO 10993, Biological Evaluation of Medical Devices. 4th ed. Geneva: International Standards Organization; 2009 October 15.

[92] Dash SN, Dash NR, Guru B, Mohapatra PC. Towards reaching the target: clinical 4 application of mesenchymal stem cells for diabetic foot ulcers. Rejuvenation Research, Mary Ann Liebert, Inc, New Rochelle, New York, United States. 5 2014 Feb 1; 17(1): 40-53. DOI: 10.1089/rej.2013.1467

[93] Chaudhary C, Garg T. Scaffolds: a novel carrier and potential wound healer. Critical Reviews™ in Therapeutic Drug Carrier Systems. 2015;32(4):277–321. DOI: 10.1615/CritRevTherDrugCarrierSyst.2015011246

[94] Abdi R, Fiorina P, Adra CN, Atkinson M, Sayegh MH. Immunomodulation by mesenchymal stem cells a potential therapeutic strategy for type 1 diabetes. Diabetes. 2008 Jul 1;57(7):1759–67. DOI: 10.2337/db08-0180

[95] Duscher D, Barrera J, Wong VW, Maan ZN, Whittam AJ, Januszyk M, Gurtner GC. Stem cells in wound healing: the future of regenerative medicine a mini-review. Gerontology. 2015 May 29;62(2):216–25. DOI: 10.1159/000381877

[96] Ezquer FE, Ezquer ME, Parrau DB, Carpio D, Yañez AJ, Conget PA. Systemic administration of multipotent mesenchymal stromal cells reverts hyperglycemia and prevents nephropathy in type 1 diabetic mice. Biology of Blood and Marrow Transplantation. 2008 Jun 30;14(6):631–40. DOI: 10.1016/j.bbmt.2008.01.006

[97] Yang M, Sheng L, Zhang TR, Li Q. Stem cell therapy for lower extremity diabetic ulcers: where do we stand?. BioMed Research International. 2013 Mar 18;2013:462179. DOI: 10.1155/2013/462179

[98] Takahashi K, Yamanaka S. Induction of pluripotent stem cells from mouse embryonic and adult fibroblast cultures by defined factors. Cell. 2006 Aug 25;126(4):663–76. DOI: 10.1016/j.cell.2006.07.024

[99] Kirby GT, Mills SJ, Cowin AJ, Smith LE. Stem cells for cutaneous wound healing. BioMed Research International. 2015 Jun 2;2015. DOI: 10.1155/2015/285869

[100] Jarow JP, Baxley JH. Medical devices: US medical device regulation. Urologic Oncology: Seminars and Original Investigations, 2015 Mar 31; 33(3): 128–132. DOI: 10.1016/j.urolonc.2014.10.004

[101] Alpert S. Cost Recovery and the Future of the Medical Device Regulation Program in Canada. Health Law Review. 2008 May 1;16(3):73–78.

Chapter 5

Cellular Therapy for Wounds: Applications of Mesenchymal Stem Cells in Wound Healing

Moyassar B. H. Al-Shaibani, Xiao-nong Wang,
Penny E. Lovat and Anne M. Dickinson

Additional information is available at the end of the chapter

http://dx.doi.org/10.5772/63963

Abstract

Despite progress in wound treatment including gene therapy, biological dresses and engineered skin equivalents, present treatment options for chronic wounds are restricted and not always effective. For example, inability to get consistent product from the introduced gene, biological covers may give rise to hypoxic conditions and engineered skin models are limited by their construction from substances which are hard to be degraded, and do not always result in complete replication into normal uninjured skin. A growing body of evidence suggests mesenchymal stem cells (MSCs), and their secreted growth factors and microvesicles, may potentiate the wound-healing process and as such their addition to novel wound-healing treatments may improve the efficacy of current therapeutic strategies. Recent studies report the ability of bone marrow-derived MSCs (BM-MSCs) to migrate and differentiate into skin cells *in vivo*.

Therefore, this chapter aims to review the important concepts of wound healing at the cellular and kinetic level and the potential therapeutic strategies of MSCs through which to improve their treatment. Focus to this chapter will begin with a description of wound types, phases of healing process, followed by an outline of the role of MSC secretions in each phase, leading to potential novel treatment strategies and the requirements for a successful healing process.

Keywords: cellular therapy, conditioned medium, growth factors, mesenchymal stem cells, skin regeneration

1. Introduction

In the United Kingdom, around 200,000 patients experience a chronic wound of varying type, ranging between ulcerations, scars, trauma and burns. Unfortunately, patient morbidity and in some cases mortality may result from such injuries for which chronic ulceration is a major factor [1–3]. One of these impacts is the reduced contribution to society by the individuals suffering from these chronic wounds including their inability to work [3]. In addition, healthcare treatment and hospitalisation for chronic wounds are costly [2] involving lengthy treatment and nursing care. In 2005 and 2006, the care of patients with a chronic wound costs the UK NHS approximately £2.3bn–£3.1bn each year, with £6.08 million in England lone being attributed to nursing care [4]. In the United States, approximately 6.5 million patients suffered from chronic wounds with expenses for wound care management exceeding US $25 billion in 2009 [5]. Furthermore, infection is inevitable, which not only negatively affect wound healing but can also be life threatening, requiring more hospitalisation and increased healthcare expenditure [6] and repetitive treatment [7]. Consequently, both the society and the health sector are negatively affected by the burden of chronic wounds. Moreover, despite great progress in wound treatment including the implementation of growth factors and biological engineering of skin equivalents, present treatment options for burns and non-healing chronic wounds are restricted and not always effective [8]. Engineered skin to aid the development of novel wound care strategies is limited by their construction from substances that are hard to be degraded, and do not always result in complete replication into normal uninjured skin. Furthermore, complete renewal of this model requires the alteration of immune responses to reduce fibrotic reactions in order to diminish scar production [9]. Gene therapy may also be limited by insufficient selection of target cells, the identification of the factors which may affect the introduction of genes or the inability to produce stable prolonged specific gene product which is the main problem with systemic gene therapy [10]. Additionally, biofilms give rise to hypoxic conditions. Therefore, there is an urgent need for new therapies for wounds with delayed healing [8]. Specific extracellular matrix (ECM) proteins equivalent to the skin, specific growth factors, mesenchymal stem cells (MSCs), fibroblasts or viable epithelial cells may, however, aid the wound-healing process, and their addition to potential wound-healing treatments may improve the efficacy of current therapeutic strategies [11]. The availability of MSCs in normal human skin [12], and their vital function in wound healing suggests that the exogenous application of such cells may represent a promising solution for the treatment of non-healing wounds [13].

Mesenchymal stem cells (MSCs) are generally defined as self-renewable, multi-potent progenitor adult stem cells present in peripheral blood. *In vivo*, they have the ability to differentiate widely into many mesenchymal lineages such as cartilage, bone, muscle and adipose tissues [14]. Furthermore, MSCs have the ability to migrate from the bone marrow to an injured site and differentiate into functional skin cells [15]. *In vitro* they can be defined as fibroblast-like cells capable of self-renewal with the ability to adhere to plastic and subsequently differentiate into adipose, bone, cartilage tissue [16] as well as a multi-layered epidermis-like structure [17]. Paracrine factors secreted by MSCs are considered the principle factors with therapeutic potential for tissue wound healing [18] including growth factors, cytokines and chemokines which promote angiogenesis and wound repair [19–22]. Moreover, MSCs produce soluble factors that regulate cellular responses, angiogenesis formation and tissue remodelling [23] and play a vital role in each of the five phases of wound-healing process including haemostasis, inflammation, proliferation, contraction and remodelling [11]. In addition, MSCs exert antimicrobial activity via the secretion of the antimicrobial peptide LL-37 thereby preventing wound infection [24]. Furthermore, Tamama and Kerpedjieva [25] report that conditioned medium derived from the cell culture of MSCs (MSC-CM) contains all the effector molecules secreted by MSCs which could be effectively utilised in tissue regeneration and wound healing. Collectively these data thus suggest that MSC-CM may represent a novel therapeutic strategy for wound therapy, but the mechanisms mediating these events and exactly how MSCs contribute in skin regeneration remain undefined.

2. Skin wounds and healing process

Generally, wounds are classified on the basis of location, depth and tissue loss into three categories: superficial wounds where damage affects the epidermis only; partial thickness wounds when both the epidermis and dermis are involved; and full thickness wounds which involve the dermis, subcutaneous fats and sometimes, bones. However, depending on normal healing trajectory, there are two principal categories of skin wounds: acute and chronic wounds [26, 27].

2.1. Acute wounds

Acute wounds arise either as a result of surgical incision or following traumatic accidents including abrasions, superficial burns and partial thickness injuries with significant loss of tissues. Irrespective to their causes, the healing process of acute wounds is complex and utilises different types of cells and cytokines [26].

2.2. Chronic skin wounds

Wounds are defined as chronic when they fail to heal during one or all of the phases of the healing process causing an injury that cannot be repaired within the expected time period of normal wound repairs [11]. Chronic wounds mainly accompany disorders such as pressure ulcers, diabetes, burns, vascular insufficiency and vasculitis [5]. The chronic state of non-healing wounds is exacerbated by many factors including tissue hypoxia, microbial infection, necrosis, exudates and an elevated ratio of inflammatory cytokines during the different healing stages [28]. Neutrophils also contribute by releasing excessive amounts of collagenase which leads to break down the ECM [29] and enzyme elastase destroying important healing factors such as PDGF and transforming growth factor-beta (TGF-β). Chronic wounds do not respond to therapeutic methods unless the prolonged inflammation is targeted [11]. Consequently, human skin with its limited abilities will fail to heal itself in cases of wounds penetrating the epidermis [30] due to the deficiency in growth factors and cytokines which are depleted during the healing process [31, 32]

2.3. Phases of wound-healing process

Each wound undergoes a series of successive events for repairing and healing. These processes take from several minutes such as coagulation, several days such as inflammation to several months or years such as remodelling and can be divided into three, four or five overlapping phases and stages. Monaco and Lawrence [26] state the wound-healing process consists of five distinct phases: (a) haemostasis, (b) inflammation, (c) cellular migration and proliferation, (d) protein synthesis and wound contraction and (e) remodelling, while Gosain and DiPietro [33] and Zhou et al. [34] describe the healing process as consisting of four highly integrated and overlapping phases: (a) haemostasis, (b) inflammation, (c) proliferation and (d) tissue remodelling or resolution [7]. A normal wound-healing mechanism is a dynamic and complex process involving a series of coordinated events, including (a) bleeding and coagulation, (b) acute inflammation, (c) cell migration, (d) proliferation, (e) differentiation, (f) angiogenesis, re-epithelialisation and (g) synthesis and remodelling of ECM. Conversely, Maxson et al. [11] report that the healing process is a complex event occurring in three overlapping phases: (a) inflammatory, (b) proliferative and (c) remodelling. These phases and their biophysiological functions must occur in the proper sequence, at a specific time, and continue for a specific duration and intensity [35]. There are many factors that can affect wound healing which interfere with one or more phases in this process, thus causing improper or impaired tissue repair [28]. All in all, a successful healing process cannot be accomplished without any one of these processes; haemostasis, inflammation, angiogenesis, proliferation, contraction, re-epithelialisation and remodelling [36]. To better understand the healing process, we will discuss the five phases and how they overlap.

2.3.1. Haemostasis phase (coagulation)

During blood circulation in an intact blood vessel, endothelial cells of the blood vessel secrete coagulation and aggregation inhibitors, that is they release heparin-like molecules to prevent blood coagulation and thrombomodulin to prevent platelet aggregation. Prostacyclin and nitric oxide are also involved in this process [37]. In contrast, the endothelial cells of broken blood vessels replace the secretions of clot inhibitors with a blood glycoprotein called von Willebrand factor (vWF) which initiates haemostasis [37, 38].

Haemostasis is the first phase of wound healing and consists of three successive steps: vasoconstriction, blockage the wound by platelet aggregation and blood coagulation. When skin is injured, a blood extravasation begins to fill the injured site. Immediately after the skin injury and bleeding, the blood vessel contracts and reduces the blood flow to the wounded site thereby keeping the blood within the damaged vessel and causing bleeding to stop [38, 39]. Not only do vessel contractions stop haemorrhage, but also blood changing from a liquid phase to a gel phase forming a blood clot (coagulation) and platelet aggregation generates a haemostatic buffer (plasma) which is rich in fibrin, thereby stopping the haemorrhage and restoring a barrier protecting the wound from infection by invading microorganisms. This process constitutes a matrix what encourages cell migration [40, 41]. In this phase, the role of platelets is not only restricted to blocking the damaged area and in clot formation, but also in the formation of a transient extracellular matrix by secreting adhesion molecules such as fibronectin and thrombospondin, as well as growth factors such as epidermal growth factor (EGF), platelet-derived growth factor (PDGF), transforming growth factor-alpha (TGF-α) and beta (TGF-β), and vascular endothelial growth factor (VEGF) [42]. This matrix serves as a reservoir for growth factors and cytokines critical to subsequent healing phases [41]. Collectively, the matrix, activated cascade coagulation and parenchymatous cells make the injured vessel a chemotactic environment to attract inflammatory cells at the wound site and initiate the start of inflammatory phase [43].

2.3.2. Inflammation phase

An inflammatory reaction begins soon after the haemorrhage stops at the site of injury. This reaction promotes mobility of various cells toward the injured tissue giving rise to a multitude of complicated and successive series of reactions ending with rebuilding of a tissue-like structure [44]. The main advantages of this phase are isolating the injured tissues from the surrounding contaminated environment, cleaning out cell debris and damaged tissues and the initiation of the healing process [45]. The main reactivity observed in this phase is an increased migration of inflammatory cells from intravascular tissue towards the extracellular wound site due to increased vascular permeability. This permeability increases due to vasodilation when both fibrin and thrombin are activated by the coagulation cascade. Meanwhile, clot formation and their stimuli are dissipated and plasminogen converted to plasmin [46]. Three main cell types are involved in the inflammatory phase: neutrophils, macrophages and lymphocytes whose activity is initiated within hours of injury [44, 45]. Neutrophils seem to be the most dominant cell type during the first 48 hours, cleaning the wound site from bacteria, cell debris and damaged tissue by releasing free radicals; however, they are not essential for the healing process [40, 41, 47]. Approximately 48 hours following the injury, stimuli for neutrophils no longer persist and neutrophil numbers cease when macrophages (monocyte-derived macrophage) then penetrate the wound site via the blood and become the dominant cellular component of the inflammatory phase by phagocytosing cell debris and bacteria including expended neutrophils. Macrophages also secrete collagenases and elastases to break down the damaged tissues [48]. In contrast to neutrophils, the role of macrophages is not restricted to cleaning of the tissues as they also play a crucial role in the healing process by secreting prostaglandins, which act as vasodilators increasing microvessel permeability and attracting other inflammatory cells into the wounded site [41, 49, 50]. In addition, macrophages secrete fibroblast growth factor (FGF), PDGF, TGF-α and VEGF which are important for proliferation and migration of fibroblasts as well as cytokines, which attract endothelial cells to the injury site promoting their proliferation and the development of a new tissue [48, 49, 51]. Within three days of the inflammatory phase, T lymphocytes home to the injury site by the activity of interlukin-1 and secret lymphokines such heparin-binding epidermal growth factor (HB-EGF) and basic fibroblast growth factor (bFGF), promoting fibroblast proliferation [52].

2.3.3. Proliferation phase (epithelialisation)

The proliferation phase (epithelial proliferation phase) represents the main phase responsible for actual wound closure. In the case of skin wounds, endothelial non-inflammatory cells such as keratinocytes and fibroblasts start to proliferate and migrate towards the edges of the wound-producing collagen for the development of new tissues [53–55]. Within a few hours (between 6 and 24 hours) of injury, TGF-β and EGF act as mitogenic and chemotactic stimulators attracting keratinocytes which migrate towards the wound and start epithelialisation [54]. Fibroblasts are activated and start to differentiate into myofibroblasts which participate in reducing the wound size by contracting and secreting extracellular matrix (ECM) proteins giving rise to healing of the connective tissue [56, 57]. Meanwhile, angiogenesis progresses, coordinating the transfer of nutrients and oxygen from newly formed capillaries to the wound site enhancing metabolic activity [58]. Epithelisation, fibroplasia and angiogenesis collectively comprise granulation tissue which covers the damaged tissues within four days of injury [55].

2.3.4. Contraction phase

Wound contraction could be defined as mobility of wound margins towards the wound core to facilitate closure; this phase begins when fibroblasts stop proliferating and undergo apoptosis within 5–15 days post-injury which occurs concurrently with collagen synthesis [59, 60]. The rate of movement of wound edges depends on tissue laxity and wound shape; for instance, the looser tissues tend to contract more rapidly than the compact tissues and squared wounds contract more quickly than rounded wounds. The contraction rate also depends on the availability of myofibroblast and their proliferation and connection to the surrounding extracellular matrix [61].

2.3.5. Remodelling phase (resolution)

Remodelling or resolution is the last phase of the wound-healing process. The biological processes observed in this step involve gradual resolution of the inflammatory phase, collagen deposition, complete coverage of the injured site by the new tissues and formation of scar tissue [62]. Successful remodelling requires stable collagen content; therefore, the important step in this phase is controlling collagen remodelling [34]. Although collagen synthesis is continuing during this phase, its level is restricted due to the activity of collagenases and metalloproteinases which aid in removing the excess collagen [63, 64]. For optimal remodelling, collagen levels need to be balanced by the activity of metalloproteinases inhibitors secreted by tissue arresting the collagenolytic enzymes and balancing the production of new collagen with that of the removed old collagen [64]. The outcome of this process is that collagen type III is replaced by collagen type I, hence replacing both hyaluronic acid and glycosaminoglycans by proteoglycans and the disappearance of fibronectin as well as resorbing water from scar tissues. These events start approximately 3 weeks after the injury and may last indefinitely as collagen fibres stack closer to each other decreasing scar thickness and increasing wound bursting strength 'resistance to rupture' [65].

As described above, the main issues in the wound-healing process are how cells are attracted to the site of injury site and how to enhance their proliferation and differentiate at the wounded region. These cells include inflammatory cells (neutrophils, macrophages and lymphocytes) and epithelial cells (fibroblasts and keratinocytes). All these activities are mainly regulated by growth factors and cytokines. In many cases, these cells fail to migrate, proliferate and

http://dx.doi.org/10.5772/63963

differentiate due to deficiency in growth factors and cytokines; consequently, the healing process will be impaired and chronic wounds will arise [54]. Therefore, in order to improve wound healing, there is a need for an alternative source of healing cytokines and growth factors to enrich the injury site. MSC-CM acts as a rich source of 36 growth factors, cytokines and chemokines which collected from MSC *in vitro* under good manufacturing practice could be used as therapy for wounds in the future [66]. The main events and phases of the wound-healing process are summarised in **Table 1**.

Phase	**Haemostasis**	**Inflammation**	**Proliferation migration**	**Contraction**	**Remodelling**
Starts post-injury	Immediately	First hours	Day 4	Day 5	Day 20
Duration	(minutes–hour)	(3 days to 14 days)	(21 days)	(10 days to 20 days)	(Months to 2 years)
	Haemorrhage	Phagocytosis	Endothelial cells migration	Fibroblast apoptosis	Collagen control remodelling
	Vasoconstriction	Growth factors secretion	Epithelialisation	Wound edges pull	Replacing collagen type III by type I
	Platelet aggregation	Cytokines secretion	Fibroblast differentiate into myofibroblasts	Wound closure	Disappearance of fibronectin
Events	Blood coagulation	Synthesis of preliminary ECM	ECM production	Scar maturation	
		Immunomodulation by T lymphocytes	Angiogenesis	Collagen fibre cross-linking	
	Migration of inflammatory cells		Collagen production		
	Activation of coagulation cascade		Granulation		
		Fibroblast migration			
		Fibroplasia			
Healing progress	**(a) Wound initiated**	**(b) Healing not initiated**	**(c) Progressive healing**	**(d) Healed**	**(e) Healing complete**

This table shows the main phases and events of the wound-healing process which are divided into five overlapping phases. For example, the phase (a) indicates that the wound is not healed and there is a possibility to reach a chronic state if the coagulation phase failed. The phase (b) indicates that the wound is still not healed, but it is progressing towards healing; however, if the inflammation is not terminated, a chronic condition has a chance to be initiated. The phase (c) indicates that the active healing process has been initiated. The phase (d) represents further development of the healing process with less chance of progression to a chronic condition. The phase (e) represents the complete healing and remodelling.

Table 1. The main phases and events of the wound-healing process.

3. Utilisation of mesenchymal stem cells in wound healing

3.1. Definition of mesenchymal stem cells

MSCs can be defined as a heterogeneous population of cells which are non-hematopoietic stem cells with the potential capacity to differentiate into various somatic lineages and tissues of both mesenchymal and non-mesenchymal origin [67]. Song et al. [68] have defined MSCs as a type of stem cell population capable of self-renewing and differentiating into different cell types with pluripotent potential. On the other hand, MSCs have also been termed marrow stromal cells, or fibroblastoid colony-forming unit (FCFU) [69], mesenchymal stem cells, multipotent mesenchymal stromal cells or stromal progenitor cells [23]. MSCs can be isolated from different tissues; however, they share the major criteria defining MSCs with minor differences related to their differentiation capacity and cell surface expression profile [67, 70]. These differences have challenged the definition of MSCs. In 2006, the International Society for Cellular Therapy (ISCT) attempted to demystify the nomenclature of MSCs suggesting that the term mesenchymal stem cells should only be referred to the cells which are characterised by the specific criteria, while the nomenclature of multipotent mesenchymal stromal cells should be used to describe the fibroblast-like plastic-adherent population irrespective of their source of origin [16, 23, 71]. Three minimal criteria have been agreed to become consensus characteristics shared by human MSCs [16, 23, 72, 73]. These criteria are:

1. The isolated MSCs should possess plastic adherence ability.

2. More than 95 % of the isolated MSCs must express CD73 (SH3), CD90 and CD105 (HS2), and more than 98 % of the isolated MSCs do not express CD14, D19, CD34, CD45, CD11b, CD79a and HLA-DR surface molecules.

3. The isolated MSCs have the capacity to differentiate into osteoblastic, chondrogenic and adipogenic lineages under *in vitro* standard differentiation conditions.

3.2. Clinical applications of mesenchymal stem cells

MSCs have been considered as safe irrespective to therapeutics since there is no critical inverse or side effect of MSCs has been detected on disease conditions [74, 75]. The characteristics of MSCs make them good candidates for regenerative medicine and tissue engineering [8, 25]. The most popular application of MSCs in regenerative medicine is in wound healing and skin regeneration [76]. However, MSCs have other clinical applications including ameliorating tissue damage in nearly all the major organs in the body such as skin regeneration, cardiac therapy, hepatic cirrhosis [23, 77, 78], brain, lung and kidney repair [23, 77]. In addition, MSCs can be used for pancreatic regeneration, neurological defects, limb ischemia, graft-versus-host disease (GvHD), rheumatoid arthritis, osteoarthritis (OA) and other bone and cartilage disorders [78]. The availability of MSCs in normal human skin suggests that these cells potentiate vital functions in wound healing and could be a promising solution for the treatment of chronic wounds [8, 25].

http://dx.doi.org/10.5772/63963

3.3. Mesenchymal stem cells in skin regeneration

Wounding in mammals evokes two types of biological responses: tissue regeneration and wound repair. Recently, skin regeneration especially cutaneous regeneration via MSCs leads to accelerated wound closure, re-epithelialisation and angiogenesis [7]. BM-MSCs transplanted into the injury site expressing keratinocyte-specific protein (KSP) form glandular structures [79, 80]. One of these successful studies is the induction of BM-MSCs to acquire phenotypic characteristics of sweat gland cells (SGCs) *in vitro* followed by re-transplantation of these cells into fresh wounds in five patients and resulted in recovery of functional sweat gland participating in perspiration function during 2 to 12 months follow-up [81]. Another study focusing on chronic diabetic foot ulcers showed that injection of a biografts consisting of a combination of MSCs and autologous skin fibroblasts resulted in increase of both dermal thickness and vascularity and decreased wound size [82, 83]. Another study has showed that MSCs acquire phenotypic characteristics of epidermal cells or vascular endothelial cells after *in vitro* culture in media supplemented with EGF or VEGF, respectively [82]. MSCs also undergo trans-differentiation into keratinocytes enabling them to interact with the original epidermal cells suggesting that MSCs can participate directly in tissue regeneration of both dermal and epidermal cells [30]. These characteristics, collectively, reveal the plasticity of MSCs and suggesting them promising therapeutic for the regeneration of skin and consequently wound healing [81].

3.4. Modes of action of mesenchymal stem cells in wound healing

The wound-healing process requires interaction between cells, extracellular matrix proteins (EMP) and biomolecules such as growth factors, cytokines and chemokines in which MSCs are a pivotal player in the coordination of the repair processes [11, 84]. Differentiation and

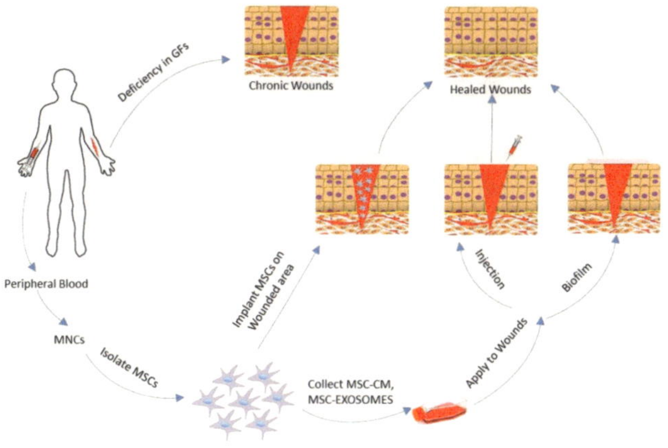

Figure 1. Potential applications of MSCs in wound healing. MSC therapy contributes to skin wound healing via two mechanisms: (1) Differentiation into skin-like cells, thereby compensating for the loss cells due to damaged tissue. (2) Promote proliferation and migration of skin cells into the injury site by secreting soluble factors and macrovesicles. MSC secretions represented by MSC-CM and MSC-EXOSOME can be either injected onto the wounded skin area or applied on skin wound using biofilm dressings.

paracrine signalling have both been implicated as mechanisms by which MSCs recruit other host cells in all steps of healing process to improve tissue repair [23]. To better understand the role of MSCs in wound healing, we have divided their participation in repair into two major mechanisms: (1) cell-mediated repair and (2) secretory-mediated repair (**Figure 1**).

3.4.1. Cell-mediated repair

In vitro studies have shown that MSCs possess phenotypic properties resembling native dermal fibroblasts or myoblasts [85]. Furthermore, BM-MSCs may accelerate wound closure by differentiating into epidermal keratinocytes and other skin cells [15, 23, 79, 86, 87]. Recent studies have shown that MSCs undergo trans-differentiation into keratinocyte, epidermal cells and microvascular endothelial cells when cultured under defined culture conditions [30] and express keratinocyte-specific protein (KSP) [79, 88, 89]. MSCs therefore could be utilised for wound healing by transplanting aggregated MSCs into the injured tissue to increase collagen deposition and improve epithelisation [80]. They can also differentiate into other skin cells such as endothelial cells, keratin 14-positive cells and pericytes, when localised to blood vessels and dermis [86], sebaceous glands and hair follicles [23].

3.4.2. Secretory-mediated repair–role of mesenchymal stem cell-conditioned media (MSC-CM)

Paracrine signalling of BM-MSCs is the major mechanism by which these cells contribute to wound repair, in which their secretory products impact on inflammation, fibrotic proliferation and angiogenesis [18]. Many studies have reported that MSC-CM is the supernatant from MSC *in vitro culture* significantly promotes wound healing by affecting the pivotal steps of the repair process. The components of MSC-CM have accelerated epithelialisation and via chemotaxis recruit endothelial cells and macrophages to the injured site *in vivo* [21]. The MSC-CM recruits both epidermal keratinocytes and dermal fibroblasts to the wound site *in vitro* [21, 23]. As well as to its activity as chemoattractant, MSC paracrine secretions serve as regulators for cell migration in response to wounding leading to faster wound closure by regulating dermal fibroblast migration [90]. MSC secretory mitogenic molecules stimulate the proliferation of keratinocytes, dermal fibroblasts and endothelial cells [91]. Conditioned medium derived from the cell culture of MSCs (MSC-CM) contains all the effector biomolecules which could be effectively utilised in tissue regeneration and wound healing by promoting migration, proliferation and differentiation of human skin cells such as fibroblast and keratinocytes. Collectively, these data suggest MSC-CM may represent a novel therapeutic strategy for wound therapy [25].

3.5. Biologically active substances secreted by mesenchymal stem cells

The potential of MSCs in regenerative medicine and wound healing has been reflected by their secretion of biomolecules including growth factors, cytokines and chemokines [18, 21, 25]. Some 36 biomolecules have been reported to be released by human MSCs (h-MSCs) which act in concert to promote the wound-healing process [66].

3.5.1. Growth factors

Human MSCs secrete a wide range of growth factors that play a significant role in the wound-healing process. These are angiopoietins (ANGPT), connective tissue growth factors (CTGFs), epidermal growth factor (EGF), fibroblast growth factors (FGFs), insulin-like growth factors (IGF), keratinocyte growth factor (KGF), nerve growth factor (NGF), platelet-derived growth factor (PDGF), transforming growth factor (TGF), vascular endothelial growth factor (VEGF) and scatter factors which are a family of growth factors also known as plasminogen-related growth factors (PRGFs), which include two members: hepatocyte growth factor (HGF) also referred to as plasminogen-related growth factor-1 (PRGF-1) and macrophage-stimulating protein (MSP) which is also known as scatter factor-2 (SF-2) or hepatocyte growth factor-like protein (HGFL) (**Table 2**).

Growth factors	**Function(s)**	**References**
ANGPT	ANGPT-1 is responsible for the stabilisation of blood vessels and promotes wound closure	[21, 22]
	ANGPT-2 causes vessel destabilisation and remodelling	[40]
CTGFs	Stimulation of chemotaxis, proliferation of fibroblasts and the induction of extracellular matrix proteins including fibronectin and collagen type I	[40]
	Promote endothelial angiogenesis, survival, migration, proliferation and adhesion	[92]
EGF	Re-epithelialisation of skin wounds and	[40]
	promotion of wound closure	[22]
FGFs	Exert a cytoprotective function in would repair, supporting cell survival under stress conditions	[93]
	Promotes mitogenic activity for keratinocytes and fibroblasts at the wound site. FGF1 and FGF2 stimulate angiogenesis. Basic fibroblast growth factor (bFGF) enhances the proliferation of endothelial cells and smooth muscle cells	[94]
IGF	In association with HB-EGF, IGF enhances the proliferation of keratinocyte *in vitro*. Mitogenesis and survival of many cells are stimulated by IGF-I and IGF-II, promotes wound closure	[40]
KGF	Promotes wound closure in two ways:	[21, 22]
	(1) It serves as a transporter for alveolar epithelial fluid	[94]
	(2) It plays a role in tissue remodelling	[11]
NGF	Involved in fibroblast migration, increasing expression of actin by smooth muscle and collagen gel contraction by these cells	[95]
	Performs two functions in wound healing: (1) it stimulates proliferation of keratinocytes and inhibits apoptosis *in vitro*, (2) it supports the proliferation of human dermal	[40]

Growth factors	Function(s)	References
	microvascular endothelial cells and their adherence molecule expression	
PDGF	Stimulates DNA synthesis, attracts fibroblasts to wound sites, enhances their production of collagenase, collagen and glycosaminoglycan	[96]
	The first chemotactic growth factor participating in migration of fibroblasts, monocytes and neutrophils into the skin wound, subsequently stimulating the production of extracellular matrix and the induction of a myofibroblast phenotype	[97]
HGF or PRGF-1	It inhibits fibrosis and promotes re-epithelialisation	[98]
	Enhances keratinocytes to migrate, proliferate and produce matrix metalloproteinase and stimulates new blood vessel formation	[99]
MSP	Accelerates cell migration and proliferation with regulation of proliferation and differentiation of keratinocytes and macrophages. plays an integral role in inflammation, proliferation and the remodelling phases of the healing process	[40, 100]
TGF	Enhances proliferation of epithelial cells, expression of antimicrobial peptides and release of chemotactic cytokines	[40]
	TGF-β1 activates keratinocytes and macrophages, while suppressing T lymphocytes	[94]
	TGF-β3 stimulates remodelling	[11]
	Activins which are members of TGF-β family act as enhancers for granulation tissue fibroblasts and the induction of extracellular matrix deposition	[40]
	Activin B supports wound repair and regeneration of hair follicles, promotes wound closure	[21, 22]
VEGF	Regulates angiogenesis	[20, 40]
	VEGF-α promotes wound closure	[21, 22]
	Promotes proliferation of endothelial cells	[11]

MSCs secrete a wide spectrum of growth factors. These biological substances participate in wound healing from early stages starting with haemostasis and coagulation and ending with remodelling. These growth factors promote angiogenesis, accelerate proliferation and also migration of endothelial cells. In addition, they are involved in the contraction phase, ending at the last stages of remodelling, leading to wound healing in the absence of scar formation.

Table 2. The main growth factors secreted by MSCs and their roles and functions in the wound-healing process.

3.5.2. Cytokines

Cytokines are small proteins secreted by many cell types which affect the activity of other cells including immune cells; they include interleukins, lymphokines and other signalling biomolecules including interferons and tumour necrosis factor [40]. Here, they are categorised into groups depending on their role in the wound-healing process (**Table 3**).

Cytokines	Function(s)	References
Pro-inflammatory cytokines		
IL-1α	They influence the inflammatory phase	[101–103]
IL-1β IL-6 TNF-β	They promote wound healing by controlling the proliferation of fibroblast and keratinocyte and regulate the synthesis and breakdown of extracellular matrix proteins. They also control fibroblast chemotaxis and regulate the immune response	[40]
Anti-inflammatory cytokines		
PGE2 IL-1 IL-4	They play a primary role in limitation and termination of inflammatory responses	[11, 40, 102–106]
LL-37	It acts as antimicrobial peptide and reduce inflammation	[24]
Proliferative cytokines		
IL-6	Plays an axial role in wound healing by regulating cellular responses	[8, 23]
	Promotes epithelial cell migration	[25]
	Promotes angiogenesis formation	[8, 25, 107]
	Regulates leukocyte recruitment and infiltration to the inflammatory sites and regulates collagen deposition	[107]
	Possess both pro-inflammatory and anti-inflammatory activities under different conditions of the wound-healing process	[25, 105]
IL-10	Regulates differentiation and/or growth of keratinocytes, endothelial and various immune cells	[108]
	Regulates the infiltration of macrophage-derived neutrophils into the wound site, promotes the expression of pro-inflammatory cytokines and reduces matrix deposition and thereby inhibiting scar formation	[40]
GM-CSF	Enhances wound healing either indirectly via stimulating secondary cytokines such as TGF-β1	[109]
	Directly via its mitogenic activity for keratinocytes, and the stimulation of endothelial cell proliferation and migration	[40]
	Regulating angiogenesis formation, cellular responses and tissue remodelling	[8]

MSCs secrete a wide range of cytokines. These secretions initiate and terminate the inflammatory phase and accelerate proliferation and also migration of endothelial cells. In addition, they are involved in the contraction phase, ending at the last stages of remodelling, leading to wound healing in the absence of scar formation.

Table 3. The main cytokines secreted by MSCs and their roles and functions in the wound-healing process.

3.5.3. Chemokines

Chemokines are a subtype of small cytokines responsible for stimulating chemotaxis and extravasation of leukocytes; hence, referred to as so, they are called chemotactic cytokines [40]. Human MSCs release several chemokines that participate in wound healing such as IL-8 and its receptor (CXCL8), macrophage chemoattractant protein-1 (MCP-1) and its receptor (CCL2), macrophage inflammatory protein-1-alpha and macrophage inflammatory protein-1-beta (MIP-1α and MIP-1β) and stromal-derived factor 1 (SDF-1) (**Table 4**).

Chemokines	Function(s)	References
IL-8	Increases keratinocyte proliferation and stimulate re-epithelialisation in human skin grafts, both in *vitro* and in *vivo*. IL-8 and its receptor (CXCL8) act as a chemoattractant for neutrophils	[110]
	Enhances the migration of epithelial cells *in vitro*	[25, 111]
MCP-1	MCP-1 and its receptor (CCL2) are primarily involved in macrophage infiltration	[66, 105]
	Inflammation regulatory chemokines in the wound-healing process	[40]
MIP-1	MIP-1α and MIP-1β promote wound closure	[21, 22]
	MIP-1α and MIP-1β increase macrophage trafficking	[105]
SDF-1	Plays a role in regulating skin homeostasis and tissue remodelling	[40]
	Promotes wound closure	[21, 22]
	Induces cell migration	[74]

MSCs secrete some chemokines. These biological substances participate in wound healing from early stages starting with haemostasis and coagulation and ending with remodelling. They also participate in the inflammatory phase and accelerate proliferation and also migration of endothelial cells. In addition, they are involved in the contraction phase, ending at the last stages of remodelling, leading to wound healing in the absence of scar formation.

Table 4. The main chemokines secreted by MSCs and their roles and functions in the wound-healing process.

3.5.4. Mesenchymal stem cell exosomes (MSC-EXOSOME)

Exosomes are tiny vesicles (30–100 nm in diameter) present in blood and urine and perhaps all other biological fluids that may also be collected from *in vitro* cell culture [112, 113]. Originating from endosomal sections and released from the plasma membrane into the extracellular environment these vesicles participate in coagulation, intracellular communication and signalling and cytoplasmic cleaning [112–115]. It has been reported that MSC-EXOSOME repair renal injury indicating that MSC-EXOSOME as a potential mechanism that could be harnessed for wound healing [116, 117]. With respect to wound healing, MSC-EXOSOME plays an important role in collagen synthesis, the acceleration of cell migration and proliferation and in the formation of new and mature blood vessel [113]. Exosome healing action could be attributed to its ability to transfer RNA, miRNA and proteins such as Wint-4 into the injured tissues which participate in skin repair by promoting re-epithelialisation and cell proliferation as well as through the activation of β-catenin which plays a pivotal role in skin development and wound healing [116]. Additionally, MSC-EXOSOME has been shown to accelerate wound healing through mediating pathway signalling of some genes such as Akt, ERK and STAT3 as well as by enhancing the expression of important growth factors, Such as;

http://dx.doi.org/10.5772/63963

HGF, IGF-1, NGF and SDF-1 which collectively accelerate migration and proliferation of fibroblasts in normal and diabetic wounds [118]. Moreover, MSC-EXOSOME reduces levels of pro-apoptotic Bax thereby inhibiting apoptosis of skin cells such keratinocytes and fibroblasts [117, 119]. Collectively, these data suggest the MSC-EXOSOMES thus play a significant role in wound healing.

The application of MSC-CM or MSC-EXOSOME onto chronic wounds either by direct injection or by designing biological dressings enriched with MSC-CM collected from autologous MSCs may therefore provide a valuable therapeutic strategy.

The participation of MSC secretions in wound healing is summarised in **Figure 2**.

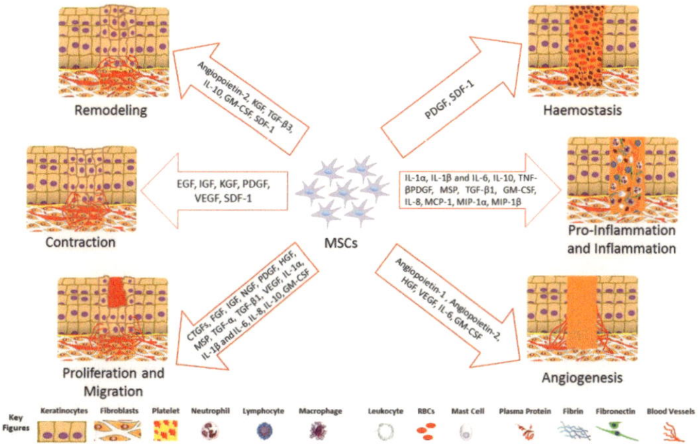

Figure 2. Participation of MSC secretions in wound-healing phases and events. MSCs secrete a wide spectrum of growth factors, cytokines and chemokines. These biological substances participate in wound healing from early stages starting with haemostasis and coagulation and ending with remodelling. These secretions initiate and terminate the inflammatory phase and promote angiogenesis, accelerate proliferation and also migration of endothelial cells. In addition, they are involved in the contraction phase, ending at the last stages of remodelling, leading to wound healing in the absence of scar formation.

3.6. Benefits of the use of mesenchymal stem cells in treating wounds

As we previously mentioned, MSCs have been considered safe irrespective their use in different clinical indications, since no critical adverse or side effect of MSCs has been shown when used therapeutically in humans [74, 75, 120]. Interestingly, patients with conditions such as sepsis [106], acute limb ischemia, acute GvHD [78, 120], critical myocardial infarction, Crohn's disease, acute tubular necrosis and multiple sclerosis can obtain benefit from the use of MSC therapies with no reported contraindications [120].

3.6.1. Immunomodulatory features of MSCs

In 2000, Liechty et al. [121] were the first to recognise that MSCs possess unique immunologic features allowing them to persist in a xenogeneic environment and modulate the immune response. They have the potential to reduce inflammation and enhance repair wounds [122]. The exact mechanism by which MSCs modulate the immune system is not fully understood. The potential mechanism includes cell-to-cell direct contact and by the secretion of immune suppressive factors, interacting with other immune cells such as T lymphocytes, B lymphocytes, dendritic cells (DC) and natural killer cells (NKCs) [123]. In 2013, Patel et al. [74] reported that MSCs suppress both the activation and proliferation of lymphocytes in response to allogeneic antigens as well as enhancing the development of CD8+ regulatory T cells (Treg) in the suppression of an allogeneic lymphocyte response. Additional immune suppressive activities of MSC include inhibition of differentiation of peripheral blood monocyte progenitor cells and CD34+ haematopoietic progenitor cells (HPCs) into antigen-presenting cells (APCs) [124]. MSCs also inhibit the proliferation of NK cells mediated by IL-2 or IL-15 [125]. MSCs have been shown to exert other immunomodulatory activities including altering the proliferation and activation of B cells, IgG production, antibody secretion, chemoattractant behaviour, and reducing the expression of CD40, and CD86 and major histocompatibility complex class II (MHC-II) [126].

The ability of MSCs to modulate T cell and their proliferation, participation and activity [127] and suppress the proliferation of B cells [128] and NK cells [125] is well documented. By attenuating the function of these cells, MSCs reduce the pro-fibrotic process [129]. Importantly, by the secretion of Prostaglandin E2 (PGE2) [102, 103] and 1L-10 [11, 40, 106], MSCs regulate macrophage and lymphocyte function [30]. For instance, PGE2 attenuates mitogenesis and proliferation of T cells in the wound [124] acting as co-parameter in regulating the transition from T_{h1} cells into T_{h2} cells [130]. On the other hand, IL-10 prevents the deposition of excessive collagen and inhibits the invasion of neutrophils into the wound and their release of reactive oxygen species (ROS) factors, which collectively participate in the prevention of scar tissue formation [30].

3.6.2. Migration and engraftment capacity

Various studies have reported the capability of MSCs to selectively migrate to and engraft into the wound site and exert local functional effects on inflammatory reactions regardless of tissue type [30, 73]. In this context, murine studies have shown that MSCs can home to the lung, adopting phenotypic characteristics of epithelium-like cells and reducing inflammation in response to injury [131]. Another study in mdx mice, a strain of mice arising from a spontaneous mutation (mdx) in inbred C57BL mice showed that MSCs may migrate to muscle tissues [132]. MSC migration has been shown to be regulated by a multitude of signals [133] ranging from growth factors such as PDGF and IGF-1, cytokine such as SDF-1, chemokine such as CCL5 and chemokine receptors, including CCR2, CCR3 and CCR4 [73, 134].

3.6.3. Wound closure acceleration

MSCs play a role not only in wound healing but also in accelerating the healing process by increasing the strength of wound and by reducing scaring [23]. The effects of MSCs during wound healing include acceleration of epithelialisation, an increase in angiogenesis and the formation of granulation tissue [11]. These activities are attributed to the ability of MSCs to produce biologically active substances capable of accelerating the regeneration process [135] including IL-8 and CXCL1, responsible for stimulating the migration of epithelial cells and accelerating wound closure [111].

3.6.4. Antimicrobial activity

Conditioned medium of hBM-MSCs is capable of inhibiting bacterial growth directly indicating the ability of MSCs to produce and release substantial amounts of antibacterial substances known as human cathelicidin peptide-18 (hCAP-18) or LL-37 peptide which are characterised by their ability to retard *in vitro* growth of *Pseudomonas aeruginosa* and *Escherichia coli* [24], thus avoiding wound contamination and infections complications which exacerbate the healing process [28].

3.6.5. Prevent chronic condition

Besides having immune modulatory activities, the effective biomolecules secreted by MSCs can prevent wounds from reaching a chronic state by their angiogenic and antiapoptotic characteristics [105]. For instance, transplantation of hMSCs intramyocardially has the ability to improve cardiac function via enhancing myogenesis and angiogenesis in the ischemic myocardium [136]. Also, MSCs enable a wound to progress to healing beyond the inflammation stage and not regress into a chronic state [11].

3.6.6. Attenuation of scar formation

The tissues in the scar have many disadvantages including their undesirable visual appearance and lack of structures that are present in the native skin such as hair follicles, sebaceous glands and sensory nerve receptors [30]. In addition, scar tissue weakens the skin making it more susceptible for re-injury [137]. MSCs have been shown to overcome these disadvantages via attenuating scar formation [138].

3.6.7. Neutralising the reactive oxygen species (ROS)

Although IL-10 participates in preventing the invasion of neutrophils into the site of tissue injury and the enhancement of collagen deposition, the penetrations of some populations result in the release of ROS, which are oxygen molecules have an unpaired electron making them extremely reactive such as superoxide, hydrogen peroxide and alkyl peroxides [139]. Many tissues are susceptible to attack by ROS contributing to dangerous diseases including heart disease and cancer. Also, prolonged persistence of ROS induces fibrogenesis and the accumulation of fibrotic tissues [30]. To counter act such effects, MSCs significantly upregulate the expression of nitric oxide synthase [140] which alters the ROS balance preventing the formation of fibrotic tissues [141].

3.6.8. Producing antifibrotic factors

MSCs release growth factors and cytokines characterised by their antifibrotic activities such as HGF and IL-10 [142]. HGF has been shown to downregulate the expression of collagen type

I and type III by fibroblasts therefore attenuating fibrosis and scar formation [143]. Moreover, HGF impacts on the keratinocyte behaviour by promoting their migration, proliferation and expression of VEGF-A, thereby generating a well-granulated tissue with a high degree of vascularisation and re-epithelialisation [30].

3.6.9. Enhancing dermal fibroblast function

In response to the wounding process, fibroblasts present at the injury site produce additional quantities of ECM to restore the integrity of the skin leading to scarred tissue [144]. Also, many endothelial cells undergo epithelial-to-mesenchymal transition (EMT) under the effect of TGF-β1 and become wound-healing myofibroblasts [138]. Both of these actions affect the function of dermal fibroblasts. Therefore, MSCs present in the wound site enhance dermal fibroblast function by producing HGF and PGE2 which both play a role in inhibiting EMT [145] and secrete biomolecules promoting the function of dermal fibroblast in wound healing [90]. MSCs therefore enable the cells present in the wound site to release ECM similar to those produced by neighbouring dermal cells [30].

3.6.10. Promoting angiogenesis and vascular stability

It has been well documented that BM-MSCs play a major role in angiogenesis and microvascularisation via promoting proliferation, migration and differentiation of microvascular endothelial cells by producing basic FGF and VEGF-A [146].

3.7. Requirements for the healing process

3.7.1. Infection fighting

Open wounds are at risk of infections by bacteria and other microorganisms causing serious conditions such tetanus and gangrene and giving rise to chronic wounds, bone necrosis, long-term disabilities and death. Unfortunately, in some wound types, the necrotic tissues exudate secretions which act as a medium for bacterial growth inside the wound and protect the bacteria from the host's immune defence [147]. The use of disinfectant is useless, because they damage the injured tissues and arrest wound contraction. Also, they are easily suppressed by the inorganic substances present in the wound including blood components and other tissue secretions [148]. Therefore, appropriate care is required to protect open wounds and reduce the possibility of bacterial infection. Included in such cares are the treatments of wounds with topical antibiotics to kill the invading bacteria and moisturise the wounded area [149, 150], accelerate the healing process [151] and modulate inflammation [152]. Failure of antibiotic treatment leads to non-healing wounds in which bacteria thrive on dead tissue giving rise to uncontrolled infection leading to additional complicated treatments including draining and removal of dead tissues from the injured site or even amputation in the case of diabetic ulcers [147, 150].

3.7.2. Prevention of ischemia and hypoxia

Ischemia is defined as the failure of blood to reach the target tissue and characterised by insufficient nutrient and oxygen supply resulting in turn in hypoxia and the insufficient availability or very low oxygen concentration at the injury site [153]. Therefore, the prevention of such circumstances is critical to the acceleration of wound-healing process [154]. Cold environment causes continuous constriction of blood vessels thereby reducing blood flow into the injury site and causing ischemia. Therefore, keeping tissue warm will dilate blood vessels facilitating blood flow and decrease the probability of ischemia initiation; however, hyperthermia is not recommended as this increases the likelihood of post-surgical infection [147]. In some cases of diabetic ulcers and venous ulcers, surgery is required to treat ischemia by revascularisation the veins and arteries to correct their function [155]. Another approaches to combat ischemia include pressure-assisted treatment or negative pressure wound therapy (NPWT), involving the creation of a vacuum to drain and remove wound exudate and their bacterial component, reducing tissue swelling, enhancing cell proliferation at the wounded site and the production of extracellular matrix thereby improving the healing process [156, 157]. Hypoxemia could arise due to vascular disease that arrests oxygen transfer, high demand for oxygen by tissue metabolism at the injured site and the formation of reactive oxygen species (ROS) [153]. The best therapy for hypoxemia is increasing the oxygenation of injured tissue by hyperbaric oxygen therapy (HBOT) to compensate oxygen limitations [155]. Also, higher oxygen content results in bacterial death, the acceleration of growth factor production, the enhancement of fibroblast growth and the promotion of angiogenesis [155, 157]. Another method to treat hypoxemia is the use of antioxidants to reduce the presence of oxidant substances [32].

MSCs could potentially be used to treat ischemia and hypoxia because they release angiogenic and mitogenic factors such as VEGF, IGF-1 and HGF which are well known to induce angiogenesis and myogenesis [158]. Intravenous (IV) administration of BM-MSCs increased the activity of matrix metalloproteinase-2 and decreased the activity of matrix metalloproteinase-9 resulting in improved cardiac function in a rat model of diabetic cardiomyopathy [159]. Wang et al. [160] showed that MSCs secrete hypoxia-regulated haem oxygenase-1, frizzled-related protein-2, hypoxic Akt-regulated stem cell factor, heat-shock protein-20, adrenomedullin (AM) and SDF which collectively contribute to regeneration, neovascularisation and remodelling. MSCs were also be used to treat diabetic limb ischemia in the ischemic hind limb of type II diabetic mice due to the secretion of proangiogenic factors including hypoxia-inducible factor and VEGF, responsible for vasculogenesis, blood flow regulation [161] and improvement of arterial perfusion in type 1 diabetic patients with gangrene [162]. A pilot study carried on patients of critical limb ischemia, who did not respond to other therapies, showed that multiple intramuscular injections of MSCs induced formation of vascular networks across the closed arteries, resulting in successful improvement of limb ischemia in terms of pain reduction and claudication [163]. In another study using a pig model of stenotic kidney blood flow, administration of MSCs improved the architecture of microvessels in term of size and density [164].

3.7.3. Regulation of growth factors and hormones

As previously described, growth mediatory factors play pivotal roles in wound healing. Therefore, more quantities of these growth factors are required to progress the healing process, in particular in case of chronic wounds, so they should be continuously upregulated [31, 32]. Several methodologies have been proposed to maintain efficient concentrations of growth factors at the injury site. Direct application of such biomolecules, however, requires large quantities and repetitive application. Spreading autologous platelets over the injury site which later secrete growth factors such as EGF, IGF-1, IGF-2, TGF-β and VEGF has been proposed [165] as has the utilisation of keratinocytes and fibroblasts on a collagen matrix to enhance further secretion of growth factors when applied on the wound [32, 166]. Another potential way to protect efficient concentrations of growth factors at the wound site is through the prevention of their breakdown by analytical enzymes and thereby preventing the formation of proteases such as elastase [31, 32]. Oestrogen and prostaglandins have also been showed to play a role in the healing process; maintenance of their concentration at efficient levels may thus prevent excess neutrophils from reaching the injury site and produce more elastase [41, 49, 50, 167].

3.8. Limitations of using MSCs for wound healing

MSCs can be considered as a promising tool for treating non-healing wounds; however, some aspects of MSC biology need to be intensively studied before use in clinical application. One of these is the problem of finding a source of MSC isolation with no invasive procedure for autologous treatment, for example isolation of MSCs from peripheral blood instead of bone marrow. Other questions include the following: What is the ideal number and timing of MSC administration/implantation? How long can MSCs survive at the injury site after implantation? Are multiple administrations or implantations required for successful healing? When do the implanted MSCs start releasing their soluble secretions after implantation/administration? And finally, are the secretions of MSCs controllable? Answers to these questions are important and essential for the therapeutic use of MSCs and a safer and a more effective treatment for non-healing wounds.

4. Conclusion

Mesenchymal stem cells (MSCs) and their secretions are promising therapeutics for use in accelerating wound healing. Ease of availability, isolation and *in vitro* expansion make MSCs the best candidates for wound-healing therapies in comparison with other stem cells including embryonic stem cells (ESCs). Two main strategies could be used in the application of MSCs to the treatment of non-healing wounds. MSCs show the ability to differentiate into different cells of the epidermis. Also, MSC secretions collected from their *in vitro* cultures (MSC-CM) and their small vesicles (MSC-EXOSOME) are important for promoting proliferation and migration of skin cells, such as keratinocytes and fibroblasts, into the injury site. MSC-CM contains a wide range of at least 36 known growth factors, and cytokines work in synergy to accelerate wound healing. These characteristics make MSCs unique when compared to other cells, such as keratinocytes and fibroblasts, since keratinocytes are unable to migrate by themselves without growth factors and cytokines and fibroblasts cannot differentiate into skin-like cells. Therefore, MSCs are bi-functional combining wound healing and skin regeneration. MSC-CM and MSC-EXOSOME if developed into a medicinal product could potentially be applied directly onto the wounded area either by injection or by enriching biological dressings with these growth factors and exosomes and aid in combating the problems of non-healing wounds.

Author details

Moyassar B. H. Al-Shaibani[1,2*], Xiao-nong Wang[1], Penny E. Lovat[1] and Anne M. Dickinson[1]

*Address all correspondence to: m.b.h.al-shaibani@newcastle.ac.uk

1 Faculty of Medical Sciences, Institute of Cellular Medicine, Newcastle University, Newcastle upon Tyne, UK

2 Department of Medical Biotechnology, College of Biotechnology, Al-Nahrain University, Baghdad, Iraq

References

[1] Franks PJ, Morgan PA. Health-related quality of life with chronic leg ulceration. Expert Rev Pharmacoecon Outcomes Res. 2003; 3(5): 611-622. DOI:10.1586/14737167.3.5.611

[2] Posnett J, Franks PJ. The burden of chronic wounds in the UK. Nurs Times. 2008; 104(3): 44-45. PMID: 18293879

[3] White B. National best practice and evidence based guidelines for wound management. Kelly E, Tierney S, Apelqvist J, Dealey C. (Reviewers). HSE. Dublin: Ireland. 2009; ISBN 978-1-906218-29-4 URI: http://hdl.handle.net/10147/92646

[4] Drew P, Posnett J, Rusling L. The cost of wound care for a local population in England. Int Wound J. 2007; 4(2): 149-155. DOI: 10.1111/j.1742-481X.2007.00337.x

[5] Sen CK, et al., Human skin wounds: a major and snowballing threat to public health and the economy. Wound Repair Regen. 2009; 17(6): 763-771. DOI: 10.1111/j.1524-475X.2009.00543.x

[6] Cook L, Ousey K. Demystifying wound infection: identification and management. Practice Nurs. 2011; 22(8): 424-428. DOI: 10.12968/pnur.2011.22.8.424

[7] Marfia G, et al., Mesenchymal stem cells: potential for therapy and treatment of chronic non-healing skin wounds. Organogenesis. 2015; 11(4): 183-206. DOI: 10.1080/15476278.2015.1126018

[8] Hocking AM. Mesenchymal stem cell therapy for cutaneous wounds. Adv Wound Care (New Rochelle). 2012; 1(4): 166-171. DOI: 10.1089/wound.2011.0294

[9] Metcalfe AD, Ferguson MWJ. Tissue engineering of replacement skin: the crossroads of biomaterials, wound healing, embryonic development, stem cells and regeneration. J Royal Soc Interface. 2007; 4(14): 413-437. DOI: 10.1098/rsif.2006.0179

[10] Branski LK, et al., A review of gene and stem cell therapy in cutaneous wound healing. Burns. 2009; 35(2): 171-180. DOI:10.1016/j.burns.2008.03.009

[11] Maxson S, et al., Concise review: role of mesenchymal stem cells in wound repair. Stem Cells Transl Med. 2012; 1(2): 142-149.DOI: 10.5966/sctm.2011-0018

[12] Hoogduijn MJ, Dor FJMF. Mesenchymal stem cells: are we ready for clinical application in transplantation and tissue regeneration? Front Immunol. 2013; 4 (144): 1-2. DOI: 10.3389/fimmu.2013.00144

[13] Paquet-Fifield S, et al., A role for pericytes as microenvironmental regulators of human skin tissue regeneration. J Clin Invest. 2009; 119(9): 2795-806. DOI 10.1172/JCI38535

[14] Kadir RA, et al., Molecular characterisation of human peripheral blood stem cells. South African J Sci. 2012; 108: 67-73. DOI:10.4102/sajs.v108i5/6.939

[15] Badiavas EV, et al., Participation of bone marrow derived cells in cutaneous wound healing. J Cellular Physiol. 2003; 196(2): 245-250. DOI: 10.1002/jcp.10260

[16] Dominici M, et al., Minimal criteria for defining multipotent mesenchymal stromal cells. The International Society for Cellular Therapy position statement. Cytotherapy. 2006; 8(4): 315-317. DOI: 10.1080/14653240600855905

[17] Ma K, et al., Differentiation of bone marrow-derived mesenchymal stem cells into multi-layered epidermis-like cells in 3D organotypic coculture. Biomaterials. 2009; 30(19): 3251-3258. DOI:10.1016/j.biomaterials.2009.02.025

[18] Gnecchi M, et al., Paracrine mechanisms in adult stem cell signaling and therapy. Circ Res. 2008; 103(11): 1204-1219. DOI: 10.1161/CIRCRESAHA

[19] Alfaro MP, et al., A physiological role for connective tissue growth factor in early wound healing. Lab Invest. 2013; 93(1): 81-95. DOI: 10.1161/CIRCRESAHA.108.176826.

[20] Caplan AI. Why are MSCs therapeutic? New data: new insight. J Pathol. 2009; 217(2): 318-324. DOI: 10.1002/path.2469

[21] Chen L, et al., Paracrine factors of mesenchymal stem cells recruit macrophages and endothelial lineage cells and enhance wound healing. PLoS One. 2008; 3(4): e1886. DOI: 10.1371/journal.pone.0001886

[22] Barrientos S, et al., Growth factors and cytokines in wound healing. Wound Repair Regen. 2008; 16(5): 585-601. DOI: 10.1111/j.1524-475X.2008.00410.x.

[23] Hocking AM, Gibran NS. Mesenchymal stem cells: paracrine signaling and differentiation during cutaneous wound repair. Exp Cell Res. 2010; 316(14): 2213-2219. DOI: 10.1016/j.yexcr.2010.05.009

[24] Krasnodembskaya A, et al., Antibacterial effect of human mesenchymal stem cells is mediated in part from secretion of the antimicrobial peptide LL-37. Stem Cells. 2010; 28(12): 2229-2238. DOI:10.1002/stem.544

[25] Tamama K, Kerpedjieva SS. Acceleration of wound healing by multiple growth factors and cytokines secreted from multipotential stromal cells/mesenchymal stem cells. Adv Wound Care (New Rochelle). 2012; 1(4): 177-182. DOI: 10.1089/wound.2011.0296

[26] Monaco JL, Lawrence WT. Acute wound healing an overview. Clin Plast Surg. 2003; 30(1): 1-12. DOI: 10.1016/S0094-1298(02)00070-6

[27] Whitney JD. Overview: acute and chronic wounds. Nurs Clinics of North Am. 2005; 40(2): 191-205. DOI: 10.1016/j.cnur.2004.09.002

[28] Guo S, DiPietro LA. Critical review in oral biology & medicine: factors affecting wound healing. J Dental Res. 2010; 89(3): 219-229. DOI: 10.1186/scrt363

[29] Diegelmann RF, Evans MC. Wound healing: an overview of acute, fibrotic and delayed healing. Front Biosci. 2004; 9: 283-289. DOI: 10.2741/1184

[30] Jackson W, Nesti L, Tuan R. Mesenchymal stem cell therapy for attenuation of scar formation during wound healing. Stem Cell Res Ther. 2012; 3(3): 20. DOI:10.1186/scrt111.

[31] Edwards JV, Howley P, Cohen IK. In vitro inhibition of human neutrophil elastase by oleic acid albumin formulations from derivatized cotton wound dressings. Int J Pharmaceutics. 2004; 284(1–2): 1-12. DOI:10.1016/j.ijpharm.2004.06.003

[32] Schönfelder U, et al., Influence of selected wound dressings on PMN elastase in chronic wound fluid and their antioxidative potential in vitro. Biomaterials. 2005; 26(33): 6664-6673. DOI:10.1016/j.biomaterials.2005.04.030

[33] Gosain A, DiPietro LA. Aging and wound healing. World J Surg. 2004; 28(3): 321-326. DOI: 10.1007/s00268-003-7397-6

[34] Zhou, S., et al., Increased collagen synthesis rate during wound healing in muscle. PLoS One. 2013; 8(3): e58324. DOI:10.1371/journal.pone.0058324

[35] Mathieu D, Linke J-C, Wattel F. Non-healing wounds, in Handbook on Hyperbaric Medicine, D. Mathieu, Editor. Netherlands: Springer. 2006; 401-428. DOI: 10.1007/1-4020-4448-8.

[36] Jorgensen LN, et al., Increased collagen deposition in an uncomplicated surgical wound compared to a minimal subcutaneous test wound. Wound Repair Regen. 2001; 9(3): 194-199. DOI: 10.1046/j.1524-475x.2001.00194.x

[37] Mendonça RJd, Coutinho-Netto J. Cellular aspects of wound healing. Braz Ann Dermatol. 2009; 84: 257-262. DOI: 10.1590/S0365-05962009000300007

[38] Rasche H. Haemostasis and thrombosis: an overview. European Heart J Suppl. 2001; 3(suppl Q): Q3-Q7. DOI: 10.1016/S1520-765X(01)90034-3

[39] Versteeg HH, et al., New fundamentals in hemostasis. Physiol Rev. 2013; 93(1): 327-358. DOI: 10.1152/physrev.00016.2011

[40] Werner S, Grose R. Regulation of wound healing by growth factors and cytokines. Physiol Rev 2003; 83(3): 835-870. DOI:10.1152/physrev.00032.2002

[41] Eming SA, et al., Accelerated wound closure in mice deficient for interleukin-10. Am J Pathol. 2007; 170(1): 188-202. DOI: 10.2353/ajpath.2007.060370

[42] Streit M, et al., Thrombospondin-1 suppresses wound healing and granulation tissue formation in the skin of transgenic mice. EMBO J. 2000; 19(13): 3272-3282. DOI: 10.1093/emboj/19.13.3272

[43] Cohen J. The Molecular and Cellular Biology of Wound Repair. 2nd ed. Clark RAF, editor. Plenum: New York. 1996. 611 p. DOI: org/10.1016/S0741-5214(97)70244-1

[44] Midwood KS, Williams LV, Schwarzbauer JE. Tissue repair and the dynamics of the extracellular matrix. Inte J Biochem Cell Biol. 2004; 36(6): 1031-1037. DOI:10.1016/j.biocel.2003.12.003

[45] Abbas AK, Lichtman AH. Basic Immunology: Functions and Disorders of the Immune System. 2010, Philadelphia, PA: Saunders. DOI: 10.1002/bmb.2004.494032069999

[46] Sherwood ER, Toliver-Kinsky T. Mechanisms of the inflammatory response. Best Practice Res Clin Anaesthesiol. 2004; 18(3): 385-405. DOI:10.1016/j.bpa.2003.12.002

[47] Wright HL, et al., Neutrophil function in inflammation and inflammatory diseases. Rheumatol. 2010; 49(9): 1618-1631. DOI:10.1093/rheumatology/keq045

[48] Ariel A, et al., Macrophages in inflammation and its resolution. Front Immunol. 2012; 3: 324. DOI: 10.3389/fimmu.2012.00324

[49] Singer AJ, Clark RAF. Cutaneous wound healing. New Eng J Med. 1999; 341(10): 738-746. DOI: 10.1056/NEJM199909023411006

[50] Tonnesen MG, Feng X, Clark RAF. Angiogenesis in wound healing. J Investig Dermatol Symp Proc. 2000; 5(1): 40-46. DOI:10.1046/j.1087-0024.2000.00014.x

[51] Swirski FK, et al., Identification of splenic reservoir monocytes and their deployment to inflammatory sites. Science. 2009; 325(5940): 612-616. DOI: 10.1126/science.1175202

[52] Ross R. The role of T lymphocytes in inflammation. Proc Natl Acad Sci USA. 1994; 91(8): 2879. DOI: 10.1073/pnas.91.8.2879

[53] Santoro MM, Gaudino G. Cellular and molecular facets of keratinocyte reepithelization during wound healing. Exp Cell Res. 2005; 304(1): 274-286. DOI:10.1016/j.yexcr.2004.10.033

[54] Usui ML, et al., Keratinocyte migration, proliferation, and differentiation in chronic ulcers from patients with diabetes and normal wounds. J Histochem Cytochem. 2008; 56(7): 687-696. DOI: 10.1369/jhc.2008.951194

[55] Bellayr IH, Walters TJ, Li Y. Scarless wound healing. J Am College of Cert Wound Specialists. 2010; 2(2): 40-43. DOI: 10.1016/j.jcws.2010.05.001

[56] Li B, Wang JHC. Fibroblasts and myofibroblasts in wound healing: force generation and measurement. J Tissue Viability. 2011; 20(4): 108-120. DOI:10.1016/j.jtv.2009.11.004

[57] Li L, Fukunaga-Kalabis M, Herlyn M. The three-dimensional human skin reconstruct model: a tool to study normal skin and melanoma progression. J Vis Exp. 2011; (54): e2937-e2940. DOI:10.3791/2937

[58] Dvorak HF. Vascular permeability factor/vascular endothelial growth factor: a critical cytokine in tumor angiogenesis and a potential target for diagnosis and therapy. J Clin Oncol. 2002; 20(21): 4368-4380. DOI: 10.1200/JCO.2002.10.088

[59] Eichler MJ, Carlson MA. Modeling dermal granulation tissue with the linear fibroblast-populated collagen matrix: a comparison with the round matrix model. J Dermatol Sci. 2006; 41(2): 97-108. DOI:10.1016/j.jdermsci.2005.09.002

[60] Hinz B. Masters and servants of the force: The role of matrix adhesions in myofibroblast force perception and transmission. European J Cell Biol. 2006; 85(3–4): 175-181. DOI: 10.1016/j.ejcb.2005.09.004

[61] Newton PM, et al., Macrophages restrain contraction of an in vitro wound healing model. Inflammation. 2004; 28(4): 207-214. DOI: 10.1023/B:IFLA0000049045.41784.59

[62] Mora S, Pessin JE. An adipocentric view of signaling and intracellular trafficking. Diabetes/Metabolism Res Rev. 2002; 18(5): 345-356. DOI: 10.1002/dmrr.321

[63] Greenhalgh DG. The role of apoptosis in wound healing. Int J Biochem Cell Biol. 1998; 30(9): 1019-1030. DOI:10.1016/S1357-2725(98)00058-2

[64] Ruszczak Z. Effect of collagen matrices on dermal wound healing. Adv Drug Delivery Rev. 2003; 55(12): 1595-1611. DOI:10.1016/j.addr.2003.08.003

[65] McDougall S, et al., Fibroblast migration and collagen deposition during dermal wound healing: mathematical modelling and clinical implications. Philos Trans A Math Phys Eng Sci. 2006; 364(1843): 1385-1405. DOI: 10.1098/rsta.2006.1773

[66] Hwang JH, et al., Comparison of cytokine expression in mesenchymal stem cells from human placenta, cord blood, and bone marrow. J Korean Med Sci. 2009; 24(4): 547-554. DOI: 10.3346/jkms.2009.24.4.547

[67] Rastegar F, et al., Mesenchymal stem cells: molecular characteristics and clinical applications. World J Stem Cells. 2010; 2(4): 67-80. DOI: 10.4252/wjsc.v2.i4.67

[68] Song YS, et al., Potential differentiation of human mesenchymal stem cell transplanted in rat corpus cavernosum toward endothelial or smooth muscle cells. Int J Impot Res. 2007; 19(4): 378-385. DOI:10.1038/sj.ijir.3901539

[69] Gregory CA, Prockop DJ, Spees JL. Non-hematopoietic bone marrow stem cells: molecular control of expansion and differentiation. Exp Cell Res. 2005; 306(2): 330-335. DOI:10.1016/j.yexcr.2005.03.018

[70] Wagner W, et al., Comparative characteristics of mesenchymal stem cells from human bone marrow, adipose tissue, and umbilical cord blood. Exp Hematol. 2005; 33(11): 1402-1416. DOI:10.1016/j.exphem.2005.07.003

[71] Horwitz EM, et al., Clarification of the nomenclature for MSC: the International Society for Cellular Therapy position statement. Cytotherapy. 2005; 7(5): 393-395.DOI: 10.1080/14653240500319234

[72] Oswald J, et al., Mesenchymal stem cells can be differentiated into endothelial cells in vitro. Stem Cells. 2004; 22(3): 377-384. DOI: 10.1634/stemcells.22-3-377

[73] Wang S, Qu X, Zhao R. Clinical applications of mesenchymal stem cells. J Hematol Oncol. 2012; 5(1): 19. DOI: 10.1186/1756-8722-5-19

[74] Patel DM, Shah J, Srivastava AS. Therapeutic potential of mesenchymal stem cells in regenerative medicine. Stem Cells Int. 2013; 2013: 15. DOI: 10.1155/2013/496218

[75] Jin HJ, et al., Comparative analysis of human mesenchymal stem cells from bone marrow, adipose tissue, and umbilical cord blood as sources of cell therapy. Int J Mol Sci. 2013; 14(9): 17986-18001. DOI: 10.3390/ijms140917986

[76] Yeum CE, et al., Quantification of MSCs involved in wound healing: use of SIS to transfer MSCs to wound site and quantification of MSCs involved in skin wound healing. J Tissue Eng Regen Med. 2013; 7(4): 279-291. DOI: 10.1002/term.521

[77] Lau K, et al., Exploring the role of stem cells in cutaneous wound healing. Exp Dermatol. 2009; 18(11): 921-933. DOI: 10.1111/j.1600-0625.2009.00942.x

[78] Si YL, et al., MSCs: biological characteristics, clinical applications and their outstanding concerns. Ageing Res Rev. 2011; 10(1): 93-103. DOI: 10.1016/j.arr.2010.08.005

[79] Wu Y, et al., Mesenchymal stem cells enhance wound healing through differentiation and angiogenesis. Stem Cells. 2007; 25(10): 2648-2659. DOI: 10.1634/stemcells.2007-0226

[80] An Y, et al., Bone marrow mesenchymal stem cell aggregate: an optimal cell therapy for full-layer cutaneous wound vascularization and regeneration. Scient Rep. 2015; 5: 17036. DOI: 10.1038/srep17036

[81] Sheng Z, et al., Regeneration of functional sweat gland-like structures by transplanted differentiated bone marrow mesenchymal stem cells. Wound Repair Regen. 2009; 17(3): 427-435. DOI: 10.1111/j.1524-475X.2009.00474.x

[82] Fu X, Li H. Mesenchymal stem cells and skin wound repair and regeneration: possibilities and questions. Cell Tissue Res. 2009; 335(2): 317-321. DOI: 10.1007/s00441-008-0724-3

[83] Vojtassak J, et al., Autologous biograft and mesenchymal stem cells in treatment of the diabetic foot. Neuro Endocrinol Lett. 2006; 27(suppl 2): 134-7. PMID: 17159798

[84] Zahorec P, et al., Mesenchymal stem cells for chronic wounds therapy. Cell Tissue Bank. 2015; 16(1): 19-26.DOI: 10.1007/s10561-014-9440-2

[85] Yamaguchi Y, et al., Bone marrow cells differentiate into wound myofibroblasts and accelerate the healing of wounds with exposed bones when combined with an occlusive dressing. Br J Dermatol. 2005; 152(4): 616-622. DOI: 10.1111/j.1365-2133.2005.06402.x

[86] Sasaki M, et al., Mesenchymal stem cells are recruited into wounded skin and contribute to wound repair by transdifferentiation into multiple skin cell type. J Immunol. 2008; 180(4): 2581-2587. DOI: 10.4049/?jimmunol.180.4.2581

[87] Chen L, et al., Analysis of allogenicity of mesenchymal stem cells in engraftment and wound healing in mice. PLoS One. 2009; 4(9): e7119. DOI: 10.1371/journal.pone.0007119

[88] Alfaro MP, et al., The Wnt modulator sFRP2 enhances mesenchymal stem cell engraftment, granulation tissue formation and myocardial repair. Proc Natl Acad Sci USA. 2008; 105(47): 18366-18371. DOI: 10.1073/pnas.0803437105

[89] Chen D, et al., Transdifferentiation of umbilical cord–derived mesenchymal stem cells into epidermal-like cells by the mimicking skin microenvironment. Int J Lower Extremity Wounds. 2015; 14(2): 136-145. DOI: 10.1177/1534734615569913

[90] Smith AN, et al., Mesenchymal stem cells induce dermal fibroblast responses to injury. Exp Cell Res. 2010; 316(1): 48-54. DOI: 10.1016/j.yexcr.2009.08.001

[91] Kim WS, et al., Wound healing effect of adipose-derived stem cells: a critical role of secretory factors on human dermal fibroblasts. J Dermatol Sci. 2007; 48(1): 15-24. DOI: 10.1016/j.jdermsci.2007.05.018

[92] Shimo T, et al., Connective tissue growth factor induces the proliferation, migration, and tube formation of vascular endothelial cells in vitro, and angiogenesis in vivo. J Biochem. 1999; 126(1): 137-145. DOI: 10.1093/oxfordjournals.jbchem.a022414

[93] Ornitz DM, Itoh N. Fibroblast growth factors. Genome Biol. 2001; 2(3): REVIEWS3005. DOI: 10.1186/gb-2001-2-3-reviews3005

[94] Wang Z, et al., Enhanced keratinocyte proliferation and migration in co-culture with fibroblasts. PLoS One. 2012; 7(7): e40951. DOI: 10.1371/journal.pone.0040951

[95] Micera A, et al, Nerve growth factor displays stimulatory effects on human skin and lung fibroblasts, demonstrating a direct role for this factor in tissue repair. Proc Natl Acad Sci USA. 2001. 98(11): 6162-6167. DOI: 10.1073/pnas.101130898

[96] Lynch SE, et al., Role of platelet-derived growth factor in wound healing: synergistic effects with other growth factors. Proc Natl Acad Sci USA. 1987; 84(21): 7696-7700. DOI: 10.1073/pnas.84.21.7696

[97] Heldin C-H, Westermark B. Mechanism of action and in vivo role of platelet-derived growth factor. Physiol Rev. 1999; 79(4): 1283-1316. PMID: 10508235

[98] Chen M, et al., Effects of hepatocyte growth factor on wound healing of rabbit maxillary sinus mucosa. J Otolaryngol Head Neck Surg. 2012; 41(4): 253-258. DOI: 10.2310/7070.2012.00033

[99] van de Kamp J, et al., Hepatocyte growth factor-loaded biomaterials for mesenchymal stem cell recruitment. Stem Cells Int. 2013; 2013: 892065. DOI: 10.1155/2013/892065

[100] Cowin AJ, et al., Hepatocyte growth factor and macrophage-stimulating protein are upregulated during excisional wound repair in rats. Cell Tissue Res. 2001; 306(2): 239-250. DOI: 10.1007/s004410100443

[101] Grellner W. Time-dependent immunohistochemical detection of proinflammatory cytokines (IL-1beta, IL-6, TNF-alpha) in human skin wounds. Forensic Sci Int. 2002; 130(2-3): 90-96. DOI:10.1016/S0379-0738(02)00342-0

[102] Zhang M, et al., Activin B promotes BM-MSC-mediated cutaneous wound healing by regulating cell migration via the JNK-ERK signaling pathway. Cell Transplant. 2013; DOI: 10.3727/096368913X666999

[103] Foraker JE, et al., Cross-talk between human mesenchymal stem/progenitor cells (MSCs) and rat hippocampal slices in LPS-stimulated cocultures: the MSCs are activated to secrete prostaglandin E2. J Neurochem. 2011; 119(5): 1052-1063. DOI: 10.1111/j.1471-4159.2011.07511.x

[104] Ortiz LA, et al., Interleukin 1 receptor antagonist mediates the antiinflammatory and antifibrotic effect of mesenchymal stem cells during lung injury. Proc Natl Acad Sci USA. 2007; 104(26): 11002-11007. DOI: 10.1073/pnas.0704421104

[105] Blaber S, et al., Analysis of in vitro secretion profiles from adipose-derived cell populations. J Transl Med. 2012; 10(1): 172. DOI: 10.1186/1479-5876-10-172

[106] Nemeth K, et al., Bone marrow stromal cells attenuate sepsis via prostaglandin E(2)-dependent reprogramming of host macrophages to increase their interleukin-10 production. Nat Med. 2009; 15(1): 42-49. DOI:10.1038/nm.1905

[107] Lin Z-Q, et al., Essential involvement of IL-6 in the skin wound-healing process as evidenced by delayed wound healing in IL-6-deficient mice. J Leukocyte Biol. 2003; 73(6): 713-721. DOI:10.1189/jlb.0802397

[108] Moore KW, et al., Interleukin-10 and the interleukin-10 receptor. Annu Rev Immunol. 2001; 19: 683-765. DOI: 10.1146/annurev.immunol.19.1.683

[109] Mann A, et al., Keratinocyte-derived granulocyte-macrophage colony stimulating factor accelerates wound healing: stimulation of keratinocyte proliferation, granulation tissue formation, and vascularization. J Invest Dermatol. 2001; 117(6): 1382-1390. DOI: 10.1046/j.0022-202x.2001.01600.x

[110] Rennekampff HO, et al., Bioactive interleukin-8 is expressed in wounds and enhances wound healing. J Surg Res. 2000; 93(1): 41-54. DOI:10.1006/jsre.2000.5892

[111] Yew TL, et al., Enhancement of wound healing by human multipotent stromal cell conditioned medium: the paracrine factors and p38 MAPK activation. Cell Transplant. 2011; 20(5): 693-706. DOI: 10.3727/096368910X550198

[112] Booth AM, et al., Exosomes and HIV Gag bud from endosome-like domains of the T cell plasma membrane. J Cell Biol. 2006; 172(6): 923-935. DOI: 10.1083/jcb.200508014

[113] Zhang J, et al., Exosomes released from human induced pluripotent stem cells-derived MSCs facilitate cutaneous wound healing by promoting collagen synthesis and angiogenesis. J Transl Med. 2015; 13(1): 1-14. DOI:10.1186/s12967-015-0417-0

[114] Muralidharan-Chari V, et al., Microvesicles: mediators of extracellular communication during cancer progression. J Cell Sci. 2010; 123(10): 1603-1611. DOI: 10.1242/jcs.064386

[115] Keller S, et al., Exosomes: from biogenesis and secretion to biological function. Immunol Lett. 2006; 107(2): 102-108. DOI:10.1016/j.imlet.2006.09.005

[116] Li T, et al., Exosomes derived from human umbilical cord mesenchymal stem cells alleviate liver fibrosis. Stem Cells Dev. 2013; 22. DOI: 10.1089/scd.2012.0395

[117] Zhang B, et al., HucMSC-exosome mediated-Wnt4 signaling is required for cutaneous wound healing. Stem Cells. 2015; 33(7): 2158-2168. DOI: 10.1002/stem.1771

[118] Shabbir A, et al., Mesenchymal stem cell exosomes induce proliferation and migration of normal and chronic wound fibroblasts, and enhance angiogenesis in vitro. Stem Cells Dev. 2015; 24(14): 1635-1647. DOI: 10.1089/scd.2014.0316

[119] Rani S, Ritter T. The exosome – a naturally secreted nanoparticle and its application to wound healing. Adv Materials. 2015; n/a-n/a. DOI: 10.1002/adma.201504009

[120] Tyndall A, Pistoia V. Mesenchymal stem cells combat sepsis. Nat Med. 2009; 15(1): 18-20. DOI:10.1038/nm0109-18

[121] Liechty KW, et al., Human mesenchymal stem cells engraft and demonstrate site-specific differentiation after in utero transplantation in sheep. Nat Med. 2000; 6(11): 1282-1286. DOI:10.1038/81395

[122] Nuschke A. Activity of mesenchymal stem cells in therapies for chronic skin wound healing. Organogenesis. 2014; 10(1): 29-37. DOI: 10.4161/org.27405

[123] Popp FC, et al., Mesenchymal stem cells can induce long-term acceptance of solid organ allografts in synergy with low-dose mycophenolate. Transpl Immunol. 2008; 20(1-2): 55-60. DOI: 10.1016/j.trim.2008.08.004

[124] Djouad F, et al., Mesenchymal stem cells inhibit the differentiation of dendritic cells through an interleukin-6-dependent mechanism. Stem Cells. 2007; 25(8): 2025-2032. DOI: 10.1634/stemcells.2006-0548

[125] Sotiropoulou PA, et al., Interactions between human mesenchymal stem cells and natural killer cells. Stem Cells. 2006; 24(1): 74-85. DOI: 10.1634/stemcells.2004-0359

[126] Petrie Aronin CE, Tuan RS. Therapeutic potential of the immunomodulatory activities of adult mesenchymal stem cells. Birth Defects Res C Embryo Today. 2010; 90(1): 67-74. DOI: 10.1002/bdrc.20174

[127] Chamberlain G, et al., Concise review: mesenchymal stem cells: their phenotype, differentiation capacity, immunological features, and potential for homing. Stem Cells. 2007; 25(11): 2739-2749. DOI: 10.1634/stemcells.2007-0197

[128] Corcione A, et al., Human mesenchymal stem cells modulate B-cell functions. Blood. 2006; 107(1): 367-372. DOI: 10.1182/blood-2005-07-2657

[129] Redd MJ, et al., Wound healing and inflammation: embryos reveal the way to perfect repair. Philos Trans Royal Soc Lond B Biol Sci. 2004; 359(1445): 777-784. DOI: 10.1098/rstb.2004.1466

[130] Zanone MM, et al., Human mesenchymal stem cells modulate cellular immune response to islet antigen glutamic acid decarboxylase in type 1 diabetes. J Clin Endocrinol Metab. 2010; 95(8): 3788-3797. DOI: 10.1210/jc.2009-2350

[131] Ortiz LA, et al., Mesenchymal stem cell engraftment in lung is enhanced in response to bleomycin exposure and ameliorates its fibrotic effects. Proc Natl Acad Sci USA. 2003; 100(14): 8407-8411. DOI: 10.1073/pnas.1432929100

[132] Liu Y, et al., Flk-1+ adipose-derived mesenchymal stem cells differentiate into skeletal muscle satellite cells and ameliorate muscular dystrophy in mdx mice. Stem Cells Dev. 2007; 16(5): 695-706. DOI:10.1089/scd.2006.0118

[133] Spaeth E, et al., Inflammation and tumor microenvironments: defining the migratory itinerary of mesenchymal stem cells. Gene Ther. 2008; 15(10): 730-738. DOI:10.1038/gt.2008.39

[134] Yagi H, et al., Mesenchymal stem cells: Mechanisms of immunomodulation and homing. Cell Transplant. 2010; 19(6): 667-679. DOI: 10.3727/096368910X508762

[135] Mishra PJ, Banerjee D. Cell-free derivatives from mesenchymal stem cells are effective in wound therapy. World J Stem Cells. 2012; 4(5): 35-43. DOI: 10.4252/wjsc.v4.i5.35

[136] Liu JF, et al., Human mesenchymal stem cells improve myocardial performance in a splenectomized rat model of chronic myocardial infarction. J Formos Med Assoc. 2008; 107(2): 165-174. DOI:10.1016/S0929-6646(08)60130-8

[137] Buchanan EP, Longaker MT, Lorenz HP. Fetal skin wound healing. Adv Clin Chem, 2009. 48: p. 137-161. PMID: 19803418

[138] Jackson WM, Nesti LJ, Tuan RS. Mesenchymal stem cell therapy for attenuation of scar formation during wound healing. Stem Cell Res Ther. 2012; 3(3): 20. DOI: 10.1186/scrt111

[139] Poli G. Pathogenesis of liver fibrosis: role of oxidative stress. Mol Aspects Med. 2000; 21(3): 49-98. DOI:10.1016/S0098-2997(00)00004-2

[140] Sato K, et al., Nitric oxide plays a critical role in suppression of T-cell proliferation by mesenchymal stem cells. Blood. 2007; 109(1): 228-234. DOI: 10.1182/blood-2006-02-002246

[141] Ferrini MG, et al., Antifibrotic role of inducible nitric oxide synthase. Nitric Oxide. 2002; 6(3): 283-294. DOI:10.1006/niox.2001.0421

[142] Li L, et al., Paracrine action mediate the antifibrotic effect of transplanted mesenchymal stem cells in a rat model of global heart failure. Mol Biol Rep. 2009; 36(4): 725-731. DOI: 10.1007/s11033-008-9235-2

[143] Mou S, et al., Hepatocyte growth factor suppresses transforming growth factor-beta-1 and type III collagen in human primary renal fibroblasts. Kaohsiung J Med Sci. 2009; 25(11): 577-587. DOI:10.1016/S1607-551X(09)70560-1

[144] McAnulty RJ, Fibroblasts and myofibroblasts: their source, function and role in disease. Int J Biochem Cell Biol. 2007; 39(4): 666-671. DOI:10.1016/j.biocel.2006.11.005

[145] Zhang A, et al., Prostaglandin E2 is a potent inhibitor of epithelial-to-mesenchymal transition: interaction with hepatocyte growth factor. Am J Physiol Renal Physiol. 2006; 291(6): F1323-F1331. DOI: 10.1152/ajprenal.00480.2005

[146] Renault MA, et al., The hedgehog transcription factor Gli3 modulates angiogenesis. Circ Res. 2009; 105(8): 818-626. DOI: 10.1161/CIRCRESAHA.109.206706

[147] Mustoe T. Understanding chronic wounds: a unifying hypothesis on their pathogenesis and implications for therapy. The Am J Surg. 2004; 187(5, suppl 1): S65-S70. DOI: 10.1016/S0002-9610(03)00306-4

[148] Rubin RH. Surgical wound infection: epidemiology, pathogenesis, diagnosis and management. BMC Infec Dis. 2006; 6: 171-171. DOI: 10.1186/1471-2334-6-171

[149] Brem H, et al., Mechanism of sustained release of vascular endothelial growth factor in accelerating experimental diabetic healing. J Invest Dermatol. 2009; 129(9): 2275-2287. DOI:10.1038/jid.2009.26

[150] Brem H, Kirsner RS, Falanga V. Protocol for the successful treatment of venous ulcers. Am J Surg. 2004; 188(1, suppl 1): 1-8. DOI: 10.1016/S0002-9610(03)00284-8

[151] Taylor JE, et al., Extent of iron pick-up in deforoxamine-coupled polyurethane materials for therapy of chronic wounds. Biomaterials. 2005; 26(30): 6024-6033. DOI:10.1016/j.biomaterials.2005.03.015

[152] Dhall S, et al., A novel model of chronic wounds: importance of redox imbalance and biofilm-forming bacteria for establishment of chronicity. PLoS One. 2014; 9(10): e109848. DOI: 10.1371/journal.pone.0109848

[153] Sen CK. Wound healing essentials: let there be oxygen. Wound Repair and Regen (official publication of the Wound Healing Soc [and] The Eur Tissue Repair Soc). 2009; 17(1): 1-18. DOI: 10.1111/j.1524-475X.2008.00436.x

[154] Kumari R, et al., Impaired wound healing after cerebral hypoxia-ischemia in the diabetic mouse. J Cereb Blood Flow Metab. 2006; 27(4): 710-718. DOI: 10.1038/sj.jcbfm.9600382

[155] Alleva R, et al., α-Lipoic acid supplementation inhibits oxidative damage, accelerating chronic wound healing in patients undergoing hyperbaric oxygen therapy. Biochem Biophys Res Commu. 2005; 333(2): 404-410. DOI:10.1016/j.bbrc.2005.05.119

[156] Moreo K. Understanding and overcoming the challenges of effective case management for patients with chronic wounds. The Case Manager. 2005; 16(2): 62-67. DOI:10.1016/j.casemgr.2005.01.014

[157] Snyder RJ. Treatment of nonhealing ulcers with allografts. Clinics in Dermatol. 2005; 23(4): 388-395. DOI:10.1016/j.clindermatol.2004.07.020

[158] Volarevic V, Lako M, Stojkovic M. Mesenchymal Stem cells for diabetes and related complications, in Essentials of Mesenchymal Stem Cell Biology and Its Clinical Translation, C.R. Zhao, Editor. Dordrecht, Netherlands: Springer. 2013; 207-227. DOI: 10.1007/978-94-007-6716-4_14

[159] Zhang N, et al., Bone marrow mesenchymal stem cells induce angiogenesis and attenuate the remodeling of diabetic cardiomyopathy. Exp Clin Endocrinol Diabetes. 2008; 116(2): 104-111. doi: 10.1055/s-2007-985154.

[160] Crovetti G, et al., Platelet gel for healing cutaneous chronic wounds. Transfusion and Apheresis Sci. 2004; 30(2): 145-151. DOI: 10.1016/j.transci.2004.01.004

[161] Amin AH, et al., Modified multipotent stromal cells with epidermal growth factor restore vasculogenesis and blood flow in ischemic hind-limb of type II diabetic mice. Lab. Invest J Tech Meth Pathol. 2010; 90(7): 985-996. DOI: 10.1038/labinvest.2010.86

[162] Comerota AJ, et al., Upper extremity ischemia treated with tissue repair cells from adult bone marrow. J Vascular Surg. 2010; 52(3): 723-729. DOI: org/10.1016/j.jvs.2010.04.020

[163] Lee HC, et al., Safety and effect of adipose tissue-derived stem cell implantation in patients with critical limb ischemia: a pilot study. Circulation J. 2012; 76(7): 1750-1760. DOI:10.1253/circj.CJ-11-1135

[164] Eirin A, et al., Adipose tissue-derived mesenchymal stem cells improve revascularization outcomes to restore renal function in swine atherosclerotic renal artery stenosis. Stem Cells (Dayton, Ohio). 2012; 30(5): 1030-1041. DOI: 10.1002/stem.1047

[165] Crovetti G, et al., Platelet gel for healing cutaneous chronic wounds. Transfusion and Apheresis Sci. 2004; 30(2): 145-151. DOI: 10.1016/j.transci.2004.01.004

[166] Lai J-Y, et al., Mitosis increases levels of secretory leukocyte protease inhibitor in keratinocytes. Biochem Biophys Res Commu. 2004; 316(2): 407-410. DOI:10.1016/j.bbrc.2004.02.065

[167] Wysocki AB, Staiano-Coico L, Grinnell F. Wound fluid from chronic leg ulcers contains elevated levels of metalloproteinases MMP-2 and MMP-9. J Investig Dermatol; 1993; 101(1): 64-68. DOI:10.1111/1523-1747.ep12359590

Chapter 6

The Role of Actin Remodelling Proteins in Wound Healing and Tissue Regeneration

Zlatko Kopecki and Allison J Cowin

Additional information is available at the end of the chapter

http://dx.doi.org/10.5772/64673

Abstract

The actin cytoskeleton is an essential network of filaments that is found in all cells and has an important role in regulating cellular activities. The dynamic regulation of cytoskeletal synthesis, remodelling and function is critical for many physiological processes and is integral for the successful repair of wounds. Wound healing relies on the fine balance between cellular proliferation, adhesion and migration, resulting in tightly controlled equilibrium between tissue regeneration and fibrosis. The actin cytoskeleton regulates all these processes and is therefore an important factor contributing to the re-establishment of the skin barrier function, restoration of the skin anatomical structure and wound repair; however, it also inevitably results in scar formation. Regulation of the actin cytoskeleton is tightly controlled by several large protein families, which are discussed in this chapter. Members of the FERM superfamily of proteins, the filamin and tropomyosin families of actin-associated proteins as well as the gelsolin family of actin remodelling proteins are all important regulators of the actin cytoskeleton, which can affect different stages of wound healing. Targeted therapies against different proteins involved in cytoskeletal regulation may lead to novel therapeutic interventions aimed at improving wound healing and reducing scar formation.

Keywords: actin cytoskeleton, wound healing, skin regeneration, fibrosis

1. Introduction

The actin cytoskeleton is made up of a complex network of microtubules, actin filaments, intermediate filaments and stress fibres, providing a cellular engine that drives motility, adhesion and contraction downstream of complex signalling pathways. The actin cytoskeleton is also involved in modulating cell signalling, growth, differentiation and gene expression, while components of the actin cytoskeleton further work in synergy to provide stronger cell stability during stress [1, 2].

Cutaneous wound repair is a dynamic process triggered in response to tissue injury, which aims to restore the skin barrier function, and involves a sequence of events including acute inflammation, reepithelialisation, collagen deposition and contraction and remodelling [3]. Common to all tissue repair processes is the migration of cells into the wound space including fibroblasts, epithelial cells and endothelial cells. It is the active assembly and disassembly of the filamentous actin and reorganisation of its networks that underpins the important cell processes, which occur during wound healing.

Changes in the distribution of actin-associated proteins during epidermal wound healing in vivo were first reported in 1992 [4]. Filamentous actin was found in all the living epidermal layers before, after and during wound healing while different actin-associated proteins, namely talin, filamin and gelsolin, showed a reduced expression at the leading edge of migrating epidermis, which returned to normal levels once the epidermis has reformed [4].

The precise orchestration of actin polymers into filaments and their interactions with various proteins regulating actin remodelling, stability, branching and bundling is what underpins cellular migration and outcomes of wound healing. Central to the ability of fibroblasts and keratinocytes to move into the wounded area is a dynamic and responsive actin cytoskeleton and the molecules that regulate actin filament dynamics and change the rate of cell migration can also alter the rate of wound healing [5]. Understanding the role of the actin cytoskeleton in cellular functions vital for tissue repair and regeneration and how different regulators of the actin cytoskeleton control this intricate balance between actin polymerisation and disassembly will be critical for the development of novel therapeutic approaches. New therapies that can regulate the actin cytoskeleton could lead to improved wound healing outcomes. Here, we will focus on describing the role of different actin cytoskeleton regulators and how they are able to modulate the cytoskeleton and influence different stages of wound healing.

2. Actin dynamics during wound healing

Actin-based cell motility relies on the balanced activity of specific actin-binding proteins that drive the dynamics of the actin system and govern its special organisation [6]. A number of different structural and dynamic aspects of cell behaviour are dependent on the actin cytoskeleton, including cell morphology, polarity, adhesion complex formation, vesicle trafficking and phagocytosis, cytokinesis and movement [7]. Actin microfilaments are the smallest components of the actin cytoskeletal network and play a role in cellular motility, structure and division [6]. Two types of actin microfilaments have been categorised; individual non-polymerised globular actin subunits termed G-actin and long filamentous polymerised fibres termed F-actin assembled from individual G-actin subunits. Microfilament actin (F-actin) exists in equilibrium with a soluble monomeric actin (G-actin) and this balance is often shifted in response to changes in cellular environment, cellular migration, adhesion and wound repair [8]. During wound healing, activation of neutrophils during the inflammatory phase of wound repair induces changes in cell shape, migration, degranulation and phagocytic responses, all of which require cytoskeletal restructuring. In addition, the reestablishment of the skin barrier function as well as endothelial vessel integrity in wounds is dependent on actin cytoskeleton integrity [9]. Microtubules and intermediate filaments are larger structures of the cytoskeleton composed of α and β tubulin dimers which function in both cellular movement and division [6]. Intermediate filaments are involved in the formation of adhesion complexes namely hemidesmosomes, desmosomes and focal adhesions and directly interact with proteins of the extracellular matrix [10]. Key roles of the intermediate filaments include signal transduction, cytoskeletal crosstalk between the organelles in the cytoplasm and organisation of the cytoplasm [11].

Stress fibres are also a component of the actin cytoskeleton network allowing a cell to modulate its responses to tissue injury. Mammalian cells contain three types of stress fibres: ventral stress fibres attached to focal adhesions at both ends, dorsal stress fibres attached to focal adhesions at one end, and transverse arcs which are the acto-myosin bundles that do not attach to focal adhesions directly [12]. The major role of stress fibres is to maintain a balance between contraction and adhesion. This balance results in stable actin bundles, which maintain a constant length under tension, especially in ventral stress fibres attached to the extracellular matrix on both sides [13].

Changes in cell shape, adhesion and migration properties are all regulated by the continuous remodelling of the actin cytoskeleton. Cell motility is powered by controlled assembly and disassembly of the actin cytoskeleton, and the migration speed is dependent on the membrane tension created by the coalescence of the actin filaments growing against the tense membrane [14]. In order to migrate in response to extracellular signals, cells first assemble actin at the cell front driving the extension of membrane protrusions called lamellipodia and filopodia [15]. At the leading edge of the cell, adhesions are formed with the extracellular matrix, hence anchoring the protrusions to move the cell body. The combination of the acto-myosin contractibility and disassembly of the adhesion structures at the rear of the cell allows the cell body to move forward [8]. Lamellipodia, filopodia and membrane ruffles are components of the actin cytoskeleton involved in both cell motility and cell-matrix adhesions [16]. Lamellipodia consist of a network of branched actin filaments that produce the force for cell protrusions at the leading edge. The assembly of actin-based projections is regulated by GTPases of the Rho family, which link the surface receptors to the organisation of the actin cytoskeleton. While Rho GTPase is instrumental in formation of stress fibre and focal adhesion formation, Rac1 and Cdc42 signal the formation of lamellipodia and filopodia, respectively.

Filapodia are thin cellular processes consisting of long parallel actin filaments arranged into tight bundles. Membrane ruffling is characterised by the dynamic movement of the membrane protrusions, consisting of lamellipodia and filopodia, in response to the extracellular signals. Away from the leading edge of the cell at the site of slow actin turnover, lamellas are formed and are characterised by proteins involved in the movement of stress fibres, namely tropomyosin and myosin II [8]. Initial integrin mediated cell-matrix adhesions, termed focal complexes, develop underneath lamellipodia and are driven by actin polymerisation. These are highly dynamic structures that exist for a limited time. A proportion of the stable focal complexes develop into elongated focal adhesions, which are associated with contractile stress fibres [17]. A vital function of focal adhesions is the anchoring of polymerised actin filament stress fibres into bundles, which provide contractile force required for effective translocation of a cell body during cellular migration [18]. Different components of the actin cytoskeleton of the moving cell and adhesion sites formed in response to GTPase signalling in fibroblasts are shown in **Figure 1**. The main changes in the actin cytoskeleton during wound healing include lamellipodia remodelling during keratinocyte migration and wound reepithelialisation, infiltration of inflammatory cells and migration of fibroblasts required for the deposition and remodelling of the extracellular matrix and dermal wound contraction [19, 20].

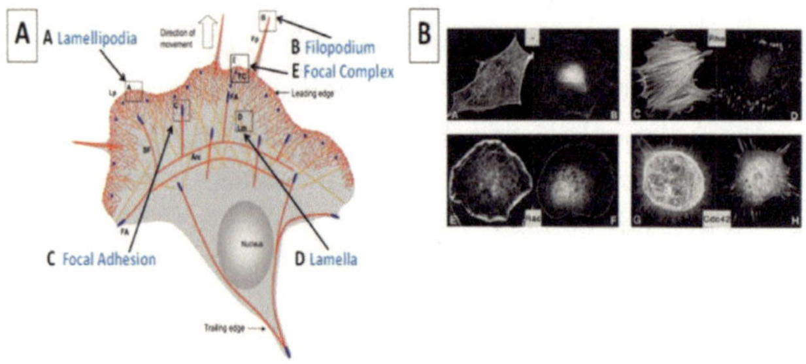

Figure 1. Actin cytoskeleton of the moving cell. (A) Arrangement of the actin cytoskeleton in a moving cell A lamellipodia, B filopodium, C focal adhesion, D lamella, E focal complex. (B) Formation of different actin cytoskeleton components in response to GTPase signalling in fibroblasts. Actin filaments visualised with phalloidin staining in A, C, E and G and adhesion complexes visualised with an anti-vinculin antibody in B, D, F and H. Quiescent fibroblasts in A and B show few organised actin filaments or adhesion complexes. In response to Rho stress fibre formation C and adhesion complex formation D is evident. Microinjection of Rac induces lamellipodia E and associated focal adhesion complexes, while microinjection of Cdc42 induces filopodia formation G and associated adhesion complexes H. Figure adapted from [8, 25].

In resting cells, there is little actin turnover, and fast-growing actin ends are blocked, with large pools of actin monomers in a complex with polymerising-inhibiting or sequestering proteins. In response to wounding, a local increase in actin polymerisation is initiated by uncapping the actin ends and by severing existing filaments leading to *de novo* polymerisation. The barbed ends of the actin filament are the hotspots for the majority of biochemical reactions that control filament assembly and a number of actin remodelling, capping, severing and sequestering proteins modulate their affinity for barbed ends in a spatial and temporal manner [21]. Some actin remodelling proteins also affect the actin filament barbed ends by indirect activity and control of the flux of actin monomers available at the barded end [22]. Signal transduction networks that translate environmental signals into intracellular changes govern actin dynamics and interplay between extracellular environment and cell motility. Many actin-binding proteins accumulate at sites of actin-rich lamella and have been shown to regulate actin dynamics in motile keratinocytes [23]. Focal adhesion formation in fibroblasts is a complex process initiated by the ligation and clustering of the integrin subunits and signalling via

RhoGTPases, which influence both actomyosin contractibility and actin stress fibre formation [24].

For cellular migration, dynamic rearrangements of the actin cytoskeleton occur to form protrusive structures and generate intracellular forces required for cell movement. The actin-based motility is best described in four steps: polarisation, protrusion of lamellipodia, formation of attachment sites and retraction of cell rear end [6]. Fibroblast locomotion during wound healing is the result of series of coordinated cellular events and main motor protein involved in mediating formation of lamellipodia of migrating cells is Myosin I. However, during wound healing, Myosin II, motor protein, is involved in the contraction of transverse actin fibres during lamellar contractile phase of wound healing [26]. In addition, release of Myosin II contractibility accelerates the healing of large wounds in long term by mobilisation of large cell sheet or rows of cells behind the leading edge [27].

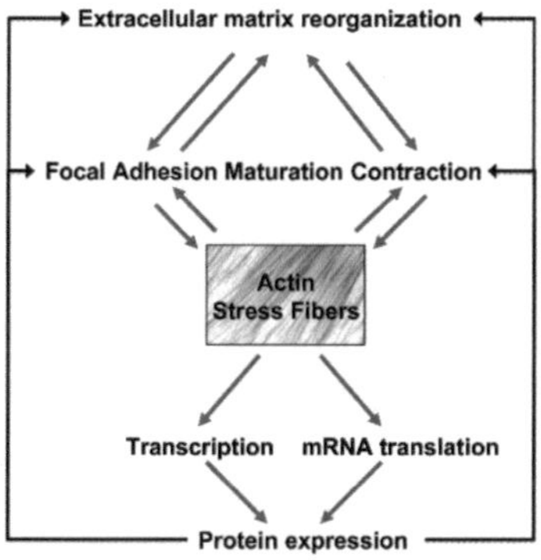

Figure 2. The role of actin cytoskeleton in regulating myofibroblast function. Actin cytoskeleton involvement in bidirectional signalling augmenting extracellular matrix organisation, focal adhesion turnover and contraction as well as transcriptional regulation of proteins instrumental in these processes vital for outcomes of wound repair. Figure adapted from [24].

Myofibroblasts are modified fibroblasts characterised by the presence of the contractile apparatus and formation of robust stress fibres. These cells are involved in the contraction and remodelling of the extracellular matrix but are also found in aberrant tissue remodelling in fibrotic disorders. The actin cytoskeleton regulates several mechanical functions during myofibroblast differentiation including focal adhesion formation, contraction and matrix remodelling and simultaneously regulates transcription of genes involved in the same mechanical functions and therefore plays an important role in amplifying the signal leading to myofibroblast differentiation. The bidirectional signalling between matrix stiffness, focal adhesion augmentation and stress fibre formation during actin cytoskeletal regulation of myofibroblast function is illustrated in **Figure 2** [28].

2.1. Scar-free foetal and adult wound healing

Whereas adult wound keratinocytes crawl forwards over the exposed substratum closing the deficit, a wound in embryonic epidermis is closed by contraction of an actin purse string. Blocking the assembly of this actin cable in chick and mouse embryos by drugs or by inactivation of small GTPase Rho severely hinders the reepithelialisation process [29]. Foetal wounds reepithelialise quickly via contraction of actin-myosin fibres in a "purse-string" like manner drawing the edges of the wound together. This is facilitated by the rapid polymerisation of the F-actin some five to six cells back from wound edge and is anchored by the E-cadherin at the leading edge to facilitate coordinated movement [30]. Foetal wound fibroblasts do not express alpha smooth muscle actin, suggesting that they do not change their phenotype into contractile myofibroblasts observed in adult wounds and these differences may account for differences in repair outcomes in foetal vs adults wound tissue [30]. Changes in the expression profile of proteins associated with actin cytoskeleton are indicative of the switch between scar-free regeneration and scar forming repair. Wounding has a differential effect on cytoskeletal proteins including gelsolin and paxillin associated with actin dynamics both in foetal and adult skin wounds [19, 31]. Interestingly, wounding also has an effect on the expression of filamentous F-actin. While "scar-free" foetal wounds have predominantly epidermal expression of F-actin, the "scar forming" adult wounds have predominantly dermal F-actin expression and this developmental switch in actin expression might be important in foetal wound contraction and "scar-free" wound healing [32]. The importance of the actin cytoskeleton in healing of foetal wounds was demonstrated at embryonic day E17 by the addition of cytochalasin-B, an inhibitor of actin polymerisation, which completely prevented epithelial wound closure with no actin cable structures evident while at embryonic day E19, dermal actin filaments formed spherical structures around the wound margin but did not affect already limited wound repair response (**Figure 3**) [19].

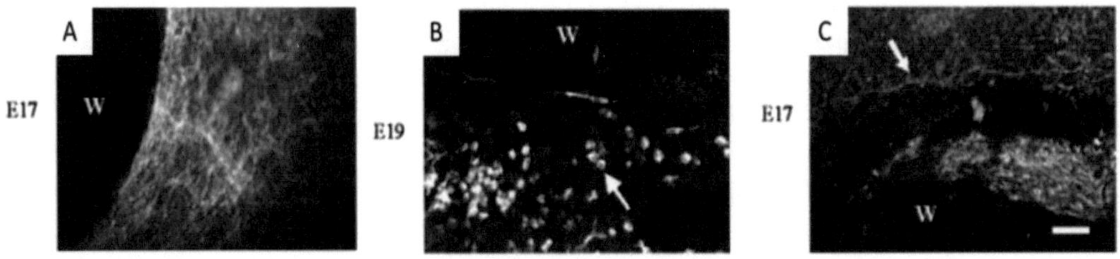

Figure 3. Effect of inhibiting actin polymerisation and protein proliferation on actin cable formation in E17 foetal wounds. Phalloidin-FITC binding to actin in E17 and E19 skins foetal skin treated with 10 μg cytochalasin-B per ml (A and B, respectively). Phalloidin-FITC binding to actin in E17 foetal skin treated with 2 mM hydroxyurea (C). Scale bar = 50 μm in (C) and applies to all images. Figure adapted from [19] and modified.

3. FERM superfamily of proteins

The FERM domain (F for 4.1protein, E for ezrin, R for radixin and M for moesin) is a widespread domain found in many cytoskeletal associated proteins at the interface between the plasma membrane and the actin cytoskeleton. The function of FERM domain is to localise the proteins to the plasma membrane, and therefore, members of the FERM superfamily of proteins mediate the linkage between the actin cytoskeleton and cell membrane and are characterised by the presence of the conserved FERM domain at the N-terminus and often an actin binding domain at the C-terminus. FERM proteins are involved in cellular motility and membrane-cytoskeletal interactions and play roles in promotion of cancer and wound healing [33]. The main members of this family include protein 4.1R, ezrin, radixin and moesin, often referred to as ERM proteins. Ezrin is a component of the microvilli of the plasma membrane, meosin is involved in binding major cytoskeletal structures to the plasma membrane, while radixin is involved in the binding of the barbed end of actin filaments to the plasma membrane [21, 34]. Earlier studies have shown that ezrin, radixin and meosin colocalise with F-actin in the endothelial cells in vitro and in vivo and play a role in formation of focal F-actin branching points, while their interaction with phosphorylated protein kinase C (PKC) has been shown to be important during wound repair [35]. Inhibition of PKC activity results in delayed wound repair, reduced association with ERM proteins and reduced F-actin branching points. In addition, phosphorylation of ERM proteins by PCK improved in vitro wound healing of cancer cells [36]. Furthermore, in vivo studies examining the healing of hepatic injury in meosin knockdown mice showed reduced inflammatory infiltrate, fibrosis and collagen deposition at the wound margins of these mice compared with control animals [37].

The role of the FERM protein superfamily during wound healing has also been demonstrated in 4.1R knockout mice (4.1R^{2013}/^{2013}) and their cultured keratinocytes. Protein 4.1R is present in the cytoplasm and the leading edge of the moving cell [34]. Absence of 4.1R protein leads to reduced adhesion, spreading and migration of keratinocytes. In addition, diminished focal adhesion complexes and reduced integrin Beta-1 expression were directly linked to absence of 4.1R protein in vitro. Using its FERM domain, 4.1R protein was shown to interact with the Ras GTPase-activating-like protein 1, a scaffolding protein that binds and cross-links actin filaments, allowing migration to take place [34]. In addition, ezrin/radixin/moesin proteins have been shown to be involved in the development of diabetes including the secretion and utilisation of insulin and may contribute to the pathogenesis and progression of diabetic angiopathy, nephropathy and cardiomyopathy [38]; all of which have been implicated in the development of diabetic ulcers. These proteins may be novel targets for therapeutic interventions aimed at preventing diabetic complications; however, further research is required to elucidate their exact mechanisms before they can be developed for specific treatments.

The FERM superfamily of proteins consists of over 30 proteins including the Kindlin family of focal adhesion proteins. Kindlin-1 and Kindlin-2 have been implicated in integrin signalling and focal adhesion turnover, while deletion of the Kindlin-1 is associated with a congenital skin disease—Kindler Syndrome, where patients experience skin atrophy, blister formation and impaired wound healing [39–42]. Kindlin-2 is an important regulator of focal adhesion stabilisation and maturation of focal adhesions and stress fibres in myofibroblasts. In addition, the upregulation of Kindlin-2 observed in myofibroblasts during wound healing suggests a role for Kindlin-2 in skin fibroblasts and tissue regeneration [41]. More recently, talin and Ehm2 have been added to the FERM superfamily both of which have roles in wound repair [21, 34].

3.1. Talin

Talin, a member of the FERM family of proteins, is concentrated in regions of cell-substrate and cell-cell contacts. Using its FERM domain, talin acts as a "hyper-activator" of integrin receptors linking the cytoplasmic tail of integrin receptors to the actin cytoskeleton and increasing the affinity of the integrin extracellular domain to the extracellular matrix, hence regulating cell adhesion-dependent processes including tissue remodelling [43]. Talin knock-out results in abnormal cellular migration and early embryonic lethality [8]. Integrin adhesion receptors connect the extracellular matrix to the actin cytoskeleton and serve as bidirectional mechanotransducers during wound healing mediating actin cytoskeletal remodelling in response to stiffening of the extracellular matrix [44]. The inside out-signalling of integrin receptors regulates the ligand binding affinity of the cell surface receptors in response to changes in environmental factors important for cell survival, including tissue injury [45]. Cytoplasmic talin is activated in response to phosphatidylinositol 4,5-biphosphate (PIP2) binding which also terminates the auto-inhibition of talin through the talin head-rod binding. Once activated, the talin subdomain interacts with the β integrin tails, forms the talin specific

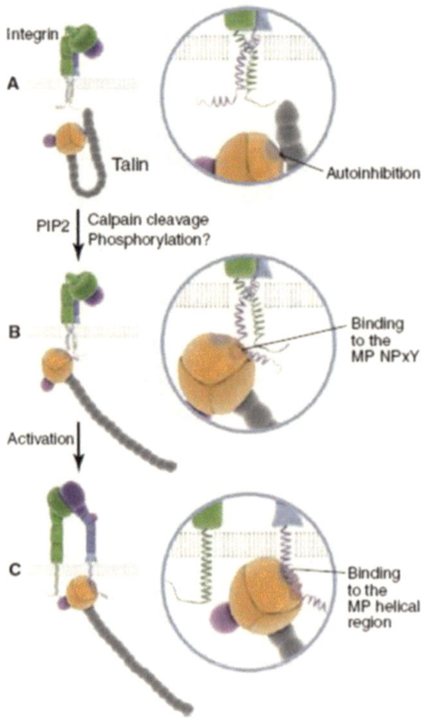

Figure 4. Talin activation of integrin receptor subunits. (A) PIP2 binding to the cytoplasmic talin activates the talin protein by ending the auto-inhibitory interaction with the rod domain. (B) Talin subdomain engages with the membrane proximal NPxY motif in the β integrin cytoplasmic tail. (C) Talin-specific loop structure forms with binding to the MP helical region of the integrin cytoplasmic chain, hence disrupting the connection between α/β subunit integrin cytoplasmic tails. Pulling forces at the β integrin tail reorient the transmembrane domains, hence disrupting the packing of the α/β transmembrane domains. Figure adapted from [46].

loop structure and disrupts the connection between the cytoplasmic tails linking the integrin receptors and the actin cytoskeleton [46]. This model of integrin activation by talin is an example of how cytoplasmic proteins can regulate activation state of integrin receptors and can transduce the biochemical signals into an array of cellular signalling transduction pathways, a crucial function for cellular adhesion, migration, angiogenesis, extracellular matrix assembly and wound remodelling [47]. **Figure 4** illustrates a schematic model of talin activation of integrin subunits; however, this process is likely to be more complex and involves spatial activation and interaction of different proteins involved in actin dynamics. Recent findings have shown that talin associates with the actin remodelling protein Flightless I (Flii) in wounded keratinocytes and this interaction may contribute to Flii regulation of adhesion-dependent signalling pathways during wound repair [48].

3.2. Ehm2

Ehm2 is a member of the FERM family that has been identified as a positive regulator of keratinocyte adhesion and motility. Ehm2 is upregulated in response to tissue injury and its levels are up to three times higher in acute wounds compared with chronic wound samples [34]. Ehm2 expression is highest in wounds undergoing active healing, where high expression was observed at the wound edge suggesting a functional role for Ehm2 during wound repair. In vitro knock-down of Ehm2 reduces NWasp protein expression and cellular adhesion, migration and motility without affecting cell growth, cell cycle or apoptosis, suggesting that Ehm2 is an important actin modulator of cell migration during healing of acute wounds [34]. Therefore, in common with other FERM family members, these findings suggest that Ehm2 promotes wound healing via the process of reepithelialisation.

4. Filamin family of proteins

The filamin (FLN) family of proteins consists of three proteins, namely Filamin-a (FLNa), Filamin-b (FLNb) and Filamin-c (FLNc). While FLNa and FLNb are enriched at the cell periphery and focal adhesions, FLNc is mainly localised in muscle Z-disc. These proteins function as actin filament cross-linking proteins and serve as scaffolds to over 90 different binding partners including channels, receptors, intracellular signalling molecules and transcription factors [49]. FLN proteins are required for the recycling, trafficking and stabilisation of membrane proteins and facilitate the signal transduction at specific locations within the cell. In addition, the FLN family of proteins act as cohesive proteins to stiffen the F-actin networks, cross-linking the filament structures and reconstituting many aspects of cell mechanics [49]. In humans, mutation in the FLNa gene results in disrupted neuronal cell migration, while FLNa overexpression also prevents migration [50]. However, genetic knockdown of FLNa in embryonic fibroblasts results in no defect in migration, suggesting a compensatory mechanism by FLNb. The main family member, FLNa, has been the predominant focus of research and has been shown to play a role in wound healing.

4.1. Filamin-a

FLNa acts as a negative regulator of integrin activation by blocking talin binding to the β integrin tail, and subsequent proteolysis and depletion of FLN. Phosphorylation of the β integrin tail dissociates FLN from integrins, hence allowing activation of integrins via talin and other members. FLNa binding with different partners leads to different outcomes in cell adhesion, spreading and migration: association with F-actin leads to formation of orthogonal F-actin networks with unique mechanical and physiological properties; interaction with Migfilin and R-Ras induces and enhances integrin activation respectively; interaction with RalA induces filopodia formation, while interaction with ROCK and Rho GTPases leads to increased actin cytoskeleton remodelling required for cell migration [49].

Human wounds heal through a combination of granulation tissue formation (via production of extracellular matrix and neovascularisation) and wound contraction (via fibroblast-mediated contraction). FLNa has been shown to protect fibroblasts against force-induced apoptosis by stabilising cell-matrix contacts [51]. Moreover, fibroblast spreading and adhesion are dependent on FLNa, consistent with its known role in cytoskeletal dynamics [52]. Studies in mice show that FLNa stabilises actin filaments in fibroblasts and mediates wound closure by promoting elastic deformation and maintenance of tension in the collagen matrix [53]. FLNa accumulates at membrane ruffles where it interacts with different binding proteins and regulates fibroblast interactions with their mechanical environment [54]. When FLNa was blocked using short hairpin RNA, fibroblasts were unable to maintain tension in collagen matrices, and they had reduced migration in vitro. In addition, FLNa-deficient fibroblasts were less able to realign collagen matrix fibres in response to tension, and they demonstrated impaired ability to form cell extensions, a deficit reversed with pharmacologic stabilisation of the actin cytoskeleton. When FLNa was deleted conditionally in dermal fibroblasts in a mouse model, full-thickness wounds healed significantly more slowly and was associated with decreased matrix deposition. No side effects or contradictions were observed in these mouse models suggesting that targeted therapies against FLNa may be worth pursuing. As researchers continue to unlock the molecular mechanisms of fibroblast mechanotransduction, novel therapies may be developed to target and manipulate fibroblast behaviour for a wide range of cutaneous diseases [55].

5. Tropomyosin family of actin-associated proteins

Members of the tropomyosin family of actin-associated proteins display a tissue-specific and time-specific expression, while their association with actin filaments impairs a isoform-specific regulation of actin filament dynamics [56]. There are over 40 different isoforms of tropomyosin and many of them have functional relevance to actin filament dynamics: Tm5NM1 and Tm3 increase actin filament resistance to actin depolymerising drugs; TmBr3 increases actin filament sensitivity to actin depolymerising drugs; TmBr3 reduces actin stress fibre formation, while Tm5a and Tm2 inhibit Arp2/3-mediated filament branching in vitro [57]. Tropomyosin proteins assemble as the polymers in the major grove of the polymerised actin filaments and this association has been shown to regulate the molecules that control actin filament turnover [58]. Specific members of the tropomyosin family of actin-associated proteins have yet to be investigated in diabetic wound healing; however, tropomyosin receptor kinase A (TrkA) has been found to be increased in diabetic patients and linked to diabetic nephropathy [59].

High levels of Tm5NM1 expression have been shown to inhibit cell migration and invasion, while loss of Tm5NM1 leads to increased cell motility [57]. Elevated Tm5NM1 expression is associated with inhibition of Src activation [57]; stabilisation of mature focal adhesions [18]; increased myosin II recruitment and actin filament tension [58]; and increased paxillin phosphorylation [18]. These findings suggested that tropomyosins may be important regulators of actin function during physiological processes dependent on cell migration, including wound healing. The effect of wounding on Tm5NM1 expression has shown that Tm5NM1/2 expression is increased in response to wounding in mice skin and inversely correlates with paxillin phosphorylation and Rac activity regulating lamellapodial protrusions [60]. In addition, the effect of Tm5NM1 and Tm5NM2 isoform knock-down on wound healing using Tm5NM1/$2^{-/-}$ mice showed an accelerated wound healing response with smaller wound area and gape at day 7 post-wounding (**Figure 5**) suggesting a negative role for tropomyosins during wound repair [60]. Increased wound healing was not associated with increased cell proliferation or matrix remodelling but increased cell migration and activation of the paxillin/Rac signalling, suggesting that tropomyosin isoform expression has an important role in temporal regulation of wound repair [60]. Understanding how different actin remodelling proteins affect wound repair may hold clues for the development of novel therapies aimed at improved wound healing outcomes.

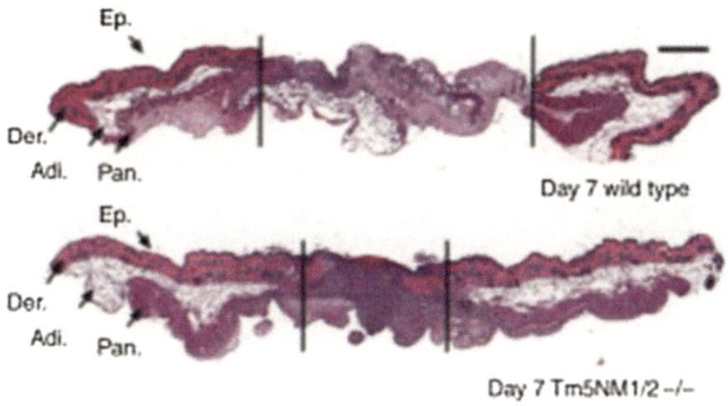

Figure 5. Cutaneous wound healing is accelerated at day 7 in Tm5NM1/$2^{-/-}$ mice. Representative H&E-stained transverse sections of full-thickness wounds after 7 days in Tm5NM1/2 and wild-type control mice (lines indicate the edges of the wound area). Adi., adipose tissue; Der., dermis; Ep., epidermis; Pan., panniculus. Bar = 500 μm. Figure adapted from [60].

6. Gelsolin family of actin remodelling proteins

The dynamic remodelling of the cytoskeleton is facilitated by the gelsolin family of remodelling proteins, which includes gelsolin, villin, adseverin, capG, advillin, supervillin and flightless I

[22]. These actin-binding proteins function in the cytoplasm of cells where they control actin organisation by severing pre-existing filaments, capping the fast-growing filament ends and nucleating or bundling actin filaments to enable filament reassembly into new cytoskeletal structures [61–64]. By remaining attached to the "barbed" ends of broken severed actin filament, these remodelling proteins prevent annealing of the broken filaments or addition of new actin monomers. Subsequently, the broken actin filaments are uncapped by interactions with phosphoinositides which results in rapid actin assembly and allows cells to reorientate the cytoskeleton and mediate the changes required for adhesion, motility and contraction [65]. The gelsolin family of actin remodelling proteins has three to six homologous gelsolin-like structural domains known as G1–G6 segmental domains, three actin binding regions and a number of calcium-independent monomer and filament binding domains. Villin, supervillin and Flii have evolved to contain additional domains allowing them to have multiple specific roles and interact with a variety of proteins. Villin contains an additional actin binding domain, termed villin head piece; supervillin contains an N-terminus domain capable of protein-protein interactions and nuclear localisation, while Flii contains a N-terminus leucine-rich repeat (LRR) domain also capable of multiple protein-protein interactions. In contrast, CapG only contains three gelsolin-like structural domains; however, it still retains full actin severing and capping ability and affects cell migration [8, 66]. There is a high homology in structure of different members of the gelsolin family; however, the differences in structure observed suggest evolutionary changes allowing specific and unique functional properties beyond actin remodelling [62, 67]. Indeed, specific functional roles have been demonstrated in cell motility, apoptosis and gene expression [68]. Several members including Flii, supervillin and gelsolin have roles in as nuclear receptor co-activators regulating gene expression [62, 69], and current studies have identified some of these proteins as new targets for improved healing and reduced scar formation [31].

6.1. Gelsolin

Gelsolin, the most abundant member of this family, is involved in regulating the dynamics of the filamentous actin by binding, severing and capping actin filaments [65]. In resting cells, gelsolin is either inactive or associated with filaments as a capping protein, while stimulation of cells or increased Ca^{2+} levels lead to an increased gelsolin activity at the plasma membrane and severing and capping of filaments resulting in increased cytoskeletal rearrangements [6]. High gelsolin levels have been associated with stress fibre formation and gelsolin was found to play a role in promoting stress fibre formation and actin stabilisation [70]. Gelsolin is also a secreted protein where its role in plasma is to "clean up" actin filaments that have been released into circulation during burn injury and cell necrosis using its gelsolin domain [27–29]. Plasma gelsolin is able to inactivate pathogen-associated molecular pattern (PAMPs) molecules, like lipopolysaccharides (LPS) and LTA (lipoteichoic acid) resulting in decreased TLR-mediated NF-kB activity [30, 31] suggesting a potential protective role for plasma gelsolin against inflammation. Gelsolin has also been shown to play a role in inflammation with studies suggesting potential clinical applications for plasma gelsolin in diagnosis and disease activity evaluation as patients with systemic lupus erythematosus (SLE) and rheumatoid arthritis (RA) who have significantly decreased plasma gelsolin levels compared with healthy controls [23,

24]. A study examining the differential effect of wounding on actin and actin-associated protein in foetal skin explants showed that it is not the migration or proliferation of cells but rather formation of the actin cable that is important in early gestation foetal wound closure [19]. In foetal skin, gelsolin was observed surrounding the actin filaments at embryonic day 19 but not at embryonic day 17 which coincided with its upregulation in embryonic day 19 foetal skin but not embryonic day 17 foetal skin [19]. In adult skin, however, gelsolin is expressed predominantly in suprabasal keratinocytes at the leading edge of migrating epidermis [71] and studies examining the effect of gelsolin on wound repair indicate that increases in cellular gelsolin levels in mouse fibroblasts enhance cellular migration and results in increased rates of wound closure [72]. Moreover, absence of gelsolin in skin fibroblasts results in a variety of actin-related defects, including decreased motility and delayed wound closure potentially due to reduction in the reorganisation of cytoskeletal actin into contractile elements [66].

6.2. Flightless I

Flightless I (Flii) is a highly conserved multifunctional protein possessing an unique structure, containing six gelsolin domains and an additional 11 tandem repeats of a 23-amino acid leucine-rich repeat (LRR) motif not present in other family members [5]. The specificity of its structure allows Flii to regulate multiple intracellular and extracellular processes [5]. Flii uses its gelsolin domain to bind and remodel (via severing, capping and bundling) cytoplasmic actin monomers (G-actin) and actin filaments (F-actin) and it possesses F-actin severing ability [67]. Unlike other members of the gelsolin family, which enhance actin polymerisation, Flii inhibits actin polymerisation [73] and associates with focal adhesions inhibiting their turnover in a Rac1-dependant manner [74]. Unique specificity of its LRR domain allows Flii to interact with multiple signalling and structural proteins including paxillin, talin, vinculin, Ras, Cdc42 and LRR Flightless Interacting proteins 1 and 2 [48, 74]. The bipartite domain structure of Flii provides capacity for it to transduce cell signalling events into remodelling of the actin cytoskeleton and Flii has been proposed to be involved in a variety of signalling pathways, many of which are important in wound healing [74–77]. In addition, Flii binds to proteins other than actin, both in the cytoplasm and in the nucleus as well as outside the cell [76, 77]. It is sequestered in the cytosol by the active form of the calmodulin-dependent protein kinase type II (CaMK-II) protein [76]. Within the nucleus, it binds to a variety of coactivator complexes and to nuclear hormone receptor molecules, thereby mediating changes in transcription [76]. Flii may therefore provide a link between cell signalling pathways and actin-dependent morphogenetic processes including proliferation, migration and adhesion [31, 74].

Flii expression is increased in response to tissue injury in fibroblasts and LPS activation in macrophages [31, 77]. Flii is found in the nucleus, cytosol, lysosomes and like gelsolin is also a secreted protein by both fibroblasts and macrophages through a late endosome/lysosome pathway regulated by Rab7 and Stx11 [5, 77, 78]. Secreted Flii has been detected in human plasma [77], and acute and chronic human wound fluids [78, 79] and this secretion allows it to affect both intracellular and extracellular TLR-mediated signalling and subsequent production of pro-inflammatory cytokines important during wound repair [77]. Like gelsolin, secreted Flii has been shown to inactivate LPS, resulting in decreased TLR activation and downstream inflammation-mediated signalling [77]. In addition, Flii has been shown to control inflammasome activation by way of direct blocking of caspase-1 and caspase-11 and by modulating their subcellular localisation [80]. These findings suggest that Flii upregulation in response to wounding may be directed towards regulating inflammation with unfortunate consequences on healing of wounded area.

Complete knockout of Flii leads to gastrulation failure and embryonic lethality [81], while Flii heterozygous and transgenic mice appear phenotypically normal [82] suggesting an important role in development. In foetal skin, Flii is transiently increased in E17 but not E19 mice skin; however, its expression is downregulated in the E17 keratinocytes immediately adjacent to the wound margin [83] suggesting that temporal regulation of Flii during healing may influence wound repair outcomes. In addition, Flii interaction with tight junction proteins Cld-4 and ZO-2 is instrumental in development of skin barrier function and recovery following injury [84]. Wound healing studies using Flii heterozygous and transgenic mice have demonstrated that reduced Flii expression results in improved rate of healing via effects on cellular migration, adhesion and proliferation [31, 48]. In contrast, Flii transgenic mice have thinner more fragile skin, reduced number of hemidesmosomes and impaired cellular migration and adhesion leading to delayed healing [31, 48]. In addition, studies using mice with an inducible fibroblast specific Flii overexpression have shown inhibited wound healing with larger wounds than non-induced controls, suggesting that fibroblast-derived Flii may have an important role during wound repair [85].

Flii impairs the turnover of focal adhesions via a Rac1-dependant mechanism and Flii interaction with Rac1-interacting proteins may be crucial to its effects on cell migration [74, 86]. In addition, Flii inhibits actin polymerisation [73] and this delicate balance of actin monomers and polymers can be altered using Flii neutralising antibodies (FnAb) raised against LRR domain of Flii [84] affecting collagen contraction, angiogenesis and wound healing outcomes [31, 87, 88].

Topical application of FnAb to wounds in preclinical models of wound repair results in a decreased wound area, a quicker rate of healing and decreased early scar formation [31, 88, 89] (**Figure 6**). Supporting these findings, both in vitro and in vivo studies have demonstrated that Flii plays a role in tissue scarring, collagen deposition and contraction [89, 90]. Using a preclinical model of porcine wound healing, studies have shown that Flii affects collagen I to collagen III ratio, impairs healing and contributes to the formation of early scars [89]. In addition, in vivo studies using human studies and animal models of bleomycin-induced hypertrophic scaring show that Flii-deficient mice exhibit reduced scarring in response to bleomycin as evident by decreased dermal thickness, smaller cross-sectional scar areas, fewer myofibroblast numbers and increased collagen I to collagen III ratios [91]. Use of FnAb in porcine models of wound healing is the first example of using antibodies in large animal in vivo to modify the regulators of actin cytoskeleton that lead to improved wound healing outcomes. No side effects, complications or contraindications were observed when FnAb was administered locally to mouse or pigs suggesting the potential for the development of this therapy for human use. Application of such approaches to regulate different modulators of actin cytoskeleton may therefore lead to novel therapies aimed at optimal tissue regeneration and decreased scar formation following injury.

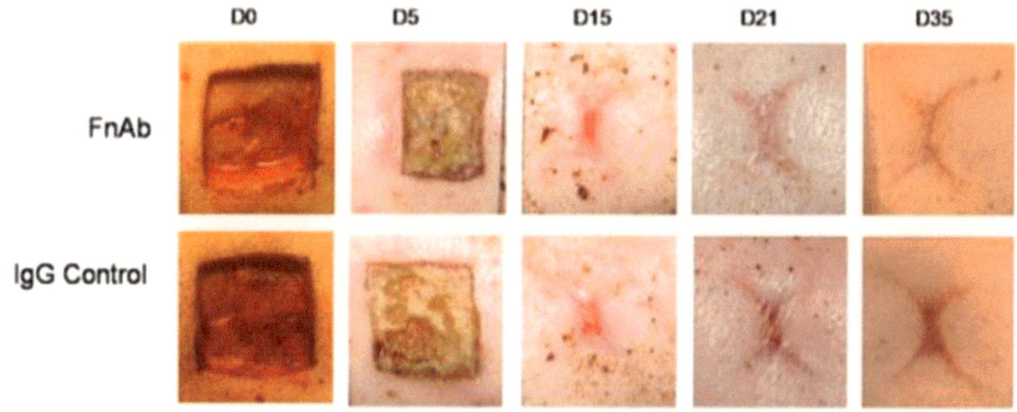

Figure 6. Treatment of excisional wounds with an FnAb improves wound healing and early scar appearance. Representative macroscopic images of wounds treated with either FnAb or a dose-matched IgG control on days 0, 5, 15, 21 and 35. These images were all taken from the same distance. The FnAb- and IgG control-treated wounds are from the same animal and the same position on either flank. Figure adapted from [89] and modified.

7. Conclusion

The actin cytoskeleton is an important regulator of numerous physiological processes that are important for efficient wound healing. Research has identified novel regulators of the actin cytoskeleton that can affect skin cell functions, tissue regeneration and repair. Identifying and understanding the role of the actin cytoskeleton and these regulating proteins will identify how they can affect outcomes of wound repair. The development of new approaches aimed at modulating actin remodelling proteins may therefore hold tremendous promise for therapeutic development and translation into clinical practice.

Author details

Zlatko Kopecki and Allison J Cowin*

*Address all correspondence to: allison.cowin@unisa.edu.au

Future Industries Institute, Regenerative Medicine, University of South Australia, Adelaide, SA, Australia

References

[1] Cairns, N.J., V.M. Lee, and J.Q. Trojanowski, *The cytoskeleton in neurodegenerative diseases*. J Pathol, 2004. 204(4): p. 438-49.

[2] Esue, O., et al., *A direct interaction between actin and vimentin filaments mediated by the tail domain of vimentin*. J Biol Chem, 2006. 281(41): p. 30393-99.

[3] Gurtner, G.C., et al., *Wound repair and regeneration*. Nature, 2008. 453(7193): p. 314-21.

[4] Kubler, M.D. and F.M. Watt, *Changes in the distribution of actin-associated proteins during epidermal wound healing*. J Invest Dermatol, 1993. 100(6): p. 785-89.

[5] Kopecki, Z. and A.J. Cowin, *Flightless I: an actin-remodelling protein and an important negative regulator of wound repair*. Int J Biochem Cell Biol, 2008. 40(8): p. 1415-19.

[6] Lambrechts, A., M. Van Troys, and C. Ampe, *The actin cytoskeleton in normal and pathological cell motility*. Int J Biochem Cell Biol, 2004. 36(10): p. 1890-909.

[7] Hall, A. and C.D. Nobes, *Rho GTPases: molecular switches that control the organization and dynamics of the actin cytoskeleton*. Philos Trans R Soc Lond B Biol Sci, 2000. 355(1399): p. 965-70.

[8] Le Clainche, C. and M.F. Carlier, *Regulation of actin assembly associated with protrusion and adhesion in cell migration*. Physiol Rev, 2008. 88(2): p. 489-513.

[9] Rogers, K.R., C.J. Morris, and D.R. Blake, *The cytoskeleton and its importance as a mediator of inflammation*. Ann Rheum Dis, 1992. 51(4): p. 565-71.

[10] Bazile, F., et al., *Complex relationship between TCTP, microtubules and actin microfilaments regulates cell shape in normal and cancer cells*. Carcinogenesis, 2009. 30(4): p. 555-65.

[11] Goldman, R.D., et al., *Intermediate filaments: versatile building blocks of cell structure*. Curr Opin Cell Biol, 2008. 20(1): p. 28-34.

[12] Naumanen, P., P. Lappalainen, and P. Hotulainen, *Mechanisms of actin stress fibre assembly*. J Microsc, 2008. 231(3): p. 446-54.

[13] Goffin, J.M., et al., *Focal adhesion size controls tension-dependent recruitment of alpha-smooth muscle actin to stress fibers*. J Cell Biol, 2006. 172(2): p. 259-68.

[14] Sens, P. and J. Plastino, *Membrane tension and cytoskeleton organization in cell motility*. J Phys Condens Matter, 2015. 27(27): p. 273103.

[15] Partridge, M.A. and E.E. Marcantonio, *Initiation of attachment and generation of mature focal adhesions by integrin-containing filopodia in cell spreading*. Mol Biol Cell, 2006. 17(10): p. 4237-48.

[16] Small, J.V., et al., *The lamellipodium: where motility begins*. Trends Cell Biol, 2002. 12(3): p. 112-20.

[17] Bershadsky, A.D., et al., *Assembly and mechanosensory function of focal adhesions: experiments and models*. Eur J Cell Biol, 2006. 85(3-4): p. 165-73.

[18] Bach, C.T., et al., *Tropomyosin isoform expression regulates the transition of adhesions to determine cell speed and direction*. Mol Cell Biol, 2009. 29(6): p. 1506-14.

[19] Cowin, A.J., et al., *Differential effect of wounding on actin and its associated proteins, paxillin and gelsolin, in fetal skin explants*. J Invest Dermatol, 2003. 120(6): p. 1118-29.

[20] Jacinto, A., A. Martinez-Arias, and P. Martin, *Mechanisms of epithelial fusion and repair*. Nat Cell Biol, 2001. 3(5): p. E117-23.

[21] Shekhar, S., J. Pernier, and M.F. Carlier, *Regulators of actin filament barbed ends at a glance*. J Cell Sci, 2016. 129(6):1085-91

[22] Carlier, M.F., et al., *Control of polarized assembly of actin filaments in cell motility*. Cell Mol Life Sci, 2015. 72(16): p. 3051-67.

[23] Hiroyasu, S., Z.T. Colburn, and J.C. Jones, *A hemidesmosomal protein regulates actin dynamics and traction forces in motile keratinocytes*. FASEB J, 2016. 30(6):2298-310

[24] Sandbo, N. and N. Dulin, *Actin cytoskeleton in myofibroblast differentiation: ultrastructure defining form and driving function*. Transl Res, 2011. 158(4): p. 181-96.

[25] Hall, A., *Rho GTPases and the actin cytoskeleton*. Science, 1998. 279(5350): p. 509-14.

[26] Conrad, P.A., et al., *Relative distribution of actin, myosin I, and myosin II during the wound healing response of fibroblasts*. J Cell Biol, 1993. 120(6): p. 1381-91.

[27] Matsubayashi, Y., W. Razzell, and P. Martin, *'White wave' analysis of epithelial scratch wound healing reveals how cells mobilise back from the leading edge in a myosin-II-dependent fashion*. J Cell Sci, 2011. 124(Pt 7): p. 1017-21.

[28] Sandbo, N., et al., *Delayed stress fiber formation mediates pulmonary myofibroblast differentiation in response to TGF-beta*. Am J Physiol Lung Cell Mol Physiol, 2011. 301(5): p. L656-66.

[29] Redd, M.J., et al., *Wound healing and inflammation: embryos reveal the way to perfect repair*. Philos Trans R Soc Lond B Biol Sci, 2004. 359(1445): p. 777-84.

[30] Strudwick, X.L. and A.J. Cowin, *Cytoskeletal regulation of dermal regeneration*. Cells, 2012. 1(4): p. 1313-27.

[31] Cowin, A., et al., *Flightless I deficiency enhances wound repair by increasing cell migration and proliferation*. J Pathol, 2007. 211(5): p. 572-81.

[32] Cowin, A.J., *Differential expression of F-actin in in utero fetal wounds*. Eur J Dermatol, 2005. 15(3): p. 133-39.

[33] Yu, H., et al., *The FERM family proteins in cancer invasion and metastasis*. Front Biosci (Landmark Ed), 2011. 16: p. 1536-50.

[34] Bosanquet, D.C., et al., *FERM family proteins and their importance in cellular movements and wound healing (review).* Int J Mol Med, 2014. 34(1): p. 3-12.

[35] Jensen, P.V. and L.I. Larsson, *Actin microdomains on endothelial cells: association with CD44, ERM proteins, and signaling molecules during quiescence and wound healing.* Histochem Cell Biol, 2004. 121(5): p. 361-69.

[36] Ng, T., et al., *Ezrin is a downstream effector of trafficking PKC-integrin complexes involved in the control of cell motility.* EMBO J, 2001. 20(11): p. 2723-41.

[37] Okayama, T., et al., *Attenuated response to liver injury in moesin-deficient mice: impaired stellate cell migration and decreased fibrosis.* Biochim Biophys Acta, 2008. 1782(9): p. 542-48.

[38] McRobert, E.A., et al., *The amino-terminal domains of the ezrin, radixin, and moesin (ERM) proteins bind advanced glycation end products, an interaction that may play a role in the development of diabetic complications.* J Biol Chem, 2003. 278(28): p. 25783-89.

[39] Bouaouina, M., et al., *A conserved lipid-binding loop in the kindlin FERM F1 domain is required for kindlin-mediated alphaIIbbeta3 integrin coactivation.* J Biol Chem, 2012. 287(10): p. 6979-90.

[40] Has, C., *Kindler syndrome. A new bullous dermatosis.* Hautarzt, 2009. 60(8): p. 622-26.

[41] He, Y., et al., *Role of kindlin-2 in fibroblast functions: implications for wound healing.* J Invest Dermatol, 2011. 131(1): p. 245-56.

[42] Karakose, E., H.B. Schiller, and R. Fassler, *The kindlins at a glance.* J Cell Sci, 2010. 123(Pt 14): p. 2353-56.

[43] Song, X., et al., *A novel membrane-dependent on/off switch mechanism of talin FERM domain at sites of cell adhesion.* Cell Res, 2012. 22(11): p. 1533-45.

[44] Balcioglu, H.E., et al., *The integrin expression profile modulates orientation and dynamics of force transmission at cell-matrix adhesions.* J Cell Sci, 2015. 128(7): p. 1316-26.

[45] Wang, J.H., *Pull and push: talin activation for integrin signaling.* Cell Res, 2012. 22(11): p. 1512-14.

[46] Moser, M., et al., *The tail of integrins, talin, and kindlins.* Science, 2009. 324(5929): p. 895-99.

[47] Campbell, I.D. and M.H. Ginsberg, *The talin-tail interaction places integrin activation on FERM ground.* Trends Biochem Sci, 2004. 29(8): p. 429-35.

[48] Kopecki, Z., et al., *Flightless I regulates hemidesmosome formation and integrin-mediated cellular adhesion and migration during wound repair.* J Invest Dermatol, 2009. 129(8): p. 2031-45.

[49] Nakamura, F., T.P. Stossel, and J.H. Hartwig, *The filamins: organizers of cell structure and function.* Cell Adh Migr, 2011. 5(2): p. 160-69.

[50] Sarkisian, M.R., et al., *MEKK4 signaling regulates filamin expression and neuronal migration*. Neuron, 2006. 52(5): p. 789-801.

[51] Pinto, V.I., et al., *Filamin A protects cells against force-induced apoptosis by stabilizing talin- and vinculin-containing cell adhesions*. FASEB J, 2014. 28(1): p. 453-63.

[52] Kim, H., et al., *Filamin A is required for vimentin-mediated cell adhesion and spreading*. Am J Physiol Cell Physiol, 2010. 298(2): p. C221-36.

[53] Gurtner, G.C. and V.W. Wong, *Filamin A mediates wound closure by promoting elastic deformation and maintenance of tension in the collagen matrix*. J Invest Dermatol, 2015. 135(11): p. 2569-71.

[54] Paudyal, P., et al., *Grb7 and Filamin-a associate and are colocalized to cell membrane ruffles upon EGF stimulation*. J Mol Recognit, 2013. 26(11): p. 532-41.

[55] Mohammadi, H., et al., *Filamin A mediates wound closure by promoting elastic deformation and maintenance of tension in the collagen matrix*. J Invest Dermatol, 2015. 135(11): p. 2852-61.

[56] Gunning, P., G. O'Neill, and E. Hardeman, *Tropomyosin-based regulation of the actin cytoskeleton in time and space*. Physiol Rev, 2008. 88(1): p. 1-35.

[57] Lees, J.G., C.T. Bach, and G.M. O'Neill, *Interior decoration: tropomyosin in actin dynamics and cell migration*. Cell Adh Migr, 2011. 5(2): p. 181-86.

[58] Bryce, N.S., et al., *Specification of actin filament function and molecular composition by tropomyosin isoforms*. Mol Biol Cell, 2003. 14(3): p. 1002-16.

[59] Fragiadaki, M., et al., *Hyperglycemia causes renal cell damage via CCN2-induced activation of the TrkA receptor: implications for diabetic nephropathy*. Diabetes, 2012. 61(9): p. 2280-88.

[60] Lees, J.G., et al., *Tropomyosin regulates cell migration during skin wound healing*. J Invest Dermatol, 2013.

[61] Kwiatkowski, D.J., *Functions of gelsolin: motility, signaling, apoptosis, cancer*. Curr Opin Cell Biol, 1999. 11(1): p. 103-8.

[62] Archer, S.K., C. Claudianos, and H.D. Campbell, *Evolution of the gelsolin family of actin-binding proteins as novel transcriptional coactivators*. Bioessays, 2005. 27(4): p. 388-96.

[63] Goshima, M., et al., *Characterization of a novel Ras-binding protein Ce-FLI-1 comprising leucine-rich repeats and gelsolin-like domains*. Biochem Biophys Res Commun, 1999. 257(1): p. 111-16.

[64] Liu, Y.T. and H.L. Yin, *Identification of the binding partners for flightless I, a novel protein bridging the leucine-rich repeat and the gelsolin superfamilies*. J Biol Chem, 1998. 273(14): p. 7920-27.

[65] Sun, H.Q., et al., *Gelsolin, a multifunctional actin regulatory protein*. J Biol Chem, 1999. 274(47): p. 33179-82.

[66] Witke, W., et al., *Comparisons of CapG and gelsolin-null macrophages: demonstration of a unique role for CapG in receptor-mediated ruffling, phagocytosis, and vesicle rocketing*. J Cell Biol, 2001. 154(4): p. 775-84.

[67] Campbell, H.D., et al., *Genomic structure, evolution, and expression of human FLII, a gelsolin and leucine-rich-repeat family member: overlap with LLGL*. Genomics, 1997. 42(1): p. 46-54.

[68] Silacci, P., et al., *Gelsolin superfamily proteins: key regulators of cellular functions*. Cell Mol Life Sci, 2004. 61(19-20): p. 2614-23.

[69] Archer, S.K., et al., *The flightless I protein and the gelsolin family in nuclear hormone receptor-mediated signalling*. Biochem Soc Trans, 2004. 32(Pt 6): p. 940-42.

[70] Arora, P.D., P.A. Janmey, and C.A. McCulloch, *A role for gelsolin in stress fiber-dependent cell contraction*. Exp Cell Res, 1999. 250(1): p. 155-67.

[71] Cowin, A., *Role of actin cytoskeleton in wound healing and scar formation*. Primary Intention: The Australian Journal of Wound Management, 2006. 14: p. 39-42.

[72] Cunningham, C.C., T.P. Stossel, and D.J. Kwiatkowski, *Enhanced motility in NIH 3T3 fibroblasts that overexpress gelsolin*. Science, 1991. 251(4998): p. 1233-36.

[73] Mohammad, I., et al., *Flightless I is a focal adhesion-associated actin-capping protein that regulates cell migration*. FASEB J, 2012. 26(8): p. 3260-72.

[74] Kopecki, Z., et al., *Regulation of focal adhesions by Flightless I involves inhibition of paxillin phosphorylation via a Rac1-dependent pathway*. J Invest Dermatol, 2011. 131(7): p. 1450-59.

[75] Dai, P., et al., *Modulation of TLR signaling by multiple MyD88-interacting partners including leucine-rich repeat Fli-I-interacting proteins*. J Immunol, 2009. 182(6): p. 3450-60.

[76] Lee, Y.H. and M.R. Stallcup, *Interplay of Fli-I and FLAP1 for regulation of beta-catenin dependent transcription*. Nucleic Acids Res, 2006. 34(18): p. 5052-59.

[77] Lei, N., et al., *Flightless, secreted through a late endosome/lysosome pathway, binds LPS and dampens cytokine secretion*. J Cell Sci, 2012. 125(Pt 18): p. 4288-96.

[78] Cowin, A.J., et al., *Lysosomal secretion of Flightless I upon injury has the potential to alter inflammation*. Commun Integr Biol, 2012. 5(6): p. 546-49.

[79] Ruzehaji, N., et al., *Cytoskeletal protein Flightless (Flii) is elevated in chronic and acute human wounds and wound fluid: neutralizing its activity in chronic but not acute wound fluid improves cellular proliferation*. Eur J Dermatol, 2012. 22(6): p. 740-50.

[80] Li, J., H.L. Yin, and J. Yuan, *Flightless-I regulates proinflammatory caspases by selectively modulating intracellular localization and caspase activity*. J Cell Biol, 2008. 181(2): p. 321-33.

[81] Campbell, H.D., et al., *Fliih, a gelsolin-related cytoskeletal regulator essential for early mammalian embryonic development*. Mol Cell Biol, 2002. 22(10): p. 3518-26.

[82] Thomsen, N., et al., *Mouse strains for the ubiquitous or conditional overexpression of the Flii gene*. Genesis, 2011. 49(8): p. 681-88.

[83] Lin, C.H., et al., *Decreased expression of Flightless I, a gelsolin family member and developmental regulator, in early-gestation fetal wounds improves healing*. Mamm Genome, 2011. 22(5-6): p. 341-52.

[84] Kopecki, Z., et al., *Flightless I over-expression impairs skin barrier development, function and recovery following skin blistering*. J Pathol, 2014. 232(5): p. 541-52.

[85] Turner, C.T., et al., *Fibroblast-specific upregulation of Flightless I impairs wound healing*. Exp Dermatol, 2015. 24(9): p. 692-97.

[86] Marei, H., et al., *Differential Rac1 signalling by guanine nucleotide exchange factors implicates FLII in regulating Rac1-driven cell migration*. Nat Commun, 2016. 7: p. 10664.

[87] Ruzehaji, N., et al., *Attenuation of flightless I improves wound healing and enhances angiogenesis in a murine model of type 1 diabetes*. Diabetologia, 2014. 57(2): p. 402-12.

[88] Kopecki, Z., et al., *Topically applied Flightless I neutralizing antibodies improve healing of blistered skin in a murine model of epidermolysis Bullosa Acquisita*. J Invest Dermatol, 2012. 133(4):1008-16

[89] Jackson, J.E., et al., *Flii neutralizing antibodies improve wound healing in porcine preclinical studies*. Wound Repair Regen, 2012. 20(4): p. 523-36.

[90] Kopecki, Z., et al., *Overexpression of the Flii gene increases dermal-epidermal blistering in an autoimmune ColVII mouse model of epidermolysis bullosa acquisita*. J Pathol, 2011. 225(3): p. 401-13.

[91] Cameron, A.M., et al., *Flightless I is a key regulator of the fibroproliferative process in hypertrophic scarring and a target for a novel anti-scarring therapy*. Br J Dermatol, 2015. 225(3):401-13

Chapter 7

Regenerative Approaches in Wound Healing: New Alternatives for Older Tools

Michele R Colonna, Lupo Flavia, Delia Gabriele and Stagno d'Alcontres Francesco

Additional information is available at the end of the chapter

http://dx.doi.org/10.5772/64133

Abstract

Critical wounds are well known to develop in elderly people and in other conditions where inflammation, vascular, and nervous disease lead to chronical inefficiency in running up healing processes. Recent researches have been focusing on microenvironment, and specific technologies have contributed to design and produce new materials (the era of biomaterials and devices in wound healing).

At present, regenerative medicine and surgery have introduced a new approach, based on cells' transplantation producing specific cytokines and stimulating healing. This is the role played by fat transplantation combining both stromal and vascular cellular progenitor lines, monocyte products, platelet-rich plasma, and glues.

New tools, such as templates and materials (comprising micro- and nanoparticles), as well as technologies, such as cell seeding and gene therapy, revealed promising in this direction. The authors report their experimental evidences and clinical experiences with lipografting and peripheral blood mononuclear cells in critical wounds, focusing on how to treat monocyte/macrophage cell depletion as well as insufficient vascular supply.

Keywords: adipose-derived stem cells, angiogenesis, difficult wounds, lipografting, monocytes, vascular supply

1. Introduction

Wound healing is a highly structured physiological process involving cells and signal molecules; it is known to run throughout inflammation, cell proliferation, angiogenesis, collagen deposition, and re-epithelization [1]. In the very first steps, natural immunity [2] plays an important role through aggregation of inflammasomes. The next step goes through inflammatory cell types, and messages from the first to this step together with monocyte responsivity are able to determine whether inflammation will prolong to a sort of a steady, chronically established state, which freezes the whole process transforming it into a chronic inflammation [2–6].

Monocyte/macrophage sequestration together with their lack of switch to type 2 [3, 4, 6] impairs angiogenesis and cell activities resulting in a delayed re-epithelialization, reduced call for fibroblasts and diminishing collagen deposition, as well as a decreased cell proliferation.

The aim of this chapter is to report our experience on how to modify impaired wound healing, starting from our experimental studies and concluding with our recent clinical experiences.

2. Pathophysiology

Following our studies [2] and those by Mirza et al. [4, 5], we started to focus on the role of accumulation and insufficiency of macrophages in wound healing. Macrophage dysfunction has been shown to produce prolonged inflammatory responses in critical wounds, in diabetes through local secretion of proinflammatory cytokines, such as IL-1β, TNF-α, MMP-9, and IL-6, in particular, lack of switch to a second macrophage phenotype secreting proregenerative factors, such as IL-10, IGF-1, and TGF-β [6].

The result is an important interruption of healing with persistence of inflammation, whether hyperglycemia through cascade of ROS is its cause or not.

This produces critical wounds. Obviously, single biological steps can be analyzed in experimental studies, whereas in clinical practice this single factor must often be added to other associated diseases, such as reduction of blood supply due to vascular obstruction. In the latter case, translation from experimental to clinical work must also take into account adding proangiogenetic factors even to provide a complete care.

Our clinical experience deals with persistence of inflammation through both monocyte and vascular insufficiency.

2.1. Our experimental studies on wound healing

In this section, we report our experimental evidences leading to the results about the above-mentioned inflammasome inhibition [2]. Plastic surgeons together with pharmacologists of the University of Messina have been working on wound healing for more than 15 years developing some models on rodents.

2.1.1. Animals

For these experiments adult male mice have been chosen, caged alone, and maintained under a controlled environment (12-hour light cycles day/night and 23°C room temperature, food, and water ad libitum) following Helsinki's declaration and European and Italian laws and Guidelines for Animal Laboratory Experiments.

Animals aging 8 weeks and weighing 20–25 g were used.

2.2. Model of incisional wound healing

The animals (mice) underwent general anesthesia with sodium thiopental (80 mg/kg intraperitoneal injection) were scrubbed with iodine povidone on their back – their back skin shaved and rinsed with physiological serum. Two longitudinal parallel 4 cm incisions were performed and sutured with alternate stitches placed 1 cm from one another.

Sacrifices were conducted on Days 7 and 14, respectively, and wounds were divided into three segments of 80 mm large and 120 mm long. Caudal and cranial strips were used for molecular studies, whereas the central one was used for histology and immunohistochemistry.

2.3. Model of dorsal skin flap

"Double H" flaps were described following Quirinia et al.'s classification: this model was modified and adopted [7, 8].

The animals (mice) underwent general anesthesia with sodium thiopental (80 mg/kg intraperitoneal injection) were scrubbed with iodine povidone on their back – their back skin shaved and rinsed with physiological serum. Double H flap consists of two opposite flaps: the former pedicled from the cranial side and the latter from the caudal one, both to be incised and elevated on the dorsal skin. The central horizontal wound together with the two distal parts of the flaps acts as critical ischemia-risk area. The flaps were sutured back with separate stitches in Nylon 4/0. The animals were divided into three groups and sacrifices were performed on Days 3, 6, and 12, respectively. As for incisional wounds, three flap segments were taken and processed the cranial and distal one for molecular essays, the central one for histology and immunocytochemistry

2.4. Model of burn injury

Under the same anesthesia and dorsum preparation described above, the dorsum of mice was immersed in an 80°C bath for 10 seconds to produce a scald burn. Fluid resuscitation was achieved through a subcutaneous 1 mL saline injection, treated with different agents (last used EPO Z in comparison with EPO alpha), divided into three groups, and sacrificed on Days 3, 6, and 12, respectively. Burned skin has been divided into two flaps that have been, respectively, used for molecular essays and histology.

Molecular essays are consisted in cytoplasmic protein dosage (Bio-Rad Protein Assay (Bio-Rad Lab, Richmond, CA, USA), spectrophotometry, using albumin as a standard); Western blot for GFs and cell cycle molecules; histology measured the presence of inflammatory infiltrates, necrosis, and repair in standard hematoxylin (eosin, trichromic, and immunohistochemistry were used to visualize and quantify alpha-smooth positive cells such as a response to VEGF in both neoangiogenesis and neovasculogenesis).

Statistical analysis was conducted with parametric essays for repeated measures (ANOVA) and bonferroni test was used to evaluate intergroup positivity, with a *p* ¼ 0.05 considered as statistically significant.

Our experimental studies have pointed out some important features of antioxidant molecules in impaired wound healing (diabetic mice), as well as the role of some cytokine-related molecules and endogenous products belonging to natural immunity cascade [2] in normal and impaired wound healing [9–13].

2.5. Another important contribution to the study of neoangiogenesis and biomaterials prefabrication

Our group also developed a collaboration with the group from Padriciano, International Center for Genetic Engineering and Biology, United Nations, to study a model of prefabricated flap in the groin of adult rats creating an artero-venus loop that was included into a dermal regenerative template; this new regeneration chamber was then injected with different viral vectors (AAV 156) encoding for the production of VEGF. Results were remarkable, demonstrating enhancement of neoangiogenesis and neovasculogenesis and the utility of this novel model of regeneration chamber that could act as a bioreactor and stimulate healing and even repair poor vascularized tissues [14, 15].

3. Clinical experiences

Chronic wounds are produced either by an interruption in healing processes, as an effect of lack of positive (vascular supply and neurotrophism) or of an excess of inhibitory factors (metallo proteinases in ECM, some cytokines), or by a lack of switch in inflammatory cell phenotypes, such as in diabetes.

As a final effect, wound bed does not progress beyond detersion, typically presenting itself as necrosis or debris. They are especially present in lower limbs, often as a result of complex mix of the above-mentioned factors.

Vascular and diabetic ulcers are the most common chronic wounds affecting nearly 2–5% of the general population and have received an important impact in terms of morbidity, absence from work, and social costs.

Traditional wound dressings do not restore vascular supply, which is a *sine qua non* for restarting healing.

An important role is played by vascular surgery and endovascular techniques, which act restoring the lost vascular supply or producing bypasses to revascularize the area.

At present, some novel suggestions come from regenerative surgery.

3.1. Lipograft in chronic wounds

The target is endothelial insufficiency, as documented in diabetes and vascular obstructive diseases.

It consists of poor endothelial progenitor cell mobilization and homing, with altered levels of the chemokine stromal-derived factor-1 (SDF-1) at the wound site [2, 6, 16].

The use of tissue engineering techniques such as stem-cell therapy and gene therapy to improve wound healing has proved a promising strategy [14, 15].

A well-established clinical experience with lipografting has been obtained in the early years of this century, especially in scar treatment after important fibrotic status, such as in postburn scars and in postradiation mastectomy scars [17, 18].

Since 2001, Zuk et al. documented that lipoaspirate from adipose tissue represents a source of adipose tissue-derived stem cells, which are adult mesenchymal stem cells [19].

Starting from the first regenerative approach with lipografting on fibrotic tissues, its role has been expanded to chronic wounds, applying as a rationale, and has the potential to induce angiogenesis and regeneration. The potential of ADSCs to differentiate into adipocytes, osteoblasts, chondrocytes, cardiomiocytes, and endothelial cells, in vitro and in vivo, was shown by several authors. In particular, ADSCs are able to express endothelial markers when cultured in the presence of VEGF.

The stimulatory effect of ADSC on cutaneous wound healing may be partially mediated by paracrine effects of ADSCs on other skin cells [20–27].

Application of ADSCs or ADSC-derived molecules could be an innovative therapeutic approach in the treatment of chronic wounds and other conditions; it has been proposed in association with platelet-rich plasma [28] or under particular conditions [29].

3.1.1. Procedure

The surgical procedure was performed under local anesthesia together with midazolam medication (see below). The periumbilical area and the hip were the preferred donor site because of the good quantity and quality of dermal fat graft.

With the patient in supine position, the donor area was infiltrated with 250 cc of saline solution (NaCl 0.9%), 0.5 cc adrenalin 1/1000, 10 cc of lidocain 2%, and 10 cc ropivacain 7.5%; the incision to introduce the cannula was made with a no. 11 scalpel (**Figure 1**).

Adipose tissue was harvested through the same incision by a blunt 2 mm cannula connected to a Luer-Lock syringe of 10 cc, a small amount of aspirate (about 10 cc) was sufficient.

The full syringe was placed into a sterile cup and washed with NaCl 0.9% to remove the anesthetic solution.

The authors used Coleman's technique and centrifuged the fat (3000 rpm for 3 minutes) to separate cellular blood components with infiltration solution, adipocytes with vascular stromal tissue and oil derived from the breakdown of fat cells.

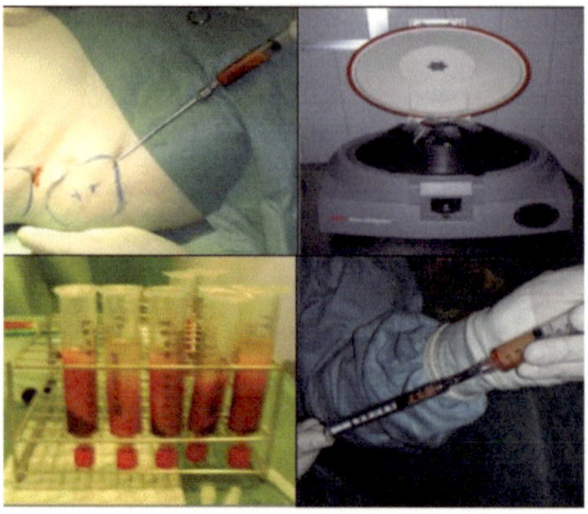

Figure 1. Lipoaspirate procedure: ADSC and VASF harvesting, centrifuge and its products on the aspirate, and harvesting of the lipograft to be implanted.

The adipose-stromal fraction was transferred from a 10 cc syringe to a 1 mL Luer-Lock syringe to allow a precise control of the amount of injected fat (**Figure 1**).

The adipose tissue fraction was then implanted with gentle care; small "pearls" of adipose tissue were placed at the dermal-hypodermal junction in the ulcer's edges and into the wound bed. Many radiating passages were made through the same incision, to place fat in different directions.

The access incisions in the donor areas were sutured with Nylon 5/0.

The treated area after surgical procedure was covered with non-adherent gauze, whereas an elastic adhesive bandage was applied to the fat donor site to prevent hematomas and seromas.

A second grafting session was performed, if needed, 3 months later.

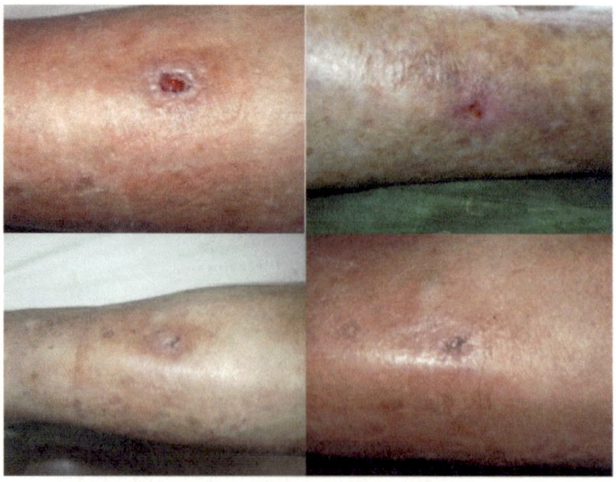

Figure 2. Chronic ulcers: before and after treatment with ADSCs.

Four patients were treated, wound closure occurred in approximately 17 days (**Figures 2** and **3**).

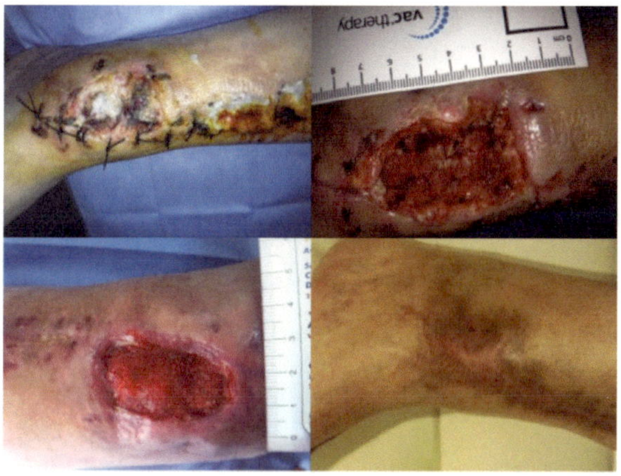

Figure 3. Lipografting in chronic posttraumatic wound in a diabetic patient. Two sessions were needed to obtain a complete closure.

3.2. Mononuclear cells in chronic wounds

Cell therapy is an innovative and promising approach for regeneration of damaged tissues. In particular, new scientific evidence shows that the total mononuclears from peripheral blood are cells with high angiogenic and vasculogenic capacity and, in general, in tissue regeneration processes.

Patients with CLI, who suffer from rest pain, nonhealing ischemic ulcers, or necrosis (Fontaine 3–4), rarely respond to standard therapy as drug therapy (e.g., prostaglandin and anticoagulant, etc.) and surgical revascularization.

The autologous transplantation of peripheral blood mononuclear cells (PBMNCs) can produce tissue regeneration and improve physiological healing process through their paracrine action, consisting in production of cytokines, especially VEGF and bFGF.

The monocells have three principal roles:

– progenitors of multipotent cells,

– angiogenesis and vasculogenesis, and

– anti-inflammatory.

The PBMNCs isolated from peripheral blood have the same differentiating and regenerating capacities as the bone marrow mononuclear cells (BMMNCs), but their isolation is simpler and minimally invasive.

Monocytes and macrophages are capable of producing a large variety of growth factors, metalloproteinases, chemokines, and vasoactive substances such as nitric oxide; all can facilitate angiogenesis and arteriogenesis [30–34].

Angiogenesis is characterized by capillary sprouting, endothelial cell migration, proliferation, and luminogenesis to generate new capillaries [14, 32–34].

Arteriogenesis is a positive remodeling of preexisting collateral channels in the limb, as the product of endothelial factors, as well as of infiltrating macrophages [15, 32–34].

During chronic inflammation, macrophages/monocells are polarized in the antimicrobial form (M1), or in the regenerative form (M2). The implantation of concentrated PBMNCs in this condition can address M1 to M2 promoting the regenerative form.

The autologous transplantation of PBMNCs can be considered a valid and safe treatment option for patients with critical wounds [30–34].

3.2.1. Procedure

In the theater, under sedation and local anesthesia of the patient, 120 mL of peripheral venous blood was drawn and added to 12 mL of ACD-A (anticoagulant by apheresis). This was then processed by the WB Pall Celeris system to obtain 12 mL of concentrated PBMNCs (**Figure 4**).

The concentrated PBMNCs were transferred to a 1 mL Luer-Lock syringe to allow a precise control during injection (**Figure 4**).

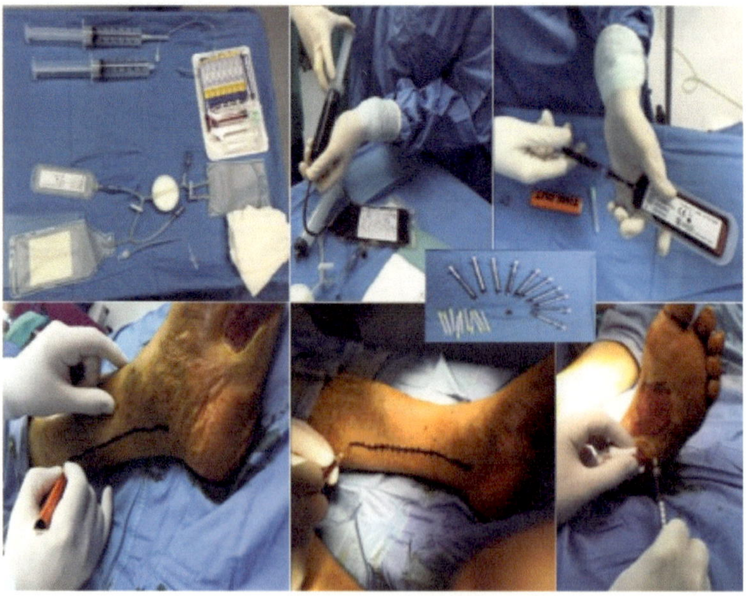

Figure 4. Mononuclear cells preparation procedure: 120 mL of peripheral venous are processed by the WB Pall Celeris system to obtain 12 mL of concentrated PBMNCs, and the posterior tibial axis is traced and the injection performed.

After an appropriate surgical cleansing of the wound bed, the concentrate was implanted into the perilesional area in a single-stage procedure with multiple local subcutaneous perilesional and intralesional injections and intramuscular injections.

The suspension was placed along the relevant damaged vascular axis too, at intervals of 1–2 cm and at a mean depth of 1.5–2 cm, using a 21G needle (**Figure 4**).

After the A-PBMNCs implant, the wound was always covered with hyaluronic acid monolayer.

This treatment was repeated three times, once a month for three months (**Figure 5**).

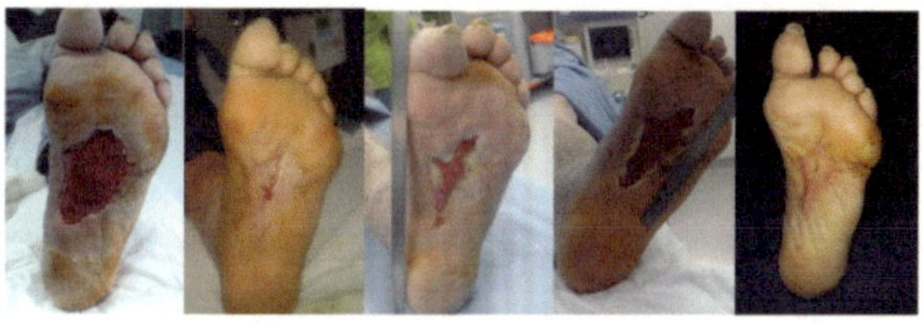

Figure 5. PBMNC injections were repeated three times, once a month for three months, and a complete healing was registered.

One month after the first treatment, the size of the ulcers of all patients were significantly reduced. At the end of the third session, ulcers seemed totally healed, the skin overlying the wound appeared perfectly normal, and the skin complexion was ruddy (**Figure 5**).

Because of their early capability to stimulate vascular ingrowth, monocell implant can be used in one step only to prepare wound bed to receive an autologous skin graft (**Figure 6**).

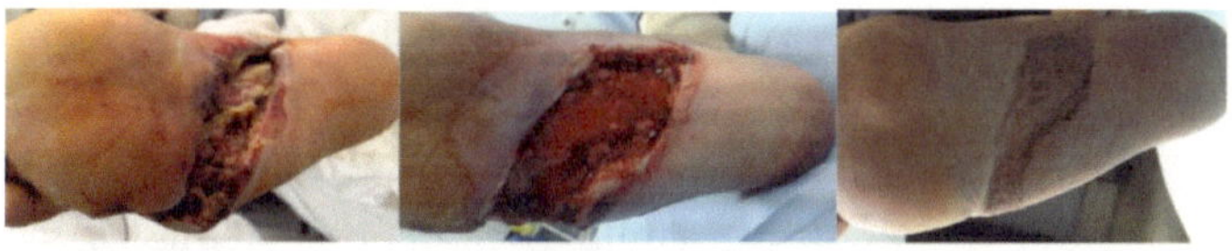

Figure 6. Monocell implants can be used in one step only to prepare wound bed to receive an autologous skin graft. In this case, a severe necrosis of the midplantar skin was excised and PBMNCs injected. A well-vascularized granulation tissue was appreciated in 12 days, allowing repair with a split thickness skin graft in this nonweight bearing area.

Author details

Michele R Colonna*, Lupo Flavia, Delia Gabriele and Stagno d'Alcontres Francesco

*Address all correspondence to: mrcolonna1@gmail.com

Department of Human Pathology and the Child's and Adolescent's Diseases, University of Messina, Messina, Italy

References

[1] Falanga V. Wound healing and its impairment in the diabetic foot. Lancet. 2005;366(9498):1736–43.

[2] Bitto A, Altavilla D, Pizzino G, Irrera N, Pallio G, Colonna MR, Squadrito F. Inhibition of inflammasome activation improves the impaired pattern of healing in genetically diabetic mice. Br J Pharmacol. 2014;171(9):2300–7. doi: 10.1111/bph.12557.

[3] Salazar JJ, Ennis WJ, Koh TJ. Diabetes medications: impact on inflammation and wound healing. J Diabetes Complications. 2015. pii:S1056-8727(15)00506-1. doi: 10.1016/j.jdiacomp.2015.12.017.

[4] Mirza RE, Fang MM, Weinheimer-Haus EM, Ennis WJ, Koh TJ. Sustained inflammasome activity in macrophages impairs wound healing in type 2 diabetic humans and mice. Diabetes. 2014;63(3):1103–14. doi: 10.2337/db13-0927.

[5] Weinheimer-Haus EM, Mirza RE, Koh TJ. Nod-like receptor protein-3 inflammasome plays an important role during early stages of wound healing. PLoS One. 2015;10(3):e0119106. doi: 0.1371/journal.pone.0119106.

[6] Koh TJ, Novak ML, Mirza RE. Assessing macrophage phenotype during tissue repair. Methods Mol Biol. 2013;1037:507–18. doi: 10.1007/978-1-62703-505-7_30.

[7] Quirinia A, Jensen FT, Viidik A. Ischemia in wound healing. I: Design of a flap model —changes in blood flow. Scand J Plast Reconstr Surg Hand Surg. 1992;26:21–8.

[8] Quirinia A, Viidik A. Ischemia in wound healing. II: Design of a flap model—biochemical properties. Scand J Plast Reconstr Surg Hand Surg. 1992;26:133–9.

[9] Irrera N, Bitto A, Pizzino G, Vaccaro M, Squadrito F, Galeano M, Stagno d'Alcontres F, Stagno d'Alcontres F, Buemi M, Minutoli L, Colonna MR, Altavilla D. Epoetin alpha and epoetin zeta: a comparative study on stimulation of angiogenesis and wound repair in an experimental model of burn injury. Biomed Res Int. 2015;2015:968927. doi: 10.1155/2015/968927.

[10] Altavilla D, Galeano M, Bitto A, Minutoli L, Squadrito G, Seminara P, Venuti FS, Torre V, Calò M,Colonna M, Lo Cascio P, Giugliano G, Scuderi N, Mioni C, Leone S, Squadrito F. Lipid peroxidation inhibition by raxofelast improves angiogenesis and wound healing in experimental burn wounds. Shock. 2005;24(1):85–91.

[11] Galeano M, Deodato B, Altavilla D, Squadrito G, Seminara P, Marini H, Stagno d'Alcontres F, Colonna M, Calò M, Lo Cascio P, Torre V, Giacca M, Venuti FS, Squadrito F. Effect of recombinant adeno-associated virus vector-mediated vascular endothelial growth factor gene transfer on wound healing after burn injury. Crit Care Med. 2003;31(4):1017–25.

[12] Galeano M, Torre V, Deodato B, Campo GM, Colonna M, Sturiale A, Squadrito F, Cavallari V, Cucinotta D, Buemi M, Altavilla D. Raxofelast, a hydrophilic vitamin E-

like antioxidant, stimulates wound healing in genetically diabetic mice. Surgery. 2001;129(4):467–77.

[13] Altavilla D, Saitta A, Cucinotta D, Galeano M, Deodato B, Colonna M, Torre V, Russo G, Sardella A, Urna G, Campo GM, Cavallari V, Squadrito G, Squadrito F. Inhibition of lipid peroxidation restores impaired vascular endothelial growth factor expression and stimulates wound healing and angiogenesis in the genetically diabetic mouse. Diabetes. 2001;50(3):667–74.

[14] Manasseri B, Cuccia G, Moimas S, D'Alcontres FS, Polito F, Bitto A, Altavilla D, Squadrito F, Geuna S, Pattarini L, Zentilin L, Collesi C, Puligadda U, Giacca M, Colonna MR. Microsurgical arterovenous loops and biological templates: a novel in vivo chamber for tissue engineering. Microsurgery. 2007;27(7):623–9.

[15] Moimas S, Manasseri B, Cuccia G, Stagno d'Alcontres F, Geuna S, Pattarini L, Zentilin L, Giacca M, Colonna MR. AAV vector encoding human VEGF165-transduced pectineus muscular flaps increase the formation of new tissue through induction of angiogenesis in an in vivo chamber for tissue engineering: a technique to enhance tissue and vessels in microsurgically engineered tissue. J Tissue Eng. 2015;6. doi: 10.1177/2041731415611717. eCollection 2015 Jan–Dec.

[16] Di Rocco G, Gentile A, Antonini A, Ceradini F, Wu JC, Capogrossi MC, Toietta G. Enhanced healing of diabetic wounds by topical administration of adipose tissue-derived stromal cells overexpressing stromal-derived factor-1: biodistribution and engraftment analysis by bioluminescent imaging. Stem Cells Int. 2010;2011:304562.

[17] Caviggioli F, Klinger FM, Vinci V, Cornegliani G, Klinger M. Treatment of Chronic Posttraumatic Leg Injury Using Autologous Fat Graft, Case Reports in Medicine, Volume 2012, Hindawi Publishing Corporation, Article ID 648683, 4 pp.

[18] Klinger M, Caviggioli F, Vinci V, Salval A, Villani F. Treatment of chronic posttraumatic ulcers using autologous fat graft. Plast Reconstr Surg. 2010;126(3):154e–5e.

[19] Zuk PA, Zhu M, Mizuno H, Huang J, Futrell JW, Katz AJ, Benhaim P, Lorenz HP, Hedrick MH. Multilineage cells from human adipose tissue: implications for cell-based therapies. Tissue Eng. 2001;7(2):211–28.

[20] Miranville A, Heeschen C, Sengenès C, Curat CA, Busse R, Bouloumié A. Improvement of postnatal neovascularization by human adipose tissue-derived stem cells. Circulation. 2004;110(3):349–55.

[21] Coleman SR, Mazzola R. Fat injection from filling to regeneration. QMP Missouri. 2009.

[22] Coleman SR. Structural fat graft: more than permanent filler. Plastic Reconstr Surg. 2006;118(3 Suppl):108S–20S.

[23] Seung HL, Sang YJ, Jin SS, Kyle KS, Kwang HC. Paracrine effects of adipose-derived stem cells on keratinocytes and dermal fibroblasts. Ann Dermatol. 2012;24(2):136–43.

[24] Akita S, Yoshimoto H, Ohtsuru A, Hirano A, Yamashita S. Autologous adipose-derived regenerative cells are effective for chronic intractable radiation injuries. Radiat Prot Dosimetry. 2012;151(4):656–60.

[25] Akita S, Yoshimoto H, Akino K, Ohtsuru A, Hayashida K, Hirano A, Suzuki K, Yamashita S. Early experiences with stem cells in treating chronic wounds. Clin Plast Surg. 2012;39(3):281–92.

[26] Lee SH, Jin SY, Song JS, Seo KK, Cho KH. Paracrine effects of adipose-derived stem cells on keratinocytes and dermal fibroblasts. Ann Dermatol. 2012;24(2):136–43.

[27] Tabit CJ, Slack GC, Fan K, Wan DC, Bradley JP. Fat grafting versus adipose-derived stem cell therapy: distinguishing indications, techniques, and outcomes. Aesthetic Plast Surg. 2012;36(3):704–13.

[28] Cervelli V, Gentile P, Grimaldi M. Regenerative surgery: use of fat grafting combined with platelet-rich plasma for chronic lower-extremity ulcers. Aesthetic Plast Surg. 2009 May;33(3):340–5.

[29] Waniczek D, Mikusek W, Kamiński T, Wesecki M, Lorenc Z, Cieślik-Bielecka A. The "biological chamber" method—use of autologous platelet-rich plasma (PRP) in the treatment of poorly healing lower-leg ulcers of venous origin. Pol Przegl Chir. 2015;87(6):283–9. doi: 10.1515/pjs-2015-0055.

[30] Nuschke A. Activity of mesenchymal stem cells in therapies for chronic skin wound healing. Organogenesis. 2014;10(1):29–37. Published online 2013 December.

[31] Michael BD, Amil AJ, Ambalangodage CJ. Current wound healing procedures and potential care. Mater Sci Eng C Mater Biol Appl. 2015;48:651–62.

[32] Strong AL, Bowles AC, MacCrimmon CP, Frazier TP, Lee SJ, Xiying Wu, Katz AJ, Gawronska-Kozak B, Bunnell BA, Gimble JM. Stem Cells Transl Med. 2015;4(6):632–42.

[33] Spalto G, Straino S, Gambini G, Bassetti B, Persico L, Zoli S, Zanobini M, Capogrossi MC, Spirito R, Quarti C, Pompilio G. Characterization of the pall celeris system as a point-of-care device for therapeutic angiogenesis. Cytotherapy. 2015;17:1302–13.

[34] De Angelis B, Gentile P, Orlandi F, Bocchini I, Di Pasquali C, Agovino A, Gizzi C, Patrizi F, Scioli MG, Orlandi A, Cervelli V. Limb rescue: a new autologous-peripheral blood mononuclear cells technology in critical limb ischemia and chronic ulcers. Tissue Engineering: Part C. 2015;21.

Chapter 8

Polarisation of Macrophage and Immunotherapy in the Wound Healing

Yu-Sheng Wu, Fan-Hua Nan, Sherwin Chen and Shiu-Nan Chen

Additional information is available at the end of the chapter

http://dx.doi.org/10.5772/63478

Abstract

Immune cells are involved in virtually every aspect of the wound repair process, from the initial stages where they participate in haemostasis and work to prevent infection to later stages where they drive scar formation. Immunotherapy is being developed offers some advantageous immunomodulation factors that are known in the field of alternative medicine, such as mushroom beta-glucan, anti-microbial peptides and triterpenoid; these factors represent a novel therapeutic approach for anti-inflammation to promote the wound healing.

Keywords: healing, immunotherapy, inflammation, macrophage, polarisation, wound

1. Inflammation

When an organism is injured by a wound injury or infected by a pathogen, inflammation is a crucial response. Inflammation is a complex interaction with molecular mediators; it includes the function of immune cells in a microenvironment through a response that occurs at all levels of biological organisation [1]. Following previous studies, this paper illustrates that the inflammation response involves cooperation between cells and a wide range of mediators, such as cytokines, chemokines and non-enzyme factors involved in the classical immune response. The macrophage is one of the critical inflammatory immune cells involved in the uptake and degradation of infectious agents and senescent cells and also plays critical roles in tissue growth, tissue remodelling and inflammation by producing oxidants, proteinases and anti-microbial peptides [2–4]. Activated inflammatory cells are sources of reactive oxygen species (ROS) and reactive nitrogen species (RNS) that can initiate changes in cell functions, including cell signalling pathways, transcription factor activation, mediator release and apoptosis. However, whether the ROS and RNS that are produced and released by neutrophils or macrophages are sufficient to diffuse through the extra-cellular matrix, enter epithelial cells and cross the cytoplasm is not clear [5–7]. Even the physiological roles of ROS and RNS in the cellular response are not clear [8–11]. The results obtained from experiments performed on the livers of tilapia showed that extra-cellular hydrogen peroxide (H_2O_2) attracted cell migration. These results suggested that ROS is a crucial factor in initiating the migration of macrophages that trigger cascades of phagocytic activity.

In the microenvironment of inflammation, the platelet-derived growth factor (PDGF), the tumour necrosis factors (TNF)-α and TNF-β, the hepatocyte growth factor, transforming growth factor (TGF)-β2, the epidermal growth factor (EGF) and the fibroblast growth factor all play an important role in physiological immune response. The interleukins (IL)-1, IL-6, IL-8, IL-10, and the interferon gamma (INF-γ) also detain key functions in the natural inflammatory response [12–16]. These factors hold a primordial function in fibroblast activation and regulation, also concerning reactive fibrosis that follows their continuing activation. Although these growth factors are also related to fibroblast migration and activation, particular research was recently focused on the PDGF family of growth factors and their relative receptors [17, 18]. Research has documented that PDGF exerts autocrine, mitogenic effects on keratinocytes to support epidermal proliferation and stabilisation of the epidermal junction during wound closure. In addition, it stimulates vessel maturation by recruiting and differentiating pericytes to the immature-endothelial channel [19–22]. According to these references, we investigate whether the produced ROS/RNS is related to the released factors and (if so) what type of relationship exists among ROS/RNS and these factors.

2. Reactive oxygen species production and physical response

The production and scavenging of ROS may be initiated by adverse environmental factors. Research has shown that intra-cellular levels of ROS may rapidly rise and ROS may be generated by the activation of various oxidases and peroxidases in response to certain environmental changes [23]. ROS forms through energy transfer or through electron transfer reactions. ROS formation causes the formation of singlet oxygen, which results in sequential reduction to superoxide, H_2O_2 and hydroxyl radicals [24]. Mitochondria are a crucial source of ROS production in most cells. This ROS production contributes to mitochondrial stress and plays a critical role in redox signalling from the organelles [25]. Mitochondria have a 4-layer structure composed of the outer mitochondrial membrane, intermembrane space, inner mitochondrial membrane and matrix [26]. NADPH oxidase is an enzymatic source in the mitochondrial structure that generates ROS and plays a fundamental role in maintaining normal cell functions. Recent research has focussed on the influence of this enzyme to cellular oxidative stress that may contribute to various pathophysiological conditions and diseases [27, 28]. A crucial function of NADPH oxidase is modulating multiple redox-sensitive intra-cellular signalling pathways; NADPH modulates these pathways by generating ROS molecules, inhibiting protein tyrosine phosphatases and activating certain redox-sensitive transcription factors. Moreover, the ROS consist of numerous molecular species, including H_2O_2, oxide ions (O_2) and hydroxide (OH^-) [29]. Molecular oxygen is a biradical, containing two unpaired electrons in the outer structure; because these two electrons have the same spin, oxygen can only react with one electron; therefore it is not very reactive when these two electrons have the same spin. Oxygen's unpaired electrons can become excited and can change the spin of one electron. This transforms oxygen into a powerful oxidant because the two electrons with opposing spins can rapidly react with other pairs of electrons [30]. Electrons can be contributed from NADH and FADH2 enzymes and can pass through the electron transport chain, generating superoxide (O_2^-) at complexes I and III. This generated superoxide can be reduced to H_2O_2 by superoxide dismutase and can be completely reduced into water by glutathione peroxidase, as presented in **Figure 1**.

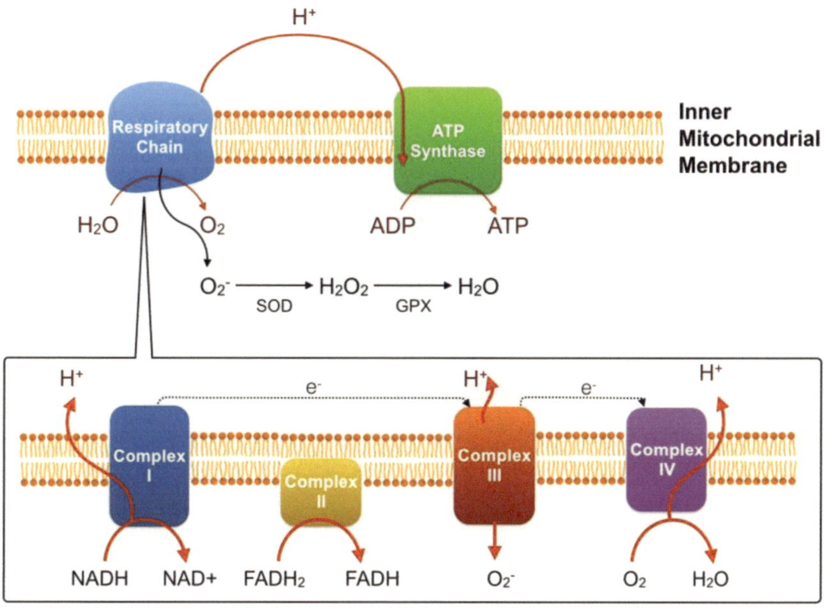

Figure 1. ROS are produced from the electron transport pathway to form superoxide (O_2^-) at complex I and complex III released into the matrix and reduced O_2 to form H_2O at complex IV. Following, the generated O_2^- is transferred to the form of H_2O_2 by superoxide dismutase (SOD) and completely reduced to water (H_2O) by glutathione peroxidase (GPX).

Research has shown that ROS consist of numerous molecular species, including H_2O_2, oxide ions (O_2^-) and OH^{-29}. These molecular species act as signalling molecules in the migration of profibrogenic cells [31] and peripheral blood monocytes [23, 32]. One of the crucial physiological functions of ROS is the modulation of ion channels. Research has illustrated that ROS may act through Ca^{2+} as an intra-cellular second messenger involved in regulating diverse functions, such as fertilisation, electrical signalling, contraction, secretion, memory, gene transcription and cell death [33, 34]. Furthermore, studies have reported that H_2O_2 may affect cell energy stores [35], induce DNA strand breaks [36], enhance cell adhesion [37], increase endothelial tissue permeability [38] and stimulate the release of cytokines.

In the research presented in **Figure 2**, the concentration of ROS seems to be considered the concentration of a crucial signalling molecule. Low concentrations of generated ROS are believed to be critical for metabolic adaptation in the organelle. Moderate concentrations of ROS can be produced and released by stress; pathogen-infected and bacterial endotoxin lipopolysaccharide (LPS) are involved in the inflammatory response. The high concentration of ROS in the induced apoptosis/autophagy process can cause cell death [39] and initiate self-healing [40].

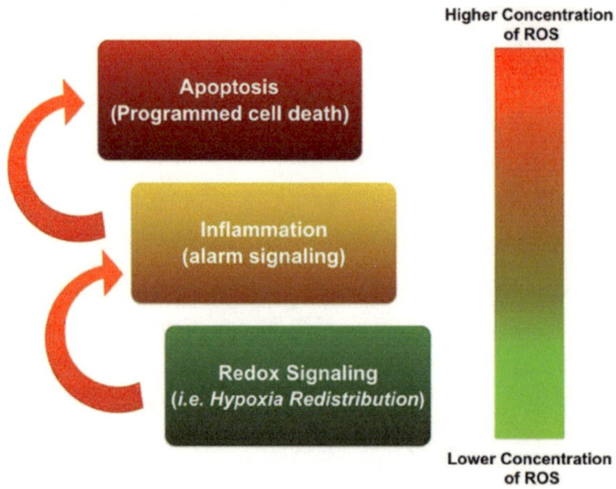

Figure 2. Concentration of generated ROS may involve in the different physiological response. At the low concentration, the ROS regulate in the redox signalling, and at the moderate concentration of induced ROS which participated in the inflammation process. At the high level of ROS concentration increased and was to be involved in the cellular apoptosis.

3. Tissue resident macrophages

Macrophages, which are present in almost all body tissue and display distinct location-specific phenotypes and gene expression profiles, display remarkable functional diversity in innate immune responses, tissue development and tissue homeostasis [41]. In different organs, the resident macrophages are given various appellations: microglia cells have fundamental importance in assessing the pathogenetic significance of perivascular inflammatory phenomena within the brain [42]; Kupffer cells are resident and recruited macrophages that play major roles in the homeostatic function of the liver and in its response to tissue damage [43]; alveolar macrophages are key determinants pulmonary immune responses and in the lung inflammation caused by asthma [44]. Previously, it was hypothesised that tissue macrophages were recruited from circulating blood monocytes. Recent studies have demonstrated that tissue macrophages such as microglia, Kupffer cells and Langerhans cells are established prenatally and arise independently of the hematopoietic transcription factor Myb [45]. Myb is required for developing hematopoietic stem cells (HSCs) and all $CD11b^{high}$ monocytes and macrophages but is not required for yolk sac (YS) macrophages and for developing YS-derived $F4/80^{bright}$ macrophages. Such macrophages can persist independently of HSCs in several types of tissue in adult mice [46]. Kupffer cells as well as other resident macrophages (e.g., microglia) originate from the YS in a colony-stimulating factor-1/receptor (CSF-1R)-dependent and Myb-independent manner. Researchers have suggested that these macrophages are maintained by local proliferation, which results in extensive mitosis after stress or an exchanged tissue microenvironment [43, 47].

Macrophages are the most crucial and abundant immune cells. They can be categorised into two primary types according to function and differentiation: classically activated macrophages (M1 macrophages) and alternatively activated macrophages (M2 macrophages) [48]. Macrophages are relevant to innate resistance and to the relationship between inflammation and autoimmune disease. In mouse models, macrophages present CD11b, F4/80 and CSF-1R, with F4/80 being the surface proteins for M1 and M2 macrophages [49, 50]. When pathogens enter the organism from the intestinal portal vein, circulating monocytes (surrounding the pathogens and present in the peripheral blood) respond to chemokines (e.g., CCL2) and are exposed to antigens. While interacting with pattern recognition receptors (PRRs), antigens may exert either M1 or M2 polarising activities, depending on the Th1 (IFN-γ) and Th2 (IL-4 and IL-13) cytokines and immune factors [51, 52].

4. Inflammation and macrophages

Inflammation is an important adaptive physiological response of the organism. Inflammation response embodies a complicated interaction among molecular mediators and cells. It globally affects the leukocytes, also the lymphocytes in their micro-environmental function and organisation [48]. Throughout their response, numerous factors are involved in the classical immune response. Macrophages detain a critical role in the uptake and degradation of infectious agents and senescent cells; they also play crucial roles in tissue growth, tissue remodelling and inflammation by producing oxidants, proteinases and anti-microbial peptide [40].

Resident macrophages sense exogenous or endogenous danger signals (e.g., bacterial products or necrotic cell debris) through PRRs. In response to Toll-like receptor (TLR) ligands and interferon-gamma (IFN-γ) or IL-4/IL-13, macrophages undergo M1 (classical) or M2 (alternative) activation. The activation of M1 and M2 macrophages mirrors TH1-TH2 polarisation; M1 and M2 activation span the extremes of a continuum. M1 macrophages, which display a morphology that depends on their tissue location, develop in response to stimulation with IFN-γ and microbial products such as LPS. M1 macrophages can secrete substantial amounts of pro-inflammatory cytokines, such as IL-1β, IL-15, IL-18, TNF-α and IL-12 [53]. M2 macrophages adapt to similarities and differences between IL-4, TLR ligands with IL-10 and glucocorticoids [54].

The phenotypes of M1 and M2 macrophages exhibit observable differences. The M1 phenotype is characterised by the expression of high levels of pro-inflammatory cytokines, high production of reactive nitrogen and oxygen intermediates, promotion of Th1 response and anti-microbial and tumour-inhibiting activity [43]. The M2 macrophage uses immune inhibitory effects to secrete large amounts of IL-10, TGF-β, and C-C motif chemokine ligands 17 (CCL17) and CCL22. Moreover, the M2 macrophage attracts non-cytotoxic T_{reg} and Type 2 T-helper cells (TH2 cells) to aggregate in tumour tissue, inhibit T-cell differentiation and function, lower cytotoxic T-cell function, induce T-cell apoptosis, secrete CCL18 and attract naive T cells [55].

Macrophage	M1	M2
Transcription factor		
Interferon regulatory factor (IRF)	IRF-3 [61, 62]	IRF-4 [63]
	IRF-5 [64]	
	IRF-8 [65]	
Nuclear factor	NF-κB [43]	
Signal transducer and activator of transcription (STAT)	STAT-1 [66]	STAT-3 [43]
		STAT-5 [67]
		SATA-6 [68]
Suppressor of cytokine signalling (SOCS)	SOCS-1 SOCS-2 SOCS-3 (controversial) [58]	
Phenotype	iNOS [69, 70]	YM-1 [71]
	IL-6 [72]	Arg-1 [73, 74]
	TNF-α [75]	Fizz-1 [76]
		IL-10 [77]

Table 1. Regulators in the M1 and M2 macrophage.

Macrophage polarisation is highly related to expressions of various TLRs on macrophages [56, 57]. The evidence indicates that TLR signalling (e.g., TLR4), which is activated by LPS and other microbial ligands, drives macrophages to prefer the M1 phenotype. In this reaction, MyD88 and TRIF activate a cascade of kinases, including IRAK4, TRAF6 and IKKβ; this results in the activation of nuclear factor kappa B (NF-κB), which drives the macrophage forward to the M1 phenotype. By contrast, IL-4 and IL-13 drive the macrophage's phenotype forward to M2. Activation of STAT6 through the IL-4 receptor alpha (IL-4Rα) and IL-10 induce activation of STAT3 through receptor IL-10R, which activates JAK1 and JAK3 (38), causing STAT6 activation [58, 59]. IL-10, TGF-β, IL-4 and IL-13 enhance inflammation and cellular immune response with NO, which is generated through IFN-γ-induced iNOS and is reduced in macrophages by Arg1 interactions with mast cells, basophils, eosinophils, NKT cells, IgE and selected subclasses of IgG. This promotes allergies and hypersensitivity [60] (**Table 1**).

5. Inflammation and disease

Accumulating evidence indicates that chronic low-grade inflammation contributes to the systemic metabolic dysfunction that is associated with inflammation disorders [78]. Cytokines and pathogen-associated molecular patterns have been shown to co-stimulate cell surface receptors, including TLRs, to initiate intra-cellular signalling that activates NF-κB. NF-κB activation was thought to induce the target gene's expression to promote cellular proliferation and to activate the immune response. However, research has revealed that NF-κB activation can occur in most cell types; recent reports have demonstrated that high level activation of NF-κB signalling pathways in the liver, adipose tissue and central nervous system (CNS) is involved in the development of inflammation-associated metabolic diseases [79]. The mutants of the brain-specific serpin, neuroserpin, also form ordered polymers that accumulate within the ER of neurons; these mutations cause an autosomal-dominant type of dementia known as familial encephalopathy with neuroserpin inclusion bodies, which is believed to be an inflammation disorder [80, 81].

Research has shown that, in specific tissue lesions, extra-cellular lipid droplets are forming a core region surrounded by smooth muscle cells and collagen-rich matrix. Lymphocytes as the T cells, monocyte, macrophages and mast cells are infiltrating in the lesion particularly in regions where the atheroma grows. These immune cells also generate important signals in the defence cascade by producing the inflammatory cytokines, largely involved in the athero-sclerotic process [82]. A case report indicated that Alzheimer's disease (AD) inflammation appears to arise from within the CNS. Little or no involvement of lymphocytes or monocytes in AD was observed beyond their normal brain surveillance. This observation has placed AD outside the realm of conventional neuroimmunologic studies that largely focus on humoral aspects of such CNS inflammatory disorders as multiple sclerosis [83]. Judging from published reports, we believe that metabolic disorders and even neuronal diseases are highly related to abnormal inflammation.

6. Macrophage and T-cell differentiation

In pathogen infection, dendritic cells (DCs) and macrophages primarily act as phagocytotic antigen-presenting cells (APCs) that degrade infected pathogens into fragments, and then move those fragments to the nearby lymphoid organs. The pathogen fragments combine with cell surface histocompatibility complex (major histocompatibility complex) to activate and differentiate T cells. **Figure 3** displays the cooperation of the antigen-presenting cells, co-stimulatory molecules and cytokines.

The metabolic organs, such as the liver, pancreas and adipose tissue, are composed of paren-chymal and stromal cells, which include macrophages to maintain metabolic homeostasis. Bacterial infection innately activates macrophages, causing the secretion of proinflammatory cytokines, such as TNF-α, IL-6 and IL-1β. This promotes peripheral insulin resistance and reduces nutrient storage during the metabolic reaction. Furthermore, some additional physiological mechanism can lead to the activation of macrophages. For these latest, the regulatory T cells (T_{reg}), the Fcγ receptors, the apoptotic cells and the prostaglandins are increasing the number of macrophages involved in the regulation of inflammation and anti-tumour defences [84]. These inflammatory mediators are involved in activating anti-microbial defence mechanisms, including oxidative processes that contribute to killing pathogens and the secreted IL-12 and IL-23. These direct the differentiation and expansion of anti-microbial T_H1 and T_H17 cells that help to drive inflammatory responses [85]. Recent research shows that intestinal antigen-presenting cells can be divided into $CD11c^+CD11b^-$, $CD11c^+CD11b^+$ and $CD11c^{dull}CD11b^+$ categories. Particularly, the $CD11c^{dull}CD11b^+$ cells are $CD103^-F4/80^+$macrophages, with efficient role in inducing the $Foxp3^+$ regulatory T (T_{reg}) cells [86]. Tumour cells affect the surrounding cellular environment by promoting tumour growth and metastasis by establishing a tumour microenvironment that is conducive to tumour development [87–90]. In the tumour microenvironment, tumour cells secrete inflammatory cytokines, such as TGF-β and IL-10. These cytokines stimulate differentiation of regulatory T and T_{reg} cells [91, 92] as well as differentiation of tumour-associated macrophages (TAMs) into M2 macrophages. This causes the host immune system to locate and attack cancer cells, which generates subsequent tumour cell evasion of this immune surveillance and attack, which enhances tumour growth and metastasis [87, 93–98]. Various cytokines, chemokines and growth factors in the tumour microenvironment are the primary elements that affect the host's anti-tumour ability and evasion of tumour cells [89, 99]. Tumour microenvironments are complicated cellular microcosms [89, 97], and numerous immune cells are located throughout tumour microenvironments. Macrophages are the most crucial and abundant immune cells in the tumour microenvironment. The two most critical types of macrophages, based on function and differentiation, are M1 and M2 macrophages. M1 macrophages are characterised by tumour

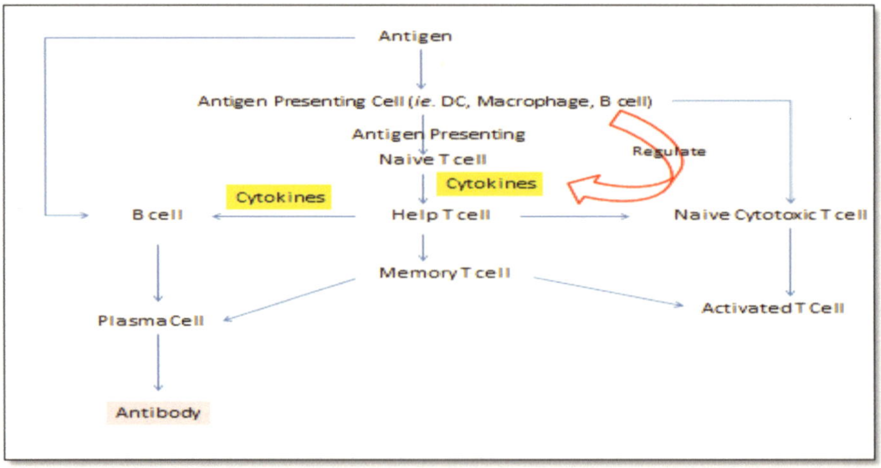

Figure 3. The cooperation of the antigen-presenting cells, costimulatory molecules, and cytokines. Bacterial infection innately activates macrophages, causing the secretion of pro-inflammatory cytokines, such as TNF-α, IL-6, and IL-1β. This promotes peripheral insulin resistance and reduces nutrient storage during the metabolic reaction. Furthermore, several additional mechanisms can also contribute to the activation of macrophages for immune-regulatory activity.

resistance, whereas M2 macrophages are characterised by tumour promotion [98, 100]. In mouse models, macrophages present CD11b, F4/80, CSF-1R and F4/80 as the surface proteins for M1 and M2 macrophages [93, 101]. Recent studies have noted large quantities of TAMs in tumour tissue. TAMs are the most abundant and critical immune cells in the tumour microenvironment [102–104] and are the main factors that enable the tumour microenvironment to exert immune inhibitory effects [101, 102]. In the tumour microenvironment, tumour cells and the surrounding stoma cells secrete cytokines and growth factors that stimulate TAMs and activate the various expression, function, receptor regulation and secretion types of chemokines [103, 105], including anti-tumour M1 macrophages and pro-tumour M2 macrophages [98, 106–108]. In the tumour microenvironment, the proportions of M1 and M2 macrophages are unequal. Tumour microenvironments contain large amounts of transmitters, such as M-CSF, IL-6, IL-10, TGF-β and COX-2, that induce transformation of TAMs into M2 macrophages that secrete immune inhibitory chemokines and have poor antigen-presenting and cytotoxic abilities, which generates tumour growth and metastasis [49, 98, 102–104, 109–114]. M2 macrophages and TAMs have protumour and immune inhibitory effects, secrete large amounts of IL-10, TGF-β, CCL17 and CCL22, attract non-cytotoxic T_{reg} and TH2 cells to aggregate in tumour tissue, inhibit T-cell differentiation and function, lower cytotoxic T-cell function, induce T-cell apoptosis, secrete CCL18 and attract naïve T cells [49, 98, 115]. NADPH oxidase is a major enzymatic source of cellular ROS. NADPH plays a fundamental role in maintaining normal cell functions. Recent research has focussed on this enzyme's role in cellular oxidative stress, which may eventually contribute to various pathophysiological conditions and diseases [27, 28]. Studies have found that NADPH oxidase modulates multiple redox-sensitive intra-cellular signalling pathways by generating ROS molecules. This modulation includes inhibition of protein tyrosine phosphatases and activation of certain redox-sensitive transcription factors [116, 117]. ROS consist of numerous molecular species, including H_2O_2, oxide ions (O_2^-) and OH^{-29}, that act as signalling molecules involved in the migration of hepatic profibrogenic cells [118] and the functioning of peripheral blood monocytes [119]. ROS and RNS, generated endogenously or in response to environmental stress, have long been implicated in tissue injury for a variety of disease states [120, 121]. Stimulation of the mitochondrial apoptotic pathway through ROS and mitochondrial DNA damage promotes outer membrane permeabilisation, which triggers caspase-dependent or caspase-independent cytosolic signalling events [122]. Activated inflammatory cells serve as sources of ROS and RNS that can initiate the alteration of the cell function, gathering specific cellular signalling, transcription factor activation, physiological factors release, the apoptosis process and compensatory cell proliferation. However, it remains unclear whether the ROS or the RNS production and release through neutrophils or macrophages enhance sufficient diffusion into the intra-cellular cytoplasm as to affect the cellular response [123, 124].

7. Wound healing

Immune cells are involved in virtually every aspect of the wound repair process, from the initial stages, where they participate in haemostasis and work to prevent infection, to later stages where they drive scar formation [125, 126]. T lymphocytes exercise crucial in vivo effects on various parameters of healing [127–129]. Neutrophils help control infection during wound healing, but they also release harmful enzymes that damage healthy tissue surrounding the wound site [130–132]. Recent researchers have noted that several specific proteins produced by wound macrophages at the site of injury are involved: (1) in the recruitment and activation of additional macrophages infiltrating in the wound; (2) in the production of growth factors that promote cellular proliferation and tissue recovery synthesis; (3) in stimulating proteases and extra-cellular matrix growth and (4) in the process of tissue remodelling [133]. β-catenin-dependent Wnt pathways, which are classified according to their ability to promote stabilisation of β-catenin in the cytoplasm, act as cellular signals through cytoplasmic stabilisation and accumulation of β-catenin in the nucleus to activate gene transcription [134]. This could enhance wound healing by lymphocytes [135, 136]. Nicotinamide adenine dinucleotide phosphate (NADPH) oxidase modulates multiple redox-sensitive intra-cellular signalling pathways by generating ROS molecules. This includes inhibiting protein tyrosine phosphatases and activating certain redox-sensitive transcription factors [116, 137, 138]. This shows that ROS regulate the expression of key chemical mediators that further modulate the inflammatory response in animal models; it has also been reported that these redox-sensitive processes may include cytokine action, angiogenesis, cell motility and extra-cellular matrix formation [139–141]; this can enable reliable estimates of wound-healing capacity, which is altered by various conditions, such as inflammation. Furthermore, research on one of the ROS has indicated that H_2O_2 plays a critical role in wound repair, inflammation and anti-inflammation mechanisms [142, 143]. Our published research also showed that the production of ROS (i.e., H_2O_2 after an injury has occurred) may cause healing to generate inflammation through the apoptosis of the cell. Over-inhibition of NADPH oxidase activity may reduce the normal progress of apoptosis under the wound and might delay healing [29].

Inflammation enhances vascular permeability, active migration of blood cells and the passage of plasma constituents into the injured tissue [144]. Blood leukocytes actively participate in the defence and inflammation responses, being activated since the earliest phases of atherosclerosis process. Inflammation and atherosclerosis shelter intricate mechanisms relied to leukocytes recruitment [145]. Neuro-inflammation mediators are described to be closely related to brain cells functioning (such as microglia and astrocytes), to the complement system activation and to cytokines, and chemokines production [146]. Regarding cancer development [147], pro-inflammatory cytokines, including IL-1α, IL-1β, IL-6, IL-8, IL-18, chemokines, matrix metallopeptidase-9 and vascular endothelial growth factor, are primarily regulated by the transcription NF-κB, which is active in most tumours and is induced by carcinogens [148]. Cutaneous wound repair is a tightly regulated and dynamic process involving blood clotting, inflammation, formation of new tissue and tissue remodelling [149]. Thrombin is the protease involved in blood coagulation. Its deregulation can cause haemostatic abnormalities, which range from subtle subclinical problems to serious life-threatening coagulopathies (i.e., during septicaemia) [150]. Inflammation and coagulation are both parts of the natural mechanism that protects the organism against infection. The endothelial cells and the platelets are capable to react in the acute, also in the chronic inflammatory environment. They release pro-inflammatory mediators that produce adhesion of molecules, proteases and clotting factors associated to leukocytes recruitment [151]. The elements of the PAR family serve as sensors that detect blood-clotting serine proteinases in the inflamed target cells. Activation of PAR-1 by thrombin and of PAR-2 by other factors on the membrane of endothelial cells generates rapid expression and exposure of adhesive proteins that mediate an acute inflammatory reaction and of the tissue factor that initiates the blood coagulation cascade [152] as presented as **Figure 4**.

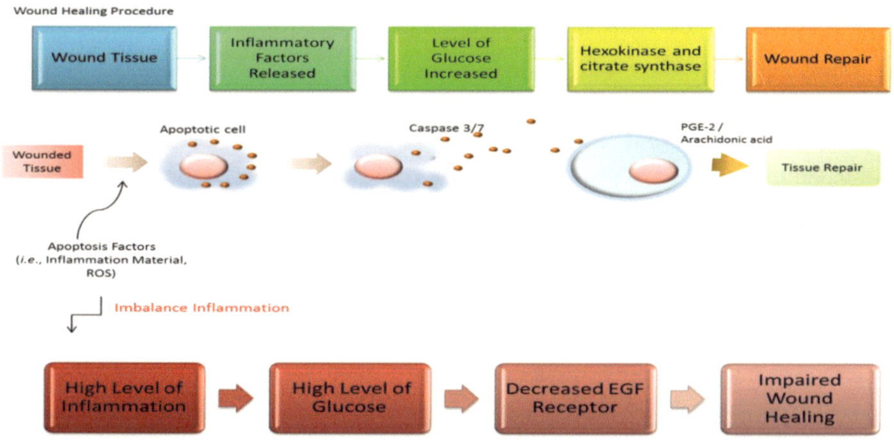

Figure 4. Wound healing was initiated after the injury of the cell, tissue even the organ. In the early stage of the healing, the damaged tissue producing a lot of ROS leading to neighbour cells into the apoptosis, following the apoptotic cells collapsed and released caspases were able to induce the tissue repair. However, the imbalance inflammatory may induce over-production of blood glucose that is leading to decrease the EGF receptor expression further to impair the wound healing.

8. Immunomodulation in anti-inflammation therapy

Nakanishi et al. found that celecoxib can alter the immune inhibitory effects of the tumour microenvironment by promoting transformation of TAMs into M1 macrophages, inhibiting tumour growth [153]. In 1968, Ikekawa et al. found that the fruiting body extracts from *Lentinus edodes*, *Trametes versicolor*, *Ganoderma tsugae*, *Flammulina velutiper* and *Tricholoma matsutake* demonstrated substantial anti-tumour activities towards transplanted tumour cells of Sarcoma 180 [154, 155]. *Autrodia comphorata*-derived beta-glucan inhibited tumour growth for Sarcoma 37, Sarcoma 180, Erlich ascites sarcoma and Yoshida sarcoma as well as inhibited LLC1 transplanted tumour growth [156]. Daily intake of *A. comphorata*-derived beta-glucan for 18 consecutive days was demonstrated to slow tumour growth and reduce the rate of metastasis [157]. Cytotoxic T-cell activity and tumour occurrence rates were observed, and the results illustrated that daily oral intake of *Grifola frondosua*-derived beta-glucan or Lentinan can enhance cytotoxic T-cell activity and reduce tumour occurrence rates [158]. The addition of a conditioned medium along with tumour cells into the progenitor cells of DCs was found to further inhibit maturation of DCs and lower the antigen-presenting capability of the DCs [159]. Tumour cells were found to secrete M-CSF, inhibiting dendritic and T-cell differentiation and anti-tumour ability [87, 159–161]. In the inflammation environment, the amounts of M1 and M2 macrophages are not equal [162]. The tumour environment contains vast quantities of transmitters such as M-CSF, IL-6, IL-10, TGF-β and COX-2 that induce tumour megakaryocytes to differentiate into M2 macrophages, which, in addition to having inferior antigen-presenting and cytotoxic abilities, also secrete factors that inhibit immune cells, resulting in enhanced immune inhibitory effects in the tumour environment [49, 98, 102–104, 109–114]. M2 macrophages in tumour bearing mice enhance tumour growth and immune inhibitory effects. They also secrete cytokines, such as IL-10 and TGF-β, in high quantities, which attract non-cytotoxic T_{reg} cells and TH2 cells to congregate in tumour tissue; those cells inhibit the differentiation and normal function of T cells, including their cytotoxic ability, and further promote T-cell apoptosis [49, 98, 115, 163, 164]. The polarisation of TH1 and TH2 is built on cytokine patterns; polarisation begins when the antigen-presenting cells interact with naive T cells; they polarise into Type 1 (TH1) and TH2 cells in response to the type of antigen encountered [165]. TH1 and TH2 cells secrete different cytokines; TH1 cells rely on IL-2, IFN-γ and TNF, which are involved in cell-mediated immunity against pathogens, but TH2 cells depend mostly on IL-4 and IL-5, which stimulate the production of IgE antibodies and eosinophil responses, resulting in allergic diseases [166, 167]. Although an imbalanced TH1/TH2 immune response is linked to certain hypersensitivity disorders such as allergies, asthma and hay fever [168], studies have suggested that using a biological response modifier to restore the balance between TH1 and TH2 immune response can be a potential treatment option for IgE-dependent hypersensitivity [169]. *Ganoderma lucidum* is a medicinal mushroom that has been widely used as a folk medicine in Asian countries such as China and Japan for hundreds of years for its immunomodulating and anti-tumour effects. Numerous biologically available substances with immunity enhancement effects, particularly polysaccharides, have been isolated from the extract of *G. lucidum* [170].

Anti-microbial peptides are effective components of innate immunity that exist widely in biological systems. One of the specific anti-microbial peptides, hepcidin, is a 25-amino acid antibiotic peptide synthesised in the liver. Hepcidin is responsible for regulating iron balance and recycling iron in humans and mice. Studies have reported 0–100 μg/ml concentrations of hepcidin incubated with HT1080, Hep-G2 and HeLa for 24 h. The results have indicated higher growth inhibition ratios after 70 μg/ml treatment with hepcidin in HT1080 cells; the treatment has been very effective in inhibiting the growth of fibrosarcoma cells [171, 172]. Tachyplesin is an anti-microbial peptide present in the leukocytes of the horseshoe crab (*Tachypleus tridentatus*); it inhibited the growth of TSU tumour cells on the CAM of chicken embryos as well as the growth of B16 tumour cells in syngenic mice; moreover, it blocked the proliferation of both tumour and endothelial cells in culture in a dose-dependent manner, whereas proliferation was relatively unaffected in non-tumourigenic cell lines Cos-7 and NIH-3T3 [173]. D-K4R2L9 is a peptide comprised of Leu, Lys and Arg residues, totalling 15 amino acid residues that bind to and lyse B16-F10 mouse melanoma cells in culture at concentrations that do not harm normal 3T3 fibroblasts or erythrocytes; this can be conducted to prevent intravenous-injected D122 lung carcinoma cells from forming lung tumours in mice [174, 175]. Bovine lactoferricin (LfcinB), an anti-microbial peptide, is a 25-amino acid long highly basic peptide with a disulfide bridge between two cysteines, thus giving it a cyclic twisted anti-parallel β-sheet solution structure. LfcinB has been tested on neuroblastoma growth *in vivo*; nude rats carrying SH-SY-5Y xenografts were given injections of 1.0 or 2.0 mg LfcinB; these rats' cancer was significantly inhibited after LfcinB treatment, compared with untreated controls [176]. Anti-microbial peptides can activate specific innate immune responses and immunomodulatory effects in the host, even if the host is at risk or has been damaged. Furthermore, researchers have proposed that anti-microbial peptides can modulate the host's immune system through inflammatory responses and can stimulate beneficial inflammation; anti-microbial peptides might be able to inhibit tumour growth.

9. Conclusion

From the injury to the wound recovery, there are a series of physiological responses that occur in relation to immune cells. Polarisation of the macrophage is an important response in wound healing. A series of inflammatory factors are cited having notable function in the differentiation from novel macrophage into the classical macrophage (M1). The cellular mechanism involved in the regulation of classical macrophage (M1) and alternative macrophage (M2) was documented in the wound healing process. At the present time, the M1/M2 differentiation was studied for selected immune responses. However, future studies may allow possible therapeutic targets considering this process in wound healing.

The immunotherapy that is being developed offers some advantageous immunomodulation factors that are known in the field of alternative medicine, such as mushroom beta-glucan, anti-microbial peptides and triterpenoid; these factors represent a novel therapeutic approach for anti-inflammation. These factors may be a viable alternative approach to the problem of drug resistance. Recent insights into wound healing and anti-inflammation are promising; however, exploiting these insights is complex because it involves chemistry, biology, instrumentation science and formulation science. Discovering new methods that are more effective in targets is difficult. Immunotherapy might be an alternative therapy that can be applied in the early phases of clinical therapy. Similarly, immunomodulation might be applicable in the early phases of immune disease.

Author details

Yu-Sheng Wu[1], Fan-Hua Nan[2], Sherwin Chen[1] and Shiu-Nan Chen[1*]

*Address all correspondence to: d97b45004@ntu.edu.tw; snchen@ntu.edu.tw

1 College of Life Science, National Taiwan University, Taipei, Taiwan

2 Department of Aquaculture, National Taiwan Ocean University, Keelung, Taiwan

References

[1] P. Allavena, A. Sica, G. Solinas *et al.*, "The inflammatory micro-environment in tumor progression: the role of tumor-associated macrophages," *Critical Reviews in Oncology/Hematology*, vol. 66, no. 1, pp. 1–9, 2008.

[2] S. S. Choe, K. C. Shin, S. Ka *et al.*, "Macrophage HIF-2alpha ameliorates adipose tissue inflammation and insulin resistance in obesity," *Diabetes*, vol. 63, no. 10, pp. 3359–71, 2014.

[3] Y. Enoki, T. Sato, S. Tanaka *et al.*, "Netrin-4 derived from murine vascular endothelial cells inhibits osteoclast differentiation in vitro and prevents bone loss in vivo," *FEBS Letters*, vol. 588, no. 14, pp. 2262–9, 2014.

[4] B. Gore, M. Izikki, O. Mercier *et al.*, "Key role of the endothelial TGF-beta/ALK1/endoglin signaling pathway in humans and rodents pulmonary hypertension," *PLoS One*, vol. 9, no. 6, p. e100310, 2014.

[5] G. Poschmann, M. Grzendowski, A. Stefanski *et al.*, "Redox proteomics reveal stress responsive proteins linking peroxiredoxin-1 status in glioma to chemosensitivity and oxidative stress," *Biochimica et Biophysica Acta*, 2014.

[6] L. Wu, H. Chen, C. Curtis *et al.*, "Go in for the kill," *Virulence*, vol. 5, no. 7, pp. 710–21, 2014.

[7] J. H. Yu, and H. Kim, "Oxidative stress and inflammatory signaling in cerulein pancreatitis," *World Journal of Gastroenterology*, vol. 20, no. 46, pp. 17324–9, 2014.

[8] E. Y. Choi, H. J. Kim, and J. S. Han, "Anti-inflammatory effects of calcium citrate in RAW 264.7cells via suppression of NF-kappaB activation," *Environmental Toxicology and Pharmacology*, vol. 39, no. 1, pp. 27–34, 2014.

[9] C. S. Luo, J. R. Liang, Q. Lin *et al.*, "Cellular responses associated with ROS production and cell fate decision in early stress response to iron limitation in the diatom *Thalassiosira pseudonana*," *Journal of Proteome Research*, vol. 13, no. 12, pp. 5510–23, 2014.

[10] E. McNeill, M. J. Crabtree, N. Sahgal *et al.*, "Regulation of iNOS function and cellular redox state by macrophage Gch1 reveals specific requirements for tetrahydrobiopterin in NRF2 activation," *Free Radical Biology & Medicine*, vol. 79C, pp. 206–16, 2014.

[11] K. A. Redgrove, and E. A. McLaughlin, "The role of the immune response in *Chlamydia trachomatis* infection of the male genital tract: a double-edged sword," *Frontiers in Immunology*, vol. 5, p. 534, 2014.

[12] F. Morescalchi, S. Duse, E. Gambicorti *et al.*, "Proliferative vitreoretinopathy after eye injuries: an overexpression of growth factors and cytokines leading to a retinal keloid," *Mediators Inflammation*, vol. 2013, p. 269787, 2013.

[13] M. J. Kipanyula, P. F. Seke Etet, L. Vecchio *et al.*, "Signaling pathways bridging microbial-triggered inflammation and cancer," *Cellular Signalling*, vol. 25, no. 2, pp. 403–16, 2013.

[14] R. Kisielewski, A. Tolwinska, A. Mazurek *et al.*, "Inflammation and ovarian cancer—current views," *Ginekologia Polska*, vol. 84, no. 4, pp. 293–7, 2013.

[15] E. Przybyt, M. J. van Luyn, and M. C. Harmsen, "Extracellular matrix components of adipose derived stromal cells promote alignment, organization, and maturation of cardiomyocytes in vitro," *Journal of Biomedical Materials Research Part A*, , 2014.

[16] R. Roshani, F. McCarthy, and T. Hagemann, "Inflammatory cytokines in human pancreatic cancer," *Cancer Letters*, vol. 345, no. 2, pp. 157–63, 2014.

[17] R. Nemenoff, "Activation of PPARgamma in myeloid cells promotes lung cancer progression and metastasis," *Oncoimmunology*, vol. 1, no. 3, pp. 403–4, 2012.

[18] R. Nemenoff, "Wound healing: a role for HDACs in inhibition of fibroblast proliferation through repression of PDGF receptor-alpha. Focus on ""Repression of PDGF-R-alpha after cellular injury involves TNF-alpha, formation of a c-Fos-YY1 complex, and negative regulation by HDAC"," *American Journal of Physiology – Cell Physiology*, vol. 302, no. 11, p. C1588–9, 2012.

[19] C. Hellberg, A. Ostman, and C. H. Heldin, "PDGF and vessel maturation," *Recent Results in Cancer Research*, vol. 180, pp. 103–14, 2010.

[20] C. Liu, W. Zhao, W. Meng *et al.*, "Platelet-derived growth factor blockade on cardiac remodeling following infarction," *Molecular and Cellular Biochemistry*, vol. 397, no. 1–2, pp. 295–304, 2014.

[21] S. Shimizu, H. Kouzaki, T. Ogawa *et al.*, "Eosinophil-epithelial cell interactions stimulate the production of MUC5AC mucin and profibrotic cytokines involved in airway tissue remodeling," *American Journal of Rhinology & Allergy*, vol. 28, no. 2, pp. 103–9, – 2014.

[22] K. L. Spiller, R. R. Anfang, K. J. Spiller *et al.*, "The role of macrophage phenotype in vascularization of tissue engineering scaffolds," *Biomaterials*, vol. 35, no. 15, pp. 4477–88, 2014.

[23] K. Apel, and H. Hirt, "Reactive oxygen species: metabolism, oxidative stress, and signal transduction," *Annual Review of Plant Biology*, vol. 55, pp. 373–99, 2004.

[24] L. O. Klotz, "Oxidant-induced signaling: effects of peroxynitrite and singlet oxygen," *Biological Chemistry*, vol. 383, no. 3–4, pp. 443–56, 2002.

[25] A. Y. Andreyev, Y. E. Kushnareva, and A. A. Starkov, "Mitochondrial metabolism of reactive oxygen species," *Biochemistry (Moscow)*, vol. 70, no. 2, pp. 200–14, 2005.

[26] X. Li, P. Fang, J. Mai *et al.*, "Targeting mitochondrial reactive oxygen species as novel therapy for inflammatory diseases and cancers," *Journal of Hematology & Oncology*, vol. 6, pp. 19, 2013.

[27] E. C. Chan, F. Jiang, H. M. Peshavariya *et al.*, "Regulation of cell proliferation by NADPH oxidase-mediated signaling: potential roles in tissue repair, regenerative medicine and tissue engineering," *Pharmacology & Therapeutics*, vol. 122, no. 2, pp. 97–108, 2009.

[28] F. Jiang, Y. Zhang, and G. J. Dusting, "NADPH oxidase-mediated redox signaling: roles in cellular stress response, stress tolerance, and tissue repair," *Pharmacolical Reviews*, vol. 63, no. 1, pp. 218–42, 2011.

[29] Y. S. Wu, S. L. Huang, F. H. Nan *et al.*, "Over-inhibition of NADPH oxidase reduce the wound healing in liver of finfish," *Fish and Shellfish Immunology*, vol. 40, no. 1, pp. 174–81, 2014.

[30] J. F. Turrens, "Mitochondrial formation of reactive oxygen species," *Journal of Physiology*, vol. 552, no. Pt 2, pp. 335–44, 2003.

[31] E. Novo, C. Busletta, L. V. Bonzo *et al.*, "Intracellular reactive oxygen species are required for directional migration of resident and bone marrow-derived hepatic profibrogenic cells," *Journal of Hepatology*, vol. 54, no. 5, pp. 964–74, 2011.

[32] A. Van der Goes, D. Wouters, S. M. Van Der Pol *et al.*, "Reactive oxygen species enhance the migration of monocytes across the blood-brain barrier in vitro," *FASEB Journal*, vol. 15, no. 10, pp. 1852–4, 2001.

[33] A. Ghosh, and M. E. Greenberg, "Calcium signaling in neurons: molecular mechanisms and cellular consequences," *Science*, vol. 268, no. 5208, pp. 239–47, 1995.

[34] S. Orrenius, B. Zhivotovsky, and P. Nicotera, "Regulation of cell death: the calcium-apoptosis link," *Nature Reviews Molecular Cell Biology*, vol. 4, no. 7, pp. 552–65, 2003.

[35] R. G. Spragg, D. B. Hinshaw, P. A. Hyslop *et al.*, "Alterations in adenosine triphosphate and energy charge in cultured endothelial and P388D1 cells after oxidant injury," *Journal of Clinical Investigation*, vol. 76, no. 4, pp. 1471–6, 1985.

[36] R. G. Spragg, "DNA strand break formation following exposure of bovine pulmonary artery and aortic endothelial cells to reactive oxygen products," *American Journal of Respiratory Cell and Molecular Biology*, vol. 4, no. 1, pp. 4–10, 1991.

[37] A. C. Gasic, G. McGuire, S. Krater *et al.*, "Hydrogen peroxide pretreatment of perfused canine vessels induces ICAM-1 and CD18-dependent neutrophil adherence," *Circulation*, vol. 84, no. 5, pp. 2154–66, 1991.

[38] A. Siflinger-Birnboim, H. Lum, P. D. Vecchio *et al.*, "Involvement of Ca2+ in the H2O2-induced increase in endothelial permeability," *American Journal of Physiology–Lung Cellular and Molecular Physiology*, vol. 14, no. 6, pp. L973, 1996.

[39] T. Finkel, "Signal transduction by mitochondrial oxidants," *Journal of Biological Chemistry*, vol. 287, no. 7, pp. 4434–40, 2012.

[40] Y.-S. Wu, and S.-N. Chen, "Apoptotic cell: linkage of inflammation and wound healing," *Frontiers in Pharmacology*, vol. 5, 2014.

[41] M. Haldar, and K. M. Murphy, "Origin, development, and homeostasis of tissue-resident macrophages," *Immunological Reviews*, vol. 262, no. 1, pp. 25–35, 2014.

[42] G. J. Guillemin, and B. J. Brew, "Microglia, macrophages, perivascular macrophages, and pericytes: a review of function and identification," *Journal of Leukocyte Biology*, vol. 75, no. 3, pp. 388–97, 2004.

[43] A. Sica, P. Invernizzi, and A. Mantovani, "Macrophage plasticity and polarization in liver homeostasis and pathology," *Hepatology*, vol. 59, no. 5, pp. 2034–42, 2014.

[44] S. Przybranowski, C. Wilke, N. Van Rooijen *et al.*, "Resident alveolar macrophages suppress while recruited macrophages promote allergic lung inflammation in murine models of asthma," *American Journal of Respiratory and Critical Care Medicine*, vol. 189, pp. A3685, 2014.

[45] S. Epelman, K. J. Lavine, A. E. Beaudin *et al.*, "Embryonic and adult-derived resident cardiac macrophages are maintained through distinct mechanisms at steady state and during inflammation," *Immunity*, vol. 40, no. 1, pp. 91–104, 2014.

[46] C. Schulz, E. G. Perdiguero, L. Chorro *et al.*, "A lineage of myeloid cells independent of Myb and hematopoietic stem cells," *Science*, vol. 336, no. 6077, pp. 86–90, 2012.

[47] J.-J. Widmann, and H. Fahimi, "Proliferation of mononuclear phagocytes (Kupffer cells) and endothelial cells in regenerating rat liver. A light and electron microscopic cytochemical study," *The American Journal of Pathology*, vol. 80, no. 3, pp. 349, 1975.

[48] W.-J. Wang, Y.-S. Wu, S. Chen *et al.*, "Mushroom β-glucan may immunomodulate the tumor-associated macrophages in the Lewis lung carcinoma," *BioMed Research International*, 2014.

[49] F. O. Martinez, L. Helming, and S. Gordon, "Alternative activation of macrophages: an immunologic functional perspective," *Annual Review of Immunology*, vol. 27, pp. 451–83, 2009.

[50] R. A. Flavell, S. Sanjabi, S. H. Wrzesinski *et al.*, "The polarization of immune cells in the tumour environment by TGFβ," *Nature Reviews Immunology*, vol. 10, no. 8, pp. 554–67, 2010.

[51] A. Sica, and A. Mantovani, "Macrophage plasticity and polarization: in vivo veritas," *The Journal of Clinical Investigation*, vol. 122, no. 3, pp. 787–95, 2012.

[52] A. Mantovani, S. K. Biswas, M. R. Galdiero *et al.*, "Macrophage plasticity and polarization in tissue repair and remodelling," *The Journal of Pathology*, vol. 229, no. 2, pp. 176–85, 2013.

[53] F. O. Martinez, A. Sica, A. Mantovani *et al.*, "Macrophage activation and polarization," *Frontiers in Bioscience: A Journal and Virtual Library*, vol. 13, pp. 453–61, 2007.

[54] A. Mantovani, S. Sozzani, M. Locati *et al.*, "Macrophage polarization: tumor-associated macrophages as a paradigm for polarized M2 mononuclear phagocytes," *Trends in Immunology*, vol. 23, no. 11, pp. 549–55, 2002.

[55] F. R. Smiderle, G. Alquini, M. Z. Tadra-Sfeir *et al.*, "*Agaricus bisporus* and *Agaricus brasiliensis* (1→6)-β-d-glucans show immunostimulatory activity on human THP-1 derived macrophages," *Carbohydrate Polymers*, vol. 94, no. 1, pp. 91–9, 2013.

[56] R.-S. Sauer, D. Hackel, L. Morschel *et al.*, "Toll like receptor (TLR)-4 as a regulator of peripheral endogenous opioid-mediated analgesia in inflammation," *Molecular Pain*, vol. 10, no. 1, pp. 10, 2014.

[57] J. S. Orr, M. J. Puglisi, K. L. Ellacott *et al.*, "Toll-like receptor 4 deficiency promotes the alternative activation of adipose tissue macrophages," *Diabetes*, vol. 61, no. 11, pp. 2718–27, 2012.

[58] N. Wang, H. Liang, and K. Zen, "Molecular mechanisms that influence the macrophage M1–M2 polarization balance," *Frontiers in Immunology*, vol. 5, 2014.

[59] C. S. Whyte, E. T. Bishop, D. Rückerl *et al.*, "Suppressor of cytokine signaling (SOCS) 1 is a key determinant of differential macrophage activation and function," *Journal of Leukocyte Biology*, vol. 90, no. 5, pp. 845–54, 2011.

[60] S. Gordon, and F. O. Martinez, "Alternative activation of macrophages: mechanism and functions," *Immunity*, vol. 32, no. 5, pp. 593–604, 2010.

[61] H. Zhou, J. Liao, J. Aloor *et al.*, "CD11b/CD18 (Mac-1) is a novel surface receptor for extracellular double-stranded RNA to mediate cellular inflammatory responses," *The Journal of Immunology*, vol. 190, no. 1, pp. 115–25, 2013.

[62] Y. S. Schwartz, and A. Svistelnik, "Functional phenotypes of macrophages and the M1-M2 polarization concept. Part I. Proinflammatory phenotype," *Biochemistry (Moscow)*, vol. 77, no. 3, pp. 246–60, 2012.

[63] U. S. Rangaswamy, and S. H. Speck, "Murine gammaherpesvirus M2 protein induction of IRF4 via the NFAT pathway leads to IL-10 expression in B cells," *PLoS Pathogens*, vol. 10, no. 1, pp. e1003858, 2014.

[64] I. A. Udalova, T. Krausgruber, T. Smallie *et al.*, "IRF5 promotes inflammatory macrophage polarization and Th1/Th17 response," *Nature Immunology*, 2011.

[65] H. Xu, J. Zhu, S. Smith *et al.*, "Notch-RBP-J signaling regulates the transcription factor IRF8 to promote inflammatory macrophage polarization," *Nature Immunology*, vol. 13, no. 7, pp. 642–50, 2012.

[66] H. J. Lee, Y. K. Oh, M. Rhee *et al.*, "The role of STAT1/IRF-1 on synergistic ROS production and loss of mitochondrial transmembrane potential during hepatic cell death induced by LPS/d-GalN," *Journal of Molecular Biology*, vol. 369, no. 4, pp. 967–84, 2007.

[67] W. Xiao, H. Hong, Y. Kawakami *et al.*, "Regulation of myeloproliferation and M2 macrophage programming in mice by Lyn/Hck, SHIP, and Stat5," *The Journal of Clinical Investigation*, vol. 118, no. 3, pp. 924, 2008.

[68] Y. Ji, S. Sun, A. Xu *et al.*, "Activation of natural killer T cells promotes M2 macrophage polarization in adipose tissue and improves systemic glucose tolerance via interleukin-4 (IL-4)/STAT6 protein signaling axis in obesity," *Journal of Biological Chemistry*, vol. 287, no. 17, pp. 13561–71, 2012.

[69] J. Wan, M. Benkdane, F. Teixeira-Clerc *et al.*, "M2 Kupffer cells promote M1 Kupffer cell apoptosis: a protective mechanism against alcoholic and nonalcoholic fatty liver disease," *Hepatology*, vol. 59, no. 1, pp. 130–42, 2014.

[70] M. Heusinkveld, P. J. d. V. van Steenwijk, R. Goedemans *et al.*, "M2 macrophages induced by prostaglandin E2 and IL-6 from cervical carcinoma are switched to activated M1 macrophages by CD4+ Th1 cells," *The Journal of Immunology*, vol. 187, no. 3, pp. 1157–65, 2011.

[71] D. Zhou, C. Huang, Z. Lin *et al.*, "Macrophage polarization and function with emphasis on the evolving roles of coordinated regulation of cellular signaling pathways," *Cellular Signalling*, vol. 26, no. 2, pp. 192–7, 2014.

[72] A. J. Covarrubias, and T. Horng, "IL-6 strikes a balance in metabolic inflammation," *Cell Metabolism*, vol. 19, no. 6, pp. 898–9, 2014.

[73] P. Kell, T. Ennis, K. Chang *et al.*, "Macrophages mediate the ability of the receptor for advanced glycation end products to prevent formation of abdominal aortic aneurysm in a murine model," *Arteriosclerosis, Thrombosis, and Vascular Biology*, vol. 34, no. Suppl 1, p. A114, 2014.

[74] A. Gal, T. T. Tapmeier, and R. J. Muschel, "Plasticity of tumor associated macrophages in a metastatic melanoma model in the mouse," *Cancer Research*, vol. 72, no. 8 Suppl, pp. 402, 2012.

[75] K. L. Spiller, S. Nassiri, C. E. Witherel *et al.*, "Sequential delivery of immunomodulatory cytokines to facilitate the M1-to-M2 transition of macrophages and enhance vascularization of bone scaffolds," *Biomaterials*, vol. 37, pp. 194–207, 2015.

[76] X. Cai, Y. Yin, N. Li *et al.*, "Re-polarization of tumor-associated macrophages to pro-inflammatory M1 macrophages by microRNA-155," *Journal of Molecular Cell Biology*, vol. 4, no. 5, pp. 341–3, 2012.

[77] J.-H. Lee, G. T. Lee, S. H. Woo *et al.*, "BMP-6 in renal cell carcinoma promotes tumor proliferation through IL-10–dependent M2 polarization of tumor-associated macrophages," *Cancer Research*, vol. 73, no. 12, pp. 3604–14, 2013.

[78] N. Ouchi, J. L. Parker, J. J. Lugus *et al.*, "Adipokines in inflammation and metabolic disease," *Nature Reviews Immunology*, vol. 11, no. 2, pp. 85–97, 2011.

[79] R. G. Baker, M. S. Hayden, and S. Ghosh, "NF-κB, inflammation, and metabolic disease," *Cell Metabolism*, vol. 13, no. 1, pp. 11–22, 2011.

[80] B. Gooptu, and D. A. Lomas, "Polymers and inflammation: disease mechanisms of the serpinopathies," *The Journal of Experimental Medicine*, vol. 205, no. 7, pp. 1529–34, 2008.

[81] R. L. Davis, A. E. Shrimpton, P. D. Holohan *et al.*, "Familial dementia caused by polymerization of mutant neuroserpin," *Nature*, vol. 401, no. 6751, pp. 376–9, 1999.

[82] G. K. Hansson, "Inflammation, atherosclerosis, and coronary artery disease," *New England Journal of Medicine*, vol. 352, no. 16, pp. 1685–95, 2005.

[83] H. Akiyama, S. Barger, S. Barnum *et al.*, "Inflammation and Alzheimer's disease," *Neurobiology of Aging*, vol. 21, no. 3, pp. 383–421, 2000.

[84] T. A. Wynn, A. Chawla, and J. W. Pollard, "Macrophage biology in development, homeostasis and disease," *Nature*, vol. 496, no. 7446, pp. 445–55, 2013.

[85] A. Sica, and A. Mantovani, "Macrophage plasticity and polarization: in vivo veritas," *Journal of Clinical Investigation*, vol. 122, no. 3, pp. 787–95, 2012.

[86] T. L. Denning, B. A. Norris, O. Medina-Contreras *et al.*, "Functional specializations of intestinal dendritic cell and macrophage subsets that control Th17 and regulatory T cell responses are dependent on the T cell/APC ratio, source of mouse strain, and regional localization," *The Journal of Immunology*, vol. 187, no. 2, pp. 733–47, 2011.

[87] J. A. Joyce, and J. W. Pollard, "Microenvironmental regulation of metastasis," *Nature Reviews Cancer*, vol. 9, pp. 239–52, 2009.

[88] L. M. Coussens, and Z. Werb, "Inflammation and cancer," *Nature*, vol. 420, pp. 860–67, 2002.

[89] G. Baronzio, G. Fiorentini, and C. R. Cogle, *Cancer microenvironment and therapeutic implications*. Springer, 2009.

[90] F. Xing, J. Saidou, and K. Watabe, "Cancer associated fibroblasts (CAFs) in tumor microenvironment," *Frontiers in Bioscience (Landmark Ed)*, vol. 15, pp. 166–79, 2010.

[91] G. Castello, S. Scala, G. Palmieri *et al.*, "HCV-related hepatocellular carcinoma: From chronic inflammation to cancer," *Clinical Immunology*, vol. 134, pp. 237–50, 2010.

[92] C. A. Janeway, M. Walport, and P. Travers, *Immunobiology: the immune system in health and disease*. Garland Science, 2005.

[93] D. I. Gabrilovich, and A. A. Hurwitz, *Tumor-induced immune suppression*. Springer, 2008.

[94] W. Zou, "Immunosuppressive networks in the tumour environment and their therapeutic relevance," *Nature Reviews Cancer*, vol. 5, pp. 263–74, 2005.

[95] G. P. Dunn, A. T. Bruce, H. Ikeda *et al.*, "Cancer immunoediting: from immunosurveillance to tumor escape," *Nature Immunology*, vol. 3, pp. 991–8, 2002.

[96] G. P. Dunn, L. J. Old, and R. D. Schreiber, "The immunobiology of cancer immunosurveillance and immunoediting," *Immunity*, vol. 21, pp. 137–48, 2004.

[97] B. Z. Qian, and J. W. Pollard, "Macrophage diversity enhances tumor progression and metastasis," *Cell*, vol. 141, pp. 39–51, 2010.

[98] D. W. Siemann, "*Tumor microenvironment*. Wiley Online Library, 2011.

[99] N. Mach, S. Gillessen, S. B. Wilson *et al.*, "Differences in dendritic cells stimulated *in vivo* by tumors engineered to secrete granulocyte-macrophage colony-stimulating factor of flt3-ligand," *Cancer Research*, vol. 60, pp. 3239–46, 2000.

[100] S. K. Biswas, and A. Mantovani, "Macrophage plasticity and interaction with lymphocyte subsets: cancer as a paradigm," *Nature Immunology*, vol. 11, pp. 889–96, 2010.

[101] B. Ruffell, N. I. Affara, and L. M. Coussens, "Differential macrophage programming in the tumor microenvironment," *Trends in Immunology*, vol. 33, pp. 119–126, 2012.

[102] R. A. Flavell, S. Sanjabi, S. H. Wrzesinski *et al.*, "The polarization of immune cells in the tumour environment by TGFbeta," *Nature Reviews Immunology*, vol. 10, pp. 554–67, 2010.

[103] L. Bingle, N. J. Brown, and C. E. Lewis, "The role of tumour-associated macrophages in tumour progression: implications for new anticancer therapies," *The Journal of Pathology*, vol. 196, pp. 254–65, 2002.

[104] J. W. Pollard, "Tumour-educated macrophages promote tumour progression and metastasis," *Nature Reviews Cancer*, vol. 4, pp. 71–78, 2004.

[105] A. Mantovani, A. Sica, S. Sozzani *et al.*, "The chemokine system in diverse forms of macrophage activation and polarization," *Trends in Immunology*, vol. 25, pp. 677–86, 2004.

[106] A. Mantovani, and A. Sica, "Macrophages, innate immunity and cancer: balance, tolerance, and diversity," *Current Opinion in Immunology*, vol. 22, pp. 231–7, 2010.

[107] A. Mantovani, A. Sica, P. Allavena *et al.*, "Tumor-associated macrophages and the related myeloid-derived suppressor cells as a paradigm of the diversity of macrophage activation," *Human Immunology*, vol. 70, pp. 325–30, 2009.

[108] C. Steidl, T. Lee, S. P. Shah *et al.*, "Tumor-associated macrophages and survival in classic Hodgkin's Lymphoma," *The New England Journal of Medicine*, vol. 362, pp. 875–85, 2010.

[109] K. D. Elgert, D. G. Alleva, and D. W. Mullins, "Tumor-induced immune dysfunction: the macrophage connection," *Journal of Leukocyte Biology*, vol. 64, pp. 275–90, 1998.

[110] C. Sunderkötter, M. Goebeler, K. Schulze-Osthoff *et al.*, "Macrophage-derived angiogenesis factors," *Pharmacology & Therapeutics*, vol. 51, pp. 195–216, 1991.

[111] E. Giraudo, M. Inoue, and D. Hanahan, "An amino-bisphosphonate targets MMP-9-expressing macrophages and angiogenesis to impair cervical carcinogenesis," *The Journal of Clinical Investigation*, vol. 114, pp. 623–33, 2004.

[112] A. Ben-Baruch, "Inflammation-associated immune suppression in cancer: the roles played by cytokines, chemokines and additional mediators," *Seminars in Cancer Biology*, vol. 16, pp. 38–52, 2006.

[113] M. Mitsuhashi, J. Liu, S. Cao *et al.*, "Regulation of interleukin-12 gene expression and its anti-tumor activities by prostaglandin E2 derived from mammary carcinomas," *Journal of Leukocyte Biology*, vol. 76, pp. 322–32, 2004.

[114] A. Mantovani, S. Sozzani, M. Locati *et al.*, "Macrophage polarization: tumor-associated macrophages as a paradigm for polarized M2 mononuclear phagocytes," *Trends in Immunology* vol. 23, pp. 549–55, 2002.

[115] G. Solinas, G. Germano, A. Mantovani *et al.*, "Tumor-associated macrophages (TAM) as major players of the cancer-related inflammation," *Journal of Leukocyte Biology*, vol. 86, pp. 1065–73, 2009.

[116] M. P. Fink, "Role of reactive oxygen and nitrogen species in acute respiratory distress syndrome," *Current Opinion in Critical Care*, vol. 8, no. 1, pp. 6–11, 2002.

[117] F. Dong, X. C. Zhang, S. Y. Li *et al.*, "Possible involvement of NADPH oxidase and JNK in homocysteine-induced oxidative stress and apoptosis in human umbilical vein endothelial cells," *Cardiovascular Toxicology*, vol. 5, no. 1, pp. 9–20, 2005.

[118] E. Novo, C. Busletta, L. V. Bonzo *et al.*, "Intracellular reactive oxygen species are required for directional migration of resident and bone marrow-derived hepatic pro-fibrogenic cells," *Journal of Hepatology*, vol. 54, no. 5, pp. 964–74, 2011.

[119] A. Van der Goes, D. Wouters, S. M. Van Der Pol *et al.*, "Reactive oxygen species enhance the migration of monocytes across the blood-brain barrier in vitro," *FASEB Journal : Official Publication of the Federation of American Societies for Experimental Biology*, vol. 15, no. 10, pp. 1852–4, 2001.

[120] J. W. Park, S. W. Ryter, and A. M. Choi, "Functional significance of apoptosis in chronic obstructive pulmonary disease," *COPD*, vol. 4, no. 4, pp. 347–53, 2007.

[121] S. W. Ryter, H. P. Kim, A. Hoetzel *et al.*, "Mechanisms of cell death in oxidative stress," *Antioxid Redox Signal*, vol. 9, no. 1, pp. 49–89, 2007.

[122] M. L. Circu, and T. Y. Aw, "Reactive oxygen species, cellular redox systems, and apoptosis," *Free Radical Biology and Medicine*, vol. 48, no. 6, pp. 749–62, 2010.

[123] B. T. Mossman, "Introduction to serial reviews on the role of reactive oxygen and nitrogen species (ROS/RNS) in lung injury and diseases," *Free Radical Biology and Medicine*, vol. 34, no. 9, pp. 1115–6, 2003.

[124] S. I. Grivennikov, F. R. Greten, and M. Karin, "Immunity, Inflammation, and Cancer," *Cell*, vol. 140, no. 6, pp. 883–899, 2010.

[125] T. A. Wilgus, "Immune cells in the healing skin wound: influential players at each stage of repair," *Pharmacological Research*, vol. 58, no. 2, pp. 112–6, 2008.

[126] R. Alinovi, M. Goldoni, S. Pinelli *et al.*, "Oxidative and pro-inflammatory effects of cobalt and titanium oxide nanoparticles on aortic and venous endothelial cells," *Toxicology In Vitro*, vol. 29, no. 3, pp. 426–37, 2014.

[127] G. Pellegrini, G. Rasperini, G. Obot *et al.*, "Soft tissue healing in alveolar socket preservation technique: histologic evaluations," *International Journal of Periodontics Restorative Dent*, vol. 34, no. 4, pp. 531–9, –2014.

[128] V. Kumar, "Innate lymphoid cells: new paradigm in immunology of inflammation," *Immunology Letters*, vol. 157, no. 1–2, pp. 23–37, 2014.

[129] A. Barbul, and M. C. Regan, "The regulatory role of T lymphocytes in wound healing," *Journal of Trauma*, vol. 30, no. 12 Suppl, pp. S97–100, 1990.

[130] T. A. Petrie, N. S. Strand, C. Tsung-Yang *et al.*, "Macrophages modulate adult zebrafish tail fin regeneration," *Development*, vol. 141, no. 13, pp. 2581–91, 2014.

[131] M. Sugaya, "Chemokines and skin diseases," *Archivum Immunologiae et Therapia Experimentalis (Warsz)*, 2014.

[132] S. Zhang, S. Dehn, M. DeBerge *et al.*, "Phagocyte-myocyte interactions and consequences during hypoxic wound healing," *Cellular Immunology*, vol. 291, no. 1–2, pp. 65–73, 2014.

[133] L. A. DiPietro, "Wound healing: the role of the macrophage and other immune cells," *Shock*, vol. 4, no. 4, pp. 233–40, 1995.

[134] C. Fathke, L. Wilson, K. Shah *et al.*, "Wnt signaling induces epithelial differentiation during cutaneous wound healing," *BMC Cell Biology*, vol. 7, pp. 4, 2006.

[135] M.-K. Song, Y.-K. Park, and J.-C. Ryu, "Polycyclic aromatic hydrocarbon (PAH)-mediated upregulation of hepatic microRNA-181 family promotes cancer cell migration by targeting MAPK phosphatase-5, regulating the activation of p38 MAPK," *Toxicology and Applied Pharmacology*, vol. 273, no. 1, pp. 130–9, 2013.

[136] Y. Wang, Y. Zhou, and D. T. Graves, "FOXO transcription factors: their clinical significance and regulation," *BioMed Research International*, vol. 2014, 2014.

[137] C. W. Chow, M. T. Herrera Abreu, T. Suzuki *et al.*, "Oxidative stress and acute lung injury," *American Journal of Respiratory Cell and Molecular Biology*, vol. 29, no. 4, pp. 427–31, 2003.

[138] C. Yang, H. Moriuchi, J. Takase *et al.*, "Oxidative stress in early stage of acute lung injury induced with oleic acid in guinea pigs," *Biological and Pharmaceutical Bulletin*, vol. 26, no. 4, pp. 424–8, 2003.

[139] V. Patel, I. V. Chivukula, S. Roy *et al.*, "Oxygen: from the benefits of inducing VEGF expression to managing the risk of hyperbaric stress," *Antioxidants & Redox Signaling*, vol. 7, no. 9–10, pp. 1377–87, 2005.

[140] A. C. Bulua, A. Simon, R. Maddipati *et al.*, "Mitochondrial reactive oxygen species promote production of proinflammatory cytokines and are elevated in TNFR1-associated periodic syndrome (TRAPS)," *The Journal of Experimental Medicine*, vol. 208, no. 3, pp. 519–33, 2011.

[141] R. J. Aitken, K. T. Jones, and S. A. Robertson, "Reactive oxygen species and sperm function—in sickness and in health," *Journal of Andrology*, vol. 33, no. 6, pp. 1096–1106, 2012.

[142] S. Eligini, I. Arenaz, S. S. Barbieri *et al.*, "Cyclooxygenase-2 mediates hydrogen peroxide-induced wound repair in human endothelial cells," *Free Radical Biology and Medicine*, vol. 46, no. 10, pp. 1428–36, 2009.

[143] M. Iizuka, and S. Konno, "Wound healing of intestinal epithelial cells," *World Journal of Gastroenterology: WJG*, vol. 17, no. 17, pp. 2161, 2011.

[144] D. Maslinska, and M. Gajewski, "Some aspects of the inflammatory process," *Folia Neuropathologica*, vol. 36, no. 4, pp. 199–204, 1998.

[145] P. Libby, P. M. Ridker, and A. Maseri, "Inflammation and atherosclerosis," *Circulation*, vol. 105, no. 9, pp. 1135–43, 2002.

[146] J. M. Rubio-Perez, and J. M. Morillas-Ruiz, "A review: inflammatory process in Alzheimer's disease, role of cytokines," *Scientific World Journal*, 2012.

[147] C. D. Gregory, "Inflammation and cancer revisited: an hypothesis on the oncogenic potential of the apoptotic tumor cell," *Autoimmunity*, vol. 46, no. 5, pp. 312–6, 2013.

[148] B. B. Aggarwal, S. Shishodia, S. K. Sandur *et al.*, "Inflammation and cancer: how hot is the link?," *Biochemical Pharmacology*, vol. 72, no. 11, pp. 1605–21, 2006.

[149] A. K. Muller, M. Meyer, and S. Werner, "The roles of receptor tyrosine kinases and their ligands in the wound repair process," *Seminars in Cell & Developmental Biology*, vol. 23, no. 9, pp. 963–70, 2012.

[150] S. Danckwardt, M. W. Hentze, and A. E. Kulozik, "Pathologies at the nexus of blood coagulation and inflammation: thrombin in hemostasis, cancer, and beyond," *Journal of Molecular Medicine: JMM*, vol. 91, no. 11, pp. 1257–71, 2013.

[151] S. Strukova, "Blood coagulation-dependent inflammation. Coagulation-dependent inflammation and inflammation-dependent thrombosis," *Frontiers in Bioscience*, vol. 11, pp. 59–80, 2006.

[152] T. N. Dugina, E. V. Kiseleva, I. V. Chistov *et al.*, "Receptors of the PAR-family as a link between blood coagulation and inflammation," *Biochemistry (Moscow)*, vol. 67, no. 1, pp. 65–74, 2002.

[153] Y. Nakanishi, M. Nakatsuji, H. Seno *et al.*, "COX-2 inhibition alters the phenotype of tumor-associated macrophages from M2 to M1 in ApcMin/+ mouse polyps," *Carcinogenesis*, vol. 32, pp. 1333–9, 2011.

[154] T. lkekawa, "Enokitake, *Flammulina velutipes*: host-mediated antitumor polysaccharides," *Food Reviews International*, vol. 11, pp. 203–6, 1995.

[155] T. Ikekawa, N. Uehara, Y. Maeda *et al.*, "Antitumor activity of aqueous extracts of edible mushrooms," *Cancer Research*, vol. 29, pp. 734–5, 1969.

[156] S. P. Wasser, "Medicinal mushrooms as a source of antitumor and immunomodulating polysaccharides," *Applied Microbiology and Biotechnology*, vol. 60, pp. 258–74, 2002.

[157] T. Inomata, G. B. Goodman, C. J. Fryer *et al.*, "Immune reaction induced by X-rays and pions and its stimulation by schizophyllan (SPG)," *The British Journal of Cancer*, vol. 27, pp. 122–5, 1996.

[158] H. Nanba, and K. Kubo, "Effect of Maitake D-fraction on cancer prevention," *Cancer*, vol. 833, pp. 204–7, 1997.

[159] C. Menetrier-Caux, G. Montmain, M. C. Dieu *et al.*, "Inhibition of the differentiation of dendritic cells from $CD34^+$ progenitors by tumor cells: role of interleukin-6 and macrophage colony-stimulating factor," *Blood*, vol. 92, pp. 4778–91, 1998.

[160] E. Y. Lin, V. Gouon-Evans, A. V. Nquyen *et al.*, "The macrophage growth factor CSF-1 in mammary gland development and tumor progression," *Journal of Mammary Gland Biology and Neoplasia*, vol. 7, pp. 147–62, 2002.

[161] C. E. Lewis, and J. W. Pollard, "Distinct role of macrophages in different tumor microenvironment," *Cancer Research*, vol. 66, pp. 605–12, 2006.

[162] E. S. Ch'ng, H. Jaafar, and S. E. Tuan Sharif, "Breast tumor angiogenesis and tumor-associated macrophages: histopathologist's perspective," *Pathology Research International*, vol. 2011, pp. 1–13, 2011.

[163] T. J. Standiford, R. Kuick, U. Bhan *et al.*, "TGF-β-induced IRAK-M expression in tumor-associated macrophages regulates lung tumor growth," *Oncogene*, vol. 30, pp. 2475–84, 2011.

[164] K. Murphy, P. Travers, and M. Walport, *Immunobiology*, 7th ed. Graland Science, 2008.

[165] T. R. Mosmann, H. Cherwinski, M. W. Bond *et al.*, "Two types of murine helper T cell clone. I. Definition according to profiles of lymphokine activities and secreted proteins. 1986," *Journal of Immunology*, vol. 175, no. 1, pp. 5–14, 2005.

[166] T. R. Mosmann, and R. L. Coffman, "TH1 and TH2 cells: different patterns of lymphokine secretion lead to different functional properties," *Annual Review of Immunology*, vol. 7, pp. 145–73, 1989.

[167] E. Maggi, "The TH1/TH2 paradigm in allergy," *Immunotechnology*, vol. 3, no. 4, pp. 233–44, 1998.

[168] P. Kidd, "Th1/Th2 balance: the hypothesis, its limitations, and implications for health and disease," *Alternative Medicine Review*, vol. 8, no. 3, pp. 223–46, 2003.

[169] M. E. Stern, K. F. Siemasko, and J. Y. Niederkorn, "The Th1/Th2 paradigm in ocular allergy," *Current Opinion in Allergy and Clinical Immunology*, vol. 5, no. 5, pp. 446–50, 2005.

[170] Z. B. Lin, and H. N. Zhang, "Anti-tumor and immunoregulatory activities of Ganoderma lucidum and its possible mechanisms," *Acta Pharmacologica Sinica*, vol. 25, no. 11, pp. 1387–95, 2004.

[171] J. S. Shi, and A. C. Camus, "Hepcidins in amphibians and fishes: antimicrobial peptides or iron-regulatory hormones?" *Developmental and Comparative Immunology*, vol. 30, no. 9, pp. 746–55, 2006.

[172] J. Y. Chen, W. J. Lin, and T. L. Lin, "A fish antimicrobial peptide, tilapia hepcidin TH2-3, shows potent antitumor activity against human fibrosarcoma cells," *Peptides*, vol. 30, no. 9, pp. 1636–42, 2009.

[173] Y. X. Chen, X. M. Xu, S. G. Hong *et al.*, "RGD-tachyplesin inhibits tumor growth," *Cancer Research*, vol. 61, no. 6, pp. 2434–38, 2001.

[174] D. W. Hoskin, and A. Ramamoorthy, "Studies on anticancer activities of antimicrobial peptides," *Biochimica et Biophysica Acta–Biomembranes*, vol. 1778, no. 2, pp. 357–75, 2008.

[175] N. Papo, M. Shahar, L. Eisenbach *et al.*, "A novel lytic peptide composed of DL-amino acids selectively kills cancer cells in culture and in mice," *Journal of Biological Chemistry*, vol. 278, no. 23, pp. 21018–23, 2003.

[176] L. T. Eliassen, G. Berge, A. Leknessund *et al.*, "The antimicrobial peptide, Lactoferricin B, is cytotoxic to neuroblastoma cells in vitro and inhibits xenograft growth in vivo," *International Journal of Cancer*, vol. 119, no. 3, pp. 493–500, 2006.

Chapter 9

How Plasma Membrane and Cytoskeletal Dynamics Influence Single-Cell Wound Healing: Mechanotransduction, Tension and Tensegrity

Eric Boucher, Tatsuya Kato and Craig A. Mandato

Additional information is available at the end of the chapter

http://dx.doi.org/10.5772/63765

Abstract

Organisms are able to recover from injuries by replacing damaged tissues, which recover by replacing damaged cells and extracellular structures. Similarly, a cell recovers from injuries by replacing damaged components of its structural integrity: its plasma membrane and cytoskeletal structures. Cells can be thought of as tensegral structures, their structural integrity relying on the interplay between tensile forces generated within and without the cell, and the compressive elements that counteracts them. As such, direct or indirect insults to the plasma membrane or cytoskeleton of a cell may not only result in the temporary loss of structural integrity, but also directly impact its ability to respond to its environment. This chapter will focus on the various aspects linking tensile forces and single-cell wound healing: where and how are they generated, how does the cell counteract them and how does the cell return to its previous tensegrity state? These questions will be explored using ubiquitous and cell-type specific examples of single-cell repair processes. Special attention will be given to changes in plasma membrane composition and area to cytoskeletal dynamics, and how these factor each other to influence and effect single-cell repair.

Keywords: single-cell wound healing, tensegrity, plasmalemma dynamics, cytoskeleton dynamics, mechanotransduction

1. Introduction

Cells are neither amorphous blobs nor rigid, unchanging structures. They are able to sense, react and most of the time recover from many types of physical insults ranging from pores created by osmotic shock or bacterial toxins to mechanical damages of various origins and intensity. Whatever the origin, the loss of barrier function provided by the plasmalemma leads to many potentially harmful effects including, but not limited to, the loss of intracellular content, the uncontrolled entry of Ca^{2+} and exposure of the intracellular milieu to reactive oxygen species (ROS), all of which may lead to a broad range of diminished cellular function, or even cell death. The negative effects of cellular injury are not limited to biochemical processes, they also directly affect the cell's structural integrity. As such, single-cell repair is as much a return to normal cell function as it is a return to structural integrity.

While they share common general steps of wound stabilization, resealing of plasmalemma damage and cytoskeletal remodeling, wound-healing mechanisms have been shown to vary widely according to the types of injury and cell-types. This chapter, using ubiquitous and injury- and cell-specific examples, aims to present an overview of the different mechanisms proposed for wound healing. Particular focus is put on how mechanotransduction, tension and tensegrity influences single-cell wound healing.

2. Background

2.1. Cells are tensegral structures

In eukaryotic cells, structural integrity is achieved and maintained through tensegrity [1], a term originally coined by the architect R. Buckminster Fuller as a portmanteau of "tensile integrity." Tensegrity describes stable structures achieved through prestress and the interaction of opposing stretch and compression elements [2]. In the cell, cytoskeletal actin filaments act as the main stretch-generating elements and microtubules are the main compression-bearing elements [3]. The role of intermediate filaments is not as well defined, as vimentin has been suggested to act principally as a major component that allows chondrocytes to withstand compressive loading, its contribution to the regulation of cytoskeletal tension and elastic modulus being relatively minor [4, 5]. While tensegrity is mainly achieved through these cytoskeletal elements, the plasma membrane has also been shown to play a key role in the cell's tensegrity [6]. Indeed, the composition and shape of the plasma membrane [7, 8], its intrinsic in-plane tension and membrane-to-cortex attachments (MCAs) [6] and the various external forces that may act on a cell's plasma membrane [9–11] have all been suggested to contribute to cellular tensegrity. The terminology surrounding these forces can be somewhat opaque and as such are defined in greater detail in **Figure 1**.

2.2. Plasma membrane disruptions, tensegrity and spontaneous repair

Early observations of lipid bilayers [12], liposomes [13] and erythrocyte ghosts [14] have shown that resealing of small lesions (<1 nm) are thermodynamically favored events [14]. Disruption of lipid membranes leads to the loss of barrier function of the plasma membrane, which may lead to uncontrolled changes in osmolality and hydrostatic pressure. These changes may be sufficient to alter the wounded cell's apparent membrane tension and thus its tensegrity state [11].

Apparent membrane tension

The force required to effectively deform liposomal membranes has historically been referred simply as "membrane tension". The plasma membrane of cells also contains relatively high amounts of proteins that specifically or non-specifically link them to cytoskeletal structures and therefore require higher amounts of energy to deform than lipid vesicles. As such, it is more accurate to use "apparent membrane tension" in the case of cells since it is the sum of the tensile forces produced by the intrinsic in-plane tension and the membrane-to-cortex attachments (MCAs).

a. In-plane tension of the plasma membrane

In-plane tension of the plasma membrane is generated by the osmotically controlled difference in hydrostatic pressures between the cytosol and extracellular fluid directly acting on the plasmalemma [11, 12] and on the attached cytoskeleton [13]. In-plane tension is thus a factor of the mechanical and viscoelastic properties of the plasmalemma and can be influenced by variations in plasmalemma area [12, 14], shape [7, 8, 15] and composition [7, 16].

b. Membrane-to-cortex attachments (MCAs).

In eukaryotic cells, adhesion between the plasma membrane and the relatively stiffer cortical cytoskeleton significantly contributes to a cell's apparent membrane tension [17]. Whereas in-plane tension is usually considered to be uniform across the membrane, MCA is able to vary across the cell surface, thereby creating areas of high and low apparent membrane tension in polarized cells [18], as well as membrane blebs in areas of low MCA. The specifics of MCA regulations are still unclear, but involves several membrane associated proteins such as filamin, spectrin, ankyrin, and affixin, as well as involving inner leaflet PIP_2, as it is known to bind to or affects a great number of actin binding and remodeling proteins such as MARCKS, cofilin, profilin, gelsolin, vinculin, talin, α-actinin, WASP, Arp2/3, and the Rho family of GTPases (reviewed in [19]).

c. Focal adhesions and Stress-fibers

External parameters such as the forces generated via cell-matrix adhesion are partly mediated by integrins, a group of heterodimeric transmembrane proteins that bind a variety of extra-cellular matrix (ECM) proteins. Integrins connect to the actin cytoskeleton via numerous intracellular linker proteins such as talin and vinculin. Uneven distribution of these adhesion complexes into "focal adhesions" can therefore influence cytoskeletal and apparent membrane tension, but their assembly and disassembly can also induce variations in apparent membrane tension. Indeed, focal adhesions [20, 21] and stress fibers [22] can act as mechanosensors and induce actin depolymerization through a variety of processes including mechanosensitive ion channels, RhoA signaling or directly via F-actin and cofilin (reviewed in [20]).

Figure 1. Tensile forces in the unwounded cell.

Immediately following its disruption, the plasma membrane also loses its asymmetry [15] and individual membrane phospholipids become disordered around the wound edge, which creates edge tension [16]. Indeed, plasma membrane damage directly alters the membrane composition, shape, and its physical properties. Mechanical damage also exposes hydrophobic domains of phospholipid molecules to the comparatively aqueous environment of the newly formed wound edge, which in turn creates a difference in chemical potential between the phospholipids of the wound edge and those of the planar membrane [13]. It is this so-called edge tension [16] that along with the line tension [17] present on the wound edge, provides the driving force necessary for the lateral movement of phospholipids [18, 19] and spontaneous resealing of phospholipid membranes. Rates of spontaneous resealing of these relatively simple systems have been shown to depend on a variety of factors that also affect single-cell wound healing: bilayer composition [19], Ca^{2+} concentration [20] and disruption radius [13]. On the contrary, liposomes, erythrocytes and erythrocyte ghosts membranes are associated with a variety of proteins such as spectrin, which diminish overall phospholipid lateral movement and lead to high tension at the wound edge [21]. As such, neither large liposomes, nor erythrocyte ghosts possess the machinery necessary to actively respond to the dramatic loss of tensegrity and changes in localized tensions that are created by large membrane disruption. Consequently, large erythrocyte ghosts' wounds do not spontaneously reseal under physiological conditions [14]. This has been attributed to a number of factors, including the presence of strong MCAs [19] and the lack of endomembranes [22] (**Figure 1**).

Finally, plasma membrane disruption also exposes the cell to high levels of ROS and Ca^{2+} ions, either of which can be detrimental to normal cell function. Numerous pathways involving membrane dynamics such as the capacitation [23] and acrosomal reaction [24] steps of sperm maturation (reviewed in [25]) involve Ca^{2+}-dependent signaling. Exocytosis events, such as surfactant secretion [26–28], as well as neuroendocrine [29], synapses [30–32] and auditory cells exocytosis [33, 34], are similarly Ca^{2+} dependent. These events are mediated by a variety of Ca^{2+}-binding proteins such as calpains, annexins and synaptotagmins. Unsurprisingly, the uncontrolled Ca^{2+} entry that accompanies plasma membrane damage has been shown to activate the same families of Ca^{2+}-binding proteins (reviewed in [35]). The downstream effects of Ca^{2+} entry will eventually lead to an overall diminution of apparent membrane tension.

3. Early events of single-cell wound healing are mechanically driven processes

Single-cell repair proper is an active process, requiring dynamic and concerted manipulations of the cell's membrane and cytoskeletal compartments. Most of these processes, however, take place relatively late following injury or are dependent on preliminary disruption of cytoskeletal structures. In this subchapter, we present the principal wound mitigation events that are activated in the moments immediately following injury and facilitate the subsequent exocytosis-, endocytosis- or membrane-shedding-mediated wound-healing processes.

3.1. Caveolae-mediated decrease of in-plane membrane tension

Caveolae are plasma membrane invaginations with a diameter of 50–80 nm and specific flask-like morphology [36]. Caveolae have long been known to flatten in response to mechanically induced membrane deformation stretch [37]. Indeed, the preincubation of cells with methyl-β-cyclodextrin diminishes the time to cell lysis upon hypotonic challenge [38]. Methyl-β-cyclodextrin is a cholesterol-depleting compound that has also been shown to severely reduce the number of caveolae at the cell surface [39], probably by limiting the recruitment of caveolin oligomers to the plasma membrane. Caveolae can thus be viewed as a "membrane buffer" that limits injury-induced increases in apparent membrane tension by diminishing the in-plane tension without the need of additional membrane components from Ca^{2+}-dependent exocytosis (**Figure 1**). Instead, additional membrane area is produced by the rapid flattening and disassembling of caveolae upon mechanical stress, which are rapidly reassembled upon mechanical stress release [40].

The exact molecular events leading to caveolae assembly and disassembly is still somewhat unclear, the specifics of which go beyond the scope of this chapter. Briefly, their assembly is initiated by the clustering and further recruitment of phosphatidylinositol 4,5-bisphosphate (PIP_2), phosphatidylserine (PS) and cholesterol with caveolin oligomers. Recruitment of various cavins oligomers will further increase the local concentration of negatively charged lipid, which in turn nucleates membrane curvature and formation of caveolae structure by the way of electrostatic cavins-cavins or cavins-membrane interactions (reviewed in [41, 42]).

While caveolin-3-deficient mice exhibit robust muscular degeneration [43], the relative contribution of caveolae in protection against stretch-induced mechanical deformation is therefore difficult to judge. An attractive, albeit speculative, hypothesis is that caveolae are involved in both wound prevention and healing. Firstly, they can act as a membrane reserve that buffers the cell against local or global increases in in-plane membrane tension. Secondly, they can passively potentiate plasma membrane repair by releasing apparent membrane tension near the wound edge, a site of initial high membrane tension because of both high line tension and MCA-related tether forces. Finally, caveolae are also known to play central roles in dysferlin-mediated exocytosis (see Section 4.1.3.1) and the endocytic removal of bacterial pores ([44, 45]; see Section 4.2.1) and small mechanical lesions ([45]; see Section 4.1.3.2).

3.2. Protein array-mediated wound site stabilization

Most of the wound-healing mechanisms described to date (see Section 4) require a substantial lowering of apparent membrane tension. This is achieved in a number of ways, including the disruptions of MCAs through both Ca^{2+}-dependent and Ca^{2+}-independent membrane repair mechanisms (see Section 4). These Ca^{2+}- and mechanosensor-mediated disruption of the MCAs and cytoskeletons have been shown to occur in large areas surrounding the wounds or throughout the cell and therefore only help to stabilize the wound indirectly.

The annexins form a large family of Ca^{2+}-sensitive, negatively charged phospholipid-binding proteins (reviewed in [46]). Upon wounding, annexin V translocate to the internal leaflet of the damaged membrane where it binds to the newly exposed phosphatidylserine residues on the wound edge and self-assembles into two-dimensional (2D) arrays [47]. These arrays have been shown to be able to cluster phospholipids, thereby reducing the lateral diffusion of phospholipids [48]. As such, these arrays may help stabilize the wound site until the apparent membrane tension has sufficiently been lowered by other wound-healing mechanisms (reviewed in [35]; see Section 3.1) Indeed, laser ablation experiments performed on murine perivascular cells have shown that the formation of annexin V arrays was necessary for normal wound healing and cell survival [49]. Similar wound stabilization arrays have also been proposed to involve mitsugumin 53 (MG53) oligomers, mini-dysferlinC72 and caveolins [50].

3.3. Cytoskeletal and MCA dynamics and wound healing

The cytoskeleton constitutes a substantial component of apparent membrane tension in eukaryotic cells through MCAs (**Figure 1**). Consequently, cortical cytoskeleton dynamics can also reduce apparent membrane tension and constitutes an important preliminary step of single-cell wound healing. Indeed, actin destabilization has been demonstrated to enhance active membrane resealing in a variety of cell types, including 3T3 fibroblasts [51], septal neurons [52] and RGM1 gastric epithelial cells [53].

3.3.1. Direct and indirect regulation of single-cell injury by cytoskeleton dynamics

Considering actin's importance for wound healing, it is not surprising that cellular injury affects actin dynamics in several ways. Changes of tensegrity experienced by damaged cells may lead to cytoskeletal remodeling either directly or through mechanotransductive signals. Indeed, sonoporation experiments showed that disruptions of existent plasmalemmal and adjacent cytoskeletal structures were enough to elicit a sustained and broad secondary disruption of the actin cytoskeleton [54]. As previously stated, actin filament bundles are the main providers of tensile forces necessary for a cell's tensegrity ([1]; **Figure 1**). Cells usually respond to external changes in tensile forces by modulating the sizes, numbers and distributions of F-actin and stress fibers in order to preserve mechanical homeostasis (reviewed in [55]). This is exemplified by experiments performed on endothelial cells [56] and osteoblasts [57] in which compression-induced stress fiber collapse through buckling, followed by actin disassembly events [56, 58]. Computer-assisted modeling strongly suggests that the loss of tensile force within the actin fiber upon its buckling is sufficient to induce actin disassembly [59, 60]. Whether a similar phenomenon contributes to actin fiber disassembly following mechanical damage is intriguing, as it would mean that actin filaments are able to act as their own mechanosensor. Indeed, a series of experiments showed that the tension state of individual actin filaments were inversely proportional to the binding affinity and actin filament-severing activity of cofilin [61–63]. Cofilin is an actin-binding protein that is known to accelerate actin depolymerization at the pointed end, which is also able to sever F-actin [64, 65]. This type of mechanosensing is especially attractive in the context of single-cell wound healing, as it is more sensitive and could induce downstream signals much faster than other traditional mechanosensors such as mechanosensitive ion channels [66], integrins, talin, or other F-actin-localized mechanosensors (reviewed in [62]).

Aside from mechanically related disruptions, cortical and cytoskeletal actin filaments are also disrupted in a variety of Ca^{2+}-dependent manners. Indeed, permeabilization of cells by bacterial pores, such as streptolysin O (SLO), leads to an increase in intracellular Ca^{2+} without substantial direct damage to the plasmalemma or subjacent actin cytoskeleton and also incites actin depolymerization [67]. While Ca^{2+} is able to disrupt actin filaments on its own [68, 69], the effect of Ca^{2+} on the disruption of normal cytoskeletal architecture is probably best exemplified by its activation of calpains. Calpains are Ca^{2+}-dependent, intracellular cysteine proteases that are known for their relative specificity [70]. Among others, calpains have been shown to cleave talin [71] into a large globular head domain that directly binds integrins, PIP_2 and focal adhesion kinases, and a rod domain that binds vinculin and actin. Its degradation by calpains upon wounding would therefore be compatible with the cytoskeletal remodeling that follows membrane disruptions.

3.3.2. Cytoskeletal dynamics is at the center of single-cell wound healing processes

Aside from its role in reducing apparent membrane tension, cytoskeleton remodeling is further required for single-cell wound healing as several plasma-resealing processes involve exocytosis of various vesicles such as lysosomes, MG53-positive vesicles and AHNAK-positive vesicles (reviewed in [35]; see Sections 4.1.2 and 4.1.3.1). As such, these intracellular vesicles must undergo actin- or microtubule-mediated transport to the wound site. An intact cortical cytoskeleton would therefore hinder not only transport and fusion of these vesicles, but also the subsequent removal of the damaged portions of the plasma membrane through endocytosis, blebbing or membrane-shedding processes. However, it should be noted that active repair mechanisms, such as exocytosis, cannot occur with just a minimal actin structure [67]. Reorganization of the cytoskeleton needs to be balanced in such a way that vesicles from intracellular pools are able to cross the actin barrier layer [53], then undergo docking to the wound site facilitated by remaining actin filaments [72] and the kinesin and myosin motor proteins [73].

4. Archetypes of single-cell repair: influence of injury type and cell type

As previously stated, disruptions of the plasma membrane or cytoskeletal structures may lead to local or global increases in apparent membrane tension that prohibits spontaneous resealing to occur. Furthermore, plasma membrane damage can be accompanied by direct or indirect disruptions of the cytoskeleton, which worsen the damaged cell structural integrity. In contrast, plasma membrane disruptions generated by pore-forming toxins (PFTs) have little to no immediate impact on local in-plane membrane tension. As such, Ca^{2+}-mediated exocytosis (see Section 4.1.2) and cytoskeletal remodeling (see Section 3.3) and cell-type (**Table 1**) may have profoundly different impacts depending on the type and size of the injury and may determine the healing pathway that is available to the cell (**Figure 2**) (reviewed in [35, 74]). Indeed, while uncontrolled entry of Ca^{2+} is a hallmark of all injury types, its intensity and distribution, together with the nature and size of the wound, as well as tissular context may control how the wound is repaired (**Figure 2**). The following section aims to present each wound-healing processes in the cellular context of which they were first identified. As it will become apparent in the next subsection, some processes, such as exocytosis, are quasi-ubiquitous, albeit with slight variations in vesicle species or molecular players involved. On the other hand, other processes, such as ESCRT-mediated membrane shedding (see Section 4.2.2) seem to be heavily dependent on wound size.

Cell type	Repair mechanism	Experimental wound type(s)	Major molecular players	Reference(s)
Germ cells				
Oocytes	"Membrane patch" formation	Mechanical wounding; laser wounding	Yolk granules; syntaxins; SNAP-25	[22, 75]

Cell type	Repair mechanism	Experimental wound type(s)	Major molecular players	Reference(s)
	Synaptotagmin-mediated exocytosis and "vertex fusion"	Mechanical wounding; laser wounding	Yolk granules; synaptobrevin; synaptotagmin VII; SNAP-25	[76–82]
	Actomyosin contractile ring	Mechanical wounding; laser wounding	RhoA; Cdc42; F-actin; myosin II; microtubules	[83–89]
Somatic cells				
Neuronal cells	Synaptotagmin-mediated exocytosis	Axon transection	Lysosomes; synaptotagmin I; syntaxin I;	[90, 91]
	Calpain-mediated vesicle fusion	Axon transection	Calpains	[52, 92–94]
Fibroblasts	Synaptotagmin-mediated exocytosis	Mechanical wounding	Lysosomes; synaptotagmin I; Synaptotagmin VII; VAMP-7; Syntaxin-4; SNAP-23	[76, 77, 95]
	Facilitated resealing	Laser wounding	Predocked TGN-vesicles; myosin IIA; PKC	[51, 96–98]
	Potentiated resealing	Laser wounding	PKG; CREB	[99]
Muscle cells	"Membrane patch" formation; Dysferlin-mediated exocytosis	Mechanical wounding; laser wounding	Lysosomes; calpains; mini-dysferlinC72; MG53; KIF5B; AHNAK; S100A10; Annexin II	[50, 100–107]
	Caveolae-mediated endocytic repair	Mechanical wounding	ASM[2]; Caveolin-3; annexin I	[108–113]
Epithelial cells	Caveolae-mediated endocytosis	PFTs[1]	ASM; Caveolin-3; annexin I	[45, 108, 110]
	ESCRT-mediated shedding	PFTs	ALG-2; ESCRT-III; ALIX; Vps4	[74, 114]

PFTs: Pore-forming toxins; ASM: Acid Sphingomyelinase

Table 1. Wound healing mechanisms according to cell-type.

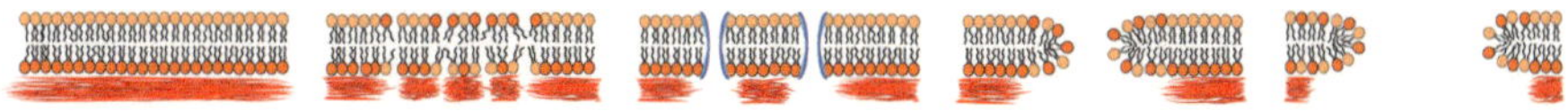

Wound type	*Unwounded plasma membrane*	*Very small wounds* *(electroporation, osmotic shock)*	*PFTs*	*Small mechanical wounds*	*Large mechanical wounds*
Effect of wound on:					
Calcium entry	-	Small uniform entry	Highly localized to pore site	Localized and restricted at wound site	Localized and restricted at wound site
Apparent Membrane Tension	-	None to small increase	None	Small increase	Large increase
In-plane membrane tension	-	None	None	Small increase	Large increase
MCAs	-	Small uniform	Disruptions localized at pore-sites	Disruptions localized at wound-sites	Disruptions over large areas and wound-site
Role of exocytosis	-	-↑ membrane area	-↑ membrane area **-ASM delivery to outer leaflet**	-↑ **membrane area** -ASM delivery to outer leaflet	-↑ **membrane area** **-ASM delivery to outer leaflet**
Possible wound healing mechanism(s)	-	-Spontaneous resealing -Caveolae flattening	-Endocytic degradation -Ectocytosis	-Exocytic repair -Facilitated repair -Endocytic repair *(Caveolae-mediated repair)* -Blebbing and membrane shedding *(ESCRT, Annexin II:S100A10, etc.)*	-"Membrane patch" -Endocytic repair *(Caveolae-mediated repair)*

Figure 2. Schematic (top) depicts lateral sections of the plasma membrane before and after different types of wounding (individual phospholipids represented as orange and beige heads with hairpin-like tails; cortical actin network represented as red lines; toxic pores represented in blue). Table (bottom) lists changes to wound-type-dependent factors of Ca^{2+} influx and tension, role of exocytosis and possible wound healing mechanisms upon different types of wounding. MCAs: membrane-to-cortex attachments; PFTs: pore-forming toxins.

4.1. Large wounds: exocytic repair, membrane patches and endocytic repair

4.1.1. Oocytes

Oocytes of *Xenopus laevis* and sea urchins are large, easily accessible and manipulable cells. While their size and lack of adhesive and cell-cell contact-derived tension distinguish them from mammalian somatic cells, these characteristics also provide a simpler platform which helped to elaborate the first models of single-cell wound healing. Oocytes have been observed to recover form very large mechanical disruptions of both the plasma membrane and cytoskeleton (>1000 μm²) [75].

4.1.1.1. "Membrane patch"-mediated resealing

In addition to providing essential amino acids and other nutrients for oocyte development, yolk platelets also act as vesicle reservoirs upon plasma membrane injury of oocytes in a variety of species [22, 75]. Upon wounding, there is a rapid influx of Ca^{2+} from the extracellular milieu to the intracellular space, which favors rapid homotypic fusions of yolk granules [75]. These homotypic vesicular fusogenic events lead to the formation of a large "membrane patch" that eventually covers the gap present at the wound site [75–77]. It is perhaps best to think of the "membrane patch" model of wound healing as a somewhat oocyte-specific process. Indeed, this model relies almost entirely on homotypic fusions [75], and yolk granules offer a pool of readily available vesicle reserves that is incomparable with those available to somatic cells [78]. Also, while the "membrane patch" model of single-cell repair has also initially been proposed for the repair of large wounds in somatic cells [79, 80], it now appears that large somatic cell membrane disruptions are directly removed by endocytosis, which heavily relies on exocytosis and heterotypic fusion events (reviewed in [35, 81]; see Section 4.1.3.2). Whether these apparent differences are an intrinsic property of oocytes, a direct consequence of the wound size involved, larger wounds exposing larger areas of the intracellular space to Ca^{2+}, or of the higher density of available vesicles in oocytes, remains open for interpretation.

While the mechanism behind membrane patch formation is sufficient to block unregulated exchanges between extra- and intracellular spaces, it does not technically reseal the membrane, or restore membrane continuity or normal plasma membrane composition and shape. The way this resealing is achieved is still somewhat unclear and is the subject of two alternate but compatible models. The first states that heterotypic fusion events between intracellular vesicles, the membrane patch and the borders of the wounded plasma membrane first restore membrane continuity, after which contraction of an actomyosin ring restores normal plasma membrane composition and shape ([82]; see Section 4.1.1.2). The so-called "vertex fusion" model relies on the same heterotypic fusion events but states that multiple fusion pores would form around the periphery of the wounded region. Expansion of these fusion pores may cause shedding of a membrane fragment containing both wound residual portions of the patch vesicle, in a mechanism reminiscent of the one observed for yeast vacuoles ([83, 84]; reviewed in [81]).

4.1.1.2. Actomyosin contractile ring

As previously discussed, disruptions of the plasma membrane may be accompanied by, as well as induce direct and indirect cytoskeletal disruptions. Restoration of the local cytoskeleton is primarily driven by the contraction of a purse-string structure primarily assembled from F-actin and myosin II [82]. This actomyosin ring is anchored to the plasma membrane at frequent points along its border [82], and its closure has been shown to restore normal membrane composition and shape [82].

Formation of the actomyosin array is controlled by the Ca^{2+}-dependent recruitment and activation of Rho family GTPase proteins [85]. In *Xenopus* oocytes, activated Rho GTPases Ras homolog family member A (RhoA) and cell division control protein 42 homolog (Cdc42) localize to exclusive, concentric zones around the wound [86, 87]. These GTPases influence the activities of, among many other downstream targets, myosin light-chain kinase (MLCK) and myosin phosphatase [88, 89]. Through the above effectors, RhoA indirectly regulate the phosphorylation levels of myosin II light chains, mediating the assembly and contraction of the actomyosin ring (reviewed in [85]). As for Cdc42, its interactions with neural Wiskott-Aldrich syndrome protein (N-WASP) and actin-related protein 2/3 (Arp2/3) [90–92] induce construction of highly dynamic, branched F-actin networks [86]. Binding of Arp2/3 with the C terminus of N-WASP, which is activated by Cdc42, stimulates Arp2/3's actin nucleation activity [91], accelerating production of actin networks critically involved in actomyosin ring assembly. The formation of contractile arrays has been demonstrated to also be regulated by an underlying "signaling treadmill" [93] in which gradients of Rho GTPase activities influence F-actin turnover. RhoA is preferentially activated and maintains its zone of high activity at the leading edge of the wound [93], while active Cdc42 encircles the inner RhoA zone [86]. The processes leading to the establishment of these concentric zones is still somewhat unclear, but a recent study by Vaughan et al. [94] has led to some interesting insights. They observed that wounding induced the formation of micrometer-scale PIP_{2}-, phosphatidylinositol 3,4,5-trisphosphate (PIP_3)- and phosphatidylserine (PS)-, phosphatidic acid (PA)- and diacylglycerol (DAG)-enriched domains. This is of particular interest as PS moved to a zone closest to the wound edge, near to an area of high RhoA activity, whereas PIP_2 and PIP_3 were observed to be associated with the so-called Cdc42 zone. As for DAG and PA, both of them were shown to immediately segregate in a zone overlapping that of which of RhoA and Cdc42 activity. Since DAG is known to be able to recruit PKCβ and PKCη [95], the authors suggested that generation of DAG at the wound site could therefore act as an upstream signal for the regulation of RhoA and Cdc42. Whether a similar signal cascade exist for somatic cells is still unclear, but cell-lifting experiments done of primary epithelial cells induced phospholipase D (PLD) activation was transient, consistent with a possible role in membrane repair and PLD inhibitors inhibited membrane resealing upon laser injury [96].

Whether such a contractile ring can form in the smaller wounds associated with somatic cells is unclear, but the formation of strikingly similar concentric zones of Rho1, Cdc42 and Rac have been shown to form in *Drosophila* syncytial embryos following plasma membrane wounding (reviewed in [97]).

4.1.2. *Neuronal cells and fibroblasts: insights into exocytic repair*

Neuronal cells have markedly polarized membranes, with extreme distances between axons and the cell soma. The elongated morphology of axons make them particularly susceptible to shear stress injury and offering a challenge to vesicle trafficking. Fibroblasts, on the other hand, offer a relatively simpler platform for the study of single-cell wound healing.

While the repair of oocytes relies on homotypic fusion of abundant yolk granules (see Section 4.1.1.1), repair of mammalian cells has long been observed to depend on the Ca^{2+}-dependent exocytosis of intracellular vesicles [98]. Conventional lysosomes are not only the major vesicles responsible for Ca^{2+}-dependent exocytosis in non-neuronal and non-secretory cells [99], but also occupy a central role in the exocytic [100] and endocytic models of single-cell repair (see Section 4.1.3.2). The lysosomes involved in plasmalemma repair can be defined as lysosomal-associated membrane protein 1 (LAMP-1)-positive [100], acid sphingomyelinase (ASM)-containing intracellular vesicles [101].

Exocytosis-mediated repair attracted considerable interest when Steinhardt et al. [98] specified the mechanistic similarities with Ca^{2+}-triggered synaptic exocytosis, both of which are dependent on Ca^{2+} [102, 103] and actin cytoskeleton dynamics [104–106]. Ca^{2+}-triggered synaptic exocytosis involves the interaction of synaptotagmin I, a C2 domains-containing protein present in exocytic vesicles and the soluble N-ethylmaleimide-sensitive factor (NSF) attachment protein receptor (SNARE) complexes of the synaptic membrane (reviewed in [107]). Interestingly, neurotransmission inhibitors botulinum neurotoxin A and B also negatively affected or completely blocked membrane healing in sea urchin embryos and Swiss 3T3 fibroblasts [98]. Similarly, treatment with an antibody targeting the active synaptotagmin I C2A domain was observed to prevent membrane resealing of squid and crayfish giant axons [108], 3T3 fibroblasts [100] and rat PC12 cells [109]. In contrast to the neuron-specific synaptotagmin I [110], synaptotagmin VII is ubiquitously expressed and has been found to also influence exocytic membrane repair of other cell types such as sea urchin embryos [98, 103], Chinese hamster ovary cells [100], Swiss 3T3 fibroblasts [98, 100, 111], mouse embryonic fibroblasts [112] and epithelial cells [113–115]. Indeed, embryonic fibroblasts of synaptotagmin VII-deficient mice were observed to have defects in lysosome exocytosis and wound resealing [112]. The mechanism involves the Ca^{2+}-dependent activation and recruitment of synaptotagmin VIII-positive vesicles [111], which are then transported to the wound site via microtubule-dependent trafficking [116]. Once at the plasma membrane, lysosome-bound synaptotagmin VII interacts with the SNARE formed by vesicle-associated membrane protein 7 (VAMP-7), syntaxin-4 and synaptosomal-associated proteins (SNAPs), such as SNAP-23, which leads to heterologous fusion of the lysosome with the plasma membrane [115].

As opposed to the "membrane-patch" model that relies on predominantly homotypic fusions, the exocytic model of single-cell repair assumes the predominance of heterotypic fusion events with the plasma membrane. Indeed, early microneedle-wounding experiments clearly showed a punctate distribution of lysosomal marker LAMP-1 around the wound site [100]. These heterotypic fusion events were initially thought to promote resealing by increasing plasma membrane surface area [100, 117], thereby lowering in-plane membrane tension (see Section 3.1), which could theoretically favor spontaneous resealing events between the two wound edges of with nearby vesicles [118]. Indeed, inhibiting the lowering of in-plane membrane tension via actin stabilization, or by inhibiting exocytosis via neurotoxins A and B ([51, 118] inhibits successful cell repair but is rescued by artificially reducing in-plane tension via the addition of surface active Pluronic F68 NF [51]).

As previously stated, the in-plane tension lowering effect of exocytosis indubitably has been shown to be crucial for plasma membrane repair of a variety of wounds (reviewed in [35, 119]), several lines of evidence have shown that they are not the last process in the resealing of plasma membranes. Indeed, aside from the notable exceptions of facilitated membrane repair that involves recruitment of additional vesicles originating from the transgolgi network (TGN) [120], there is little to no evidence that large micrometer size wounds are repaired via purely exocytic means. Rather, it seems that exocytosis acts as a preliminary step of other wound-healing process (see Section 4.1.3.2). In fact, there is debate as to whether conclusions made in earlier studies of exocytosis were misinterpretations of endocytic vesicles as an exocytic patch or vesicles, due to the studies being performed in the absence of extracellular endocytic tracers [121]. Similarly, there is also considerable evidence that the synaptotagmin VII/SNARE system may not be the only, or even the main, fusogenic system that mediates Ca^{2+}-dependent exocytosis following injury, at least in cells that are under constant mechanical assault such as muscle fibers and muscle cells (see Section 4.1.3).

4.1.3. Muscle cells

4.1.3.1. Dysferlin-mediated exocytosis

Muscle fibers are highly mechanically active and endure constant mechanical stresses from movement and exercise, and therefore are prone to stress-related injury. Indeed, their tubular morphology further facilitates the generation of shear stress along the long axis upon eccentric contraction, in which the muscle fiber lengthens while its constituent sarcomeres contract [122]. T-tubules are invaginations of the sarcolemma that run perpendicular to the overall muscle fiber's long axis. These invaginations penetrate deep into the muscle fiber and mediate depolarization of membrane potential required for proper muscle contraction via excitation-contraction coupling. High levels of normal stress exerted on T-tubules upon eccentric contraction may rupture them, thereby severely disrupting the local sarcolemma [123, 124]. As such, muscle cells, especially muscle fibers, evolved potent single-cell repair mechanisms to cope with the constant duress under which they find themselves. For this reason, muscle cells and muscle fibers were instrumental in the study of mechanisms responsible for mammalian somatic single-cell repair.

Dysferlin was initially identified as genetic causes of limb-girdle muscular dystrophy 2B (LGMD2B) [125] and Miyoshi myopathy [126], and dysferlin has since been shown to be ubiquitously expressed with particularly high levels in skeletal muscle, heart and kidney [127]. Its prominence in muscle membrane repair was experimentally demonstrated when dysferlin-null mice were observed to develop progressive limb-girdle muscular dystrophy 2B due to defects in Ca^{2+}-dependent sarcolemma resealing [128]. Dysferlin is a member of the C2-domain-containing ferlin family, which are known regulators of Ca^{2+}-dependent vesicle fusion for auditory neurotransmission [34, 129, 130] and are believe to be functionally similar to synaptotagmin I [131]. Dysferlin's localization at the sarcolemma [132] has led to its research in the context of sarcolemma repair. Indeed, it appears that in muscle cells, dysferlin is at the center of Ca^{2+}-dependent exocytosis following injury, after which intracellular membranes are delivered to the plasma membrane, and ASM released to the outer leaflet [133].

Molecular events involved in dysferlin-mediated exocytosis are a lot more complex than the one involved in synaptotagmin VII/SNAREs-mediated fusions. Indeed, dysferlin has been shown to bind to or be associated with a relatively high number of proteins including MG53 [134, 135], caveolin-3 [134], annexin I [136] and many others (reviewed in [137]). However, a study of human myoblasts by Lek et al. [50] led to the discovery that a calpain-cleaved product of dysferlin played a direct role in the sarcolemma's exocytic repair mechanism. Briefly, calpains activated by injury-induced Ca^{2+} influx cleave dysferlin, which releases its C-term fragment mini-dysferlinC72 [50, 138, 139]. Following vesicle packaging, mini-dysferlinC72-containing cytoplasmic vesicles are then transported to the wound site. Once localized, mini-dysferlinC72 interacts with MG53 compartments to form an array, which has been proposed to promote repair by way of wound stabilization (see Section 3.2), as well as promote heterotypic fusion between intracellular vesicles [140] and the sarcolemma [50, 138, 139].

Interestingly, dysferlin has also been shown to associate with AHNAK and may be related to enlargeosome exocytosis. Enlargeosomes are small, AHNAK-positive vesicles resistant to nonionic detergents that undergo endocytosis via a nonacidic route and are supposedly distinct form other conventional vesicular compartments [141]. AHNAK [142] is a very large (≈700 KDa) protein involved in a variety of distinct functions and pathologies (reviewed in [143]). The exact nature and contribution of enlargeosomes to dysferlin-mediated repair is still somewhat ill defined and may vary according to wound severity and cell type. Indeed, their regulated exocytoses have been suggested to add significant amount of membrane components to the injured plasmalemma in neuronal cells [144] and may therefore be involved in either endocytic (see Section 4.1.3.2) or shedding-mediated repair (see Section 4.2.3) [145]. Dysferlin may also modulate plasma membrane repair via its interaction with the AHNAK/S10010A10/Annexin II complex, which is a known organizer of the actin cytoskeleton and plasma membrane architecture [146].

Hence, contrary to oocytes, dysferlin-mediated exocytosis does not exclusively lead to the formation of a "patch," which also results in diminished in-plane membrane tension and ASM release to the outer leaflet.

4.1.3.2. Caveolae-mediated endocytic repair of mechanical wounds

Exocytosis is insufficient to fully explain the repair of membrane disruptions as lesions from pore-forming proteins are readily removed from the plasma membrane (see Section 4.2.1), which is not explainable by exocytosis alone. Also, the repair of SLO and mechanical lesions has been shown not to depend on exocytosis *per se*, but on the injury-induced release of ASM. Indeed, ASM deficiency, as seen in Niemann-Pick disease (NPD) types A and B [147], is capable of Ca^{2+}-dependent exocytosis but have severely limited Ca^{2+}-dependent endocytosis and shows signs of defective plasma membrane repair, both of which can be rescued by exogenously provided ASM [101, 148]. Similarly, inhibition of ASM by desipramine inhibited both endocytosis and normal plasma membrane repair [101]. This injury-induced endocytosis had previously been described and suggested to be involved in the endocytic degradation of SLO pores and of mechanical disruptions [149]. The same study identified the endosomes involved to be Ca^{2+}- and cholesterol dependent [149], but did not offer any mechanistic insight into their formation. As previously stated, caveolae are lipid-raft-rich whose formation is dependent on cholesterol, PIP_2 and PS (see Section 3.1), and are known to be facilitated by the transient formation of ceramide on lipid rafts [150, 151]. Once released to extracellular fluid, ASM cleaves the phosphorylcholine heads of sphingomyelin leaflets on the membrane surface to generate ceramide sphingolipids [152]. The resulting ceramide-enriched domains of the phospholipid bilayer are more prone to membrane invaginations due to them encompassing a smaller molecular area relative to other membrane lipids [152], promoting caveolae's endocytic function [153–155]. Similarly, caveolin-3 deficiency causes muscle degeneration in mice [134], which mirrors the limb-girdle muscular dystrophy 1C (LGMD1C) phenotype in humans [156]. As such, exocytosis of lysosomes and dysferlin vesicles after plasma membrane injury may not heal the membrane directly, but rather facilitate membrane resealing by encouraging caveolae formation. Indeed, upon heterotypic fusion with the membrane, ASM is released to the outer surface of the membrane, which potentiates the formation of ceramide-rich platforms that have been shown to trigger invagination of the plasmalemma [157] and formation of caveolae-derived endosomes (reviewed [158]). Indeed, transmission electron microscopy (TEM) has shown that caveolae were found to be concentrated next to mechanical disruptions of muscle cells [153] and assemble into a single, large merged caveolae-like structure around the large wounds generated in primary muscle fibers [153]. As Corrotte et al. correctly pointed out, these very large endocytic vesicles and invaginations may have initially been identified as related to the exocytic "patch" that was initially proposed to cover and eventually heal wounds in muscle cells (see Section 4.1.3.1). Alternatively, Corrotte et al. [153] proposed an endocytic-mediated model of plasma membrane repair. Briefly, large caveolae-like invaginations are formed as a consequence of a combination of the lower in-plane tension provided by the exocytosis of lysosomes, dysferlin-positive vesicles, changes in plasma membrane shape that follows release of ASM, and the presence of proteins such as dysferlin and caveolins. The growth and eventual fusion of those caveolae-like invaginations provides a "constriction force" that promotes plasmalemma resealing [153].

Endocytosis leads to a decrease in total plasma membrane surface area, increasing in-plane membrane tension and providing the force necessary for the mechanical wound removal. It is, however, important to consider that exocytosis of ASM lysosomes always precedes caveolae-mediated endocytosis. The corresponding in-plane membrane tension increases likely readjusts overall apparent membrane tension back to the cell's pre-injury levels, as type-I alveolar epithelial cells are known to remediate to hypertonic shock by increased caveolae-mediated endocytosis [159]. In fact, endocytic repair seems not to be as muscle specific as it was once thought since alveolar cell repair has been suggested to be linked to MG53 and caveolin-1 [160, 161].

4.2. Small wounds: ectocytic repair, blebbing and membrane shedding

4.2.1. Ectocytic repair of pore-forming toxins and blebbing of small mechanical wounds

As previously stated, caveolae-mediated endocytosis was shown to mediate the repair of membrane disruptions created by pore-forming toxins [45]. Indeed, SLO was directly visualized entering cells within caveolar vesicles [153]. Post-internalization, the pore has been shown to be ubiquitinated and eventually degraded by lysosomal hydrolysis [45].

While endocytic repair of SLO pores is now a widely accepted mechanism, it still raises some questions as SLO pores were shown to be successfully removed from the neurites of SH-SY5Y neuroblastoma cells [162]. SH-SY5Y cells are devoid of lysosomes and hence cannot undergo caveolae-mediated endocytosis.

As discussed in Section 3.3.1, Ca^{2+} entry can lead to local actin depolymerization, which in turn leads to a diminution of apparent membrane tension, and the formation of membrane blebs [163]. Indeed, bleb formation seems to principally depend on osmotic pressure and MCAs, the contribution of in-plane tension being minimal [164, 165]. Formation of membrane blebs can be initiated by laser ablation of the cortex cytoskeletal structures [163]. This also explains why formation of membrane blebs is inhibited by drugs that leads to depolymerization [166] or stabilization [167] of the actin cytoskeleton.

SLO pores cause localized Ca^{2+} entry and actin depolymerization without creating large plasma membrane tears-related increases in membrane tension (see Section 3.3.1). As such, it is not surprising that small blebs may be involved in the removal of SLO pores [168]. It should be noted that the same observations strongly suggest that SLO pore insertion, pore assembly, pore clustering and even bleb formation may be Ca^{2+}-independent [168]. This is controversial, however, as it would imply that SLO pore insertion could possibly displace proteins responsible of the interaction of the plasmalemma with the cytoskeleton. This also poses a problem, as other teams have shown a Ca^{2+} [169] and actin disruption [162] dependence for the survival of SLO-treated cells [169], and for the shedding of SLO-laden microvesicles [162]. In this alternate model [162], pore disruption of the membrane elevates local Ca^{2+} concentration which in turn activates annexins and calpains. Calpains then disrupt the underlying actin cytoskeleton, thereby facilitating bleb formation [170] and shedding of SLO vesicles.

4.2.2. ESCRT-mediated shedding of small disruptions

The endosomal sorting complex required for transport (ESCRT) complexes are factors of the lysosomal pathway during protein processing and are involved in various membrane remodeling events such as lysosomal targeting of ubiquitinated proteins and multivesicular body biogenesis, as well as cytokinetic abscission ([171]; reviewed by Olmos and Carlton [172]). There are five currently known ESCRT complexes: ESCRT-0, ESCRT-I, ESCRT-II, ESCRT-III and ESCRT-IV. Of these, ESCRT-III has since been found to modulate much of the membrane remodeling processes, while ESCRT-0, ESCRT-I and ESCRT-II facilitate its targeting to specific cellular compartments, ESCRT-IV orchestrating the disassembly of the ESCRT-III complex for subunit recycling (reviewed in [173]). An additional function of ESCRT-III in plasma membrane repair was proposed in a recent study, which suggested that ESCRT-III is involved in the pinching out or shedding of wounded membranes in HeLa cells [74]. Indeed, injury-induced Ca^{2+} increase results in Ca^{2+} binding of apoptosis-linked gene-2 (ALG-2) around the site of disruption. Active ALG-2 initiates ESCRT machinery assembly by facilitating the accumulation of ALG-2-interacting protein X (ALIX) near the wound site, after which ALG-2 and ALIX recruit ESCRT-III and vacuolar protein sorting-associated protein 4 (Vps4) to the injured plasma membrane [74, 174]. These subunits form a complex, which cleave and shed the wound from the plasma membrane to extracellular space [174]. ESCRT-mediated shedding leads to a decrease in total plasma membrane surface area, increasing in-plane membrane tension.

5. Conclusion

Injury-induced disruptions to the plasma membrane's shape and composition directly affect the cell's tensegrity. The different active membrane repair mechanisms that have been discussed in this chapter are perhaps best seen as a single interconnected pathway, in which the type and size of the wound determine the extent and severity of factors such as tension change and Ca^{2+} entry. These factors in turn dictate the healing mechanisms being used (**Table 1** and

Figure 2). Mechanical lesions lead to high, localized levels of membrane integrity loss, tension change and Ca^{2+} influx. These physical tears of the plasma membrane are often repaired by targeted exocytosis and endocytosis. Contrastingly, smaller injuries such as those generated by electroporation and osmotic shock induce low levels of membrane disruption, tension change and Ca^{2+} influx across large membrane areas. These in turn facilitate processes such as cytoskeletal remodeling or caveolae flattening. Conversely, membranes disrupted by toxic pores do not lead to substantial increase in plane tension. As such, they can either be rapidly shed or degraded following caveolae-mediated endocytosis. Furthermore, it appears that the wound-healing mechanisms prevalent in a given cell-type fall not only in accordance with the prevalence of specific injury types (i.e., PFTs vs. tears vs. ablations), but also according to cell type-specific differences in cell tensegrity and polarity (e.g., muscle cells vs. epithelial cells).

Similar to the plasma membrane and cytoskeletal elements interact to create tensegrity in the single-cell scale, adhesive forces of single cells and the extracellular matrix (ECM) provide structural stiffness to tissues [1]. Considering the above, it should be no surprise that successful single-cell repair influences the success of tissue repair. Indeed, contrary to tissue repair, single-cell repair is largely a binary event: it either takes place allowing the cell's survival, or not, leading to lysis or apoptotic removal. While relevant to wound healing at the tissue-level, these events have little to no relevance for single-cell wound healing outside of the modification of the environment of other injured cells in the surrounding area (asymmetric binding, change in ROS, Ca^{2+} concentration, etc.). Conversely, it seems that successful repair in one cell may lead to an increased repair potential in surrounding cells [175, 176]. This "potentiated" repair has been shown to involve purinergic and nitric oxide (NO)/PKG-signaling pathways [175, 176]. Similarly, repeated insults to a cell's structural and membrane integrity presumably affect a cell's ability to undergo subsequent membrane resealing and cytoskeletal repair, which would be reflected in its long-term viability in a given tissue. Indeed, the prominent view of the origin of the phenotypes associated with muscular dystrophies point toward a heighted susceptibly to repeated mechanical wounding, leading in turn in a higher rate of single-cell repair failure (reviewed in [177, 178]).

Another parallel between single-cell and tissue wound-healing mechanisms is their reliance on contractile arrays. This similarity has been confirmed in multicellular models such as *Xenopus* embryos [179], Caco-2 intestinal epithelial monolayers [180] and Madin-Darby canine kidney (MDCK) epithelial monolayers [181].

Wound closure in epithelial sheets has been demonstrated to be driven by the coupling of actomyosin contraction and collective cell migration [182–185]. The relative contribution of each mechanism in overall re-epithelialization depends on numerous biomechanical factors, including wound geometry [182–184], wound size [182, 186], tissue stiffness [186] and ECM composition [182]. In particular, wounds of cultured bovine corneal endothelial cell monolayers in ECM-deprived conditions were observed to reseal predominantly through actomyosin activity [182]. This is intriguing since cytoskeletal dynamics greatly influence single-cell wound-healing processes (see Section 3.3) and exhibits the ECM and cytoskeleton's analogous relationship across biological scales in the context of wound healing. These observations suggest that the importance of tensegrity components in wound repair are conserved across single-cell and multicellular models.

Considering the single cell's tensegral context in future wound-healing study will help further characterize an increasingly complex unified pathway theory of plasma membrane repair.

Author details

Eric Boucher, Tatsuya Kato and Craig A. Mandato*

*Address all correspondence to: craig.mandato@mcgill.ca

Department of Anatomy and Cell Biology, Faculty of Medicine, McGill University, Montreal, Quebec, Canada

References

[1] Ingber, D.E., N. Wang, and D. Stamenovic, *Tensegrity, cellular biophysics, and the mechanics of living systems*. Rep Prog Phys, 2014. 77(4): p. 046603.

[2] Fuller, R.B., *Tensegrity*. Portfolio Art News Annu, 1961. 4: pp. 112–27, 144, 148.

[3] Wang, N., et al., *Mechanical behavior in living cells consistent with the tensegrity model*. Proc Natl Acad Sci U S A, 2001. 98(14): pp. 7765–70.

[4] Mendez, M.G., D. Restle, and P.A. Janmey, *Vimentin enhances cell elastic behavior and protects against compressive stress*. Biophys J, 2014. 107(2): pp. 314–23.

[5] Chen, C., et al., *Effects of vimentin disruption on the mechanoresponses of articular chondrocyte*. Biochem Biophys Res Commun, 2016. 469(1): pp. 132–7.

[6] Diz-Munoz, A., D.A. Fletcher, and O.D. Weiner, *Use the force: membrane tension as an organizer of cell shape and motility*. Trends Cell Biol, 2013. 23(2): pp. 47–53.

[7] Xue, F., et al., *Effect of membrane stiffness and cytoskeletal element density on mechanical stimuli within cells: an analysis of the consequences of ageing in cells*. Comput Methods Biomech Biomed Engin, 2015. 18(5): pp. 468–76.

[8] Knoll, R., *A role for membrane shape and information processing in cardiac physiology*. Pflugers Arch, 2015. 467(1): pp. 167–73.

[9] Chatterjee, S., et al., *Shear stress-related mechanosignaling with lung ischemia: lessons from basic research can inform lung transplantation*. Am J Physiol Lung Cell Mol Physiol, 2014. 307(9): pp. L668–80.

[10] Vuckovic, A., et al., *Alveolarization genes modulated by fetal tracheal occlusion in the rabbit model for congenital diaphragmatic hernia: a randomized study*. PLoS One, 2013. 8(7): p. e69210.

[11] Myers, K.A., et al., *Hydrostatic pressure sensation in cells: integration into the tensegrity model*. Biochem Cell Biol, 2007. 85(5): pp. 543–51.

[12] Parsegian, V.A., R.P. Rand, and D. Gingell, *Lessons for the study of membrane fusion from membrane interactions in phospholipid systems*. Ciba Found Symp, 1984. 103: pp. 9–27.

[13] Zhelev, D.V. and D. Needham, *Tension-stabilized pores in giant vesicles: determination of pore size and pore line tension*. Biochim Biophys Acta, 1993. 1147(1): pp. 89–104.

[14] Hoffman, J.F., *On red blood cells, hemolysis and resealed ghosts*. Adv Exp Med Biol, 1992. 326: pp. 1–15.

[15] Kay, J.G. and S. Grinstein, *Sensing phosphatidylserine in cellular membranes*. Sensors (Basel), 2011. 11(2): pp. 1744–55.

[16] Riske, K.A. and R. Dimova, *Electro-deformation and poration of giant vesicles viewed with high temporal resolution*. Biophys J, 2005. 88(2): pp. 1143–55.

[17] Gozen, I. and P. Dommersnes, *Pore dynamics in lipid membranes*. European Physical Journal-Special Topics, 2014. 223(9): pp. 1813–1829.

[18] Thompson, N.L. and D. Axelrod, *Reduced lateral mobility of a fluorescent lipid probe in cholesterol-depleted erythrocyte membrane*. Biochim Biophys Acta, 1980. 597(1): pp. 155–65.

[19] Golan, D.E., et al., *Lateral mobility of phospholipid and cholesterol in the human erythrocyte membrane: effects of protein-lipid interactions*. Biochemistry, 1984. 23(2): pp. 332–9.

[20] Rand, R.P. and V.A. Parsegian, *Physical force considerations in model and biological membranes*. Can J Biochem Cell Biol, 1984. 62(8): pp. 752–9.

[21] Johnson, R.M. and D.H. Kirkwood, *Loss of resealing ability in erythrocyte membranes. Effect of divalent cations and spectrin release*. Biochim Biophys Acta, 1978. 509(1): pp. 58–66.

[22] McNeil, P.L., K. Miyake, and S.S. Vogel, *The endomembrane requirement for cell surface repair*. Proc Natl Acad Sci U S A, 2003. 100(8): pp. 4592–7.

[23] Tsai, P.S., et al., *Syntaxin and VAMP association with lipid rafts depends on cholesterol depletion in capacitating sperm cells*. Mol Membr Biol, 2007. 24(4): pp. 313–24.

[24] Zitranski, N., et al., *The "acrosomal synapse": Subcellular organization by lipid rafts and scaffolding proteins exhibits high similarities in neurons and mammalian spermatozoa*. Commun Integr Biol, 2010. 3(6): pp. 513–21.

[25] Correia, J., F. Michelangeli, and S. Publicover, *Regulation and roles of Ca2+ stores in human sperm*. Reproduction, 2015. 150(2): pp. R65–76.

[26] Chander, A., et al., *Annexin A7 trafficking to alveolar type II cell surface: possible roles for protein insertion into membranes and lamellar body secretion*. Biochim Biophys Acta, 2013. 1833(5): pp. 1244–55.

[27] Ichimura, H., et al., *Lung surfactant secretion by interalveolar Ca2+ signaling*. Am J Physiol Lung Cell Mol Physiol, 2006. 291(4): pp. L596–601.

[28] Miklavc, P., et al., *Ca2+-dependent actin coating of lamellar bodies after exocytotic fusion: a prerequisite for content release or kiss-and-run*. Ann N Y Acad Sci, 2009. 1152: pp. 43–52.

[29] Cardenas, A.M. and F. Marengo, *How the stimulus defines the dynamics of vesicle pool recruitment, fusion mode and vesicle recycling in neuroendocrine cells*. J Neurochem, 2016. DOI: 10.1111/jnc.13565.

[30] Chung, C. and J. Raingo, *Vesicle dynamics: how synaptic proteins regulate different modes of neurotransmission*. J Neurochem, 2013. 126(2): pp. 146–54.

[31] de Jong, A.P. and D. Fioravante, *Translating neuronal activity at the synapse: presynaptic calcium sensors in short-term plasticity*. Front Cell Neurosci, 2014. 8: p. 356.

[32] Shin, O.H., *Exocytosis and synaptic vesicle function*. Compr Physiol, 2014. 4(1): pp. 149–75.

[33] Pangrsic, T., E. Reisinger, and T. Moser, *Otoferlin: a multi-C2 domain protein essential for hearing*. Trends Neurosci, 2012. 35(11): pp. 671–80.

[34] Beurg, M., et al., *Control of exocytosis by synaptotagmins and otoferlin in auditory hair cells*. J Neurosci, 2010. 30(40): pp. 13281–90.

[35] Boucher, E. and C.A. Mandato, *Plasma membrane and cytoskeleton dynamics during single-cell wound healing*. Biochim Biophys Acta, 2015. 1853(10 Pt A): pp. 2649–61.

[36] Yamada, E., *The fine structure of the gall bladder epithelium of the mouse*. J Biophys Biochem Cytol, 1955. 1(5): pp. 445–58.

[37] Dulhunty, A.F. and C. Franzini-Armstrong, *The relative contributions of the folds and caveolae to the surface membrane of frog skeletal muscle fibres at different sarcomere lengths*. J Physiol, 1975. 250(3): pp. 513–39.

[38] Kozera, L., E. White, and S. Calaghan, *Caveolae act as membrane reserves which limit mechanosensitive I(Cl,swell) channel activation during swelling in the rat ventricular myocyte*. PLoS One, 2009. 4(12): p. e8312.

[39] Calaghan, S., L. Kozera, and E. White, *Compartmentalisation of cAMP-dependent signalling by caveolae in the adult cardiac myocyte*. J Mol Cell Cardiol, 2008. 45(1): pp. 88–92.

[40] Sinha, B., et al., *Cells respond to mechanical stress by rapid disassembly of caveolae*. Cell, 2011. 144(3): pp. 402–13.

[41] Kovtun, O., et al., *Cavin family proteins and the assembly of caveolae*. J Cell Sci, 2015. 128(7): pp. 1269–78.

[42] Shvets, E., A. Ludwig, and B.J. Nichols, *News from the caves: update on the structure and function of caveolae*. Curr Opin Cell Biol, 2014. 29: pp. 99–106.

[43] Hagiwara, Y., et al., *Caveolin-3 deficiency causes muscle degeneration in mice*. Hum Mol Genet, 2000. 9(20): pp. 3047–54.

[44] Wolfmeier, H., et al., *Ca-dependent repair of pneumolysin pores: A new paradigm for host cellular defense against bacterial pore-forming toxins*. Biochim Biophys Acta, 2015. 1853 (9): p. 2045-54.

[45] Corrotte, M., et al., *Toxin pores endocytosed during plasma membrane repair traffic into the lumen of MVBs for degradation*. Traffic, 2012. 13(3): pp. 483–94.

[46] Gerke, V. and S.E. Moss, *Annexins: from structure to function*. Physiol Rev, 2002. 82(2): pp. 331–71.

[47] Voges, D., et al., *Three-dimensional structure of membrane-bound annexin V. A correlative electron microscopy-X-ray crystallography study*. J Mol Biol, 1994. 238(2): pp. 199–213.

[48] Cezanne, L., et al., *Organization and dynamics of the proteolipid complexes formed by annexin V and lipids in planar supported lipid bilayers*. Biochemistry, 1999. 38(9): pp. 2779–86.

[49] Bouter, A., et al., *Annexin-A5 assembled into two-dimensional arrays promotes cell membrane repair*. Nat Commun, 2011. 2: p. 270.

[50] Lek, A., et al., *Calpains, cleaved mini-dysferlinC72, and L-type channels underpin calcium-dependent muscle membrane repair*. J Neurosci, 2013. 33(12): pp. 5085–94.

[51] Togo, T., et al., *The mechanism of facilitated cell membrane resealing*. J Cell Sci, 1999. 112 (Pt 5): pp. 719–31.

[52] Xie, X.Y. and J.N. Barrett, *Membrane resealing in cultured rat septal neurons after neurite transection: evidence for enhancement by Ca(2+)-triggered protease activity and cytoskeletal disassembly*. J Neurosci, 1991. 11(10): pp. 3257–67.

[53] Miyake, K., et al., *An actin barrier to resealing*. J Cell Sci, 2001. 114(Pt 19): pp. 3487–94.

[54] Chen, X., et al., *Single-site sonoporation disrupts actin cytoskeleton organization*. J R Soc Interface, 2014. 11(95): p. 20140071.

[55] Deguchi, S. and M. Sato, *Biomechanical properties of actin stress fibers of non-motile cells*. Biorheology, 2009. 46(2): pp. 93–105.

[56] Sato, K., et al., *Quantitative evaluation of threshold fiber strain that induces reorganization of cytoskeletal actin fiber structure in osteoblastic cells*. J Biomech, 2005. 38(9): pp. 1895–901.

[57] Costa, K.D., W.J. Hucker, and F.C. Yin, *Buckling of actin stress fibers: a new wrinkle in the cytoskeletal tapestry*. Cell Motil Cytoskeleton, 2002. 52(4): pp. 266–74.

[58] Matsui, T.S., et al., *Non-muscle myosin II induces disassembly of actin stress fibres independently of myosin light chain dephosphorylation*. Interface Focus, 2011. 1(5): pp. 754–66.

[59] Wu, T. and J.J. Feng, *A biomechanical model for fluidization of cells under dynamic strain*. Biophys J, 2015. 108(1): pp. 43–52.

[60] De La Cruz, E.M., J.L. Martiel, and L. Blanchoin, *Mechanical heterogeneity favors fragmentation of strained actin filaments*. Biophys J, 2015. 108(9): pp. 2270–81.

[61] Hayakawa, K., H. Tatsumi, and M. Sokabe, *Mechano-sensing by actin filaments and focal adhesion proteins*. Commun Integr Biol, 2012. 5(6): pp. 572–7.

[62] Hirata, H., et al., *Non-channel mechanosensors working at focal adhesion-stress fiber complex*. Pflugers Arch, 2015. 467(1): pp. 141–55.

[63] Hayakawa, K., H. Tatsumi, and M. Sokabe, *Actin filaments function as a tension sensor by tension-dependent binding of cofilin to the filament*. J Cell Biol, 2011. 195(5): pp. 721–7.

[64] Bernstein, B.W. and J.R. Bamburg, *ADF/cofilin: a functional node in cell biology*. Trends Cell Biol, 2010. 20(4): pp. 187–95.

[65] Orlova, A., et al., *Actin-destabilizing factors disrupt filaments by means of a time reversal of polymerization*. Proc Natl Acad Sci U S A, 2004. 101(51): pp. 17664–8.

[66] Martinac, B., *Mechanosensitive ion channels: molecules of mechanotransduction*. J Cell Sci, 2004. 117(Pt 12): pp. 2449–60.

[67] Muallem, S., et al., *Actin filament disassembly is a sufficient final trigger for exocytosis in nonexcitable cells*. J Cell Biol, 1995. 128(4): pp. 589–98.

[68] Biro, E.N. and S.Y. Venyaminov, *Depolymerization of actin in concentrated solutions of divalent metal chlorides*. Acta Biochim Biophys Acad Sci Hung, 1979. 14(1–2): pp. 31–42.

[69] Zechel, K., *Stability differences of muscle F-actin in formamide in the presence of Mg2+ and Ca2+*. Biochim Biophys Acta, 1983. 742(1): pp. 135–41.

[70] Ono, Y. and H. Sorimachi, *Calpains: an elaborate proteolytic system*. Biochim Biophys Acta, 2012. 1824(1): pp. 224–36.

[71] Nayal, A., D.J. Webb, and A.F. Horwitz, *Talin: an emerging focal point of adhesion dynamics*. Curr Opin Cell Biol, 2004. 16(1): pp. 94–8.

[72] Gasman, S., et al., *Regulated exocytosis in neuroendocrine cells: a role for subplasmalemmal Cdc42/N-WASP-induced actin filaments*. Mol Biol Cell, 2004. 15(2): pp. 520–31.

[73] Goodson, H.V., C. Valetti, and T.E. Kreis, *Motors and membrane traffic*. Curr Opin Cell Biol, 1997. 9(1): pp. 18–28.

[74] Jimenez, A.J., et al., *ESCRT machinery is required for plasma membrane repair*. Science, 2014. 343(6174): p. 1247136.

[75] Terasaki, M., K. Miyake, and P.L. McNeil, *Large plasma membrane disruptions are rapidly resealed by Ca2+-dependent vesicle-vesicle fusion events*. J Cell Biol, 1997. 139(1): pp. 63–74.

[76] McNeil, P.L., et al., *Patching plasma membrane disruptions with cytoplasmic membrane.* J Cell Sci, 2000. 113 (Pt 11): pp. 1891–902.

[77] Abreu-Blanco, M.T., J.M. Verboon, and S.M. Parkhurst, *Cell wound repair in Drosophila occurs through three distinct phases of membrane and cytoskeletal remodeling.* J Cell Biol, 2011. 193(3): pp. 455–64.

[78] Karasaki, S., *Studies on amphibian yolk 1. The ultrastructure of the yolk platelet.* J Cell Biol, 1963. 18: pp. 135–51.

[79] Glover, L. and R.H. Brown, Jr., *Dysferlin in membrane trafficking and patch repair.* Traffic, 2007. 8(7): pp. 785–94.

[80] Han, R. and K.P. Campbell, *Dysferlin and muscle membrane repair.* Curr Opin Cell Biol, 2007. 19(4): pp. 409–16.

[81] Andrews, N.W., P.E. Almeida, and M. Corrotte, *Damage control: cellular mechanisms of plasma membrane repair.* Trends Cell Biol, 2014. 24(12): pp. 734–742.

[82] Mandato, C.A. and W.M. Bement, *Contraction and polymerization cooperate to assemble and close actomyosin rings around Xenopus oocyte wounds.* J Cell Biol, 2001. 154(4): pp. 785–97.

[83] Wang, L., et al., *Vacuole fusion at a ring of vertex docking sites leaves membrane fragments within the organelle.* Cell, 2002. 108(3): pp. 357–69.

[84] McNeil, P.L. and T. Kirchhausen, *An emergency response team for membrane repair.* Nat Rev Mol Cell Biol, 2005. 6(6): pp. 499–505.

[85] Darenfed, H. and C.A. Mandato, *Wound-induced contractile ring: a model for cytokinesis.* Biochem Cell Biol, 2005. 83(6): pp. 711–20.

[86] Benink, H.A. and W.M. Bement, *Concentric zones of active RhoA and Cdc42 around single cell wounds.* J Cell Biol, 2005. 168(3): pp. 429–39.

[87] Bement, W.M., H.A. Benink, and G. von Dassow, *A microtubule-dependent zone of active RhoA during cleavage plane specification.* J Cell Biol, 2005. 170(1): pp. 91–101.

[88] Kawano, Y., et al., *Phosphorylation of myosin-binding subunit (MBS) of myosin phosphatase by Rho-kinase in vivo.* J Cell Biol, 1999. 147(5): pp. 1023–38.

[89] Bishop, A.L. and A. Hall, *Rho GTPases and their effector proteins.* Biochem J, 2000. 348 Pt 2: pp. 241–55.

[90] Egile, C., et al., *Activation of the CDC42 effector N-WASP by the Shigella flexneri IcsA protein promotes actin nucleation by Arp2/3 complex and bacterial actin-based motility.* J Cell Biol, 1999. 146(6): pp. 1319–32.

[91] Rohatgi, R., et al., *The interaction between N-WASP and the Arp2/3 complex links Cdc42-dependent signals to actin assembly.* Cell, 1999. 97(2): pp. 221–231.

[92] Taunton, J., et al., *Actin-dependent propulsion of endosomes and lysosomes by recruitment of N-WASP*. J Cell Biol, 2000. 148(3): pp. 519–30.

[93] Burkel, B.M., et al., *A Rho GTPase signal treadmill backs a contractile array*. Dev Cell, 2012. 23(2): pp. 384–96.

[94] Vaughan, E.M., et al., *Lipid domain-dependent regulation of single-cell wound repair*. Mol Biol Cell, 2014. 25(12): pp. 1867–76.

[95] Yu, H.Y. and W.M. Bement, *Control of local actin assembly by membrane fusion-dependent compartment mixing*. Nat Cell Biol, 2007. 9(2): pp. 149–59.

[96] Arun, S.N., et al., *Cell wounding activates phospholipase D in primary mouse keratinocytes*. J Lipid Res, 2013. 54(3): pp. 581–91.

[97] Abreu-Blanco, M.T., J.M. Verboon, and S.M. Parkhurst, *Coordination of Rho family GTPase activities to orchestrate cytoskeleton responses during cell wound repair*. Curr Biol, 2014. 24(2): pp. 144–55.

[98] Steinhardt, R.A., G. Bi, and J.M. Alderton, *Cell membrane resealing by a vesicular mechanism similar to neurotransmitter release*. Science, 1994. 263(5145): pp. 390–3.

[99] Jaiswal, J.K., N.W. Andrews, and S.M. Simon, *Membrane proximal lysosomes are the major vesicles responsible for calcium-dependent exocytosis in nonsecretory cells*. J Cell Biol, 2002. 159(4): pp. 625–35.

[100] Reddy, A., E.V. Caler, and N.W. Andrews, *Plasma membrane repair is mediated by Ca(2+)-regulated exocytosis of lysosomes*. Cell, 2001. 106(2): pp. 157–69.

[101] Tam, C., et al., *Exocytosis of acid sphingomyelinase by wounded cells promotes endocytosis and plasma membrane repair*. J Cell Biol, 2010. 189(6): pp. 1027–38.

[102] Leitz, J. and E.T. Kavalali, *Ca2+ Dependence of synaptic vesicle endocytosis*. Neuroscientist, 2015. DOI: 10.1177/1073858415588265.

[103] Bi, G.Q., J.M. Alderton, and R.A. Steinhardt, *Calcium-regulated exocytosis is required for cell membrane resealing*. J Cell Biol, 1995. 131(6 Pt 2): pp. 1747–58.

[104] Rust, M.B., *ADF/cofilin: a crucial regulator of synapse physiology and behavior*. Cell Mol Life Sci, 2015. 72(18): pp. 3521–9.

[105] Bi, G.Q., et al., *Kinesin- and myosin-driven steps of vesicle recruitment for Ca2+-regulated exocytosis*. J Cell Biol, 1997. 138(5): pp. 999–1008.

[106] McNeil, P.L., *Repairing a torn cell surface: make way, lysosomes to the rescue*. J Cell Sci, 2002. 115(Pt 5): pp. 873–9.

[107] Rizo, J. and J. Xu, *The synaptic vesicle release machinery*. Annu Rev Biophys, 2015. 44: pp. 339–67.

[108] Detrait, E., et al., *Axolemmal repair requires proteins that mediate synaptic vesicle fusion*. J Neurobiol, 2000. 44(4): pp. 382–91.

[109] Detrait, E.R., et al., *Plasmalemmal repair of severed neurites of PC12 cells requires Ca(2+) and synaptotagmin*. J Neurosci Res, 2000. 62(4): pp. 566–73.

[110] Fox, M.A. and J.R. Sanes, *Synaptotagmin I and II are present in distinct subsets of central synapses*. J Comp Neurol, 2007. 503(2): pp. 280–96.

[111] Shen, S.S., et al., *Molecular regulation of membrane resealing in 3T3 fibroblasts*. J Biol Chem, 2005. 280(2): pp. 1652–60.

[112] Chakrabarti, S., et al., *Impaired membrane resealing and autoimmune myositis in synaptotagmin VII-deficient mice*. J Cell Biol, 2003. 162(4): pp. 543–9.

[113] Toops, K.A. and A. Lakkaraju, *Let's play a game of chutes and ladders: lysosome fusion with the epithelial plasma membrane*. Commun Integr Biol, 2013. 6(4): p. e24474.

[114] Shen, S.S. and R.A. Steinhardt, *The mechanisms of cell membrane resealing in rabbit corneal epithelial cells*. Curr Eye Res, 2005. 30(7): pp. 543–54.

[115] Rao, S.K., et al., *Identification of SNAREs involved in synaptotagmin VII-regulated lysosomal exocytosis*. J Biol Chem, 2004. 279(19): pp. 20471–9.

[116] Tardieux, I., et al., *Lysosome recruitment and fusion are early events required for trypanosome invasion of mammalian cells*. Cell, 1992. 71(7): pp. 1117–30.

[117] Miyake, K. and P.L. McNeil, *Vesicle accumulation and exocytosis at sites of plasma membrane disruption*. J Cell Biol, 1995. 131(6 Pt 2): pp. 1737–45.

[118] Togo, T., T.B. Krasieva, and R.A. Steinhardt, *A decrease in membrane tension precedes successful cell-membrane repair*. Mol Biol Cell, 2000. 11(12): pp. 4339–46.

[119] Cooper, S.T. and P.L. McNeil, *Membrane repair: mechanisms and pathophysiology*. Physiol Rev, 2015. 95(4): pp. 1205–40.

[120] Togo, T. and R.A. Steinhardt, *Nonmuscle myosin IIA and IIB have distinct functions in the exocytosis-dependent process of cell membrane repair*. Mol Biol Cell, 2004. 15(2): pp. 688–95.

[121] Andrews, N.W., M. Corrotte, and T. Castro-Gomes, *Above the fray: surface remodeling by secreted lysosomal enzymes leads to endocytosis-mediated plasma membrane repair*. Semin Cell Dev Biol, 2015. 45: pp. 10–7.

[122] Stauber, W.T., *Eccentric action of muscles: physiology, injury, and adaptation*. Exerc Sport Sci Rev, 1989. 17: pp. 157–85.

[123] Proske, U. and D.L. Morgan, *Muscle damage from eccentric exercise: mechanism, mechanical signs, adaptation and clinical applications*. J Physiol, 2001. 537(Pt 2): pp. 333–45.

[124] Takekura, H., et al., *Eccentric exercise-induced morphological changes in the membrane systems involved in excitation-contraction coupling in rat skeletal muscle*. J Physiol, 2001. 533(Pt 2): pp. 571–83.

[125] Bashir, R., et al., *A gene related to Caenorhabditis elegans spermatogenesis factor fer-1 is mutated in limb-girdle muscular dystrophy type 2B*. Nat Genet, 1998. 20(1): pp. 37–42.

[126] Liu, J., et al., *Dysferlin, a novel skeletal muscle gene, is mutated in Miyoshi myopathy and limb girdle muscular dystrophy*. Nat Genet, 1998. 20(1): pp. 31–6.

[127] Anderson, L.V., et al., *Dysferlin is a plasma membrane protein and is expressed early in human development*. Hum Mol Genet, 1999. 8(5): pp. 855–61.

[128] Bansal, D., et al., *Defective membrane repair in dysferlin-deficient muscular dystrophy*. Nature, 2003. 423(6936): pp. 168–72.

[129] Pangrsic, T., et al., *Hearing requires otoferlin-dependent efficient replenishment of synaptic vesicles in hair cells*. Nat Neurosci, 2010. 13(7): pp. 869–76.

[130] Johnson, C.P. and E.R. Chapman, *Otoferlin is a calcium sensor that directly regulates SNARE-mediated membrane fusion*. J Cell Biol, 2010. 191(1): pp. 187–97.

[131] Reisinger, E., et al., *Probing the functional equivalence of otoferlin and synaptotagmin 1 in exocytosis*. J Neurosci, 2011. 31(13): pp. 4886–95.

[132] Piccolo, F., et al., *Intracellular accumulation and reduced sarcolemmal expression of dysferlin in limb – girdle muscular dystrophies*. Ann Neurol, 2000. 48(6): pp. 902–12.

[133] McDade, J.R., A. Archambeau, and D.E. Michele, *Rapid actin-cytoskeleton-dependent recruitment of plasma membrane-derived dysferlin at wounds is critical for muscle membrane repair*. FASEB J, 2014. 28(8): pp. 3660–70.

[134] Cai, C., et al., *Membrane repair defects in muscular dystrophy are linked to altered interaction between MG53, caveolin-3, and dysferlin*. J Biol Chem, 2009. 284(23): pp. 15894–902.

[135] Matsuda, C., et al., *The C2A domain in dysferlin is important for association with MG53 (TRIM72)*. PLoS Curr, 2012. 4: p. e5035add8caff4.

[136] Waddell, L.B., et al., *Dysferlin, annexin A1, and mitsugumin 53 are upregulated in muscular dystrophy and localize to longitudinal tubules of the T-system with stretch*. J Neuropathol Exp Neurol, 2011. 70(4): pp. 302–13.

[137] Cacciottolo, M., et al., *Reverse engineering gene network identifies new dysferlin-interacting proteins*. J Biol Chem, 2011. 286(7): pp. 5404–13.

[138] Redpath, G.M., et al., *Calpain cleavage within dysferlin exon 40a releases a synaptotagmin-like module for membrane repair*. Mol Biol Cell, 2014. 25(19): pp. 3037–48.

[139] Fuson, K., et al., *Alternate splicing of dysferlin C2A confers Ca(2)(+)-dependent and Ca(2)(+)-independent binding for membrane repair*. Structure, 2014. 22(1): pp. 104–15.

[140] McDade, J.R. and D.E. Michele, *Membrane damage-induced vesicle-vesicle fusion of dysferlin-containing vesicles in muscle cells requires microtubules and kinesin*. Hum Mol Genet, 2014. 23(7): pp. 1677–86.

[141] Cocucci, E., et al., *Enlargeosome, an exocytic vesicle resistant to nonionic detergents, undergoes endocytosis via a nonacidic route*. Mol Biol Cell, 2004. 15(12): pp. 5356–68.

[142] Shtivelman, E., F.E. Cohen, and J.M. Bishop, *A human gene (AHNAK) encoding an unusually large protein with a 1.2-microns polyionic rod structure*. Proc Natl Acad Sci U S A, 1992. 89(12): pp. 5472–6.

[143] Davis, T.A., B. Loos, and A.M. Engelbrecht, *AHNAK: the giant jack of all trades*. Cell Signal, 2014. 26(12): pp. 2683–2693.

[144] Borgonovo, B., et al., *Regulated exocytosis: a novel, widely expressed system*. Nat Cell Biol, 2002. 4(12): pp. 955–62.

[145] Cocucci, E., et al., *Enlargeosome traffic: exocytosis triggered by various signals is followed by endocytosis, membrane shedding or both*. Traffic, 2007. 8(6): pp. 742–57.

[146] Benaud, C., et al., *AHNAK interaction with the annexin 2/S100A10 complex regulates cell membrane cytoarchitecture*. J Cell Biol, 2004. 164(1): pp. 133–44.

[147] Schuchman, E.H., *Acid sphingomyelinase, cell membranes and human disease: lessons from Niemann-Pick disease*. FEBS Lett, 2010. 584(9): pp. 1895–900.

[148] Zha, X., et al., *Sphingomyelinase treatment induces ATP-independent endocytosis*. J Cell Biol, 1998. 140(1): pp. 39–47.

[149] Idone, V., et al., *Repair of injured plasma membrane by rapid Ca2+-dependent endocytosis*. J Cell Biol, 2008. 180(5): pp. 905–14.

[150] Gulbins, E. and R. Kolesnick, *Raft ceramide in molecular medicine*. Oncogene, 2003. 22(45): pp. 7070–7.

[151] van Blitterswijk, W.J., et al., *Ceramide: second messenger or modulator of membrane structure and dynamics?* Biochem J, 2003. 369(Pt 2): pp. 199–211.

[152] Holopainen, J.M., M.I. Angelova, and P.K. Kinnunen, *Vectorial budding of vesicles by asymmetrical enzymatic formation of ceramide in giant liposomes*. Biophys J, 2000. 78(2): pp. 830–8.

[153] Corrotte, M., et al., *Caveolae internalization repairs wounded cells and muscle fibers*. Elife, 2013. 2: p. e00926.

[154] Nabi, I.R. and P.U. Le, *Caveolae/raft-dependent endocytosis*. J Cell Biol, 2003. 161(4): pp. 673–7.

[155] Nichols, B., *Caveosomes and endocytosis of lipid rafts*. J Cell Sci, 2003. 116(Pt 23): pp. 4707–14.

[156] Nigro, V. and M. Savarese, *Genetic basis of limb-girdle muscular dystrophies: the 2014 update*. Acta Myol, 2014. 33(3): pp. 1–12.

[157] Trajkovic, K., et al., *Ceramide triggers budding of exosome vesicles into multivesicular endosomes*. Science, 2008. 319(5867): pp. 1244–7.

[158] Draeger, A. and E.B. Babiychuk, *Ceramide in plasma membrane repair*. Handb Exp Pharmacol, 2013(216): pp. 341–53.

[159] Wang, S., et al., *Endocytic response of type I alveolar epithelial cells to hypertonic stress*. Am J Physiol Lung Cell Mol Physiol, 2011. 300(4): pp. L560–8.

[160] Kim, S.C., et al., *TRIM72 is required for effective repair of alveolar epithelial cell wounding*. Am J Physiol Lung Cell Mol Physiol, 2014. 307(6): pp. L449–59.

[161] Jia, Y., et al., *Treatment of acute lung injury by targeting MG53-mediated cell membrane repair*. Nat Commun, 2014. 5: p. 4387.

[162] Atanassoff, A.P., et al., *Microvesicle shedding and lysosomal repair fulfill divergent cellular needs during the repair of streptolysin O-induced plasmalemmal damage*. PLoS One, 2014. 9(2): p. e89743.

[163] Tinevez, J.Y., et al., *Role of cortical tension in bleb growth*. Proc Natl Acad Sci U S A, 2009. 106(44): pp. 18581–6.

[164] Charras, G.T., et al., *Life and times of a cellular bleb*. Biophys J, 2008. 94(5): pp. 1836–53.

[165] Dai, J. and M.P. Sheetz, *Membrane tether formation from blebbing cells*. Biophys J, 1999. 77(6): pp. 3363–70.

[166] Charras, G.T., et al., *Non-equilibration of hydrostatic pressure in blebbing cells*. Nature, 2005. 435(7040): pp. 365–9.

[167] Cunningham, C.C., *Actin polymerization and intracellular solvent flow in cell surface blebbing*. J Cell Biol, 1995. 129(6): pp. 1589–99.

[168] Keyel, P.A., et al., *Streptolysin O clearance through sequestration into blebs that bud passively from the plasma membrane*. J Cell Sci, 2011. 124(Pt 14): pp. 2414–23.

[169] Babiychuk, E.B., et al., *Blebbing confers resistance against cell lysis*. Cell Death Differ, 2011. 18(1): pp. 80–9.

[170] Gauthier, N.C., et al., *Temporary increase in plasma membrane tension coordinates the activation of exocytosis and contraction during cell spreading*. Proc Natl Acad Sci U S A, 2011. 108(35): pp. 14467–72.

[171] Morita, E., et al., *Human ESCRT and ALIX proteins interact with proteins of the midbody and function in cytokinesis*. EMBO J, 2007. 26(19): pp. 4215–27.

[172] Olmos, Y. and J.G. Carlton, *The ESCRT machinery: new roles at new holes*. Curr Opin Cell Biol, 2016. 38: pp. 1–11.

[173] Schuh, A.L. and A. Audhya, *The ESCRT machinery: from the plasma membrane to endosomes and back again*. Crit Rev Biochem Mol Biol, 2014. 49(3): pp. 242–61.

[174] Scheffer, L.L., et al., *Mechanism of Ca(2)(+)-triggered ESCRT assembly and regulation of cell membrane repair*. Nat Commun, 2014. 5: p. 5646.

[175] Togo, T., *Cell membrane disruption stimulates NO/PKG signaling and potentiates cell membrane repair in neighboring cells*. PLoS One, 2012. 7(8): p. e42885.

[176] Togo, T., *Short-term potentiation of membrane resealing in neighboring cells is mediated by purinergic signaling*. Purinergic Signal, 2014. 10(2): pp. 283–90.

[177] Cooper, S.T. and S.I. Head, *Membrane injury and repair in the muscular dystrophies*. Neuroscientist, 2014. 21(6): p. 653–68.

[178] Allen, D.G., N.P. Whitehead, and S.C. Froehner, *Absence of dystrophin disrupts skeletal muscle signaling: Roles of Ca2+, reactive oxygen species, and nitric oxide in the development of muscular dystrophy*. Physiol Rev, 2016. 96(1): pp. 253–305.

[179] Clark, A.G., et al., *Integration of single and multicellular wound responses*. Curr Biol, 2009. 19(16): pp. 1389–95.

[180] Russo, J.M., et al., *Distinct temporal-spatial roles for rho kinase and myosin light chain kinase in epithelial purse-string wound closure*. Gastroenterology, 2005. 128(4): pp. 987–1001.

[181] Tamada, M., et al., *Two distinct modes of myosin assembly and dynamics during epithelial wound closure*. J Cell Biol, 2007. 176(1): pp. 27–33.

[182] Grasso, S., J.A. Hernandez, and S. Chifflet, *Roles of wound geometry, wound size, and extracellular matrix in the healing response of bovine corneal endothelial cells in culture*. Am J Physiol Cell Physiol, 2007. 293(4): pp. C1327–37.

[183] Klarlund, J.K., *Dual modes of motility at the leading edge of migrating epithelial cell sheets*. Proc Natl Acad Sci U S A, 2012. 109(39): pp. 15799–804.

[184] Ravasio, A., et al., *Gap geometry dictates epithelial closure efficiency*. Nat Commun, 2015. 6: p. 7683.

[185] Brugués, A., et al., *Forces driving epithelial wound healing*. Nat Phys, 2014. 10(9): pp. 683–90.

[186] Wu, M. and M. Ben Amar, *Growth and remodelling for profound circular wounds in skin*. Biomech Model Mechanobiol, 2015. 14(2): pp. 357–70.

Chapter 10

A Potential Mechanism for Diabetic Wound Healing: Cutaneous Environmental Disorders

Junna Ye, Ting Xie, Yiwen Niu, Liang Qiao,
Ming Tian, Chun Qing and Shuliang Lu

Additional information is available at the end of the chapter

http://dx.doi.org/10.5772/64052

Abstract

Diabetes mellitus is a chronic multi-organ metabolic disorder caused by a combination of environmental and genetic factors. Diabetic complications are considered to be multifactorial with increasing evidence that one of the major pathways involved in the progression of both microvascular and macrovascular diseases is the biochemical process of advanced glycation.

We will combine in vitro and in vivo studies and other related literatures to discuss the role of advanced glycation end products (AGEs), which may exert deleterious effects in diabetes. Dr Shuliang Lu puts forward the theory of 'cutaneous environmental disorders' mediated by AGEs. The receptor for advanced glycation end products (RAGE) was first described as a signal transduction receptor for AGEs. Recent discoveries regarding AGEs-RAGE interactions expanded our understanding of the mechanisms by which RAGE evoked pathological consequences.

In this chapter, we report on the biology of AGEs, AGEs and wound healing, as well as address current strategies to interrupt the formation of AGEs and underscore strategies by which antagonism of RAGE and AGEs-RAGE crosslinks may be realized.

Keywords: diabetic wound healing, advanced glycated end products, RAGE, measurement, treatment

1. Introduction

Diabetes mellitus is characterized by chronic hyperglycemia and an altered cellular homeostasis, which lead to diffuse vascular damage and multi-organ dysfunction. Diabetic patients risk both micro- and macro-vascular complications: the former result from damage to retinal, renal, and neural tissues, which is the cause of blindness, end-stage renal failure, and non-traumatic lower limb amputation, respectively [1]. Here, we will focus on diabetic wound. Impaired wound healing is associated with increased morbidity and mortality in diabetes mellitus. The majority of non-healing wounds often lead to amputation, increasing the direct costs of their care, rehabilitation, and lost productivity [2].

According to a national survey, the prevalence of chronic cutaneous wounds among hospitalized patients was 1.7% in China. The leading causes were diabetes (31.3% men, 35.3% women) and trauma (26.4% men, 19.2% women). Therefore, diabetes has recently become the leading cause of chronic cutaneous wounds in China [3]. In Shuliang Lu's study, it was indicated that new diabetic foot ulcers were already in poor condition when patients first visited the diabetic foot clinic. Concomitantly, patients had worse health-related quality of life compared with the general population [4].

Several mechanisms have played a role in this condition, such as neuropathy, peripheral arterial disease, biomechanical factors, infection, and wound healing. Brownlee identifies the production of reactive oxygen species (ROS) as the unifying mechanism behind the main pathological pathways triggered by hyperglycemia, one of which leads to the formation of heterogeneous moieties called advanced glycation end products (AGEs) via non-enzymatic glycation and glycoxidation processes [5]. AGEs affect the wound healing process either directly by their interference with various components involved or indirectly through their association with diabetic neuropathy or angiopathy [6, 7]. In addition, RAGE was discovered as a receptor for AGEs, such as carboxymethyl lysine (CML) [8]. RAGE has been postulated to contribute to the development of diabetic complications [9]. The mechanism of RAGE has also been widely discussed.

In this chapter, we will present data regarding the formation and the metabolism of AGEs, the role of RAGE involved in diabetic conditions, evidence emerging from in vitro and in vivo studies as well as studies using anti-AGEs and other related agents to support a pathogenic role for AGEs in the impaired process of diabetic wound healing.

2. AGEs formation

It was not until 1980 that the pathophysiological significance of AGEs emerged in medical science, particularly in relation to diabetic complications [10]. AGEs are a heterogeneous group of molecules that form from the non-enzymatic addition of sugar moieties onto arginine and lysine residues of proteins, free amino groups on lipids, or guanine nucleic acids [11]. Glycation has to be distinguished from glycosylation, which is an enzymatic reaction. First described by Louis Camille Maillard in the 1900s, non-enzymatic glycation involves condensation reaction of the carbonyl group of sugar aldehydes with the N-terminus or free-amino groups of proteins via a nucleophilic addition, resulting first in the rapid formation of a Schiff base. The physiological consequences of the Maillard reaction in the etiology of a range of important diabetic complications have already been indicated [12]. The Schiff base then goes through rearrangements to form the more stable Amadori products. Among most cellular and plasma proteins, Amadori products can change with glucose. That is to say, the levels of Amadori products will rise and fall depending on the levels of glucose. The most well-known example of an Amadori product is hemoglobin A1c (HbA1c), a naturally occurring modification to the N-terminal valine amino group of the β chain of hemoglobin [13]. Schiff bases and Amadori products are reversible reaction products. However, they can react irreversibly with amino acid residues of peptides or proteins to form protein adducts or protein crosslinks [14] (**Figure 1**).

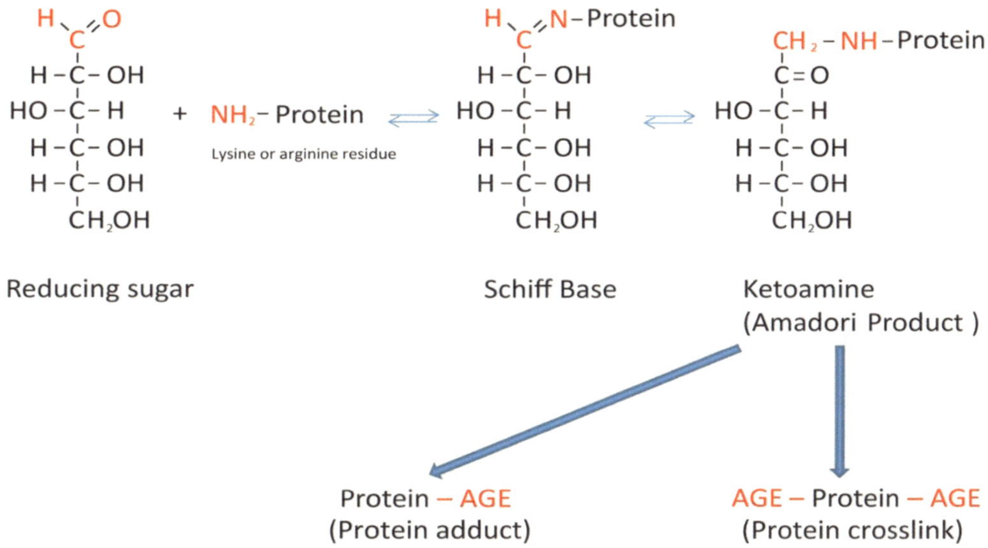

Figure 1. Schematic presentation of the Maillard reaction. Reactive carbonyl groups of a reducing sugar react with neutrophilic free amino groups of proteins to form a reversible Schiff base. Through rearrangement, a more stable Amadori product is formed. Depending on the nature of these early glycation end products, protein adducts or protein crosslinks are formed. (Illustrated from Ref. [54]).

In the context of intracellular glycation, it is important to note that glucose has the slowest rate in the glycation reaction of any sugar [15]. Because of the slow formation, it is believed that AGEs accumulate only on long-lived extracellular proteins. However, later a rapid extracellular AGEs formation on short-lived proteins and intracellular AGEs formation by reactive dicarbonyl compounds have attracted attention [16]. Thus, glycolytic intermediates such as dihydroxyacetone-phosphate, glyceraldehyde-3-phosphate and the dicarbonyl compounds glyoxal, methylglyoxal, and 3-deoxyglucosone are important for the intracellular Maillard reaction [17]. Among these compounds, methylglyoxal is regarded as the most potent glycating agent [18]. The transformation of glyceraldehyde-3-phosphate and dihydroxyacetone-phosphate formed methylglyoxal [19]. It could be detoxified by the conversion to S-Dlactoylglutathione and D-lactate, catalyzed in the cytosol of all cells by glyoxalase I and II. It has been reported that overexpression of glyoxalase I in endothelial cells completely prevented AGEs formation, thus indicating the importance of methylglyoxal to form AGEs [20]. Moreover, several studies on different animal models have established that dietary AGEs could play an important role in the pathogenesis of various pathologic conditions and their complications, such as type 1 diabetes mellitus in non-obese diabetic mice [21], atherosclerosis in apoE-deficient mice [22], type 2 diabetes, and impaired wound healing in db/db (+/+) mice [23]. It should be emphasized that a large portion of AGEs in the human body is derived from exogenous sources, e.g. from regular food, smoking, etc. [24]. Much attention has been paid to the so-called exogenous AGEs, harmful products of "browning" (or the Maillard reaction) in various foods. Together with endogenous AGEs, these compounds form the majority of glycation-free adducts. Among the various food processing methods, heating, sterilizing, and microwaves contribute to the generation of exogenous AGEs, all of which tend to accelerate the non-enzymatic addition of non-reducing sugars to free NH2 groups of proteins and lipids [25].

3. RAGE

AGEs could exert their actions not only directly but also through a receptor system, which includes two types of cell surface AGEs receptors: first type is that binds AGEs and initiates cell activation and second type is that binds and degrades AGEs. Receptor for AGEs (RAGE) is one receptor of the first type; it recognizes AGEs and initiates oxidative stress. The second type of receptors consists of AGER1, AGER3, and CD36 [26, 27]. However, it is noteworthy that there are other AGE receptors, such as the macrophage scavenger receptor and the galectin-3 receptor, which might have similar deleterious effects to RAGE when they interact with AGEs [28].

RAGE is a multi-ligand receptor of the immunoglobulin superfamily of cell surface molecules acting as a receptor not only for several molecules including AGEs but also for S100/calgranulins and amyloid. Circulating isoforms of RAGE include soluble RAGE (sRAGE) that has been cleaved from the cell surface by matrix metalloproteinases and endogenous secretory RAGE (esRAGE), and a splice variant of RAGE that is secreted into blood. Both sRAGE and esRAGE protect body against the AGEs-elicited tissue damage by acting as a decoy receptor for AGEs [29, 30]. The ligands of RAGE have a common feature that they accumulate in tissues during aging, inflammation, and degenerative diseases. Engagement of RAGE results in intracellular signaling that leads to the activation of NF-kB, a pro-inflammatory transcription factor, which is then translocated to the nucleus and subsequently activates the transcription of target genes [31]. These include genes of cytokines, adhesion molecules, and prothrombotic and vasoconstrictive products. The activation of NF-kB results in upregulation of the receptors in return. In addition, cellular-signaling cascades such as the ERK signaling pathway and PI-3 kinases are activated by the binding of ligands with RAGE [32].

In the skin, RAGE expression was observed in both epidermis and dermis, and it was increased in sun-exposed compared with UV irradiation-protected areas [33]. Not only in vivo, but also in vitro, various skin cells types have been shown to express RAGE [34–36], such as keratinocytes, fibroblasts, dendritic cells, and to a lesser extent endothelial cells and lymphocytes. Patients with diabetes also exhibit increased immunoreactivity for RAGE and AGEs. For example, in sural nerve biopsies, AGE-RAGE interaction was found which suggests it may have a clinical role in neuronal dysfunction that leads to neuropathy [37].

According to these reactions, researchers have put forward mechanisms by which AGEs lead to diabetic complications: (1) the accumulation of AGEs in the extracellular matrix causing aberrant crosslinking, resulting in a decrease of elasticity of vessels; (2) intracellular AGEs formation leading to quenching of nitric oxide and impaired function of growth factors [20]; (3) the binding of AGEs to AGE-receptors on different cell types and activation of key cell signaling pathways such as NF-kB activation with subsequent modulation of gene expression in vascular cells such as endothelial cells, smooth muscle cells, and macrophages [38].

4. AGEs and wound healing

It is generally believed that wound healing is impaired in diabetes. Wound healing is a complex process in which several pathophysiological processes are involved. They include inflammation, repair, and regeneration. Until now, there is evidence from experimental studies that glycation is involved in wound healing in diabetes.

4.1. AGEs and inflammation phase in a diabetic wound

In this part, the interaction between AGEs and RAGE could not be neglected. Data support that it negatively affects various aspects of inflammatory response in diabetic wound. Increased RAGE expression has been found in wound tissues from diabetic mice in parallel with increased AGEs accumulation and increased inflammation [39]. In Shuliang Lu's study [40], compared with the controls, enhanced expression of RAGE and accelerated cell apoptosis were observed in the burned skin of diabetic rats. The altered expression pattern of inflammatory cytokines and oxidative markers between diabetic and control groups revealed delayed neutrophil chemotaxis and respiratory burst. Furthermore, the results in vitro showed that exposure to AGEs inhibited the viability of neutrophils, promoted RAGE production and cell apoptosis, which was consistent with the findings in vivo. Besides, the mice fed with a rich AGEs diet demonstrated an increased and sustained inflammatory phase compared with those fed with a low AGEs diet [41]. In vitro, human neutrophils were isolated and treated with AGE-human serum albumin. Cell viability and reactive oxygen species levels were increased [42].

In keratinocytes, AGEs decrease cell viability and migration and induce the expression of proinflammatory mediators as well [43]. Various growth factors or proteins significant for cellular functions may be glycated inhibiting their functions [44]. Furthermore, treatment of murine macrophages with AGEs resulted in increased levels of iNOS, which has been found to be increased in diabetic wounds [45]. Macrophages play a critical role in wound healing and can be activated to two distinctive phenotypes in vitro: M1 and M2 [46]. It demonstrated insufficient M1 in the early stage but excessive M2 in the later proliferative phase. The macrophage activation markers were correlated with the instructive T helper cell type 1 (Th1)/

Th2 cytokines in both groups. Other studies suggested that RAGE expression has been strongly linked to the expression of matrix metalloproteinases (MMP)-1, MMP-3, MMP-9, mainly through RAGE engagement by AGEs [47]. In addition, AGEs induced the production of oxygen-reactive intermediates from inflammatory and endothelial cells via NADPH activation probably through their receptors, promoting further cellular activation and proinflammatory cytokine expression [48].

4.2. AGEs and proliferation phase in the diabetic wound

It has been reported that the presence of AGEs not only affected the interaction of the fibroblasts with the extracellular matrix but also reduced the amount of the extracellular matrix as well. This effect would influence almost all the cells involved in the proliferative process. In vitro incubation of human dermal fibroblasts with pentosidine or pyrraline resulted in reduction of the extracellular matrix content, which was collagen and proteoglycan [49]. In vitro study showed that type I collagen synthesis from fibroblasts was not affected in AGEs; however, the synthesis of hyaluronic acid was significantly reduced [50]. It also showed a direct effect of AGEs on fibroblast synthetic capacity and explained the decreased extracellular matrix in the diabetic wound. Because hyaluronic acid is associated with cellular locomotion, migration, and proliferation, decreased content in the matrix could result in disturbance of the proliferative phase of the healing process. Besides, histological evaluation of wound sections from diabetic rats demonstrated absence of actively migrating inflammatory cells toward the central region of the wound, reduced angiogenesis, a decrease in the secretion of extracellular matrix, and then poor granulation tissue formation [51].

AGEs may also change the action of the wound-associated cytokines and growth factors, by affecting the growth factors or their receptors. Glycation of bFGF, after its incubation with glucose-6-phosphate (G6P) or fructose, resulted in decreased heparin-binding capacity, which is necessary for the binding of bFGF to its receptor. A reduction in its mitogenic activity was also observed compared with the control bFGF group [45]. In addition, incubation of FGF2 with G6P resulted in glycation of FGF2. Bovine aortic endothelial cells incubated with the glycated FGF2 showed a reduction of proliferation, decreased mean capillary length and new blood vessel formation, a weaker increase in tyrosine-phosphorylated proteins, especially ERK-1 and ERK-2 [52] .While ECV304 cells were incubated with glyoxal proteins, a significant reduction in the free amino acid groups of the EGF receptors was found. It also showed that the EGF-induced recruitment and activation of the downstream effectors of the EGF receptor pathway PLCg1 and ERK1/2 was inhibited by AGEs [53]. Furthermore, an animal study using rats with subcutaneous implantation of sponge disks showed that pretreatment of animals with D-glucose resulted in a reduction in the angiogenesis measured by the hemoglobin content of the implanted disks and a reduction in the granulomatous response compared with control groups.

4.3. AGEs and remodeling phase in the diabetic wound

Every stage of normal wound healing appears to be disrupted in the diabetic patients. A derangement in wound contraction and remodeling is expectable. A large body of evidence supports the effects of AGEs on the phenotype, invasiveness, behavior, and survival of the cells and cell membrane interactions with extracellular matrix. Animal data showed that diabetic mice with lower circulating and tissue-bound AGEs as a result of exposure to a diet low in AGEs, showed improved reepithelialization, granulation tissue formation and angiogenesis compared with the group fed with a diet high in AGEs [54].

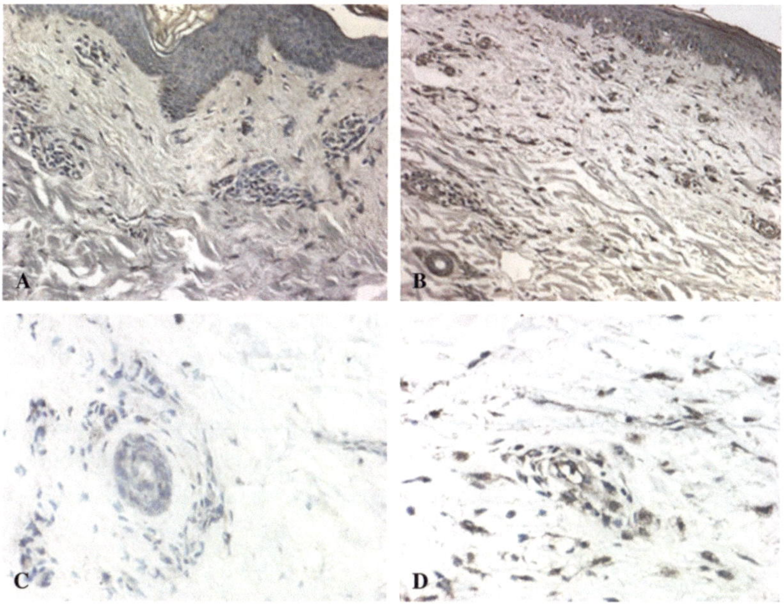

Figure 2. Immunohistochemical localization of AGE and RAGE proteins in dermis is shown. A, B, The distribution of AGE in normal skin tissue (A) and in diabetic skin tissue (B). AGE protein staining was expressed faintly at dermal matrices and cells in control skin but was prominent at the dermal matrices, cells, and basement membrane of vessels in the diabetic skin. C, D, The distribution of RAGE in normal skin tissue (C) and in diabetic skin tissue (D). RAGE-positive cells appear brown, and a light hematoxylin counter stain was used to visualize nuclei. More positive cells were detected in diabetic dermal layer than in control. [Original magnification, ×200 (A, B); original magnification, ×400 (C, D)]. (Illustrated from Ref. [55]).

The balance between proliferation and apoptosis of skin cells is responsible for the success of the wound healing process. Recent reports have shown that AGEs formation participates in dermatologic problems in diabetes. Shuliang Lu's group reported that effects of dermal micro-environment glycosylation. Histology and immunohistochemical staining were performed on type 2 diabetic and nondiabetic skin specimens to determine the distributions of proliferating cell nuclear antigen, apoptotic cells, AGEs and RAGE. Diabetic skin has degenerative, loosely arranged collagen and increased apoptotic cells compared with normal skin. Expression of AGEs and RAGE were increased in diabetic skin. Glycosylated matrix induced cell cycle arrest and apoptosis of cultured dermal fibroblasts, whereas application of RAGE-blocking antibodies redressed these changes [55] (**Figure 2**).

AGEs may alter the signaling of the wound cytokines and growth factors by disrupting the structure of either the growth factors or their receptors. Glycation of fibroblast growth factor (bFGF), after its incubation with intracellular sugars resulted in decreased heparin-binding capacity, which is essential for the ligation of bFGF to its receptor [56]. Bovine aortic endothelial cells incubated with the glycated FGF-2 showed a reduction in the proliferation, decreased mean capillary length and overall new blood vessel formation as well as a clearly weaker increase in tyrosine phosphorylated proteins, particularly ERK-1 and ERK-2 [57]. It has also been shown that the epidermal growth factor (EGF)-induced recruitment and activation of the downstream effectors of the EGF receptor pathway, the serine-threonine kinases ERK1/2, was inhibited by glyoxal and methylglyoxal [58]. Moreover, diabetic rats exhibited poor TGF-β1 expression in fibroblasts [20]. The effects of TGF-β1 on extracellular matrix synthesis and cellular phenotypes are crucial for the final stage of wound healing, suppression of MMP secretion, differentiation of fibroblasts into contractile myofibroblasts, and cellular programmed death. The increased levels of MMPs and proinflammatory cytokines in the context of a vicious self-perpetuating cycle of an inappropriately inflammatory response may be responsible for the derangement of the remodeling stage [42].

Literature data also support that in the presence of AGEs, not only the interaction of the fibroblasts with the extracellular matrix is affected, but also the amount of the extracellular matrix constituents normally secreted by cells is reduced. This effect would deprive almost all the cells involved in the proliferative process of the extracellular scaffold [59]. In vitro, studies showed a direct effect of AGEs on fibroblast survival and synthetic capacity, which might partially explain the decreased extracellular matrix density in the diabetic non-healing wounds. Human adult primary skin fibroblasts treated with CML-collagen (glycated collagen) showed a time- and dose-dependent apoptosis, which was threefold compared with that of control collagen-treated fibroblasts [60]. An insight has been gained into the mechanisms that underlie the AGEs-promoted cell apoptosis. The proapoptotic intracellular signaling consists of involving a chain of events, such as the generation of intracellular reactive oxygen species, which cause the activation of mitogen-activated protein kinase (MAPK) pathways and finally the induction of transcription factor FOXO1 and caspase-3. In addition, keratinocytes pretreated with glycoaldehyde and type I collagen exhibited reduced migration and an impaired adhesive capacity [61]. These effects were caused by conformational changes on the glycated collagen, which altered the effective receptor binding [62]. Furthermore, increased AGE/RAGE expression has been found in the diabetic skin. The apoptotic effects could be reversed by the application of RAGE antibodies, suggesting that AGEs and RAGE interaction played an important part in the cell dysfunction [40].

Another study of Shuliang Lu's group demonstrated that thickness of abdominal dermis from diabetic patients was reduced with obscured multilayer epithelium and disorganized collagen fibrils, as well as with chronic inflammatory cell infiltration. It was also shown that the prominent accumulation of AGEs in the diabetic skin induced an oxidative damage of fibroblasts and thus contributed to the thinner thickness of diabetic abdominal dermis. In vivo, less hydroxyproline, higher myeloperoxidase activity, and increased malondialdehyde (MDA) content were found in the diabetic skin. In vitro, the time- and dose-dependent inhibitory effects of AGE-bovine serum albumin (BSA) on fibroblast viability and the promotion of MDA production were shown [63].

http://dx.doi.org/10.5772/64052

5. Measurement of AGEs

Since the biochemistry of AGEs has been widely discussed, the effort to develop the measurement has been made as well. Blood is more accessible for repeated measurements of AGEs than tissue-requiring biopsies, but plasma AGEs assays have not yet been shown to be directly related to tissue AGEs content [64]. As tissue accumulation of AGEs proves a long-term course with low reversibility, the AGEs accumulated in long-lived tissue proteins like skin collagen may be a carrier of metabolic memory over a long period, even years [65]. Because certain AGEs have intrinsic fluorescence properties, tissue AGEs accumulation can be assessed as skin autofluorescence (SAF) by the AGE Reader™ (Diagn-Optics, Groningen, the Netherlands) easily and noninvasively [66], instead of other traditional invasive techniques (**Figure 3**). Several studies demonstrated that the SAF value obtained from the skin of the lower arm correlated with content of both fluorescent and nonfluorescent AGEs measured from skin biopsy specimens on the same site [67]. It is strongly related to AGEs accumulation in healthy subjects, and diabetic and hemodialysis patients over a broad age range [68]. There is no surprise that SAF values of the diabetic patients were significantly higher than the healthy population [69, 70], and SAF values of diabetes with complications were elevated compared with those without complications [71, 72]. So far, there have been SAF referential values and its influential factors for healthy Dutch, Slovakian, and Chinese people, and this offers the baseline values to further analyze diabetes and its chronic complications [73–75].

However, studies of SAF on predicting the diabetic vascular complications were of considerable clinical heterogeneity, and different experimental results were adjusted in different conditions [76, 77]. Recent publications have suggested that SAF serves as a marker of vascular damage [78], as well as a predictor of cardiac mortality in patients with type 1 and 2 diabetes. In Shuliang Lu's group, Liu Chuanbo et al. did a cross-sectional survey consisting of 118 consecutive hospitalized diabetic foot patients. The diabetic microvascular (retinopathy, nephropathy, and neuropathy) and macrovascular referring to coronary heart disease (CHD), cerebrovascular disease (CVD), or peripheral artery disease (PAD) complications were evaluated .The mean SAF value was 2.8 ± 0.2 AU. SAF was significantly associated with diabetes duration and blood urea nitrogen ($R2 = 62.8\%$; $P < 0.01$). Moreover, in logistic regression analysis, SAF was significantly associated with retinopathy (odds ratio [OR] = 40.11), nephropathy (OR = 8.44), CHD (OR = 44.31), CVD (OR = 80.73), and PAD (OR = 5.98×109). Therefore, SAF, reflecting tissue accumulation of AGEs is independently associated with the presence of micro-and macro-vascular complications in diabetic foot ulcer (DFU) patients [79]. Similarly, SAF values were significantly higher in type 1 diabetic patients with microvascular complications, like neuropathy, compared to those without complications [80]. Lisanne et al. reported that SAF was independently associated with all-cause mortality and fatal or non-fatal major adverse cardiovascular events in patients with peripheral artery disease after a 5-year follow-up [81].

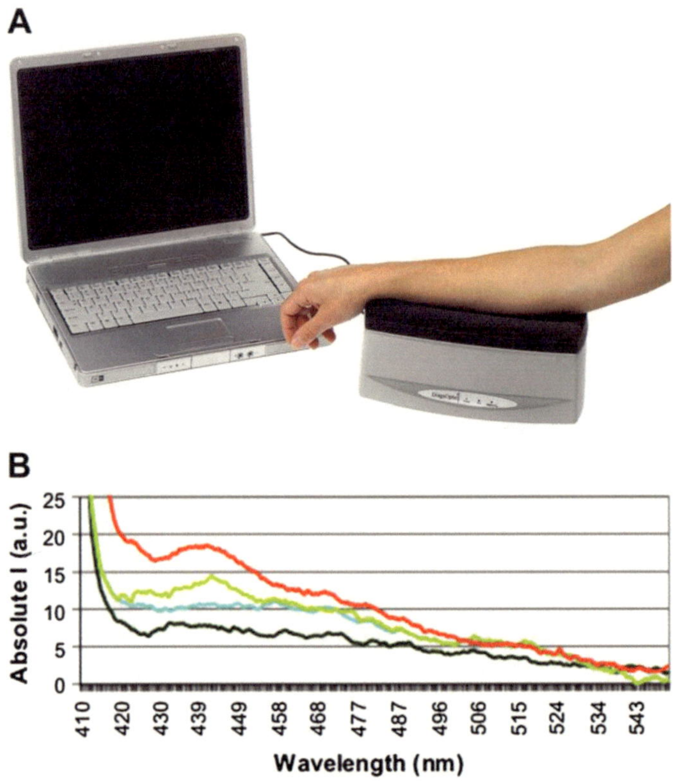

Figure 3. (A) The autofluorescence reader illuminates a skin surface with an excitation light source between 300–420 nm. Only light from the skin is measured with a spectrometer. (B) Various fluorescence spectrum results from different subjects: healthy subject (black line), diabetic patient without cardiovascular complications (blue line), diabetic patient with peripheral artery occlusive disease (green line), hemodialysis patient with recent myocardial infarction (red line). I = intensity (a.u.). (Illustrated from Meerwaldt R, van der Vaart MG, van Dam GM, et al. Clinical relevance of advanced glycation end products for vascular surgery. Eur J Vasc Endovasc Surg. 2008;36(2):125–31).

The use of SAF in the diabetic wound was also discussed. Meerwaldt et al. showed that SAF was increased and correlated with the Wagner score in DFU with neuropathy. SAF correlated inversely with nerve conduction velocity and amplitude [82]. Lapolla et al. found that AGEs were higher in type 2 diabetics with PAD compared to those without PAD; AGEs were correlated inversely to ABPI, even after correction for other cardiovascular risk factors [83]. SAF is independently associated with diabetic foot ulcerations. It might be a useful screening method for foot ulceration risk of diabetic patients [77].

Use of SAF measurement to assess foot vulnerability and to predict DFU events in high-risk patients seems to be promising. Yet, Vouillarmet et al.'s study in a subgroup of patients with an active DFU showed a nonsignificant correlation (P = 0.06) between SAF and the incidence of healing at 2 months, but the magnitude of effect is still high. Therefore, researchers deemed that the small number of patients may be the reason for the lack of statistical power. SAF method deserves attention because of its prognostic value for healing [84].

However, long-term studies validating both the specificity and sensitivity of this investigation, and its link to certain AGEs, remain to be confirmed. The importance of its use in the follow-up of DFU is not reported. Thus, AGEs might have some value as a screening tool for DFU, but there is no strong evidence for other clinical use in diabetic wound, and AGEs measurements should not be considered a replacement for HbA1c as a marker of glycemic control.

6. Anti-AGEs strategies

Since AGEs were considered as an important factor in diabetes, the development of strategies against AGEs has been of interest. Substances, which can prevent or inhibit the formation of AGEs, as well as agents that can break AGEs or antagonize their signaling have been identified.

6.1. Inhibit the formation of AGEs

The first approach is to reduce the formation of AGEs by intervention at one of the steps involved such as aminoguanidine [85]. Aminoguanidine was one of the first substances identified limiting the formation of AGEs [86]. It is a highly reactive nucleophilic reagent that prevents the formation of AGEs by reacting with the carbonyl groups as well as alpha- and beta-dicarbonyl compounds such as methylglyoxal, glyoxal, and 3-deoxyglucosone. Particularly, long-term aminoguanidine treatment improved the nerve conduction deficit and myelinated fiber pathology in diabetic rats in vivo [87]. A double-blinded, multiple-dose, placebo-controlled, randomized clinical trial of aminoguanidine in diabetic patients with overt diabetic nephropathy (ACTION) was completed in 1998; ACTION I involved 690 type 1 diabetic patients and ACTION II involved 599 type 2 diabetic patients. These studies were designed to evaluate the safety and efficacy of aminoguanidine in slowing the rate of renal disease progression in patients with overt diabetic nephropathy. However, ACTION II was terminated prematurely due to safety concerns and apparent lack of efficacy. Reported side effects included gastrointestinal disturbance, liver function abnormalities, flu-like symptoms, and a rare vasculitis [88]. Its use in clinical practice is limited due to adverse effects in clinical trials with diabetic patients. Despite the earlier promising results, aminoguanidine is unlikely to be used for therapeutic purpose due to safety concerns and lack of efficacy [89]. Studies on topical application of aminoguanidine on the skin are still lacking.

Metformin that is routinely used in the treatment of type 2 diabetic patients has some structural similarities to aminoguanidine and it was shown that in type 2 diabetes, treatment with metformin reduced levels of methylglyoxal [90]. Pyridoxamine is a natural intermediate of vitamin B6 metabolism and a potent inhibitor of the formation of AGEs [91]. Pyridoxamine traps reactive carbonyl intermediates and scavenges ROS. In addition, it inhibits post-Amadori stages of AGEs formation. Marked effects of pyridoxamine such as delayed development of nephropathy and retinopathy have been demonstrated in diabetic rats. Its oral intake could result in potent inhibition of skin collagen CML formation in diabetic rats as well [92].

6.2. Anti-RAGE

RAGE is the most studied receptor for advanced glycation end products. AGER1 has been shown to counteract AGEs-induced oxidative stress via inhibition of RAGE signaling [93]. sRAGE is a truncated splice variant of RAGE containing the ligand-binding domain but not the transmembrane domain and has been found in plasma. sRAGE is a soluble extracellular protein without signaling properties and it is considered as a natural decoy receptor of RAGE [30].

Blockage of RAGE by sRAGE may be a new target for therapeutic intervention in diabetic disorders. Potential protective effects of sRAGE have been shown in various diabetes and inflammatory models [94]. Interestingly, sRAGE could also attenuate impaired wound healing in diabetic mice. Other promising effects in various systems have been shown in vitro and in vivo with neutralizing anti-RAGE antibodies [31]. Possible approaches include gene knock-down of RAGE by siRNA or anti-sense and antagonism of RAGE with putative small molecular inhibitors against RAGE-induced signaling [95].

6.3. AGEs breakers

Chemical substances and enzymes that are able to recognize and break the Maillard reaction crosslinks have been identified. Such chemical AGEs breakers are dimethyl-3-phenayl-thiazolium chloride (ALT-711) [64], N-phenacylthiazolium and N-phenacyl-4,5-dimethylthiazolium. Promising results against diabetic cardiovascular complications have been reported, though their actual ability to cleave existing protein crosslinks in tissues has been questioned [96]. However, treatment with ALT-711 for 2 weeks had no effects on motor nerve conduction deficit, C-fiber-mediated nociceptive dysfunction, or impaired pressure-induced vasodilation in diabetic mice [97].

Interference with intrinsic AGE-detoxifying enzymes like fructosyl-amine oxidases (FAOXs), fructosamine-3-kinase (FN3K), and the enzymatic system of glyoxalase I is another interesting strategy to remove AGEs, because enzymes could recognize specific substrates [60]. It is reported that overexpression of glyoxalase I significantly inhibits hyperglycemia-induced intracellular formation of AGEs in bovine aortic endothelial cells and in mouse mesangial cells by reduction of intracellular oxidative stress and apoptosis [98]. The pharmacological induction of such enzymes could represent a novel future strategy against AGEs.

Other anti-AGE agents, including the thiazolidine derivative named OPB-9195, have been investigated [99]. OPB-9195 has been shown to prevent the progression of diabetic nephropathy in rats. It has also been demonstrated to improve motor nerve conduction slowing without affecting body weight and blood glucose levels. The improvement was associated with reduced serum AGEs levels and peripheral nerve expression of AGEs and immunoreactive 8-hydroxy-2-deoxyguanosine, which is a marker for oxidative stress-related DNA damage as well as an increase in peripheral nerve (Na+, K+)-ATPase activity [100].

Diabetic rats were found to have increased mesenteric vascular AGEs accumulation and mesenteric vascular hypertrophy, both of which were prevented by treatment with N-phenacylthiazolium bromide (PTB) [101]. A more recent study has demonstrated that although AGE-breakers such as PTB and N-phenacyl-4,5-dimethylthiazolium cleave model crosslinks in vitro, they do not significantly cleave AGE crosslinks formed in vivo in skin collagen of diabetic rats [59].

Benfotiamine, a lipophilic analogue of thiamine, is a transketolase activator that inhibits three of the four major biochemical pathways implicated in the pathogenesis of hyperglycemia-induced vascular damage: the hexosamine pathway, PKC activation, and AGEs formation [102]. In diabetic rats, nearly normalized nerve conduction velocity and inhibition of neural imidazole-type AGEs and CML formation after 6 months of benfotiamine treatment were observed [103]. In both nondiabetic and diabetic rats, benfotiamine also reduced inflammatory and neuropathic nociception [104].

6.4. Nutrient substance

An increasing list of natural antioxidants and chelating agents such as ascorbic acid, α-tocopherol, niacinamide, pyridoxal, sodium selenite, selenium yeast, trolox, rivoflavin, zinc, and manganese has been shown to inhibit glycation of albumin in vitro [105]. Many spices and herbs could inhibit glycation of albumin in vitro as well, such as ginger, cinnamon, cloves, rosemary, and tarragon [106]. Besides, green tea, vitamins C and E, and a combination of N-acetylcystein with taurine and oxerutin could inhibit skin collagen glycation in mice [107]. In healthy human subjects, supplementation of vitamin C significantly decreased serum protein glycation [108].

Alpha-lipoic acid could reverse tail tendon collagen glycation in fructose-fed rats, an effect which was attributed to its endogenous antioxidant action, its ability to recycle ascorbic acid and GSH, as well as to its positive influence on glucose uptake and glycemia [109]. Blueberry extract, an AGE-inhibitor and C-xyloside, was tested for 12 weeks in female diabetic subjects. This treatment resulted in significant improvement of skin firmness, wrinkles, and hydration. However, it failed to show a significant decrease in the cutaneous content of AGEs [110].

6.5. Molecular chaperones

Molecular chaperones like carnosine have shown promise in improving skin appearance in part by reducing the amounts of skin AGEs [111]. Yet, more studies are needed to address the accumulation of AGEs in diabetic wound.

In conclusion, AGEs are a heterogeneous group of molecules that form from the non-enzymatic addition of sugar moieties onto arginine and lysine residues of proteins, free amino groups on lipids, or guanine nucleic acids. The AGE-RAGE interactions play an important role in the diabetic wound healing process. The measurement of AGEs on the skin, namely, skin autofluorescence might have some value as a screening tool for diabetic foot ulcer, but until now, there is no strong evidence for other clinical use in diabetic wound. In addition, substances which can prevent or inhibit the formation of AGEs, as well as agents that can break AGEs or antagonize AGE/RAGE signaling have been identified.

Author details

Junna Ye[1*], Ting Xie[2], Yiwen Niu[1], Liang Qiao[1], Ming Tian[1], Chun Qing[1] and Shuliang Lu[1*]

*Address all correspondence to: 13901738685@139.com

1 Institute of Burns, Ruijin Hospital, Shanghai Jiao Tong University, Shanghai, China

2 Department of Wound Healing, Shanghai Ninth Hospital, Shanghai Jiao Tong University, Shanghai, China

References

[1] Nolan CJ, Damm P, Prentki M. Type 2 diabetes across generations: from pathophysiology to prevention and management. Lancet. 2011;378:169e81.

[2] Jeffcoate WJ, Harding KG. Diabetic foot ulcers. Lancet. 2003;361:1545–51.

[3] Jiang Y, Huang S, Fu X, et al. Epidemiology of chronic cutaneous wounds in China. Wound Repair Regen. 2011;19(2):181–8.

[4] Yao H, Ting X, Minjie W, et al. The investigation of demographic characteristics and the health-related quality of life in patients with diabetic foot ulcers at first presentation. Int J Low Extrem Wounds. 2012;11(3):187–93.

[5] Brownlee M. The pathobiology of diabetic complications: a unifying mechanism. Diabetes. 2005;54:1615e25.

[6] Armstrong DG, Lavery LA, Wu S, et al. Evaluation of removable and irremovable cast walkers in the healing of diabetic foot wounds: a randomized controlled trial. Diabetes Care. 2005;28(3):551–4.

[7] Boulton AJ, Kirsner RS, Vileikyte L. Clinical practice. Neuropathic diabetic foot ulcers. N Engl J Med. 2004;351:48–7.

[8] Kislinger T, Fu C, Huber B, et al. N(epsilon)-(carboxymethyl)lysine adducts of proteins are ligands for receptor for advanced glycation end products that activate cell signaling pathways and modulate gene expression. J Biol Chem. 1999;274(44):31740–9.

[9] Haslbeck KM, Schleicher E, Bierhaus A, et al. The AGE/RAGE/NF-(kappa)B pathway may contribute to the pathogenesis of polyneuropathy in impaired glucose tolerance (IGT). Exp Clin Endocrinol Diabetes. 2005;113(5):288–91.

[10] Monnier VM, Stevens VJ, Cerami A. Maillard reactions involving proteins and carbohydrates in vivo: relevance to diabetes mellitus and aging. Prog Food Nutr Sci. 1981;5:315–27.

[11] Peppa M, Stavroulakis P, Raptis SA. Advanced glycoxidation products and impaired diabetic wound healing. Wound Repair Regen. 2009;17:461–72.

[12] Singh R, Barden A, Mori T, et al. Advanced glycation endproducts: a review. Diabetologia. 2001;44:129–146.

[13] Ulrich P, Cerami A. Protein glycation, diabetes, and aging. Recent Prog Horm Res. 2001;56:1–21.

[14] Ahmed N. Advanced glycation endproducts – role in pathology of diabetic complications. Diab Res Clin Pract. 2005;67:3–21.

[15] Huijberts MS, Schaper NC, Schalkwijk CG. Advanced glycation end products and diabetic foot disease. Diab Metab Res Rev. 2008;24 Suppl. 1:S19–24.

[16] Giardino I, Edelstein D, Brownlee M. BCL-2 expression or antioxidants prevent hyperglycemia-induced formation of intracellular advanced glycation endproducts in bovine endothelial cells. J Clin Invest. 1996;97:1422–1428.

[17] Ruderman NB, Williamson JR, Brownlee M. Glucose and diabetic vascular disease. FASEB J. 1992;6:2905–2914.

[18] Westwood ME, Thornalley PJ. Molecular characteristics of methylglyoxal-modified bovine and human serum albumins. Comparison with glucose-derived advanced glycation endproduct-modified serum albumins. J Protein Chem. 1995;14:359–372.

[19] Phillips SA, Thornalley PJ. Formation of methylglyoxal and Dlactate in human red blood cells in vitro. Biochem Soc Trans. 1993;21:163S.

[20] Shinohara M, Thornalley PJ, Giardino I, et al. Overexpression of glyoxalase-I in bovine endothelial cells inhibits intracellular advanced glycation endproduct formation and prevents hyperglycemia-induced increases in macromolecular endocytosis. J Clin Invest. 1998;101:1142–47.

[21] Peppa M, He C, Hattori M, et al. Fetal or neonatal low-glycotoxin environment prevents autoimmune diabetes in NOD mice. Diabetes. 2003;52(6):1441–8.

[22] Lin RY, Choudhury RP, Cai W, et al. Dietary glycotoxins promote diabetic atherosclerosis in apolipoprotein E-deficient mice. Atherosclerosis. 2003;168(2):213–20.

[23] American Diabetes Association. Peripheral arterial disease in people with diabetes. Diabetes Care. 2003;26:3333–41.

[24] Koschinsky T, He CJ, Mitsuhashi T, et al. Orally absorbed reactive glycation products (glycotoxins): an environmental risk factor in diabetic nephropathy. Proc Natl Acad Sci U S A. 1997;94:6474–6479.

[25] Kankova K. Diabetic threesome (hyperglycaemia, renal function and nutrition) and advanced glycation end products: evidence for the multiple-hit agent? Proc Nutr Soc. 2008;67:60e74.

[26] Peppa M, Uribarri J, Vlassara H. Aging and glycoxidant stress. Hormones 2008;7:123–32.

[27] Cai W, He JC, Zhu L, et al. AGE-receptor-1 counteracts cellular oxidant stress induced by AGEs via negative regulation of p66shc-dependent FKHRL1 phosphorylation. Am J Physiol Cell Physiol. 2008;294:C145–52.

[28] Vlassara H. The AGE-receptor in the pathogenesis of diabetic complications. Diabetes Metab Res Rev. 2001;17:436–43.

[29] Yamagishi S, Matsui T. Soluble form of a receptor for advanced glycation end products (sRAGE) as a biomarker. Front Biosci (Elite Ed). 2010;2:1184–95.

[30] Ramasamy R, Yan SF, Schmidt AM. RAGE: therapeutic target and biomarker of the inflammatory response-the evidence mounts. J Leukoc Biol. 2009;86:505–12.

[31] Bierhaus A, Humpert PM, Morcos M, et al. Understanding RAGE, the receptor for advanced glycation end products. J Mol Med. 2005;83:876–86.

[32] Ishihara K, Tsutsumi K, Kawane S, et al. The receptor for advanced glycation end-products (RAGE) directly binds to ERK by a D-domain-like docking site. FEBS Lett. 2003;550(1–3):107–13.

[33] Loughlin DT, Artlett CM. Precursor of advanced glycation end products mediates ER-stress-induced caspase-3 activation of human dermal fibroblasts through NAD(P)H oxidase 4. PLoS One. 2010;5:e11093.

[34] Lohwasser C, Neureiter D, Weigle B, et al. The receptor for advanced glycation end products is highly expressed in the skin and upregulated by advanced glycation end products and tumor necrosis factor-alpha. J Invest Dermatol. 2006;126(2):291–9.

[35] Fujimoto E, Kobayashi T, Fujimoto N, et al. AGE-modified collagens I and III induce keratinocyte terminal differentiation through AGE receptor CD36: epidermal-dermal interaction in acquired perforating dermatosis. J Invest Dermatol. 2010;130:405–14.

[36] Zhu P, Ren M, Yang C, et al. Involvement of RAGE, MAPK and NF-kB pathways in AGEs-induced MMP-9 activation in HaCaT keratinocytes. Exp Dermatol. 2012;21:123–9.

[37] Berg TJ, Snorgaard O, Faber J, et al. Serum levels of advanced glycation end products are associated with left ventricular diastolic function in patients with type 1 diabetes. Diab. Care. 1999;22(7):1186–90.

[38] Stern DM, Yan SD, Yan SF, et al. Receptor for advanced glycation endproducts (RAGE) and the complications of diabetes. Ageing Res Rev. 2002;1:1–15.

[39] Fisher GJ, Kang S, Varani J, et al. Mechanisms of photoaging and chronological skin aging. Arch Dermatol. 2002;138:1462–70.

[40] Tian M, Qing C, Niu Y, et al. The relationship between inflammation and impaired wound healing in a diabetic rat burn model. J Burn Care Res. 2016;37(2):e115–24.

[41] Bernhard D, Moser C, Backovic A, et al. Cigarette smoke – an aging accelerator? Exp Gerontol. 2007;42(3):160–5. Epub 2006 Nov 3.

[42] Niu YW, Miao MY, Dong W, et al. Effects of advanced glycation end products and its receptor on oxidative stress in diabetic wounds. Zhonghua Shao Shang Za Zhi. 2012;28(1):32–5.

[43] Zhu P, Yang C, Chen LH, et al. Impairment of human keratinocyte mobility and proliferation by advanced glycation end productsmodified BSA. Arch Dermatol Res. 2011;303:339–50.

[44] Giardino I, Edelstein D, Brownlee M. Nonenzymatic glycosylation in vitro and in bovine endothelial cells alters basic fibroblast growth factor activity. A model for intracellular glycosylation in diabetes. J Clin Invest. 1994;94:110–7.

[45] Wondrak GT. Let the sun shine in: mechanisms and potential for therapeutics in skin photodamage. Curr Opin Investig Drugs. 2007;8:390–400.

[46] Miao M, Niu Y, Xie T, et al. Diabetes-impaired wound healing and altered macrophage activation: a possible pathophysiologic correlation. Wound Repair Regen. 2012;20(2): 203–13.

[47] Tseng JY, Ghazaryan AA, Lo W, et al. Multiphoton spectral microscopy for imaging and quantification of tissue glycation. Biomed Opt Express. 2010;2:218–30.

[48] Lee C, Yim MB, Chock PB, et al. Oxidation-reduction properties of methylglyoxal-modified protein in relation to free radical generation. J Biol Chem. 1998;273:25272–8.

[49] Kazuhiro Y, Tomohide O, Tomonobu Y, et al. Inhibitory effect of peptide free forms of advanced glycation end products on the proliferation and extracellular matrix production of cultured cells. J Health Sci. 2001;47:296–301.

[50] Alikhani Z, Alikhani M, Boyd CM, et al. Advanced glycation end products enhance expression of pro-apoptotic genes and stimulate fibroblast apoptosis through cytoplasmic and mitochondrial pathways. J Biol Chem. 2005;280:12087–95.

[51] Berlanga J, Cibrian D, Guillé;n I, et al. Methylglyoxal administration induces diabetes like microvascular changes and pertubs the healing process of cutaneous wounds. Clin Sci (Lond). 2005;109:83–95.

[52] Duraisamy Y, Slevin M, Smith N, et al. Effect of glycation on basic fibroblast growth factor induced angiogenesis and activation of associated signal transduction pathways in vascular endothelial cells: possible relevance to wound healing in diabetes. Angiogenesis. 2001;4:277–88.

[53] Teixeira AS, Andrade SP. Glucose-induced inhibition of angiogenesis in the rat sponge granuloma is prevented by aminoguanidine. Life Sci. 1999;64:655–62.

[54] Gkogkolou P, Böhm M. Advanced glycation end products: key players in skin aging? Dermatoendocrinology 2012;4(3):259–70.

[55] Niu Y, Xie T, Ge K, et al. Effects of extracellular matrix glycosylation on proliferation and apoptosis of human dermal fibroblasts via the receptor for advanced glycosylated end products. Am J Dermatopathol. 2008;30(4):344–51.

[56] Bakris GL, Bank AJ, Kass DA, et al. Advanced glycation end-product cross-link breakers. A novel approach to cardiovascular pathologies related to the aging process. Am J Hypertens. 2004;17:23S–30S.

[57] Yang S, Litchfield JE, Baynes JW. AGE-breakers cleave model compounds, but do not break Maillard crosslinks in skin and tail collagen from diabetic rats. Arch Biochem Biophys. 2003;412:42–6.

[58] Monnier VM, Wu X. Enzymatic deglycation with amadoriase enzymes from *Aspergillus* sp. as a potential strategy against the complications of diabetes and aging. Biochem Soc Trans. 2003;31:1349–53.

[59] Voziyan PA, Hudson BG. Pyridoxamine: the many virtues of a Maillard reaction inhibitor. Ann N Y Acad Sci. 2005;1043:807–16.

[60] Vasan S, Foiles P, Founds H. Therapeutic potential of breakers of advanced glycation end product-protein crosslinks. Arch Biochem Biophys. 2003;419:89–96.

[61] Smit AJ, Gerrits EG. Skin autofluorescence as a measure of advanced glycation endproduct deposition: a novel risk marker in chronic kidney disease. Curr Opin Nephrol Hypertens. 2010;19:527–33.

[62] Genuth S, Sun W, Cleary P, et al. Glycation and carboxymethyllysine levels in skin collagen predict the risk of future 10-year progression of diabetic retinopathy and nephropathy in the diabetes control and complications trial and epidemiology of diabetes interventions and complications participants with type 1 diabetes. Diabetes. 2005;54:3103–11.

[63] Niu Y, Cao X, Song F, et al. Reduced dermis thickness and AGE accumulation in diabetic abdominal skin. Int J Low Extrem Wounds. 2012;11(3):224–30.

[64] Foell D, Wittkowski H, Roth J. Mechanisms of disease: a 'DAMP' view of inflammatory arthritis. Nat Clin Pract Rheumatol. 2007;3(7):382–90.

[65] Holman RR, Paul SK, Bethel MA, et al. 10-year follow-up of intensive glucose control in type 2 diabetes. N Engl J Med. 2008;359(15):1577–89.

[66] Meerwaldt R, Graaff R, Oomen PH, et al. Simple non-invasive assessment of advanced glycation endproduct accumulation. Diabetologia. 2004;47:1324–30.

[67] Mácsai E, Takáts Z, Derzbach L, et al. Verification of skin autofluorescence values by mass spectrometry in adolescents with type 1 diabetes: brief report. Diabetes Technol Ther. 2013;15(3):269–72.

[68] Meerwaldt R, Hartog JW, Graaff R, et al. Skin autofluorescence, a measure of cumulative metabolic stress and advanced glycation end products, predicts mortality in hemodialysis patients. J Am Soc Nephrol. 2005;16(12):3687e93.

[69] Samborski P, Naskręt D, Araszkiewicz A, et al. Assessment of skin autofluorescence as a marker of advanced glycation end product accumulation in type 1 diabetes. Pol Arch Med Wewn. 2011;121(3):67–72.

[70] Tanaka K, Tani Y, Asai J, et al. Skin autofluorescence is associated with severity of vascular complications in Japanese patients with type 2 diabetes. Diabet Med. 2012;29:492–500.

[71] Noordzij MJ, Mulder DJ, Oomen PH, et al. Skin autofluorescence and risk of micro- and macrovascular complications in patients with type 2 diabetes mellitus – a multi-centre study. Diabet Med. 2012;29:1556–1561.

[72] Hu H, Han CM, Hu XL, et al. Elevated skin autofluorescence is strongly associated with foot ulcers in patients with diabetes: a cross-sectional, observational study of Chinese subjects. J Zhejiang Univ Sci B. 2012;13(5):372–7.

[73] Koetsier M, Lutgers HL, de Jonge C, et al. Reference values of skin autofluorescence. Diabetes Technol Ther. 2010;12(5):399–403.

[74] Yue X, Hu H, Koetsier M, et al. Reference values for the Chinese population of skin autofluorescence as a marker of advanced glycation end products accumulated in tissue. Diabet Med. 2011;28(7):818–23.

[75] Simon Klenovics K, Kollárová R, Hodosy J, et al. Reference values of skin autofluorescence as an estimation of tissue accumulation of advanced glycation end products in a general Slovak population. Diabet Med. 2014;31(5):581–5.

[76] Meerwaldt R, Lutgers HL, Links TP, et al. Skin autofluorescence is a strong predictor of cardiac mortality in diabetes. Diabetes Care. 2007;30:107–12.

[77] Gerrits EG, Lutgers HL, Kleefstra N, et al. Skin autofluorescence: a tool to identify type 2 diabetic patients at risk for developing microvascular complications. Diabetes Care. 2008;31:517–521.

[78] Pietzsch J, Hoppmann S. Human S100A12: a novel key player in inflammation? Amino Acids. 2009;36(3):381–9.

[79] Liu C, Xu L, Gao H, et al. The association between skin autofluorescence and vascular complications in Chinese patients with diabetic foot ulcer: an observational study done in Shanghai. Int J Low Extrem Wounds. 2015;14(1):28–36.

[80] Araszkiewicz A, Naskret D, Niedzwiecki P, et al. Increased accumulation of skin advanced glycation end products is associated with microvascular complications in type 1 diabetes. Diab Technol Ther. 2011;13(8):837–42.

[81] de Vos LC, Mulder DJ, Smit AJ, et al. Skin autofluorescence is associated with 5-year mortality and cardiovascular events in patients with peripheral artery disease. Arterioscler Thromb Vasc Biol. 2014;34(4):933–8.

[82] Meerwaldt R, Links TP, Graaff R, et al. Increased accumulation of skin advanced glycation end-products precedes and correlates with clinical manifestation of diabetic neuropathy. Diabetologia. 2005;48(8):1637–44. Epub 2005 Jul 14.

[83] Lapolla A, Piarulli F, Sartore G, et al. Advanced glycation end products and antioxidant status in type 2 diabetic patients with and without peripheral artery disease. Diab Care. 2007;30(3):670–6.

[84] Vouillarmet J, Maucort-Boulch D, Michon P, et al. Advanced glycation end products assessed by skin autofluorescence: a new marker of diabetic foot ulceration. Diab Technol Ther. 2013;15(7):601–5.

[85] Thornalley PJ. Use of aminoguanidine (Pimagedine) to prevent the formation of advanced glycation endproducts. Arch Biochem Biophys. 2003;419:31–40.

[86] Edelstein D, Brownlee M. Mechanistic studies of advanced glycosylation end product inhibition by aminoguanidine. Diabetes. 1992;41:26–9.

[87] Yagihashi S, Kamijo M, Baba M, et al. Effect of aminoguanidine on functional and structural abnormalities in peripheral nerve of STZ-induced diabetic rats. Diabetes. 1992;41(1):47–52.

[88] Freedman BI, Wuerth JP, Cartwright K, et al. Design and baseline characteristics for the aminoguanidine clinical trial in overt type 2 diabetic nephropathy (ACTION II). Control Clin Trials. 1999;20(5):493–510.

[89] Bolton WK, Cattran DC, Williams ME, et al. Randomized trial of an inhibitor of formation of advanced glycation end products in diabetic nephropathy. Am J Nephrol. 2004;24:32–40.

[90] Beisswenger P, Ruggiero-Lopez D. Metformin inhibition of glycation processes. Diab Metab. 2003;29(4 Pt 2):6S95–103.

[91] Haus JM, Carrithers JA, Trappe SW, et al. Collagen, cross-linking, and advanced glycation end products in aging human skeletal muscle. J Appl Physiol (1985). 2007;103(6):2068–76. Epub 2007 Sep 27.

[92] Degenhardt TP, Alderson NL, Arrington DD, et al. Pyridoxamine inhibits early renal disease and dyslipidemia in the streptozotocin-diabetic rat. Kidney Int. 2002;61(3):939–50.

[93] Cai W, He JC, Zhu L, et al. Oral glycotoxins determine the effects of calorie restriction on oxidant stress, age-related diseases, and lifespan. Am J Pathol. 2008;173:327–36.

[94] Yan SF, Ramasamy R, Schmidt AM. Soluble RAGE: therapy and biomarker in unraveling the RAGE axis in chronic disease and aging. Biochem Pharmacol. 2010;79:1379–86.

[95] Chen Y, Akirav EM, Chen W, et al. RAGE ligation affects T cell activation and controls T cell differentiation. J Immunol. 2008;181:4272–8.

[96] Monnier VM, Sell DR. Prevention and repair of protein damage by the Maillard reaction in vivo. Rejuvenation Res. 2006;9:264–73.

[97] Demiot C, Tartas M, Fromy B, et al. Aldose reductase pathway inhibition improved vascular and C-fiber functions, allowing for pressure-induced vasodilation restoration during severe diabetic neuropathy. Diabetes. 2006;55:1478–83.

[98] Kim KM, Kim YS, Jung DH, et al. Increased glyoxalase I levels inhibit accumulation of oxidative stress and an advanced glycation end product in mouse mesangial cells cultured in high glucose. Exp Cell Res. 2012;318:152–9.

[99] Nakamura S, Makita Z, Ishikawa S, et al. Progression of nephropathy in spontaneous diabetic rats is prevented by OPB-9195, a novel inhibitor of advanced glycation. Diabetes. 1997;46:895–9.

[100] Wada R, Nishizawa Y, Yagihashi N, et al. Effects of OPB-9195, anti-glycation agent, on experimental diabetic neuropathy. Eur J Clin Invest. 2001;31:513–20.

[101] Vasan S, Zhang X, Kapurniotu A, et al. An agent cleaving glucose-derived protein crosslinks in vitro and in vivo. Nature. 1996;382:275–8.

[102] Hammes HP, Du X, Edelstein D, et al. Benfotiamine blocks three major pathways of hyperglycemic damage and prevents experimental diabetic retinopathy. Nat Med. 2003;9:294–9.

[103] Stracke H, Hammes HP, Werkmann D, et al. Efficacy of benfotiamine versus thiamine on function and glycation products of peripheral nerves in diabetic rats. Exp Clin Endocrinol Diabetes. 2001;109:330–6.

[104] Sanchez-Ramirez GM, Caram-Salas NL, Rocha-Gonzalez HI, et al. Benfotiamine relieves inflammatory and neuropathic pain in rats. Eur J Pharmacol. 2006;530:48–53.

[105] Tarwadi KV, Agte VV. Effect of micronutrients on methylglyoxal-mediated in vitro glycation of albumin. Biol Trace Elem Res. 2011;143:717–25.

[106] Dearlove RP, Greenspan P, Hartle DK, et al. Inhibition of protein glycation by extracts of culinary herbs and spices. J Med Food. 2008;11:275–81.

[107] Odetti P, Pesce C, Traverso N, et al. Comparative trial of N-acetylcysteine, taurine, and oxerutin on skin and kidney damage in long-term experimental diabetes. Diabetes. 2003;52:499–505.

[108] Vinson JA, Howard HB. Inhibition of protein glycation and advanced glycation end products by ascorbic acid and other vitamins and nutrients. J Nutr Biochem. 1996;7:659–63.

[109] Thirunavukkarasu V, Nandhini AT, Anuradha CV. Lipoic acid prevents collagen abnormalities in tail tendon of high-fructose-fed rats. Diab Obes Metab. 2005;7:294–7.

[110] Draelos ZD, Yatskayer M, Raab S, et al. An evaluation of the effect of a topical product containing C-xyloside and blueberry extract on the appearance of type II diabetic skin. J Cosmet Dermatol. 2009;8:147–51.

[111] Babizhayev MA, Nikolayev GM, Nikolayeva JG, et al. Biologic activities of molecular chaperones and pharmacologic chaperone imidazole-containing dipeptide-based compounds: natural skin care help and the ultimate challenge: implication for adaptive responses in the skin. Am J Ther. 2012;19(2):e69–89.

Section 2

Clinical Features and New Insights in Wound Recovery

Ischemic Ulcer Healing: Does Appropriate Flow Reconstruction Stand for All That We Need?

Vlad-Adrian Alexandrescu and François Triffaux

Additional information is available at the end of the chapter

http://dx.doi.org/10.5772/64834

Abstract

During the recent decades, soaring progresses in vascular disease knowledge, particularly in critical limb ischemia (CLI) treatment, enhanced novel diagnostic and interventional strategies with high serviceableness in patient's selection, arterial recanalization, and dedicated ischemic ulcer follow-up. However, despite undeniable advances in medical technology and clinical judgment, limb salvage, the ambulation recovery, and patient's survival seem only scarcely affected in this heterogeneous CLI group, particularly concerning the diabetic and renal patients. Innovative strategies such as "*end artery occlusive disease*" treatment or "*wound-targeted revascularization*" were equally proposed by following the angiosomal anatomical distribution associating individual foot collateral assessment in a unified *macro-* and *micro*-circulatory judgment. However, despite encouraging clinical results, prospective evidence still lacks on this concern. It also appears that specific wounds could not always stand for the lowest perfusion areas according to current CLI criteria, since severe neuropathy, inflammatory swelling, local infection, and skin trauma may add complementary hindrances to tissue viability.

The present chapter endeavor to summarize main available treatment principles for ischemic ulcer recovery that every modern practitioner eventually disposes in an updated contemporary view."

Keywords: wound healing, critical limb ischemia, diabetic foot, angiosome, limb revascularization

Motto: '*Each ulcer is unique in complexity and deserves flexible understanding and control of whole individual tissue recovery challenges*' (Current clinical observation)

1. Introduction

During centuries, wound healing was believed to be part of a mysterious process that addresses only inspirational approaches of secret practitioner's experience. Outstanding scientific advances over the last 50 years revealed real complexity of this staged process, astonishing as life's unfolding itself. This natural course seems to bear thousands of overlapping and indissoluble processes [1]. Today's knowledge, beyond new high-performance techniques for revascularization and tissue engineering [1], affords additional key data about intimate mechanisms of ischemic threat, ulcer formation, and steps to wound recovery [1, 2]. In the recent decades, this proper knowledge enhanced complementary diagnostic and interventional strategies with high serviceableness in patient's selection, arterial recanalization, and dedicated ulcer follow-up [1, 3]. However, despite soaring progress in medical technology and clinical judgment for critical limb ischemia (CLI) wound treatment, limb salvage, and patient's survival seem only scarcely affected [1–3]. This assertion dwells particularly true in diabetic and renal patients who exhibit ischemic foot wounds [1, 2]. Outstanding advances in basic research and clinical management toward better tissue regeneration, unfortunately, seem to confront with parallel increasing of CLI subjects each year [1]. It becomes obvious nowadays that ischemic ulcer healing implies a convergent treatment for multifaceted presentations in patients with multiple arterial and systemic affectations [1–3].

The present chapter endeavor to summarize main treatment principles for CLI ulcer recovery that every modern practitioner eventually disposes in an updated contemporary view.

2. Historical perspectives and advancements in ischemic wounds treatment

Wound healing approaches are probably old as the history of medicine. During centuries, several significant breakthroughs, however, marked significant progress in wound repair, following thorough scientific understanding. Starting with the Ancient World, according to the oldest medical record found on a Sumerian clay tablet (2100 BC) [4], cleansing and bandaging the wound was noted to represent the central "healing gestures" to be practiced in the healing course [4]. The Ancient Egyptians (1600 BC–1550 BC) also mention the use of mixtures (honey, grease, and lint) for wound regeneration, however, without apparent etiologic segregation [5, 6]. They also displayed an impressive science of bandaging, including herbal extracts and resins (probably the first coordinated bandages ever mentioned) [5]. Hippocrates in the ancient Greece originally devised approach methods for acute and chronic wounds [6]. Later on, Cornelius A. Celsius marked a momentous step in wound care history by his original description of the "four cardinal signs of inflammation," including first "gangrenous foot" delineation in his eight-volume *Compendium of Medicine* (41 BC) [6]. A substantial contribution to ulcer's classification and healing understanding is appointed by outstanding surgical work of Ambroise Parré in the Renaissance era about the treatment of gunshot wounds including "the gangrenous battlefield limb" [7]. During the next centuries, many new ideas in wound management were unfortunately rejected by lack of validation and time-related historical tendencies. Wound healing understanding was subsequently developed by Joseph Lister's [8] and by Louis Pasteur's remarkable clinical research [8, 9] adding relevant knowledge for bacterial colonization and sepsis development, particularly in the ischemic ground [9]. More recently, notable breakthroughs in comprehending the complexity of wound healing cascade were added by Virchow [10], owning establishment of histopathology as an autonomous discipline [6, 10], and by first isolation of "epidermal growth factor" as a mitotic stimulant in 1962 [11].

Probably one of the most ponderous discoveries in the same period was the defining structure of DNA and RNA by Franklin, Watson, and Crick [6]. Parallel advances were noted in surgical and interventional revascularization techniques for *tissue healing* perceived in a hemodynamic ischemic perspective. Leading milestones in arterial flow imaging were marked by first arteriographic diagnostic reported by Brooks in 1924 [12], followed by first translumbar aortography described by Dos Santos in 1929 [13], both with considerable influence in more accurate inferior limb arterial disease diagnostic. First Doppler ultrasound assessment of atherosclerotic occlusive disease by noninvasive method was reported by Strandness [14] in 1966. All these diagnostic methods have borne huge influence first in distinguishing arterial from nonischemic wounds, and further for separating arterial from venous limb ulceration. The current ischemic injury diagnostic era yet institutes since the computed tomography (CT) scanning and magnetic resonance imaging (MRI) have become an integrated part of ongoing peripheral arterial flow evaluation [15]. For that arterial surgery enables high limb salvage nowadays, the achievement of several important steps was mandatory. The first lumbar sympathectomy in 1924 by Labat [16], the heparin use since 1937 [17], the Kunlin's first saphenous vein graft in 1951 [18] and the first Dacron [19], and polytetrafluoroethylene (PTFE) [20] prothesis utilization, all had tremendous influences in modern surgical revascularization for wound healing [1–3, 20].

Traditionally during years, open surgical bypass represented the main effective treatment strategy for tissue recovery and limb salvage [1, 21]. In addition to outstanding surgical revascularization advances, new transcatheter endovascular techniques emerged and rapidly evolved in CLI treatment arena during the last three decades [21]. They seem to improve the perioperative morbidity-mortality and the length of hospital stay, affording comparable limb preservation rates [1–3, 21]. Owning remarkable low invasiveness and reproducibility, the percutaneous transluminal angioplasty (PTA) and stenting (first promoted by Gruntzig in 1974 and by Dotter [20] in 1964) rapidly gained a wide utilization in the coronary, but also in the peripheral arterial disease (PAD) current treatment [21]. Although the "stent" term derives from Charles Stent (1807–1885), an English dentist who used this term for creating customed dental molds [21], the idea to modulate vascular lumen by diligent metallic implants had great issues in vascular practice. During the next decades, new "bare" or "covered stents" were imagined, together with new "stent grafts" originally pioneered by Volodos and Parodi in the treatment of aortic aneurysmal disease around 1985–1990s [22]. Novel "drug eluted" devices including balloons and stents have been successfully launched during the last decade with promising clinical results [1, 21].

Following parallel scientific emancipation, new strategies as to improve ischemic tissue healing were cast in parallel medical disciplines. Thus, in 1987, Taylor and Palmer initially described the "angiosome" model of human body vascularization [23] and auspiciously implemented the concept among particular plastic reconstructive surgery applications. This significant breakthrough in tissue perfusion understanding was succeeded by its first use in CLI limb salvage by Attinger and colleagues 20 years later [24], using "topographical" or angiosome-guided bypasses to the foot ischemic wounds [24]. Not surprisingly, starting with 2008–2010s, and up to the contemporary period, new endovascular "wound-directed" revascularization applications were described with promising wound healing and limb preservation results [25, 26]. All these progresses have added and undoubtedly will add complementary understanding in ischemic ulcer treatment, owning more precise revascularization selection since specific "wound-targeted" revascularization is performed [24–26].

3. Demographics, etiologic factors, and social implications of PAD with its most severe presentation represented by critical limb ischemia

Recent demographic data suggest that more than 200 million individuals worldwide suffer from varied forms of the PAD that represent a 24% increase over the last decade and concern all socioeconomic strata [27, 28]. The economic weight of PAD was proven to be ponderous [28]. It has meant that the total costs of vascular-related hospitalizations climbed to 21 billion dollars in the USA in 2004, and this threshold seems to rise each year continually [28]. Critical limb ischemia as a consequence of severe infra-inguinal atherosclerosis embodies extreme forms of PAD and currently associates rest pain and ischemic ulcers (corresponding to Fontaine stages III/IV and Rutherford categories 4-5 ischemic limb presentations) [1–3].

The term of CLI is commonly used for patients who exhibit symptoms of severe arterial hypoperfusion for more than 2 weeks [3, 27]. Elementary CLI diagnosis is made by clinical exam, anatomical stratification, and hemodynamic evaluation of flow disturbances over accessible arterial paths [1, 3, 27]. Defining and analyzing large CLI groups of patients, however, prove to be difficult [2–4].

These hindrances are mainly determined by (1) the vast heterogeneity of underlying arterial diseases [1, 27], (b) the various appended risk factors [1–3, 27], (c) the multilevel spread of arterial lesions [1, 27] (d) by concurrent systemic pathologies [27], (e) the scarce follow-up data [3, 27], and (f) the lack of synchronous macro- and microvascular apprehension for gradual hypoxic limb changes [1, 27–31]. It is known that without precocious recognition and aggressive treatment, CLI invariably inflicts significant morbidity and high rates of major amputation and mortality [1–3, 27–30].

To date, the likelihood of death within the first 6 months of CLI diagnosis has been estimated to reach 20% (all etiologies confounded) and exceeds 50% at 5 years following prime documented onset [27–32]. Contemporary studies reveal that patients with PAD (and particularly those with CLI) are more likely to experience simultaneous coronary or cerebral vascular disease, bearing a higher risk of early death [1–3, 27]. The risk for developing PAD seems

http://dx.doi.org/10.5772/64834

considerably increased in diabetic and renal patients, prone to more frequently experience systemic ischemic events compared to general population [1–3, 27–31].

Several risk factors that lead to lower limb major amputation in patients having ischemic wounds were described, including increasing age, being male, being African American, having peripheral neuropathy, and developing infected ulcers [1, 2, 27–29]. The Trans-Atlantic Inter-Society initial Consensus (TASC) II document showed that more than 15% of diabetic subjects will unfold a foot ulcer during their lifetime while 14–24% of them, unfortunately, will require amputation [3]. It is also valued that more than 170 million people suffer nowadays from diabetes mellitus, and their worldwide number is anticipated to attain 366 million by 2030 [1]. In this particular cohort of diabetic patients during the first year of CLI diagnosis, 40–50% among them may experience foot amputation while 20–25% among them will die [1, 2, 27].

Nevertheless, by applying optimal revascularization and local wound treatment as early as possible, up to 85% of amputations can be prevented [3].

The social burden of the metabolic syndrome and particularly the diabetic systemic atherosclerotic disease is tremendous for the patient, the medical care organization, and public communities [1, 2, 28, 31].

Particularly concerning *arterial* inferior limb *ulcers* (all arterial pathologies confounded), current reports document 18–29% prevalence among 60 years or older patients who interestingly bear equal rates as much younger (50-year-old) individuals associating diabetes or tobacco use [33].

4. Critical limb ischemia ulcers: do we meet the current clinical needs?

Postischemic tissue recovery implies simultaneous alignment of several distinct physiological processes [33]. Inasmuch their entire clinical signification remains only partially controlled [27, 30, 33], their unaltered unfolding dwells prerequisite. Among numerous molecular and cellular events that clearly overpass the purposes of this chapter, some practical aspects may be however useful to be highlighted and are briefly summarized in the sections below.

4.1. Leading physiological mechanisms in wound recovery and appended phases of revascularization

It is accepted that mechanisms concerning tissue regeneration are strongly influenced by the type and thickness of tissue layer affectation, also by their capacity for healing [1, 33]. The retrieval of CLI threat resets in motion the regular "cascade" of reconstructive tissue events leading in normal circumstances (absence of systemic risk factors for healing) to long-lasting tissue repair [33, 34]. Full-thickness wound regeneration following most CLI revascularizations concerns the skin, the underlying subcutaneous and the deep muscular compartments. Currently, this process is depicted in three schematic phases: the inflammatory stage (the "lag" phase), the "tissue formation" (or the "proliferative") phase, and the "tissue remodeling" phase [34]. It is important to note that this "allotment" is somewhat conventional since all three stages are commonly overlapping to some degree [33, 34]. Activating cells that participate in one phase usually produce biological triggers indispensable to interlock tissue molding into the next phase [34]. These stages are routinely *conditioned* by initial hemostasis and by intentional *arterial revascularization*, both representing fundamental activating processes [33–35]. Most details concerning these enthralling multimodal events are largely depicted in available histopathology literature and will not be further characterized in this section.

During the same sequential process, the ischemic burden relief sets in motion three parallel *hemodynamic* regenerative phases [35]. These stages are conceptualized as (1) *the initiatory* flow redistribution phase (concerning "large" remnant collaterals surrounding the ischemic wound zone), (2) *the early* or "mid-term" flow dispensation (regarding the "rescue" or "small" collaterals and arterioles), and (3) *the retarded* postischemic phase, essentially characterized by the arteriogenesis, the angiogenesis processes [33–35]. Alike most biological chain-processes, these three flow-redistribution phases exhibit specific time overlapping in their activation, according to concomitant vascular risk factors and individual patterns of arterial occlusive disease [35]. This particular knowledge may enable the clinician to choose better appropriate diagnostic and treatment methods in a timely approach for every ischemic wound follow-up [33, 35].

4.2. Main pathophysiological aspects in ischemic wound healing and related clinical presentations

To date, the exact mechanisms and time periods conducting to chronic ischemic ulceration are not completely understood [30, 31, 33, 34, 36]. Most arterial ulcers are encountered over the age of 65 as people live longer nowadays [3, 33]. Arterial ulcers are ranked to constitute about 12–19% among all leg ulcers [33, 37] while mixed venous-arterial or combined neuro-ischemic tissue defects may concern 15% [37] up to 24% [29–31] of these patients, respectively. There were described either as "spontaneous" ulcerations (typically involving the forefoot and toes as progressive collateral occlusion occurs) or as "post-minor trauma" wounds since inadequate arterial flow proves ineffective to increased oxygen demands for cicatrization [34, 38]. Bed-ridden patients with PAD represent another high-risk category to develop pressure heel ischemic ulcers on preexisting vascular impairment [37, 38]. For this particular cohort exhibiting ischemic hind foot ulcers, current guidelines emphasize that prevention by scrupulous heel elevation or soft tissue contact interposition is mandatory [3, 28, 38].

The TASC II fundamental CLI criteria [3] as absolute ankle pressure (AP) inferior to 50–70 mm Hg, or diminished toe pressure (TP) below 30–50 mm Hg are unanimously accepted [3]. A series of parallel predisposing factors for ischemic tissue damage were evinced in the last decade. They either concern the arterial perfusion (tobacco use, dyslipidemia, hypertension, weight excess, hyperglycemia, hyperhomocysteinemia, etc.), or specific foot conditions (peripheral neuropathy, inflammation, edema, infection, bedridden status, hypoalbuminemia, hyperglycemia, uremia, cortisone therapy, etc.), all with huge influence on peripheral tissue regeneration [1–3, 27, 33–35, 37, 38]. Although arterial ulcers theoretically may appear anywhere on the ischemic limb [3, 33], the presence of multilevel CLI arterial disease inflicts more distal localizations, particularly in subjects with deprived foot collateral reserve [1, 25, 29, 30].

Beyond common atherosclerotic arterial ulcers, other *arterial*-related ulcers were described such as superficial hypertensive wounds, peripheral embolic tissue defects (owning 0.01–0.2 mm. cholesterol particles), those associated with connective tissue arteritis, those affecting hypercoagulable states, or following microangiopathic lesions, within parallel to mixed nutritional, hemolytic, or neurologic disorders [33, 34, 36].

4.3. What determines ischemic tissue defects to slide toward chronicity and necrosis? Is there a conjuring threshold to consider?

It has been showed that in healthy individuals, peripheral wounds promptly tend to recover owning adapted cell's metabolism, appropriate oxygen supply, essential growth factors, cytokines, and matrix proteins inflow (Section 5.1.2.) that all endeavor to orient local tissue damage on "steady" sequential healing process [27, 33, 36].

Since initial ischemic changes last beyond local individual compensatory reserves [30, 35], the readapting mechanisms are gradually exhausted and local tissue homeostasis finally drifts toward biological extinction [36, 39, 40]. Inasmuch CLI wound onset may be commonly displayed over days or weeks [3], local infection and collateral depletion by septic thrombosis can urge irrecoverable tissue loss appearance and make it devastating [30, 32, 35]. Probably the real "tipping point" between viable or perished, for every inch of ischemic tissue around the wound relies on local collateral adaptation vigor [39]. Alike other ischemic models described in human tissues (stroke, myocardial infarction), the extent of necrosis core depends on rescue capacity inside the "penumbra" or intermediary neighboring zone [35]. For this transitional layer of undecided viability, a few factors strongly influence its fate. The timing and intensity of main ischemic threat, the type of arterial pathology, the remnant upstream arterial trunks and collaterals, and the elapsed interval to prompt debridement and revascularization, play a pivotal role in any arterial ulcer progress [30, 33, 36, 40].

Daily vascular practice proves that interventionists are more likely confronted with patients exhibiting more than one *long acting* adverse factors for tissue healing [39, 40]. These conditions can be summarized as malnutrition and hypoalbuminemia, lack of compensatory arterial collateral network, diminished arterio- and angiogenesis, peripheral edemas enhancing local compartmental syndromes, low cardiac output, and prolonged bony prominences pressure that collectively contribute as notable interferences in physiological cicatrization [34, 35, 37, 40].

4.4. Current CLI diagnostic: can we effectively assess the real ischemic burden?

A series of high-performance technologies conceived to assess tissue-related arterial disease were introduced in the last two decades. These methods afford high or low invasiveness and focus on different targets in evaluating CLI hemodynamic and tissue changes [29, 30]. With each passing year, novel or modernized diagnostic techniques strive for accurately scoring the degree of perfusion tissue impairment in mixed series of patients and arterial pathologies [1, 2, 27–32].

It has been showed that first *detailed clinical assessment* of each tissue defect is mandatory in all presentations [36, 38, 39, 40]. Basic characteristics of each ulcer (surface and depth), its precise location(s), and the appended inflammatory extensions before and after revascularization should be carefully analyzed and scored by trained clinical teams [38, 39].

The majority of available diagnostic techniques can be roughly divided into *macro-* and *microcirculatory* investigation tools. Some "routine" *noninvasive macro-vascular exams* such as the ankle-brachial index (ABI < 0.5, severe ischemia), the toe-brachial index (TBI < 0.7, presence of PAD), the ankle and toe pressure (<40 mm Hg, threat of the limb), the exercise stress testing, and the Doppler and Duplex assessments are well-documented and own undeniable benefits, and drawbacks [33–35, 37, 39]. Meticulous Doppler evaluation avails real usefulness for knowledgeable clinicians in determining antegrade versus retrograde tibial, pedal, or collateral flow toward the wound zone [24, 39]. It may also yield helpful information over the remnant "large caliber" collaterals in the targeted foot ischemic area [24, 35, 39]. A precise mapping of lower limb arteries specifying eventual stenosis, occlusions, and secondary collateral flow represents a valuable *preoperative* or *follow-up* guide for any interventionist in planning wound-directed revascularization [39].

Other low-invasiveness techniques for detecting "large" arteries and collaterals include last-generation multislice computed tomographic angiography (CTA with "Dual energy") and the magnetic resonance angiography (MRA adding "BOLD sequences") [33, 39]. The "Dual energy" CTA imaging represents a current evaluation method in our team experience for patients with normal renal function. This technology allows accurate calcific plaques removal in tibial and foot vessels and provides a true BTK "lumenograms" in these patients [39].

Despite notable progress in both techniques, these two methods host similar iodine or gadolinium-based contrast disadvantages, being contraindicated in allergic patients or for those suffering from chronic renal insufficiency [33, 39].

Unfortunately, in the daily clinical practice, most of diabetic or renal CLI patients with threatening foot ulcers often associate advanced nephropathy that challenges the use of Iodine or Gadolinium contrast agents.

Probably the most accustomed *macro-circulatory* yet *invasive* available test is represented by the digital subtraction arteriography (DSA) of the inferior limb arteries [1, 3, 28, 38].

DSA is currently recognized as a "key exam" in accurate ischemic flow assessment and classification [1–3, 38, 39]. It is cited to afford best available spatial resolution required to establish main arterial trunks and collaterals (>500 μm diameter) morphological details toward the wound zone [1, 3, 27, 35, 38]. DSA also enables appropriate diagnostic for eventual anatomical variables and their collateral network in each specific arterial pattern [1, 27, 35]. This *quantitative* information becomes essential in understanding individual vascular anatomy for performing eventual *direct* (wound targeted) or *indirect* (collateral supported) arterial revascularization to the wound zone [24–26, 39]. Peripheral angiography consequently helps in determining the most appropriate and "feasible" target vessel to be treated [23–26, 35].

It is shown that DSA affords the interventionist valuable *qualitative* information about *the severity* of distal leg ischemia (the "desert" foot presentation). It also provides accurate characteristics of run-off vessels, the integrity of foot arches, and clues about potential technical difficulties in long chronic total occlusions (CTO) recanalization (the presence of concave/convex atherosclerotic caps) [1, 21, 29, 39]. This technology provides corresponding information about extensive calcifications, tortuosities, and available arterial-arterial communicants or "blush" irrigation around the ulcer's zone [25, 26, 31, 35, 39]. Inasmuch DSA bears evoked drawbacks due to iodine contrast (allergic or renal failure reactions), it also carries the eventual access-related risk for hemorrhagic complications (0.8–3% of cases) [27, 33, 39].

Modern wound practitioners equally avail latest *micro-vascular noninvasive* diagnostic technology, with soaring applications in the last two decades. Among these methods, some showed promising results such as the consecrated transcutaneous oxygen pressure [1–3, 33, 39]; the novel vascular optical tomographic imaging (VOTI) [41]; the "real-time" Laser-Doppler skin perfusion pressure [33, 35, 39]; the continuous tissue oxygen saturation foot-mapping (StO_2); and the recent ^{99m}Tc Scintigraphic, the PET, and the single-photon emission computed tomography (SPECT) scans (owning specific CLI 3-D detection at molecular level) [35, 39]. Parallel *microcirculatory* yet, more *invasive* exploration was recently documented gathering intraoperative "Indocyanine green" angiography (ICGA) [42, 43], the "Indigo Carmine" angiography [44], and the foot "micro-oxygen sensors" (MOXYs) technology, all with encouraging applications during wound-targeted revascularization [45].

4.5. The CLI multimodal approach: a novel contemporary concern

Bell et al. first proposed the notion of critical limb ischemia in 1982 for defining severe arterial flow deprivation that currently inflicts major limb amputation threat [46]. In their original publication, the authors characterize CLI essentially on *macro-vascular hemodynamic criteria,* such as the measured AP <40 mm Hg in the presence of rest pain and <60 mm Hg when tissue necrosis is noted [46]. It should be mentioned that in the original form of this concept, the diabetic group of CLI patients was deliberately excluded since neuropathy and infection are often associated and make more complex real ischemic stratification [46]. During the next 30 years, the term of CLI was broadly, yet most of the times inappropriately, used [29–32, 47] as to characterize a much larger hierarchy of severe arterial presentations, including diabetic and renal subjects [27, 30, 46–49]. Although the particular threshold from "reversible" to "irrecoverable" limb ischemia still dwells imprecise [27, 29, 31, 34], it is accepted that CLI often implies a poor limb outcome without prompt revascularization [1–3, 27, 30, 46, 47]. An eloquent 1527 CLI subjects review analysis recently performed by Abu Dabrh et al. on the natural history of untreated "severe" or "critical" ischemic limbs revealed 22% all-cause mortality, 22% major amputation, and 35% worsening in wound evolution rates at 1 year [48]. The almost similar observation was reported in 2016 by Vallabhaneni et al. in a 443 CLI cohort assembling more than 60% diabetics and 20% dialyzed patients [49]. They found 32 and 56% mortality rate at 1 and 3 years, respectively, and 24 and 31% major amputation rates at the same time intervals [49]. The authors conclude that not all patients were encompassing current ABI- and TBI-accepted CLI *macro-vascular* criteria, obviously are at high risk for major amputation [49].

We know nowadays that CLI associates a modest quality of life to the high rate of major amputations and that about 60% of mortality is documented between 3 and 5 years following the initial diagnostic [1–3, 32, 46, 47–49].

Parallel papers focusing on equivalent *macro-vascular* hemodynamic standards (ABI, TBI, AP, TP, etc.), equally fail to explain this huge heterogeneity encountered in CLI "limb salvage" and dedicated treatments [47–49]. Struggling to provide more accurate CLI categorization, several conspicuous classifications systems were proposed in the last two decades [1, 3, 30, 47].

Owning the Bollinger angiographic scale [50], the Trans-Atlantic Inter-Society initial Consensus (TASC I and II) [3, 51], the Rutherford staging of PAD [52], and the European recommendations for CLI management [53], complementary definitions yet adding only $TcPO_2$ *microcirculatory* references were settled [27, 47, 53].

In the recent years, novel PAD classification systems were developed alike the Graziani morphologic arteriographic indexation in diabetics [54], the Toursarkissian angiographic scoring for distal limb salvage bypass [55], and the "Jenali" tibial run-off classification system, with appended below-the-knee intervention protocol [56]. This latest is based on three grades for main infragenicular arterial trunks fluency associating three levels of time-related collaterally filling (at 3–6–9 s) [56].

Undoubtedly, all abovementioned iconographic scoring systems excel in meticulous angiographic anatomy analysis, yet only partially address concomitant wound index or baseline *microcirculatory* perfusion status [30, 39].

Despite real efforts in stratifying CLI intimate mechanisms, to date, all evoked classifications add a little emphasis on coupled *macro-* and *microcirculatory* evaluation, including individual wound characteristics [30, 39].

They also fail to quantify eventual threshold [47] below which inferior limb perfusion becomes nonviable without opportune revascularization [27–30, 47]. The risk of developing CLI and ischemic wounds seems considerably increased in diabetic patients, although prone to more frequently endure systemic ischemic events compared to general population [3, 27, 31].

Contemporary clinical expertise allows better knowledge over the multifaceted "Diabetic Foot Syndrome" (DFS) presentation that gathers arteriopathy, neuropathy, sepsis, pressure injuries, and cellular and molecular metabolic disturbances, in myriads of different clinical archetypes [31, 57]. A vehement need for more specific CLI delineation in these patients was increasingly recollected in modern vascular literature.

4.6. Does healing process in diabetics follow same predictable "standards" alike other CLI patients?

Soaring progress in arterial ulcers treatment is however confronted with an exponentially increasing number of diabetic CLI subjects each year [1, 31]. To date, the prevalence of purely neuropathic, ischemic, and combined neuro-ischemic foot ulcers in patients with diabetes was estimated at 35, 15, and 50% rates, respectively [57–59].

http://dx.doi.org/10.5772/64834

Reported DFS singularities include (1) the regular tibial trunks *calcifications* [2, 30, 31, 57] that match the extent of local neuropathy [25, 31], (2) the "end-artery occlusive disease" (EAOD) concept [59], (3) an impaired *arterio-* and *angiogenesis* [60], (4) a specific *collateral deprivation* following chronic inflammation and septic thrombosis of small vessels [31, 35, 57–59], (5) intrinsic vascular or *matrix impaired regeneration* [61], and (6) characteristic neuro-ischemic *compartmental hyper pressure* foot syndromes [62].

The EAOD theory emphasizes that in the collateral-depleted diabetic limb, "each millimeter of skin" up to the "entire foot" may rely upon one particular artery with *terminal* distribution [59], while this valuable vessel may be auspiciously targeted by "wound directed" revascularization, according to the angiosome concept [24–26].

Modern diabetic ulcer understanding builds a complete design of multifaceted and potentially devastating CLI effects in these patients [2, 31, 57–62].

Enthralling scientific works in the last decade evoke a possible central mechanism playing a pivotal role in different DFS pathological changes [59, 63]. Thus, chronic hyperglycemia may enhance at the mitochondrial-level expanded free radicals production, altering normal metabolic and cellular activity [63]. This malfunction affects more particularly normal regeneration at the *microcirculatory* level (vasa-vasorum and vasa-nervorum) also the tissue binding matrix [58, 59–61].

Arteriopathy and neuropathy, albeit regular DFS features (in different proportions) [58, 59], may probably share the same pathological emergence in the vast diabetic complications puzzle [57–59, 63].

Trying to stratify main DFS characteristics, a few classification systems were proposed. It should be mentioned the "Wagner" stratification [64], the PEDIS (perfusion, extent/size, depth/tissue loss, infection, sensation/neuropathy) [65], the University of Texas (UT) [66], the sepsis, arteriopathy, denervation (SAD) scale [67], the diabetic ulcer severity score (DUSS) [68], the multiple ulceration, wound area, pedal pulse, and ulcer duration (MAID) classification [69], and the "St. Elian wound score system" [70], rejoicing unanimously recognized popularity and documented clinical benefits [57–59].

However, most of these classifications fail to provide concomitant *perfusion* information [35, 47]; individual *ulcer features* [47]; *infection, denervation*, or *gangrene* specifications [47]; systemic factors report [2, 30] (Section 4.5); and healing prognosis [2, 40, 47]. All these clinical entities seem to bear a huge interest in healing evaluation [2, 31, 37, 39].

In same effort to fully perceive each DFS presentation, the remarkable WIfI classification [47] recently brought together Wound grades, Ischemia levels, and foot Infection ranked in a unitary view, as important variables for appended wound prognosis [47]. However, diabetic neuropathy [36, 58, 71] and concurrent systemic variables influencing tissue recovery [57, 61, 72] are not included in this model of examination. In a parallel analysis, owing a consecutive 249 CLI wounds series, Azuma et al. [72] found that beyond diabetes (including neuropathy and infection), equally end-stage renal disease (ESRD), Rutherford category 6 (including or not the heel), and low albumin levels, represented significant factors in the complex tissue recovery cascade beyond prompt revascularization [72].

5. Contemporary landmarks in ischemic wounds revascularization

Expanding clinical evidence in the last three decades supports both bypass and the endovascular techniques as useful strategies in CLI revascularization [1–3, 29–31]. Providing low invasiveness, high reproducibility, and comparable limb salvage rate to open surgery [21–73], transcatheter strategies continue to evolve with new low-profile and high-performance devices in arterial reconstruction [21, 29, 74]. For most "high-risk" CLI patients [1, 2, 31, 34], new endovascular approaches and techniques were designed. In succinct overview, the "drilling," the "subintimal," or the "parallel wire" techniques via the ante- or retrograde accesses, the pedal-plantar "loop," and the femoral-femoral or transtibial collaterals angioplasties were recently described [29, 74, 75].

Not with standing with these spectacular transcatheter performances, the "classical" bypass for distal leg reperfusion is still imposed as a fundamental technique for CLI diabetic foot revascularization, tissue healing, and limb preservation [1, 3, 72, 76]. High-skill distal vein bypasses to the tibial [72], to the pedal [77], and up to the plantar or tarsal foot arteries [78] equally by targeting remote branches of pedal arteries in some particular cases [1, 76] were successfully documented. We now know that both surgical and endovascular techniques are more likely complementary than competitive techniques since each of them holds major advantages and inherent drawbacks [1, 29, 30, 79]. Endovascular techniques essentially provide minimal invasiveness, great accessibility, and reproducibility for one or multiple below-the-knee CTO recanalizations [1, 29, 73–75]. Alternatively, bypass offers a higher pressure on targeted arteries and more physiological and pulsatile flow inside collaterals around the wound zone [35, 53, 77–79]. This particularity heightens arterial-arterial collateral shear stress and enhances rising arteriogenesis [58–60] toward further tissue cicatrization [1, 29, 35, 60, 72].

Although still heterogeneously structured [1, 73, 79], increasing contemporary clinical observation documents equivalent limb salvage, clinical success, and survival outcomes for bypass versus endoluminal interventions in selected groups of CLI patients [1–3, 27, 29–31, 79, 80]. Notwithstanding with initial historical considerations [79], these two strategies appear nowadays more intricate than ever inside the conceptualized "team approach" as CLI treatment [29, 35].

Parallel advances concerning the DFS revascularization and ischemic wound healing were equally testified in the last two decades [1, 2, 75]. Beyond striking surgical arterial reconstructions [76–79], new tapered nitinol [81], drug-eluting stents (DES) [82], and original drug-eluting balloon, (DEB) [83] were imagined. Novel or redesigned directional or rotational atherectomy devices [84], together with latest "bioresorbable scaffolds" technologies [85], represent few additional of numerous achievements that challenge today ancient technical barriers [1, 29, 75, 81–86].

6. New strategies for "wound targeted revascularization"

The complex cascade of tissue regeneration needs precise circumstances to unfold [85]. Beyond high-performance techniques in reconstructing arterial flow [72–86], new strategies about "when" and "where" to perform appropriate revascularization emerge today [1, 27, 30, 35]. Contemporary practitioners equally avail key data on the molecular mechanisms generating ischemic threat and tissue regeneration [59–61]. This knowledge, part of a larger "integrated multidisciplinary medicine" [87, 88], supports new strategies in limb salvage [1, 29, 48] based on precise arterial flow mapping [23–26] and deliberate tissue healing reengineering [29–31]. A new conceptualization of ischemic wound treatment rises at present [1, 2, 33], with promising serviceableness in patient's stratification [47, 53, 57, 59], revascularization selection [35, 38], and dedicated postoperative follow-up [31].

According to this modern emphasis, novel "hybrid" surgical and endovascular techniques [89], synchronous ante- and retrograde arterial accesses [74, 90], and novel topographic "wound-directed" revascularization (WDR) [24, 35, 91–93] proved useful to save more limbs for major amputation. Alternatively, extreme venous limb arterialization [94, 95] and cell stem treatment [1, 29] parallel to rising "multidisciplinary team" practice [57, 87, 88] have also been developed and seem to revolutionize previous CLI paradigms of care [1, 29, 92–94].

6.1. The "angiosome concept" in ischemic wound healing: a succinct overview

Among all innovative strategies in CLI wound treatment, a remarkable leap was undoubtedly marked by *topographic*, or intentional, *wound directed* arterial reconstruction [23–26, 35, 72, 91–93]. This theory represents a unique clinical application of the *angiosome concept* initially pioneered in 1987 by Taylor et al. in the plastic reconstructive surgery field [23].

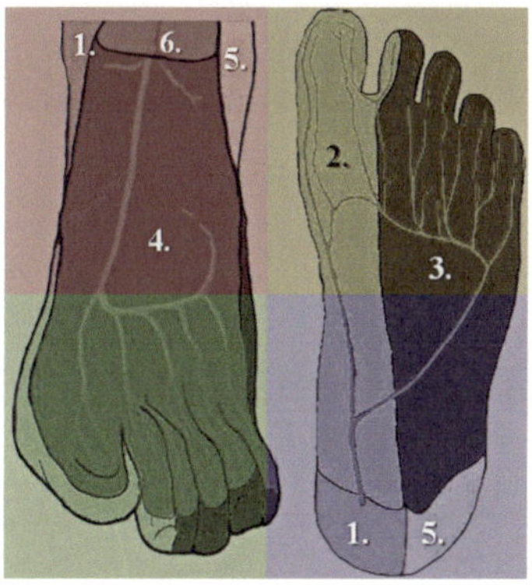

Figure 1. A schematic anatomic representation of the six angiosomes of the lower leg in a forefoot/hindfoot topographic view. (**1**) The *medial calcaneal* angiosome (from the posterior tibial artery). (**2**) The *medial plantar* angiosome (posterior tibial artery). (**3**) The *lateral plantar* angiosome (posterior tibial artery). (**4**) The *dorsalis pedis* angiosome (from the anterior tibial artery). (**5**) The *lateral calcaneal* angiosome (from the peroneal artery). (**6**) The *antero-lateral malleolar* angiosome (currently from the anterior tibial, also from the perforator branch of the peroneal artery).

The angiosome conceptualization describes more than 44 specific 3-D *tissue sectors* of the human body nourished by individual arterio-venous bundles called "the angiosomes" [23]. This anatomical representation was further referred to CLI treatment two decades later by Attinger et al. [24], owning encouraging clinical results.

The lower leg angiosome territories. The following skin and underlying tissue zones were earlier described as to nearly encompass six main *angiosomes* (**Figure 1**) of the foot and ankle [23–26, 91–93]:

- The *medial calcaneal* and appended *medial* and *lateral plantar* arteries angiosomes arising all from the *posterior tibial artery*. They supply the entire plantar heel and the medial and lateral plantar surface to the toes.
- The *dorsalis pedis* angiosome, downstream to the *anterior tibial artery* that nourishes the dorsal foot and toes areas, also ensures the upper and anterior peri-malleolar vascularization.
- The *lateral calcaneal artery* angiosome branching from the *peroneal artery* and that supplies the lateral, plantar heel.
- At a higher level of the superior ankle, other angiosomes were described, such as *the antero-lateral malleolar* owning its correspondent *antero-medial malleolar* angiosomes (both from the *anterior tibial artery*), and the *pstero-medial malleolar* angiosome following correspondent branch from the *posterior tibial artery*, respectively [23–26, 91–93].

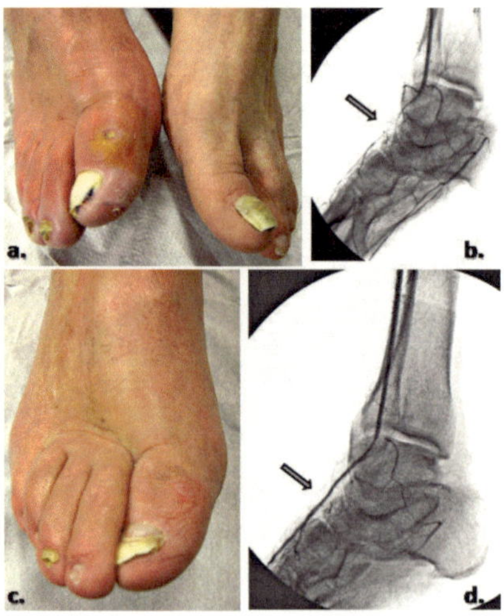

Figure 2. A diabetic neuro-ischemic ulcer associating cutaneous sepsis on the antero-medial aspect of the foot. (**a**) The initial clinical aspect (CLI, Rutherford 5). (**b**) The appended angiographic aspect showing complete occlusions of the dorsalis pedis and distal posterior tibial artery. (**c**) Healing aspect at three months, following (**d**) angiosome-targeted revascularization by deliberately opening the dorsalis pedis artery territory (arrow).

These vascular territories are closely interconnected by numerous *arterial-arterial* communicants [23, 24], whose caliber and density are strongly influenced by the age of patients, by each region's anatomy and by the manifest arterial disease triggering CLI [24, 35, 72, 96–98]. Every individual collateral system essentially assists blood supply between neighboring angiosomes. These compensatory branches the so-called "choke vessels" include *large-*, *middle-*, and *small-*sized arterial-arterial communicants, beyond the arterioles and capillary vessels in a vast "compensatory arterial foot network" [24, 29, 35]. All collateral interconnections between adjacent angiosomes are submitted to specific hemodynamic influences related to local *arterio*genesis and *angio*genesis processes [35, 59, 60].

The angiosome clinical model implies a conspicuous vascular anatomical order, although subject to specific pathophysiological changes in every CLI individual pattern. Optimal *wound-targeted revascularization* probably means correct angiosome-related anatomical evaluation associated with individual collateral-related pathophysiological judgment for each CLI presentation [30].

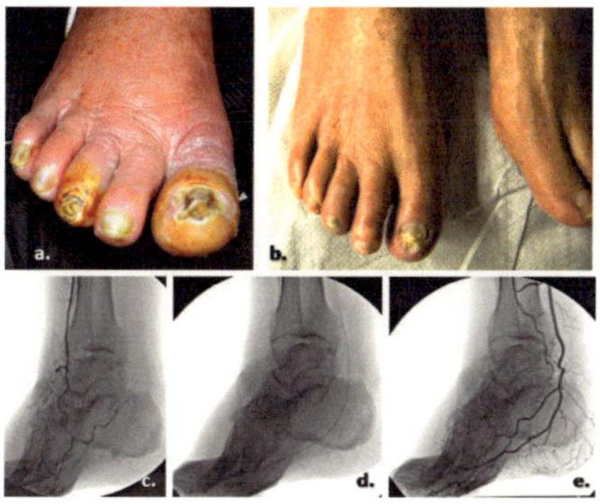

Figure 3. Wound-targeted revascularization for severe forefoot sepsis and tissue necrosis, extending to the plantar side of the hallux and toes. (**a**) The initial clinical aspect (CLI, Rutherford 5). (**b**) Healing after topographic revascularization and multidisciplinary team care at five months. (**c**) The starting angiographic image showing complete posterior tibial artery occlusion (the dominant wound territory), and the dorsalis pedis thrombosis. We can remark only a few remnant collaterals (the characteristic diabetic foot collateral deprivation) represented by two lasting diagonal arteries. (**d**) Endovascular plantar angiosomes-targeted revascularization by posterior tibial artery intentional reopening. (**e**) The end-procedural result showing the posterior tibial, the plantar arteries, and the plantar arch reperfusion in an intentional wound-directed revascularization.

In young subjects with unaltered collateral network possible post-traumatic or ischemic injuries activate unmitigated "choke-vessels" that warrant (at some point) effective compensatory blood pressure between adjacent angiosomes [24, 39, 96, 97]. Atherosclerotic, inflammatory, or local thrombotic conditions may alter this unique natural compensatory system. As previously described [23, 24], the foot angiosomes are 3-D dynamic and continuously interacting structures [30]. Although their primary anatomical distribution seems accurately reproduced in more than 90% of subjects (owing 6–9% eventual anatomival variants) [23, 24, 26, 91], their interconnections ("choke vessels") are yet submitted to continuous changes, according to each type of CLI pathology [72, 95–98].

Assessing and treating ischemic wounds in the light of the angiosome theory imposes a flexible reflection upon *how* utilizing the remnant arterial-arterial connections (**Figures 2** and **3**) at best flow benefit for the patient [88, 97].

6.2. What group of ischemic ulcers may need WDR?

Inasmuch genetic collateral network warrants a remarkable "rescue system" in non-atherosclerotic patients, it can be dramatically hindered in specific diabetic or uremic ischemic wounds [24, 35, 72, 96–98]. The interventionist should be aware of treating peculiar diabetic and ESRD *ischemic ulcers*, for that these patients may hide huge collateral decay and poor arterial-arterial connections among adjacent foot angiosomes [72, 97]. Eventual *indirect* [26] or *nonspecific* revascularization [25, 93] in these subjects may fail to afford correct arterial flow to the wound by a lack of collateral resources [25, 59, 72, 96].

Alternatively, the use of WDR principle in these cases seems to provide improved healing results [24, 39, 72, 96–98] owning scrupulous *macro-* and *microcirculatory* evaluation, planning for intervention and follow-up [39, 96, 97].

Despite encouraging tissue healing and limb salvage results for both, bypass and endovascular treatment [24–26, 91–93], uncertainty still dwells concerning the utility of angiosome-oriented revascularization in specific CLI groups of patients dysplaying different etiologies of arterial disease [35, 72, 96, 97]. Growing clinical expertise, however, seems to support WDR in "low-collateral" CLI patients such as those presenting DFS (**Figures 2** and **3**), or ESRD ischemic wounds [72, 91–93, 96–98].

6.3. Does topographic WDR allow unrestricted anatomical applications?

The angiosome-oriented revascularization theoretically offers superior chances for healing in selected ischemic wounds, yet this theory still awaits for further prospective validation in larger groups of equivalent CLI patients [92, 97].

Lower limb topographic anatomy addressed to date unnumbered ex vivo or clinical works [99–102] (most of them in the last 50 years) and their analysis largely overpasses the purposes of this chapter. However, some compelling points should be probably mentioned for better picturing this impressive graduation in the distribution of the arterial tree toward the target tissue [35, 101, 102]. The whole body vasculature can be delineated from a "fractal" point of view, as harmonious repetitive patterns of peripheral tissue irrigation [35, 101]. Particularly concerning the inferior limb vascularization, this archetype evinces some specific *levels of irrigation* [35]. A primary *level I* of perfusion contains the main arterial and venous bundles (i.e. iliac and common femoral), the *level II* gathers first rank arterial branches in the thigh and calf (i.e. the superficial and profonda femoris and the three tibial trunks), and the next *level III* features distinct ramifications for *specific skin and underlying tissue zones* in the foot [35]. This level also encompasses the *large* collaterals (around 1 mm diameter), including *the angiosomes branches*, the appended *foot arches*, and the *metatarsal perforators* [24, 35, 101], yielding specific interest in topographic revascularization [23–26, 35, 93, 100]. The next *level IV* holds the *medium-* and *small*-size (<0.5 mm) collaterals, while next microcirculatory ranks assemble *level V* that gathers *the arterioles* and the *level VI* connecting the *capillary* tier (around 8-μm diameter) [39, 101, 103]. This latest convenes several millions of small micrometric conduits in the whole human body, approximating 60,000 miles of estimated length [102].

Another parallel and more common anatomical partition used in CLI literature roughly distinguishes the *macrocirculatory* rank (that embodies previous *levels I–IV*) from the *microcirculatory* level (equivalent to other *levels V* and *VI*) of limb perfusion [1, 27, 29, 30, 103–106]. By bridging these two levels, the *medium* and *small* muscular arteries and adjacent *arterioles* contribute to a continuous *pacing system* of local tissular perfusion [103–105]. Since CLI threat appears, this function seems to be notably distorted until focused revascularization is applied [25, 60, 106].

According to the above considerations, several anatomical variants were equally described, mainly concerning level III of limb flow distribution [104, 105]. Following two recent meta-analysis gathering 7671 [107] or 5790 inferior limbs [108], and two "in vivo" analogous angiographic observations [109, 110], *native atypical leg arteries* were described in utmost 7.9–10% individuals out of general population [107–110]. Among these variants, hypoplastic or aplastic posterior tibial artery was encountered in 3.3% cases, whereas the anterior tibial trunk was absent in about 1.5% of instances [108]. The presence of highly emergent anterior tibial artery or irregular tibial trifurcation was described in 5.6–6% cases [109–110], while anomalous origins of the dorsalis pedis artery were encountered in 4.3–6% presentations [109, 111]. Aberrant first dorsal metatarsal artery and appended first toe dominant irrigation was described in 8.1% cases [112], parallel variants of the arcuate artery in 5% [113], and modified courses of the plantar arch and plantar arteries in 5% of presentations [114]. The intimate knowledge of these variants seems significant for the advised interventionist since *wound-directed revascularization* is planned [30, 100]. The presence of one anatomical popliteal variation (i.e. high origin of the anterior tibial trunk) on one side may indicate possible ipsilateral foot vessel abnormalities in about 21% of cases [107, 109], and similar contralateral leg variants in 48% of instances [109, 110]. Concomitant *acquired arterial flow disturbances* were also cited in lower leg ischemic presentations, most of them accompanying the diabetic neuro-ischemic foot syndrome [34, 53, 59]. The majority of these anomalies were represented by occlusions of at least two or all tibial arteries in more than 70% of CLI diabetic subjects [110, 115]. A higher prevalence of long (>15 cm) obstructions in the posterior tibial and plantar arteries [25, 116, 117] and extensive (type II) calcifications [25, 91] in most diabetic calf and foot arterial segments were also demonstrated [91]. Our group experience over 232 diabetic CLI limbs [91] with Wagner grade 2–4 foot wounds [64] availing *angiosome-targeted* revascularization [24, 96–98], also confirmed more frequent posterior tibial atherosclerotic occlusive disease (68% of cases versus 25% anterior tibial and 7% peroneal presentations) [91]. Moreover, the posterior tibial hypoperfusion showed significant (>90%) concordance with distinct plantar, heel and forefoot (on the plantar side) skin, and adjacent tissue trophic lesions [25–91].

Although precise below-the-knee arterial *anatomical knowledge* is of paramount importance in planning "angiosome-directed" revascularization [91–93], the skilled interventionist should also corroborate additional *hemodynamic information* enabled by each collateral pattern [24, 93, 96–98, 118].

Even in the presence of unusual anatomical variants to supply the foot, topographic revascularization still appears feasible [39] by taking advantage either on visible or on unmasked arterial branches (the "dormant" collaterals) that gradually reveal during CTO recanalization [24, 35, 56].

It becomes clearer that since all tibial trunks become occluded, the tipping point between hypoxic tissue regeneration versus chronic ulceration and necrosis hinges upon *the remnant individual collateral reserve* and ways to deliberately use it in addressing the ischemic threat [24, 30, 34, 59].

Despite encouraging results to date [91–93, 96], the angiosome concept may provide better, yet not complete, ischemic tissue control [35, 61, 72, 118].

Topographic WDR for ulcer healing remains an enthralling subject of discussion. Certainly, alike similar new openings of flourishing interest in tissue regeneration, the scarcer the available evidence, the acrider the current debate, mostly based on heterogeneous retrospective deliberations [35, 72, 92, 96–98, 118].

7. The state of foot collaterals: a key principle in modern CLI wound treatment

The TASC II recommendation [3] for prompt revascularization in CLI is generally accepted [1, 27], however, do all these interventions address similar extent of ischemic threat? Do all these interventions bear then, equivalent expectations for tissue recovery? [49] More concretely, does the modern vascular interventionist truly control all hemodynamic *macro-* and *microvascular* changes at the wound level while performing CLI revascularization? [49, 61, 97] Up-to-date research reveals that not all proven lower limb ischemic ulcers share the same TASC II/CLI criteria [3] and, consequently, harbor the corresponding amount of ischemic burden! [2, 31, 49, 61, 118, 119] Owning steady improvement in diagnostic and treatment, modern practitioners start to adapt current CLI standards to each type of arterial pathology [1, 35, 73, 107], and to resize ischemic ulcer appraisal in deeper *macro-* and *microcirculatory* perception [39, 59–61, 97, 106]. The contemporary medical community is now facing *a novel* challenge wherein specific strategies for revascularization in CLI patients *with* and *without* a convenient foot *collateral network* [92, 96–100, 119]. Thorough research in diabetic CLI treatment had already evinced good tissue cicatrization since topographic revascularization is performed in subjects having a poor collateral reserve [26, 92, 96–100, 119]. It is known that DFS currently alter common foot cutaneous, the underlying tissue and bony presentation, by iterative inflammation, scars, ischemic necrosis, sensorimotor neuropathy, and local pressure aggressions [57–60]. Even though that CLI/DFS severely distorts the "classically pictured" angiosomal foot vasculature [23–25, 96–98], *wound-targeted revascularization* using the *surviving collateral system* represents a valuable solution for better tissue regeneration [92, 96–100, 119].

Today's evidence suggests that both *macro-* and *microcirculation* evaluation should be routinely considered in each ischemic ulcer presentation toward deeper CLI understanding, as a whole limb circulatory pattern [39, 105].

http://dx.doi.org/10.5772/64834

7.1. Compensatory *collateral systems* relying the foot angiosomes and derived wound healing implications

An impressive compensatory collateral network interconnecting neighboring foot and ankle angiosomes was thoroughly documented by previous publications [23, 24, 101, 102], available as to counterbalance any possible ischemic threat [23, 24, 98].

The central *arterial-arterial* communicants relying upon different leg angiosomes encompass numerous *small* to *large* collaterals (the above-described *levels III and IV*), beyond the arterioles (*level V)* in a sequential model of perfusion [35, 101]. Numerous "large" foot collaterals hold particular importance in supplying adjacent angiosomes [24, 39, 118]. They also seem to play a pivotal role in intentional "wound-directed" revascularization and appropriate tissue regeneration [35, 96–98, 118]. These vessels assemble the *foot arches*, (acknowledging eventual 5–9% anatomical variations, Section 6.3) [108–114], the *metatarsal perforators*, the anterior *communicants*, and other sizable *arterial-arterial* branches such as the dorsal foot-to-plantar, or the peroneal-to-posterior tibial *rescue* heel collaterals (*level III* of perfusion) [35, 101].

In the same design, yet with narrow compensatory significance (Section 6.3), the *medium-* and *small*-sized muscular collateral arteries (*level IV*) [35] and *the arterioles* (*level V*), also contribute in vital tissue flow preservation [103, 105, 106]. These "rescue" connections were also implicated in the "initiatory" phase of revascularization (Section 4.1) [35, 105] and actively partake throughout the vast "choke vessels" salvage system [23, 24], before or during the angio- and arteriogenesis processes [104–106]. Regardless individual variations, the following groups of arterial-arterial collateral connections were appointed in CLI flow compensation [24, 35, 39, 102, 118]:

- The communications between the posterior tibial and peroneal arteries (via the *medial* and *lateral calcaneal branches,* also via the *posterior peroneal branch*) play an important role in *ischemic heel ulcers* supply, equally for targeted hind foot or heel intentional revascularization [24, 72, 96–98].
- The connections between the *anterior* (dorsalis pedis) and the *posterior tibial* (plantar) arteries. These branches ensure either directly via diagonal arteries or following the first *metatarsal perforators* or through the metatarsal *paired anterior* and *posterior inter-digital collaterals,* a significant compensation in *forefoot* and *toes ischemic tissue* flow preservation and eventual tarsal/metatarsal reperfusion [24, 35].
- The arterial compensation around the *peri-malleolar wounds* is reinforced by the *lateral peri-malleolar anastomoses* linking the peroneal artery (via the *anterior perforating branch*) with the anterior tibial trunk (via the *antero-lateral malleolar branch*). Following similar, but more medial connections, *the medial peri-malleolar network* (sharing similar *medial malleolar branches* from the anterior and posterior tibial arteries) represent complementarily, yet distinct, pathways for blood compensation in the ankle [24, 35].
- The communicants between *both plantar arteries* (medial and lateral, from the posterior tibial artery) and the *lateral and medial tarsal arteries* (via the anterior tibial artery) seem to enable influential compensatory flow to eventual *plantar ischemic wounds* [24, 35, 39].

All these briefly schematized *arterial-arterial* communications constitute but a small part of the whole natural foot compensatory system against ischemic aggression [23, 24, 35]. Although severely compromised in distinct CLI categories of patients (diabetes, ESRD, and inflammatory arteritis) [59–61, 104], all these "rescue branches" [35, 59, 101, 102] or "choke-vessels" [23, 24] provide noticeable flow assistance during miscellaneous ischemic injuries. Their appropriate evaluation affords valuable diagnostic and therapeutic knowledge for better tissue preservation and limb salvage [39, 56–59].

In this exhaustive "regional view" of ischemic tissue perfusion, albeit more precise than blunt angiographic assessment (Section 4.5), it appears that *not all foot areas may express similar ischemic affliction* [59–61, 104]. Even more surprisingly, the ulcer's area could not always stand for the lowest perfusion point in the ischemic limb, since severe neuropathy, inflammatory swelling, sepsis, and local skin trauma may add complementary hindrance to main CLI threat [26, 27, 31, 33].

Future diagnostic tools focusing on *superficial* and *deep* tissue "wound-oriented" arterial flow may eventually complete this unique holistic view of the neuro-ischemic diabetic foot [33, 39, 53, 59].

We know today that diabetic and renal CLI patients express serious tissue regeneration handicap, inflicted by specific infragenicular arterial collateral depletion [29–31]. This significant decay in tissue regeneration also appears proportionate with the *type* and *time* of ischemic suffering [1, 2, 27, 30, 59]. In this perspective, recent researchers advise reasonable adaptation of current revascularization indications upon individual *macro* [3, 41] and *micro-vascular* CLI characteristics [29–31, 39], weighted in patients *with* and *without* available collateral reserve [29, 39, 59].

8. The essential role of multidisciplinary approach in ischemic ulcer healing

Increasing clinical evidence suggests that despite "well-suited" revascularization efforts, at least 25% of DFS ulcers will eventually not heal, and around 28% may end however with some form of amputation [58, 120].

It appears unmistakable that no current *single* therapy can enhance *alone* profitable healing results in a majority of CLI ulcers [1, 27, 58] without concomitant management of all risk factors, including ischemic, metabolic, septic, local pressure, neuropathic, and adequate off-loading appointed treatment [1–3, 120–123]. Wound healing embodies a complex cascade of molecular and clinical events in continuous dynamic interaction [34, 48]. It was stated that because CLI wound etiology is always multidimensional [1, 27, 58], specific therapy in turns requires a parallel multidisciplinary application [1–3, 120, 121].

Every individual risk factor requires accurate identification and management and represents a fundamental task for any multidisciplinary wound center to encourage [124]. Investing

http://dx.doi.org/10.5772/64834

healing as the primary endpoint in care acts as a real benchmark for all collective therapeutic efforts [57, 87, 124].

The recent guidelines document of the Society for Vascular Surgery connecting with the American Podiatric Medical Association and the Society for Vascular Medicine acts as a great reference to current evidence of ischemic wound treatment [120]. This noteworthy analysis addresses best available proofs and guidelines to date on the following main indicators: (1) prevention of diabetic foot ulceration, (2) off-loading, (3) diagnosis of sepsis and foot osteomyelitis, (4) specific wound care, and (5) peripheral arterial disease in DFS [120].

Prevention following evidence-based program includes the patient and the referral General Practitioners (GP) as active members of the multidisciplinary group [120–123]. Knowing that peripheral neuropathy can generate about 45–65% of DFS ulcers, patients with neuropathy hold >3.5-fold complementary risk for iterative neuro-ischemic ulceration [26, 71, 87, 120]. Adequate *laboratory tests* surveillance also represents a critical method as to minimize detrimental obstacles in tissue regeneration [120–123]. It has been recorded that for every additional 1% increase in HbA_1C, there is a 0.028 cm/day healing decay in DFS wounds [120–125]. The major importance of *off-loading* devices in the global healing process is acknowledged [57, 58, 120–122]. Pressure reduction is reputed to allow superior healing effects to any revascularization strategy [2, 57, 58, 120–124]. Early diagnostic and treatment of *foot infection* also have paramount consequences in correct tissue regeneration [2, 57–59, 120–122]. Expeditious *local wound debridement* following timely reevaluation schedule bears huge implications for maintaining tissue viability, parallel to revascularization [57–59]. Since aggressively applied, early debridement can save millimeters of "time-dependent" irreversible damage [2, 57, 58, 61, 87, 120–124].

Appropriate *wound dressing* should help by maintaining a moist wound bed, providing exudate drainage, and urging granulation of tissue defect [53, 57, 120, 126].

The adapted dressing should match each specific CLI pathology, wound features and location, and individual amount of exudates, inflammation, and pain [87, 88, 120, 126].

New *complementary therapies* including negative pressure therapy, living cellular therapy, extracellular matrix products, and hyperbaric oxygen therapy were equally developed in the last years [57, 127]. Their application should follow multidisciplinary team advises [88, 120, 127] in ulcers that fail to demonstrate >50% area reduction per month, using standard therapy [120, 127].

Although revascularization still holds specific postoperative indicators [33, 39], the global efficacy of multidisciplinary approach can be timely rated by percentage reduction in wound extent as an early predictor of clinical success [120, 126]. Wound surface diminution of 10–15% per week, or >50% in 4 weeks strongly suggests increased likelihood of healing and diminished probability for amputation [120, 121, 126].

8.1. Ischemic wound healing as an integrated medicine concept

The contemporary practitioner becomes aware that every ischemic ulcer presentation should be carefully weighted and treated alike *distinct pathological prototype*. It appears reasonable that for every single ulcer puzzling (in various amounts) possible neuropathic, ischemic, hyperglycemic, uremic, venous hypoxic, septic, hypoproteic, or pressure threats, only a multimodal team approach may afford better healing expectations [121–126, 128, 129]. Every chronic ulceration case can be theoretically approached alike a 3-D graphical mold assembling in different proportions of some or the whole of the determinants mentioned above. The vital role of any multidisciplinary team is to decode each clinical presentation into basic pathological influences and treat them upon best available knowledge granted by all participant specialties [121, 123, 126].

9. Conclusions

In treating arterial ulcers it should be remembered that not all foot sectors share same ischemic affectation and that not all patients with comparable *macro*-vascular images bear same collateral reserve and related *micro*-vascular tissue recovery resources.

Contemporary research reveals astonishing multilevel anatomical and physiological intricacy of lower limb blood supply, viewed in a dynamic and time unfolding perspective. This apparent complexity represents but plausible challenges for the experienced interventionist availing high-performance macro and microcirculatory diagnostic and treatment methods for revascularization and tissue healing.

Author details

Vlad-Adrian Alexandrescu[1,2*] and François Triffaux[1]

*Address all correspondence to: v.alex@skynet.be

1 Department of General, Thoracic and Vascular Surgery, Princess Paola Hospital, IFAC/ Vivalia, Marche-en-Famenne, Belgium

2 Department of Cardio-Vascular and Thoracic Surgery, CHU Sart-Tilmant, University of Liège, Liège, Belgium

References

[1] Gulati A, Botnaru I, Garcia LA. Critical limb ischemia and its treatments: a review. *J Cardiovasc Surg (Torino)*. 2015; 56(5): 775–785.

[2] Hinchliffe RJ, Andros G, Apelqvist J, Bakker SF, Friederichs S, et al. A systematic review of the effectiveness of revascularization of the ulcerated foot in patients with diabetes and peripheral disease. *Diabetes Metab Res Rev.* 2012; 28(Suppl. 1): 179–217.

[3] Norgreen L, Hiatt WR, Dormandy JA, Nehler MR, Harris KA, et al. Inter-society consensus for the management of peripheral arterial disease (TASC II). *Eur J Vasc Endovasc Surg.* 2007; 33(Suppl 1): S1–S75.

[4] The Asu (Mesopotamia). In: Majno G: *The Healing Hand. Man and Wound in the Ancient World*, 2nd ed. 1975. Cambridge, MA: Harvard University Press: 30–67.

[5] The Swnw (Egypt). In: Majno G: *The Healing Hand. Man and Wound in the Ancient World*, 2nd ed. 1975. Cambridge, MA: Harvard University Press: 66–138.

[6] Cohen IK. The evolution of wound healing. In: Veves A: *The Diabetic Foot*, 2nd ed. 2006. New Jersey: Humana Press Inc.: 51–57.

[7] Buck AH. The development of surgery in France: Ambroise Parré. In: Buck AH: *The Growth of Medicine: From the Earliest Times to about 1800*. New Haven: Yale University Press; 1917: 499–515.

[8] Lister J. An address on the antiseptic management of wounds. *Br Med J.* 1893; 1(1): 161–162, 277–278.

[9] Wells TS. Some causes of excessive mortality after surgical operation. *Medical Times and Gazette.* 1864; 349–364.

[10] Virchow R. *Cellular Pathology.* 1860. London: John Churchill Ed.: 283–315.

[11] Cohen S. Isolation of a mouse submaxillary gland protein accelerating incisor eruption and eyelid opening in the new-born animal. *J Biol Chem.* 1962; 237: 1555–1562.

[12] Brooks B. Intraarterial injection of sodium iodine. *J Am Med Assoc.* 1024; 84: 1016.

[13] Dos Santos R, Lamas AC, Pereira-Caldas J. Arteriography of abdominal aorta, its branches and inferior limb arteries. *Bull Soc Nat Chir.* 1929; 55: 587.

[14] Strandness DE Jr, McCutcheon EP, Rushmer RF. Application of a transcutaneous Doppler flowmeter in evaluation of occlusive arterial disease. *Surg Gynecol Obstet.* 1966; 122: 1039.

[15] Jens S, Koelemay MJ, Reekers J, Bipat S. Diagnostic performance of computed tomography angiography and contrast-enhanced magnetic resonance angiography in patients with critical limb ischaemia and intermittent claudication: systematic review and meta-analysis. *Eur Radiol.* 2013; 3(11): 3104–3114.

[16] White JC, Smethwick RH. *The autonomic nervous system.* 1944. London: Macmillan Ed.

[17] Dos Santos JC. From embolectomy to endarterectomy or the fall of a myth. *J Cardiovasc Surg.* 1976; 17: 409–411.

[18] Kunlin J. Treatment of arteriopathic ischemia using long venous grafts. *Rev Chir (Paris)*. 1951; 70: 206–235.

[19] Crawford ES, De Bakey ME, Cooley DA, et al. Use of crimped knitted Dacron grafts in patients with occlusive disease of the aorta and of the iliac, femoral and popliteal arteries. In: Wesolowska SA, Denis C. *Fundamentals of Vascular Grafting*. 1963. New York: McGraw Hill: 864–872.

[20] Soyer T, Lempinen M, Cooper P, et al. A new venous prosthesis. *Surgery*. 1972; 72: 864–872.

[21] El-Sayed HF. Endovascular techniques in limb salvage: stents. *Methodist Debakey Cardiovasc J*. 2013; 9(2): 79–83.

[22] Volodos NL. The 30th anniversary of the first clinical application of endovascular stent-grafting. *Eur J Vasc Endovasc Surg*. 2015; 49(5): 495–497.

[23] Taylor GI, Palmer JH. The vascular territories (angiosomes) of the body: experimental studies and clinical applications. *Br J Plast Surg*. 1987; 40: 113–141.

[24] Attinger CE, Evans KK, Bulan E, et al. Angiosomes of the foot and ankle and clinical implications for limb salvage: reconstruction, incisions and revascularization. *Plast Reconstr Surg*. 2006; 117(7 Suppl): 261S–293S.

[25] Alexandrescu V, Hubermont G, Philips Y, et al. Selective angioplasty following an angiosome model of reperfusion in the treatment of Wagner 1-4 diabetic foot lesions: practice in a multidisciplinary diabetic limb service. *J Endovasc Ther*. 2008; 15: 580–593.

[26] Iida O, Nanto S, Uematsu M, et al. Importance of the angiosome concept for endovascular therapy in patients with critical limb ischemia. *Catheter Cardiovasc Interv*. 2010; 75: 830–836.

[27] Elsayed S, Clavijo LC. Critical limb ischemia. *Cardiol Clin*. 2015; 33(1): 37–47.

[28] Conte MS, Pomposelli FB, Clair DG, et al. Society for Vascular Surgery practice guidelines for atherosclerotic occlusive disease of the lower extremities: management of asymptomatic disease and claudication. *J Vasc Surg*. 2015; 61(Suppl): 3S–40S.

[29] Chin JA, Sumpio BE. New advances in limb salvage. *Surg Technol Int*. 2014; 25: 212–216.

[30] Alexandrescu V, Letawe A. Critical limb ischemia strategies in diabetics: present deeds and future challenges. *Curr Res Diabetes Obes J*. 2015; 1(1): 553–555.

[31] Marso SP, Hiatt WR. Peripheral arterial disease in patients with diabetes. *J Am Coll Cardiol*. 2006; 47(5): 921–929.

[32] Howell MA, Colgan MP, Seeger RW, et al. Relationship of severity of lower limb peripheral vascular disease to mortality and morbidity: a six-year follow-up study. *J Vasc Surg*. 1989; 9: 691–696.

[33] Doughty DB. Arterial ulcers. In: Bryant RA. *Acute and chronic wounds, current management concepts*. 2012. St. Louis: Elsevier Mosby: 178–194.

[34] Shai A, Maibach H. Natural course of wound repair versus impaired healing in chronic skin ulcers. In: *Wound Healing and Ulcers of the Skin, Diagnosis and Therapy*. 2005. San Francisco: Springer: 7–17.

[35] Alexandrescu VA. The angiosome concept: anatomical background and physiopathological landmarks in CLI. In: *Angiosomes Applications in Critical Limb Ischemia: In Search for Relevance*. 2012. Torino: Ed. Minerva Medica: 1–30, 71–88.

[36] Shai A, Maibach H. Etiology and mechanisms of cutaneous ulcer formation. In: *Wound Healing and Ulcers of the Skin, Diagnosis and Therapy*. 2005. San Francisco: Springer: 30–52.

[37] Hafner J. Management of arterial leg ulcers and combined (mixed) venous-arterial leg ulcers. *Curr Probl Dermatol*. 1999; 27: 211–219.

[38] Hirsch A, et al. ACC/AHA 2005 practice guidelines for management of patients with peripheral arterial disease (lower extremity, renal, mesenteric, and abdominal aortic): a collaborative report from the American Association for Vascular Surgery/raphy and Interventions, Society for Vascular Medicine and Biology, Society for Interventional Radiology, and the ACC/AHA Task Force on Practice Guidelines. *Circulation*. 2006; 113(11): 1474–1547.

[39] Alexandrescu VA, London V. Angiosomes: the cutaneous and arterial evaluation in CLI patients. Chapter 5. In: Mustapha JA: *Critical Limb Ischemia: CLI Diagnosis and Interventions*. 2015. Chicago: Ed. HMP: 71–88.

[40] Doughty DB, Sparks-DeFriese B. Wound-healing physiology. In: Bryant RA: *Acute and Chronic Wounds, Current Management Concepts*. 2012. St. Louis: Elsevier Mosby: 63–82.

[41] Khalil MA, Kim HK, Hoi JW, et al. Detection of peripheral arterial disease within the foot using vascular optical tomographic imaging: a clinical pilot study. *Eur J Vasc Endovasc Surg*. 2015; 49: 83–89.

[42] Igari K, Kudo T, Toyofuku T, et al. Quantitative evaluation of the outcomes of revascularization procedures for peripheral arterial disease using indocyanine green angiography. *Eur J Vasc Endovasc Surg*. 2013; 46(4): 460–465.

[43] Yamamoto M, Orihashi K, Nishimori H, et al. Indocyanine green angiography for intra-operative assessment in vascular surgery. *Eur J Vasc Endovasc Surg*. 2012; 43: 426–432.

[44] Higashimori A, Yokoi Y. Use of Indigo Carmine angiography to qualitatively assess adequate distal perfusion after endovascular revascularization in critical limb ischemia. *J Endovasc Ther*. 2015; 22(3): 352–355.

[45] Montero-Baker MF, Au-Yeung KY, Wisniewski NA, et al. The first-in-man "Si Se Puede" study for the use of micro-oxygen sensors (MOXYs) to determine dynamic relative oxygen indices in the feet of patients with limb-threatening ischemia during endovascular therapy. *J Vasc Surg*. 2015; 61: 1501–1510.

[46] Bell PRF, Charlesworth D, DePalma RG, et al. The definition of critical ischemia of a limb. Working Party of the International Vascular Symposium. *Br J Surg*. 1982; 69(Suppl): S2.

[47] Mills JL Sr, Conte MS, Armstrong DG, et al. The society for vascular surgery lower extremity threatened classification system: risk stratification based on Wound, Ischemia, and foot Infection (WIfI). *J Vasc Surg*. 2014; 59: 220–234.

[48] Abu Dabrh AM, Steffen MW, Undavalli C, et al. The natural history of untreated severe or critical limb ischemia. *J Vasc Surg*. 2015; 62: 1642–1651.

[49] Vallabhaneni R, Kalbaugh CA, Kouri A, et al. Current accepted hemodynamic criteria for critical limb ischemia do not accurately stratify patients at high risk for limb loss. *J Vasc Surg*. 2016; 63: 105–113.

[50] Bollinger A, Breddin K, Hess H, et al. Semiquantitative assessment of lower limb atherosclerosis from routine angiographic images. *Atherosclerosis*. 1981; 38: 339–46.

[51] Dormandy JA, Rutherford RB. Management of peripheral arterial disease (PAD). TASC Working Group: TransAtlantic Inter-Society Consensus (TASC). *J Vasc Surg*. 2000; 31(Suppl): S1–S296.

[52] Rutherford RB, Baker JD, Ernst C, et al. Recommended standards for reports dealing with lower extremity ischemia: revised version. *J Vasc Surg*. 1997; 26: 517–38.

[53] Setacci C, Ricco JB, Apelqvist J, et al. Management of critical limb ischemia and diabetic foot. *Eur J Vasc Endovasc Surg*. 2011; 42(S2): S1–S90.

[54] Graziani L, Silvestro A, Bertone V, et al. Vascular involvement in diabetic subjects with ischemic foot ulcer: a new morphologic categorization of disease severity. *Eur J Vas Endovasc Surg*. 2007; 33: 453–460.

[55] Toursarkissian B, D'Ayala M, Stefanidis D, et al. Angiographic scoring of vascular occlusive disease in the diabetic foot: relevance to bypass graft patency and limb salvage. *J Vasc Surg*. 2002; 35(3): 494–500.

[56] Mustapha JA, Heaney CM. A new approach to diagnosing and treating CLI. *Endovasc Today*. 2010; 9: 41–50.

[57] Lepantalo M, Apelqvist J, Setacci C, et al. Chapter V: diabetic foot. *Eur J Vasc Endovasc Surg*. 2011; 42(52): S60–S74.

[58] Ndip A, Jude EB. Emerging evidence for neuroischemic diabetic foot ulcers: model of care and how to adapt practice. *Int J Low Ext Wounds*. 2009; 8: 82–94.

[59] O'Neal LW. Surgical pathology of the foot and clinicopathologic correlations. In: *Levin and O'Neal's The Diabetic Foot*. 2008. Philadelphia: Mosby Elsevier: 367–401.

[60] Waltenberg J. Impaired collateral vessel development in diabetes: potential cellular mechanisms and therapeutic implications. *Cardiovasc Res*. 2001; 49: 554–560.

[61] Dangwal S, Stratmann B, Bang C, et al. Impairment of wound healing in patients with type 2 diabetes mellitus influences circulating. micro RNA patterns via inflammatory Cytokines. *Arterioscler Thromb Vasc Biol*. 2015; 35(6): 1480–1488.

[62] Alexandrescu VA, Van Espen D. Threatening inferior limb ischemia: when to consider fasciotomy and what principles to apply? *ISRN Vasc Med*. 2014; 21: 1–9.

[63] Defraigne JO. A central pathophysiological mechanism explaining diabetic complications? *Rev Med Liege*. 2005; 60(5–6): 472–478.

[64] Wagner FW Jr. The dysvascular foot: a system for diagnosis and treatment. *Foot Ankle*. 1981; 2: 64–122.

[65] Schaper NC. Diabetic foot ulcer classification system for research purposes: a progress report on criteria for including patients in research studies. *Diabet Metab Res Rev*. 2004; 20: S90–S95.

[66] Armstrong DG, Lavery LA, Harkless LB. Validation of a diabetic wound classification system. The contribution of depth, infection, and ischemia to risk of amputation. *Diabetes Care*. 1998; 21: 855–859.

[67] Macfarlane RM, Jeffcoate WJ. Classification of diabetic foot ulcers: the S(AD) SAD system. *Diabetic Foot*. 1999; 2: 123–31.

[68] Beckert S, Witte M, Wicke C, et al. A new wound-based severity score for diabetic foot ulcers: a prospective analysis of 1000 patients. *Diabetes Care*. 2006; 29: 988–992.

[69] Beckert S, Pietsch AM, Küper M, et al. M.A.I.D.: a prognostic score estimating probability of healing in chronic lower extremity wounds. *Ann Surg*. 2009; 249: 677–681.

[70] Martinez-de Jesús FR. A checklist to score healing progress of diabetic foot ulcers. *Int J Low Extrem Wounds*. 2010; 9: 74–83.

[71] Alexandrescu VA, Hubermont G. Does peripheral neuropathy have a clinical impact on the endovascular approach as a primary treatment for limb-threatening ischemic foot wounds in diabetic patients? *J Diab Metab*. 2012; S5: 006.

[72] Azuma N, Uchida H, Kokubo T, et al. Factors influencing wound healing of critical ischaemic foot after bypass surgery: is the angiosome important in selecting bypass target artery? *Eur J Vasc Endovasc Surg*. 2012; 43(3): 322–328.

[73] Jens S, Conijn AP, Koelemay MJ, et al. Randomized trials for endovascular treatment of infrainguinal arterial disease: systematic review and meta-analysis (Part 2: Below the knee). *Eur J Vasc Endovasc Surg*. 2014; 47(5): 536–544.

[74] Park SW, Kim JS, Yun IJ, et al. Clinical outcomes of endovascular treatments for critical limb ischemia with chronic total occlusive lesions limited to below-the-knee arteries. *Acta Radiol.* 2013; 54(7): 785–789.

[75] Pernès JM, Auguste M, Borie H, et al. Infrapopliteal arterial recanalization: a true advance for limb salvage in diabetics. *Diagn Interv Imaging.* 2015; 96(5): 423–434.

[76] Brochado-Neto FC, Cury MV, Bonadiman SS, et al. Vein bypass to branches of pedal arteries. *J Vasc Surg.* 2012; 55(3): 746–752.

[77] Good DW, Al Chalabi H, Hameed F, et al. Popliteo-pedal bypass surgery for critical limb ischemia. *Ir J Med Sci.* 2011; 180(4): 829–835.

[78] Hughes K, Domenig CM, Hamdan AD, et al. Bypass to plantar and tarsal arteries: an acceptable approach to limb salvage. *J Vasc Surg.* 2004; 40(6): 1149–1157.

[79] Abu Dabrh AM, Steffen MW, Asi N, et al. Bypass surgery versus endovascular interventions in severe or critical limb ischemia. *J Vasc Surg.* 2016 Jan; 63(1):244-53.e11. doi: 10.1016/j.jvs.2015.07.068. Epub 2015 Sep 11. Review.

[80] Jaff MR, White CJ, Hiatt WR, et al. An update on methods for revascularization and expansion of the TASC lesion classification to include below-the-knee arteries: a supplement to the Inter-Society Consensus for the management of peripheral arterial disease (TASC II). *J Endovasc Surg.* 2015; 22(5): 663–677.

[81] Taneja M, Tay KH, Dewan A, et al. Bare nitinol stent enabled recanalization of long-segment, chronic total occlusion of superficial femoral and adjacent proximal popliteal artery in diabetic patients presenting with critical limb ischemia. *Cardiovasc Revasc Med.* 2010; 11(4): 232–235.

[82] Spiliopoulos S, Theodosiadou V, Katsanos K, et al. Long-term clinical outcomes of infrapopliteal drug-eluting stent placement for critical limb ischemia in diabetic patients. *J Vasc Interv Radiol.* 2015; 26(10): 1423–1430.

[83] Laird JR, Schneider PA, Tepe G, et al. Durability of treatment effect using a drug-coated balloon for femoropopliteal lesions: 24-month results of IN.PACT SFA. *J Am Coll Cardiol.* 2015; 66(21): 2329–2338.

[84] Cioppa A, Stabile E, Popusoi G, et al. Combined treatment of heavy calcified femoro-popliteal lesions using directional atherectomy and a paclitaxel coated balloon: one-year single centre clinical results. Cardiovasc Revasc Med. 2012; 13(4): 219–223.

[85] Zeller T, Rastan A, Macharzina R, et al. Novel approaches to the management of advanced peripheral artery disease: perspectives on drug-coated balloons, drug-eluting stents, and bioresorbable scaffolds. *Curr Cardiol Rep.* 2015; 17(9): 624–627.

[86] Baerlocher MO, Kennedy SA, Rajebi MR, et al. Meta-analysis of drug-eluting balloon angioplasty and drug-eluting stent placement for infrainguinal peripheral arterial disease. *J Vasc Interv Radiol.* 2015; 26(4): 459–473.

[87] Rorive M, Scheen AJ, Diagnostic approach of the pathophysiological triad leading to a diabetic foot. *Rev Med Liege*. 2015; 70(9): 465–471.

[88] Alexandrescu VA, Hubermont G, Coessens V, et al. Why a multidisciplinary team may represent a key factor for lowering the inferior limb loss rate in diabetic neuro-ischaemic wounds: application in a departmental institution. *Acta Chir Belg*. 2009; 109: 79–86.

[89] Dosluoglu HH, Lall P, Cherr GS, Harris LM, Dryjski ML. Role of simple and complex hybrid revascularization procedures for symptomatic lower extremity occlusive disease. *J Vasc Surg*. 2010; 51(6): 1425–1435.

[90] Bazan HA, Le L, Donovan M, et al. Retrograde pedal access for patients with critical limb ischemia. *J Vasc Surg*. 2014; 60(2): 375–381.

[91] Alexandrescu V, Vincent G, Azdad K, et al. A reliable approach to diabetic neuroischemic foot wounds: below-the-knee angiosome-oriented angioplasty. *J Endovasc Ther*. 2011; 18: 376–387.

[92] Biancari F, Juvonen T. Angiosome-targeted lower limb revascularization for ischemic foot wounds: systematic review and meta-analysis. *Eur J Vasc Endovasc Surg*. 2014; 47(5): 517–522.

[93] Neville RF, Attinger CE, Bulan EJ, et al. Revascularization of a specific angiosome for limb salvage: does the target artery matter? *Ann Vasc Surg*. 2009; 23(3): 367–73.

[94] Houlind K, Christensen JK, Jepsen JM. Vein arterialization for lower limb revascularization. *J Cardiovasc Surg (Torino)*. 2016; 57(2): 266–272.

[95] Alexandrescu VA. Is limb loss always inevitable for critical neuro- ischemic foot wounds in diabetic patients with end stage rénal disease and unfit for vascular reconstructions? In: Sahay M, ed.: *Diseases of Renal Parenchyma*. 2012. Rijeka, Croatia: InTech Open Science: 228–246.

[96] Spillerova K, Biancari F, Leppäniemi A, et al. Differential impact of bypass surgery and angioplasty on angiosome-targeted infrapopliteal revascularization. *Eur J Vasc Endovasc Surg*. 2014; 49(4): 412–419.

[97] Alexandrescu VA. Myths and proofs of angiosome applications in CLI: where do we stand? *J Endovasc Ther*. 2014; 21: 616–624.

[98] Iida O, Takahara M, Soga Y, et al. Impact of angiosome-oriented revascularization on clinical outcomes in critical limb ischemia patients without concurrent wound infection and diabetes. *J Endovasc Ther*. 2014; 21(5): 607–615.

[99] Huang TY, Huang TS, Wang YC, et al. Direct revascularization with the angiosome concept for lower limb ischemia: a systematic review and meta-analysis. *Medicine (Baltimore)*. 2015; 94(34): 1427.

[100] Spillerova K, Sörderström M, Albäck A, et al. The feasibility of angiosome-targeted endovascular treatment in patients with critical limb ischaemia and foot ulcer. *Ann Vasc Surg*. 2015; 30: 270–276.

[101] Bouchet A, Cuilleret J. Topographic anatomy of the inferior limb. In: *Topographic Anatomy of the Human Body*. 3rd Ed. 1995. Masson, Paris: Simep Publ.: 26–97.

[102] Williams PL, Warwick R, Dyson M, et al. Angiology, blood vessels. In: *Gray's Anatomy*. 1996. Churchill Livingstone, New York: 682–694.

[103] Macchi C, Catini C, Giannelli F, et al. Collateral circulation in distal occlusion of lower limb arteries: an anatomical study and statistical research in 40 elderly subjects by echo-color-Doppler method. *Ital J Anat Embryol*. 1996; 101(4): 221–227.

[104] Lehoux S, Lévi BI. Collateral artery growth: making the most of what you have. *Circ Res*. 2006; 99: 567–569.

[105] Schaper W. Collateral circulation, past and present. *Basic Res Cardiol*. 2009; 104(1): 5–21.

[106] Ziegler MA, Distasi MR, Bills RG, et al. Marvels, mysteries and misconceptions of vascular compensation to peripheral artery occlusion. *Microcirculation*. 2010; 17(1): 3–20.

[107] Kropman RH, Kiela G, Moll FL, et al. Variations in the anatomy of the popliteal artery and its side branches. *Vasc Endovasc Surg*. 2011; 45(6): 536–540.

[108] Abou-Foul AK, Borumandi F. Anatomical variations of lower limb vasculature and implications for free fibula flap: systematic review and critical analysis. *Microsurgery*. 2016; 36(2): 165–172.

[109] Ovcharenko DV, Kaputin MI, Voronkov AA, et al. Angiographic assessment of the incidence rate of atypical variants of the development of crural and plantar arteries. *Angiol Sosud Khir*. 2012; 18(1): 57–60.

[110] Kim D, Orron DE, Slillman JJ. Surgical significance of popliteal arterial variants. A unified angiographic classification. *Ann Surg*. 1989; 210(6): 776–781.

[111] Yamada T, Gloviczki P, Bower TC, et al. Variations of the arterial anatomy of the foot. *Am J Surg*. 1993; 166(2): 130–135.

[112] Lee JH, Dauber W. Anatomic study of the dorsalis pedis-first dorsal metatarsal artery. Ann Plast Surg. 1997; 38(1): 50–55.

[113] Singh BN, Burmeister W, Machado K, et al. Variations of the origin of the arcuate artery. *J Am Podiatr Med Assoc*. 2013; 103(3): 181–184.

[114] Gabrielli C, Olave E, Mandiola E, et al. The deep plantar arch in humans: constitution and topography. *Surg Radiol Anat*. 2001; 23(4): 253–258.

[115] Karacagil S, Almgren B, Lorelius LE, et al. Angiographic runoff patterns in patients undergoing lower limb revascularization. *Acta Chir Scand*. 1989; 155(1): 19–24.

http://dx.doi.org/10.5772/64834

[116] Ciavarella A, Silletti A, Mustacchio A, et al. Angiographic evaluation of the anatomic pattern of arterial obstructions in diabetic patients with critical limb ischemia. *Diabetes Metab*. 1993; 19(6): 586–589.

[117] Santos VP, Alves CA, Fidelis C, et al. Arteriographic findings in diabetic and non-diabetic with critical limb ischemia. *Rev Assoc Med Bras*. 2013; 59(6): 557–562.

[118] Acin F, Varela C, de Maturana IL, et al. Results of infrapopliteal endovascular procedures performed in diabetic patients with critical limb ischemia and tissue loss from the perspective of an angiosome-oriented revascularization strategy. *Intern J Vasc Med*. 2014; 10: 2–15.

[119] Jörneskog G. Why critical limb ischemia criteria are not applicable to diabetic foot and what the consequences are. *J Scan Surg*. 2012; 101(2): 114–118.

[120] Hingorani A, LaMuraglia GM, Henke P, et al. The management of the diabetic foot: a clinical practice guideline by the Society for Vascular Surgery in collaboration with the American Podiatric Medical Association and the Society for Vascular Medicine. *J Vasc Surg*. 2016; 63: 3S–21S.

[121] Apelqvist J, Bakker K, van Houtum WH, et al. Practical guidelines on the management and prevention of the diabetic foot: based upon the International Consensus on the Diabetic Foot (2007) Prepared by the International Working Group on the Diabetic Foot. *Diabetes Metab Res Rev*. 2008; 24(Suppl. 1): S181–S187.

[122] Van Acker K. Importance of multidisciplinary surveillance after topographic arterial treatment for limb salvage. In: *Angiosomes Applications in Critical Limb Ischemia: In Search for Relevance*. 2012. Torino: Minerva Medica: 87–95.

[123] Van Acker K. Importance of multidisciplinary surveillance after topographic arterial treatment for limb salvage. In: *Angiosomes Applications in Critical Limb Ischemia: In Search for Relevance*. Editor : Alexandrescu VA, 2012. Torino: Minerva Medica: 87–95.

[124] Aydin K, Isildak M, Karakaya J, et al. Change in amputation predictors in diabetic foot disease: effect of multidisciplinary approach. *Endocrine*. 2010; 38: 87–92.

[125] Christman AL, Selvin E, Margolis DJ, et al. Hemoglobin A1c predicts healing rate in diabetic wounds. *J Invest Dermatol*. 2011; 131: 2121–2127.

[126] Yazdanpanah L, Nasiri M, Adarvishi S. Literature review on the management of diabetic foot ulcer. *World J Diab*. 2015; 6(1): 37–53.

[127] Elraiyah T, Apostolos T, Prutsky G, et al. A systematic review and meta-analysis of adjunctive therapies in diabetic foot ulcers. *J Vasc Surg*. 2016; 63: 46S–58S.

[128] Elraiyah T, Domecq JP, Prutsky G, et al. A systematic review and meta-analysis of debridement methods for chronic diabetic foot ulcers. *J Vasc Surg*. 2016; 63: 37S–45S.

[129] Lew EJ, Mills JL Sr, Armsrong DG. The deterioration of DFU: prioritising the risk factors to avoid amputation. *J Wound Care*. 2015; 24(5 Suppl. 2): 31–37.

Chapter 12

Venous Leg Ulceration

Aslı Aksu Çerman, İlknur Kıvanç Altunay and
Ezgi Aktaş Karabay

Additional information is available at the end of the chapter

http://dx.doi.org/10.5772/63962

Abstract

Venous leg ulcers are among the most common leg ulcerations. Advancing age, sex, race, phlebitis, family history, obesity, prolonged standing, and number of pregnancies are risk factors. Although the main pathogenetic mechanism is venous hypertension, leading to vein wall damage and thereby a cascade of events resulting in ulceration, there is no consensus about progression from venous hypertension to ulceration.

Diagnosis is based on a thorough patient history and physical examination. A typical venous ulcer is shallow and has irregular, well-defined borders with surrounding skin alterations. However, variable vascular and laboratory tests and skin biopsy may occasionally be necessary in differential diagnosis.

Although pain reduction, closure of the ulcers, and prevention of the recurrences are the main goals of the treatment, targeted therapy should be the reversal of deep venous insufficiency. Leg elevation and long-term compression therapy are essential in this context. Additionally, appropriate wound care including infection control, debridement, dressings, and antibiotics should be performed and, if needed, adjuvant therapies should be planned according to the patient.

Keywords: venous leg ulcers, lower extremity ulcers, venous insufficiency, diagnostic testing, management

1. Introduction

Venous ulcers are the most common form of leg ulcers and important medical problem, which causes significant morbidity and economic burden. Clinical findings and history are helpful in making the diagnosis, but additional diagnostic testing is helpful in confirming the diagnosis and excluding other causes of leg ulcerations. The main purpose of venous ulcer management includes healing of the ulcer and prevention of recurrence. This chapter highlights the epidemiology, pathophysiology, clinical presentation, diagnostic testing, differential diagnosis, and treatment of venous ulcers.

2. Epidemiology

Venous leg ulcers (VLUs) are the most common lower extremity ulceration and responsible for 70% of all leg ulcers, with overall prevalence ranging from 0.06 to 2% [1–4]. It occurs frequently between the ages of 60 and 80 years; however, most people have their first ulcer before the age of 60 years [5, 6]. VLUs have slight female predominance, with a female-to-male ratio ranging from 1.5:1 to 10:1 [7, 8].

Venous ulcers have a significant socioeconomic impact with reduced work productivity and quality of life. Long-term treatments are needed and recurrence is widely common, ranging from 54 to 78% of treated subjects [9]. The overall cost of VLU treatments was 1–2% of the healthcare budgets of European countries [10]. In the United States, approximately 2.5 billion dollars was expended for the treatment of VLUs per year [11].

Advancing age, sex, race, phlebitis, family history, obesity, occupation involving prolonged standing, and number of pregnancies are risk factors that have been described with chronic venous insufficiency and, subsequently, with venous ulcers [12, 13].

3. Pathogenesis

3.1. Normal venous anatomy and physiology

The venous system of the lower extremities includes the superficial veins, perforator veins, and the deep veins according to their relationship to the muscular fascia. The superficial veins comprises the reticular veins, the large (larger) and small (smaller) saphenous veins, and their tributaries. The great saphenous vein originates from where the dorsal vein of the first digit merges with the dorsal venous arch of the foot. After passing in front of the medial malleolus, it ascends the medial side of the leg. It joins the femoral vein just below the inguinal ligament. The small saphenous vein arises from the dorsal venous arch of the foot and ascends posterolaterally from behind the lateral malleolus. Usually, it drains into the popliteal vein near the popliteal fossa. The reticular veins, a network of veins parallel to the skin surface, communicate with either saphenous tributaries or the deep veins through perforators. The perforator veins connect the superficial and deep vein systems. The deep venous system is categorized as either intramuscular or intermuscular. Intermuscular veins are three paired tibial veins including, the posterior tibial vein, the anterior tibial vein, and the peroneal vein. These veins join to form the popliteal vein in the popliteal area. At the level of the adductor canal, the popliteal vein is renamed the superficial femoral vein. This vessel joins the deep femoral vein in the femoral

http://dx.doi.org/10.5772/63962

triangle to form the common femoral vein. After passing beneath the inguinal ligament to enter the pelvis, the femoral vein is renamed the common iliac vein. The superficial veins are low-pressure systems, whereas the deep veins are high-pressure systems. All three venous systems have one-way bicuspid valves, which only open toward the deep venous system and, under normal conditions, prevent reflux of blood. Normally, ambulation and the pumping action of the calf muscles propel venous blood upward toward the heart, and the valves close when pressure rises in the deep venous system, which prevents retrograde flow [4, 14, 15].

3.2. Pathophysiology

In patients with venous disease or failure, venous pressure in deep system falls less than normal during ambulation and rises in orthostatic position, and this is termed venous hypertension. In conclusion, venous hypertension in the deep veins may be transmitted to the superficial veins [4, 16]. There is no general consensus about the transition from venous hypertension to venous ulceration. Several hypotheses have been proposed.

(a) Precapillary fibrin cuffs and fibrinolytic abnormalities hypotheses:

According to this theory of Browse and Burnand [17], venous hypertension leads to distention of capillary walls and leakage of macromolecules such as fibrinogen into the dermis and subcutaneous tissues of the calf. The leaked fibrinogen polymerizes to form precapillary fibrin cuffs in the extravascular space. These precapillary cuffs were assumed to act as a physical barrier, which impede the diffusion of oxygen and nutrients, resulting in ischemia, cell death, and ulceration [17–19]. In addition, local and systemic fibrinolytic/coagulation abnormalities such as prolonged euglobulin lysis time, elevated plasma fibrinogen levels, increased levels of protein C, fibrin-related antigens, D-dimer, D-monomer, fibrin monomer, and reduction in factor XIII activity may present in patients with venous disease [20–22]. However, it is unclear whether these abnormalities are primary or secondary to venous disease.

(b) Leukocyte trapping hypothesis:

As a result of venous hypertension, there is a decreased pressure in capillary bed perfusion and capillary flux. This gives rise to erythrocyte aggregation and leukocyte plugging in the capillaries, leading to local ischemia. Moreover, these leukocytes release cytokines, tumor necrosis factor α (TNF-α), proteolytic enzymes, and free radicals which can cause increased vascular permeability resulting in the leakage of fibrinogen into the pericapillary tissues and the decreased fibrinolytic activity [23–25].

(c) The growth factor trap hypothesis:

Falanga and Eaglstein [26] recommended that macromolecules such as fibrinogen and $\alpha_2$macroglobulin, which leak into the dermis as a result of venous hypertension, bind to or trap growth factors, which then become unavailable for the maintenance of tissue integrity and repair process. The precapillary fibrin cuff of the venous ulcer contains growth factors such as transforming growth factor β (TGF-β). Trapping of growth factors can impair activation of the cells that are needed for healing process [27].

4. Diagnosis

4.1. Clinical presentation

In general, the venous ulcer is an irregularly, well-defined border and typically non-painful [4, 8]. Nevertheless, deep ulcers or small venous ulcers surrounded by atrophie blanche are highly painful [28]. The size and site of ulcers are variable, but they usually located over the medial malleolus (**Figure 1**).

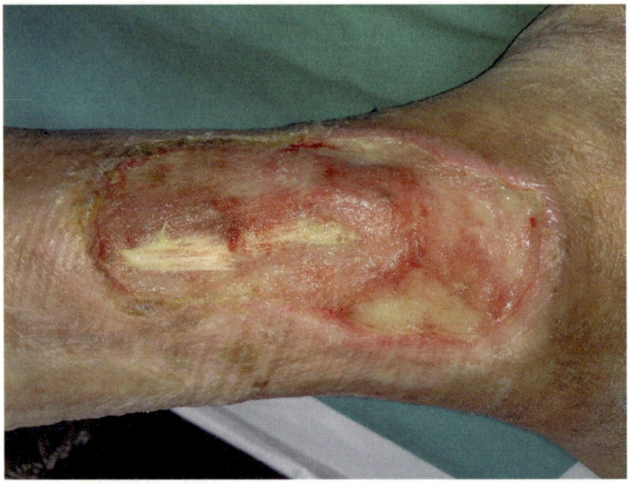

Figure 1. Typical venous ulcer over the medial malleolus.

There may be yellow fibrinous exudates on the ulcer bed. Varicose veins and ankle edema are common. The surrounding skin is erythematous or hyperpigmented with variable degrees of induration. Eczematous changes associated with venous dermatitis are commonly present. Long-standing venous disease can lead to loss of the subcutaneous fat and fibrotic changes in the skin called lipodermatosclerosis, giving the characteristic "inverted champagne-bottle" appearance of the leg [29]. The main complications of chronic venous ulcers are osteomyelitis and neoplastic transformation [4, 30]. Long-term ulcers may require biopsy at regular intervals for malignant change. If osteomyelitis is suspected, radiography, bone scanning, and bone biopsy should be considered.

4.2. Diagnostic testing

The diagnosis of venous ulcers is mainly based on patient history and clinical examination; however, there are diagnostic tests to evaluate venous anatomy and aid the diagnosis.

http://dx.doi.org/10.5772/63962

4.2.1. *Venous duplex ultrasound*

Duplex ultrasound is the first-line diagnostic test to evaluate the insufficiency in venous ulcers [31]. Continuous-wave Doppler provides information about superficial venous incompetence or obstruction; nonetheless, it can be difficult to differentiate deep from superficial venous incompetence [32, 33].

4.2.2. *Venous plethysmography*

Photoplethysmography and air plethysmography measure the degree of venous reflux and the calf muscle pump efficiency [8, 34, 35].

4.2.3. *Venous imaging*

In case of suspected venous obstruction, additional contrast imaging with computed tomography venography or magnetic resonance venography should be done; whereupon diagnosis should be confirmed by contrast venography and intravascular ultrasound [31].

4.2.4. *Laboratory testing*

Patients who have a history of venous thrombosis and thrombophilia should undergo a workup for inherited hypercoagulable factors including protein C and S, factor V Leiden, antiphospholipid antibodies, prothrombin gene mutation, homocysteine, cryoglobulins, and cryoagglutinins [8, 31].

4.2.5. *Arterial testing—Ankle Brachial Pressure Index (ABI)*

Patients with venous leg ulcers may have concomitant peripheral arterial disease component. Therefore, arterial pulse examination, Doppler ultrasound and ABI should be evaluated for the elimination of coexistent arterial disease. ABI is the ratio of the systolic blood pressure at the ankle compared with the systolic blood pressure in the arm. An ABI in the range of 0.9–1.1 is considered normal and 0.5–0.8 indicates moderate peripheral vascular disease and claudication, while less than 0.5 indicates more severe disease [4, 8, 36].

4.2.6. *Wound biopsy*

Most studies suggest wound biopsy for those that do not improve with standard wound and compression therapy after a period of 4–6 weeks of treatment. The biopsy specimen should be obtained from several sites, including the wound edge and central provisional matrix [31].

4.3. Classification

4.3.1. *CEAP*

Classification of venous ulcers, known as CEAP [clinical findings (C), etiology (E), anatomical distribution (A), and pathophysiology (P)] based on clinical findings was introduced in 1994 and revised in 2004 [37, 38] (**Table 1**).

CEAP	Definition
Clinical classification	
C0	No visible or palpable signs of venous disease
C1	Telangiectasies or reticular veins
C2	Varicose veins
C3	Edema
C4a	Pigmentation and/or eczema
C4b	Lipodermatosclerosis and/or atrophie blanche
C5	Healed venous ulcer
C6	Active venous ulcer
CS	Symptoms, including ache, pain, tightness, skin irritation, heaviness, muscle cramps, as well as other complaints attributable to venous dysfunction
CA	Asymptomatic
Etiologic classification	
Ec	Congenital
Ep	Primary
Es	Secondary (post-thrombotic)
En	No venous etiology identified
Anatomic classification	
As	Superficial veins
Ap	Perforator veins
Ad	Deep veins
An	No venous location identified
Pathophysiologic classification (basic)	
Pr	Reflux
Po	Obstruction
Pr,o	Reflux and obstruction
Pn	No venous pathophysiology identifiable

Modified from Eklöf et al. [38].

Table 1. Basic revised clinical, etiologic, anatomic, and pathophysiologic (CEAP) classification system.

The clinical findings are divided into six categories, where C_0indicates no visible or palpable signs of venous disease; C1, the presence of telangiectasies or reticular veins; C2, varicose veins; C3, edema; C4, changes in skin and subcutaneous tissue secondary to venous disease (C4a, pigmentation or eczema; C4b, lipodermatosclerosis or atrophie blanche); C5, skin changes with healed venous ulcer; C6, active venous ulcer. Each clinical class is further supplemented by (A) for asymptomatic and (S) for symptomatic presentation. Symptoms include aching, pain,

http://dx.doi.org/10.5772/63962

skin irritation, tightness, heaviness, muscle cramps, and other complaints. The etiologic classification is separated into three categories; Ec, congenital; Ep, primary; Es, secondary (post-traumatic or post-thrombotic); and En, no venous cause identified. The anatomical classification is divided into four categories: As, superficial veins; Ap, perforator veins; Ad, deep veins; and An, no venous location identified. The pathophysiologic classification is divided into four categories; Pr, reflux; Po, obstruction; Pr,o, combination of reflux and obstruction; and Pn, no venous pathophysiology identifiable.

The venous clinical severity score (VCSS) was developed because of subjective and inadequate definition of the categories in CEAP classification (**Table 2**).

	None: 0	Mild: 1	Moderate: 2	Severe: 3
Pain or other discomfort (i.e., aching, heaviness, fatigue, soreness, burning)		Occasional pain or other discomfort (i.e., not restricting regular daily activities)	Daily pain or other discomfort (i.e., interfering with but not preventing regular daily activities)	Daily pain or discomfort (i.e., limits most regular daily activities)
Presumes venous origin Varicose veins "Varicose" veins must be ≥3 mm in diameter to qualify in the standing position		Few: scattered (i.e., isolated branch varicosities or clusters) Also induces corona phlebectatica (ankle flare)	Confined to calf or thigh	Involves calf and thigh
Venous edema Presumes venous origin		Limited to foot and ankle area	Extends above ankle but below knee	Extends to knee and above
Skin pigmentation Presumes venous origin	None or focal	Limited to perimalleolar area	Diffuse over lower third of calf	Wider distribution above lower third of calf
Does not include focal pigmentation over varicose veins or pigmentation due to other chronic diseases				
Inflammation More than just recent pigmentation (i.e., erythema, cellulitis, venous eczema, dermatitis)		Limited to perimalleolar area	Diffuse over lower third of calf	Wider distribution above lower third of calf
Induration Presumes venous origin of secondary skin and subcutaneous changes (i.e., chronic edema with fibrosis,		Limited to perimalleolar area	Diffuse over lower third of calf	Wider distribution above lower third of calf

	None: 0	Mild: 1	Moderate: 2	Severe: 3
hypodermitis) Includes white atrophy and lipodermatosclerosis				
Active ulcer number	0	1	2	≥3
Active ulcer duration (longest active)	N/A	<3 months	>3 months but <1 year	Not healed for <1 year
Active ulcer size (largest active)	N/A	Diameter >2 cm	Diameter 2–6 cm	Diameter >6 cm
Use of compression therapy	0 Not used	1 Intermittent use of stockings	2 Wears stockings most days	3 Full compliance: stockings

Modified from Vasquez MA, Rabe E, McLafferty RB, Shortell CK, Marston WA, Gillespie D, et al. Revision of the venous clinical severity score: venous outcomes consensus statement: special communication of the American Venous Forum Ad Hoc Outcomes Working Group. J Vasc Surg 2010;52:1387–96.

Table 2. Revised venous clinical severity score (VCSS) system.

A VCSS may range from 0 to 30 [31, 33, 39]. A score of more than eight indicates the progression of venous problem. In addition, the VCSS has been shown to be useful to evaluate the response to treatment.

5. Differential diagnosis

5.1. Arterial ulcers

Arterial leg ulcers result from peripheral arterial occlusive disease. Arterial ulcers typically are round or punched out with a sharply demarcated border and extremely painful. A fibrous yellow base or necrotic eschar is commonly seen (**Figure 2**).

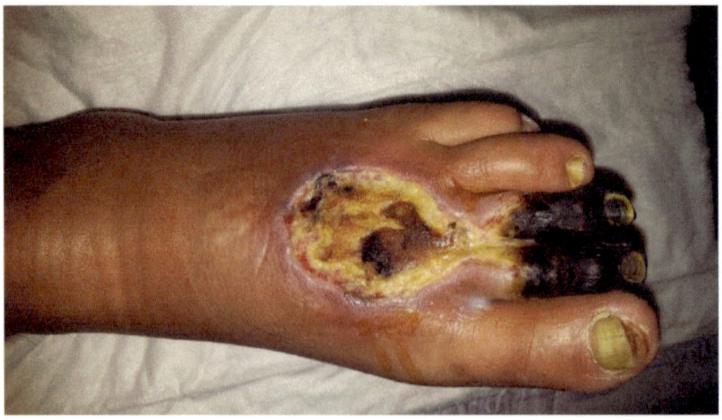

Figure 2. Arterial ulcer.

http://dx.doi.org/10.5772/63962

The surrounding skin is cool to the touch. These ulcers frequently occur at the tips of the toes and over the bony prominences. Associated findings are weak or nonexistent arteria dorsalis pedis pulse, hair loss, atrophic skin, dystrophic nails, the presence of claudication, or rest pain. The ABI of 0.5 or less indicates severe arterial disease [4, 40, 41].

5.2. Neuropathic ulcers

Neuropathic ulcers are more common in patients with diabetes mellitus (DM). Trauma and/or pressures can cause wounding and ulcer formation in patients with neuropathy [41–43]. These ulcers usually tend to be on the plantar surface of the foot. An abnormal, thickened callus develops at pressure areas, with ultimate disrupt of the tissue resulting in ulcer formation (**Figure 3**).

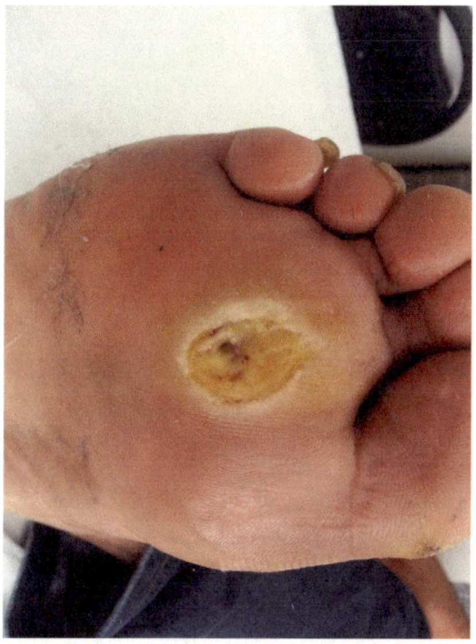

Figure 3. Diabetic neuropathic foot ulcer.

5.3. Pressure ulcers

Pressure ulcers mostly occur in patients with limited mobility. These ulcers can start to develop when soft tissue is compressed for a prolonged period of time. The main risky sites are the heel of the foot, malleoli, and sacral and trochanter areas [4, 44].

5.4. Hypertensive leg ulcer (Ulcus Cruris Hypertonicum Martorell)

Hypertensive leg ulcers are extremely painful and commonly located on the distal portion of the lower leg above the lateral malleolus. These ulcers are seen in patients with prolonged, severe, or poorly controlled hypertension [41, 42]. The ulceration is secondary to tissue ischemia caused by increased vascular resistance.

5.5. Mixed ulcer

Patients with mixed etiology ulcers have combined venous and arterial disease. Often further complicating factors such as DM, rheumatoid arthritis (RA), or lymphedema also exist [42].

5.6. Pyoderma gangrenosum

Pyoderma gangrenosum is a neutrophilic dermatosis. Clinically it starts with sterile pustules that rapidly progress and turn into painful ulcers with purplish-blue, undermined borders [42, 45]. It may be associated with inflammatory bowel disease, rheumatic, or myeloproliferative disorders [8, 12] (**Figure 4**).

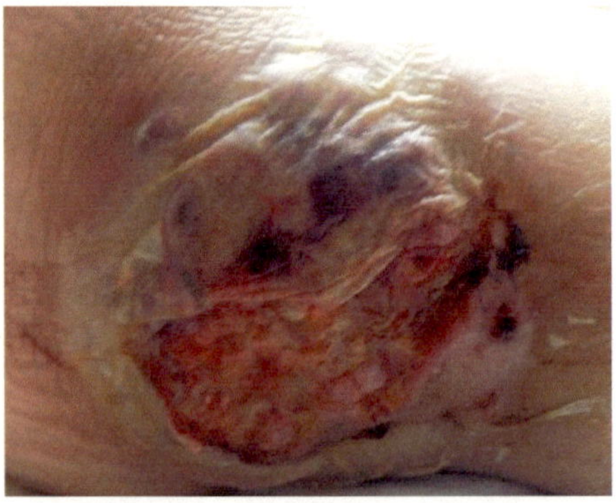

Figure 4. Pyoderma gangrenosum.

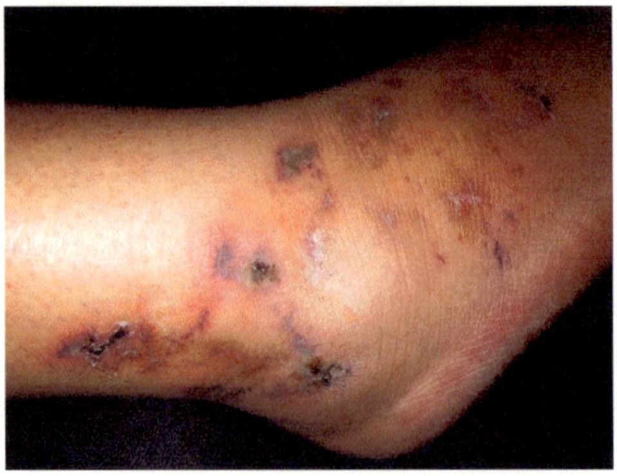

Figure 5. Livedoid vasculopathy and tiny ulcerations.

5.7. Vasculitis

Cutaneous vasculitis may present as palpable purpura, urticaria, nodule, bullae, livedo reticularis, necrotic areas, or skin ulceration. Vasculitic leg ulcers are often painful, multilocular

http://dx.doi.org/10.5772/63962

and, surrounded by livid erythema and purpura (**Figure 5**). The different types of vasculitis that can cause cutaneous ulceration include small vessel vasculitis such as leukocytoclastic vasculitis, medium-sized vessel vasculitis such as polyarteritis nodosa, microscopic polyangiitis, and Wegener granulomatosis [41, 46]. Routine blood work, sedimentation, antineutrophil cytoplasmic antibody (ANCA), urinalysis, chest X-ray, and multiple skin biopsies should be done.

Livedoid vasculopathy (LV) is characterized by irregularly shaped, recurrent perimalleolar painful ulcers overlying areas of purpura. LV typically has three phases including livedo racemosa, ulcerations, and atrophie blanche [41, 42] (**Figure 5**).

5.8. Autoimmune diseases

5.8.1. Rheumatoid ulcers

Approximately 10% of individuals with RA develop leg ulcers [41] (**Figure 6**). The cause of leg ulcerations in RA is multifactorial, including vasculitis, venous insufficiency, paraproteinemias, medications, superficial ulcerating rheumatoid necrobiosis, pyoderma gangrenosum, and Felty's syndrome [45–48](**Figure 6**).

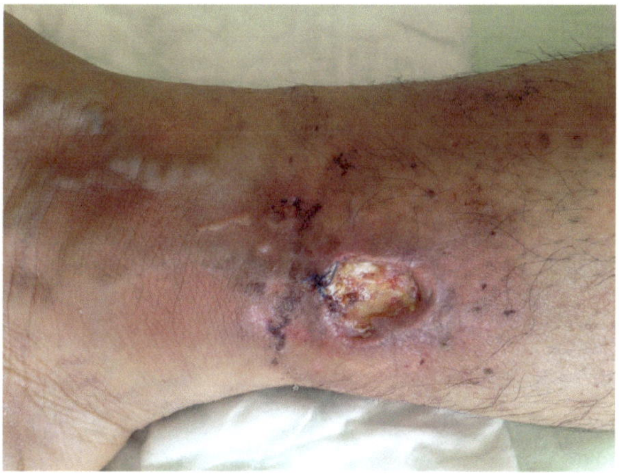

Figure 6. Rheumatoid ulcer.

5.8.2. Scleroderma

The prevalence of lower extremity ulcers in scleroderma is 3.6% and various parts of the leg can be affected [49]. These ulcers are painful and relatively refractory to standard treatment methods. Antiphospholipid antibody, fibrotic skin, vascular compromise, coagulation abnormalities, and tissue calcium deposition may have a role in their pathogenesis [45, 46, 48].

5.8.3. Systemic lupus erythematosus (SLE)

Leg ulcers of SLE are usually painful, sharply marginated, or punched out that located over the malleolar, supramalleolar, or pretibial areas [50]. Vasculitis, antiphospholipid antibody, thrombosis of vessels, venous insufficiency, lupus profundus, and drug-induced lupus syndrome have been associated with leg ulcerations.

5.8.4. Sjögren syndrome

Leg ulcerations of Sjögren syndrome have been associated with cryoglobulinemia, anticardiolipin antibody, and vasculitis [46, 51].

5.8.5. Dermatomyositis

Leg ulcers of dermatomyositis have been reported to involve calcinosis cutis and vasculitis [46].

5.8.6. Mixed connective tissue disease (MCTD)

MCTD is an overlap syndrome combining features of SLE, RA, systemic sclerosis, and dermatomyositis together with the presence of antibodies to U1-RNP. Chronic leg ulcers are not rare in MCTD and they have been reported to be due to subcutaneous calcification, vasculitis, vasospasm (Raynoud's phenomenon), vascular thrombosis, and antiphospholipid antibodies [46, 52, 53].

5.9. Infections

Numerous infections can precipitate ulcerations on the lower legs. Ecthyma, atypical mycobacterial infections, late syphilis, cutaneous leishmaniasis, actinomycoses, nocardioses, human immunodeficiency virus (HIV) infection, herpes simplex, and cytomegalovirus infections must be considered [41, 43, 54]. In addition, all chronic wounds may be secondarily contaminated with bacteria. Tissue culture will help elucidate the cause [4].

5.10. Metabolic diseases

Various metabolic factors such as diabetes mellitus, amyloidosis, hyperhomocysteinemia, prolidase deficiency, oxalosis, calciphylaxis, and gout can play a role for the lower leg ulcerations.

Necrobiosis lipoidica is a rare, chronic granulomatous disease of the skin. Clinical presentation characterized by atrophic, indurated plaques with a yellowish center and telangiectasies [42]. The lower legs, especially the shins, are the most common sites of involvement. During the course, ulcerations may occur. Necrobiosis lipoidica frequently occurs in association with diabetes mellitus (**Figure 7**).

http://dx.doi.org/10.5772/63962

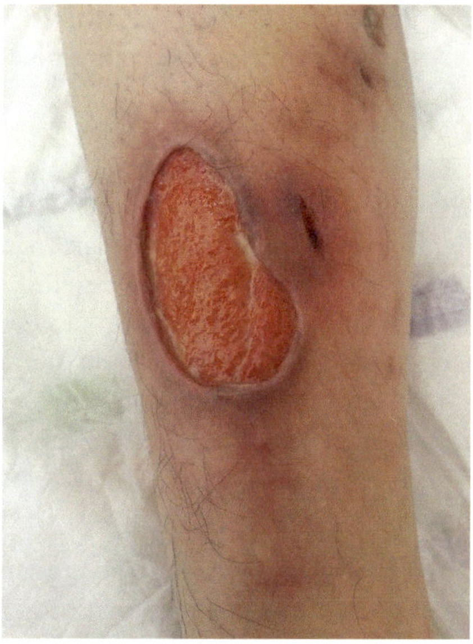

Figure 7. Necrobiosis lipoidica.

Calciphylaxis is an uncommon disorder, classically associated with renal disease and secondary parathyroidism [55]. Clinical presentation may begin as microlivedo that develop into painful ulcerations.

5.11. Hematologic diseases

Several forms of anemia (thalassemia, sickle cell anemia, hereditary spherocytosis, glucose 6 phosphate dehydrogenase deficiency), and hypercoagulable disorders (antiphospholipid antibody syndrome, antithrombin III, protein C or S deficiency, essential thrombocythemia, thrombotic thrombocytopenic purpura, polycythemia, or abnormal clotting factors such as factor V Leiden, factor II mutant) have been associated with lower leg ulceration [54].

5.12. Neoplasia

Many tumor types such as basal cell carcinoma, squamous cell carcinoma, and melanoma may present with skin ulceration. Basal cell carcinomas arising from venous ulcers appear as exuberant granulation tissue rolling onto the wound edges [4]. In addition, malignancy that presents as Marjolin's ulcers is most commonly associated with chronically inflamed, or scarred skin. Skin biopsy is necessary to identify ulcerated malignant tumors on the leg.

5.13. Medications

Hydroxyurea is a cytostatic drug used in various myeloproliferative disorders. A rare complication is the development of painful ulcers, usually localized on the malleoli or in neighboring regions [42, 54]. The coumarin derivatives, nifedipine, diltiazem, barbiturates, and erythropoietin in very rare cases, may trigger ulcer development [42].

6. Management

It is essential to treat the patients with multidisciplinary approach. The complete assessment of the chronic venous insufficiency should be evaluated together with vascular surgeons. The decision of the surgical treatment in appropriate cases should be considered with plastic surgeons. Knowledge of pathogenesis of venous ulcers and avoiding from its risk factors will be provided to choose the optimal treatment for patients with venous leg ulcers, which cause both impairment of life quality and socioeconomic burden. A multidisciplinary team of specialists will be helpful in the evaluation of venous leg ulcers and providing the most appropriate treatment.

Several treatment options are available for the management of venous ulcers. Pain reduction, closure of the ulcers, and prevention of the recurrences are the main goals of the treatment [56]. Reversing the effects of venous hypertension is the primary purpose of the treatment of venous leg ulcers. The easiest method is leg elevation [57]. Although it seems to be impractical to most of the patients, elevation of the legs above the heart level for 30 minutes, 3–4 times a day, provides the dissolution of the swelling and improves the microcirculation [58]. Leg elevation can also be performed at night by raising the foot 15–20 cm high [59]. Moreover, good nutrition and assessment with each dressing change are necessary to support the therapy. Initially and at each dressing change, the depth, width, and height of the wound bed should be measured to evaluate the improvement. Appropriate therapy of the wound must be selected patient centered. Infection control, debridement, antibiotics, dressings, compression, and adjuvant therapies will be described in this section.

6.1. Wound cleansers

Cleansers are the first and main step in preparing the wound bed. Wound cleansing with a neutral, nonirritating solution with a minimum chemical and mechanical trauma should be performed at each dressing change. Wound exudate and other debris around the wound area in venous leg ulcers must be cleansed with an appropriate solution. Although several cleansing solutions are in the market, the choice of the cleanser should have the purpose of avoiding toxicity to the viable tissue in the wound bed [31].

6.2. Debridement

Debridement during the initial evaluation is recommended to remove the necrotic tissue, excessive bacterial burden, and nonviable cells [31]. Although debridement of the wound is commonly performed to allow the formation of good granulation tissue and proper epithelialization by creating an appropriate environment to keratinocyte migration, there is a lack of evidence that routine wound debridement accelerates wound healing [31]. There are several ways of wound debridement, including autolytic, chemical, and mechanical [60].

http://dx.doi.org/10.5772/63962

6.2.1. Autolytic debridement

In venous ulcers, it is possible that wound occlusion itself promotes re-epithelialization, reduces associated pain, enhances autolytic debridement, and provides an additional barrier to bacteria [61, 62]. Hydrogels, alginates, hydrocolloids, foams, and films are the basic occlusive dressings. Wound features, exudate amount and cost of the material, and patient and physician preference affect the choice of dressing [63].

6.2.2. Chemical debridement

Several enzyme-debriding agents have been developed to promote the removal of the necrotic tissue and the formation of proper granulation tissue [64, 65]. Specific proteolytic enzyme therapies to the venous ulcers may accelerate the removal of fibrin cuffs [66]. Various enzyme-debriding agents are available, including collagenase, papain, trypsin, and tissue plasminogen activator [60, 67, 68]. Frequency of the application of the dressing may vary up to the manufacturer's recommendations. Enzymatic debridement, which does not require a trained clinician for application, has been found in several studies to remove nonviable tissue from the wound beds of venous leg ulcers, but there is no evidence that this method provides a benefit over surgical debridement [69, 70].

6.2.3. Mechanical debridement

Application of wet-to-dry dressings, hydrotherapy, irrigation, and dextranomers are some of the methods of mechanical debridement [71]. The removal of the viable tissue along with the necrotic material is the major disadvantage of mechanical debridement [72]. Hydrosurgical debridement was showed to have a shorter procedure time but requires additional cost and a trained clinician [73, 74]. Furthermore, it may be associated with a significant periprocedural pain [69]. Dextranomer's hydrophilic structure that provides a high absorptive capacity makes it useful for wounds with heavy exudate. The possibility of dehydration of the wound bed demands caution [4]. Surgical debridement, which may be performed with a curette, forceps, scalpel, or sharp scissors, is another way to remove necrotic tissue. As venous ulcers do not comprise frank necrosis or eschar tissue, this method is rarely used in venous ulcers [75]. During surgical debridement, local infiltrative, regional block, or general anesthesia may be required according to the extensity of the wound [31].

6.3. Antibiotics

Antimicrobial therapy is suggested in venous ulcers with $>1 \times 10^6$colony-forming unit (CFU)/g of bacteria on quantitative culture and clinical evidence of infection. Systemic antibiotic therapy, guided by sensitivities performed on wound culture, is recommended. Oral antibiotics are preferred in the beginning of the therapy duration and should be limited to 2 weeks [31]. Combination of mechanical debridement and antibiotic therapy is thought to be successful in eradicating infection in venous leg ulcer. In case of cellulitis, beta-lactam and non beta-lactam antibiotics may be treatment options. Trimethoprim-sulfamethoxazole and clindamycin are recommended as initial empiric therapy if methicillin-resistant Staphylococcus aureus is the suspected reason of cellulitis [76]. The use of topical silver for infected venous ulcers is controversial [31]. Recently, cadexomer iodine is reported to shorten the healing time of venous ulcers [77].

It is likely to be an increased risk of contact dermatitis in patients with chronic venous insufficiency, so in these patients any topical preparation must be used carefully [4]. There is a lack of evidence of the positive effects of topical antimicrobials in the healing of venous ulcers [31].

6.4. Periulcer skin management

It is important to keep the periulcer skin healthy to provide improvement in venous ulcers. Management of dermatitis and other abnormalities in periulcer skin accomplishes other therapy strategies in venous ulcers [31]. As mentioned above, contact dermatitis related to topical agents and dressings used in the treatment of venous ulcers are very common. In severe contact dermatitis, a short term of systemic steroids may be needed [4, 31]. Skin lubricants will be helpful in the terms of dermatitis in the calf and ankle due to venous hypertension [31]. Care of the periulcer skin will improve the venous wound healing; therefore, it is necessary to recognize the abnormalities in this area and start the appropriate treatment.

6.5. Dressing

Several types of wound dressings including gauzes, films, gels, foams, hydrocolloids, alginates, hydrogels, and other polymers are being used beneath compression bandages. Some of the dressings show biological activity on its own, while some provide the release of bioactive constituents. Different types of wound dressings such as hydrogels, hydrocolloids, foams, films, and wafers may comprise of antimicrobials, anti-inflammatory agents, analgesics, growth factors, and proteins, which would be useful in different problems of wound healing [78, 79]. During the choice of the wound dressing type, features of the ulcer should be considered and the mostly desired function of the dressing (such as cleaning, absorbing, regulating, creating a moist environment, and the possibility of adding medication, protecting the periulcer skin) should be decided [80]. Of course, the patient's needs and cost-effectiveness are other factors affecting the dressing choice [81]. The optimal wound dressing should absorb the exudate and also maintain a moist, warm wound bed and protect the periulcer skin [31, 76]. Routine use of topical antimicrobial dressings is not recommended [31]. While using wound dressings, risk of allergy should be kept in mind in venous ulcers. In conclusion, topical wound dressings are recommended as a part of the standard therapy in venous ulcers [31].

6.6. Compression

Compression therapy remains the mainstay treatment of venous leg ulcers [76]. Compression is a kind of mechanical therapy, which is simply based on applying pressure to the limb [31]. There is a significant improvement in ulcer healing and reduction in recurrence rates with an appropriate compression therapy [4, 82]. Compression therapy corrects the venous hypertension by improving venous pumping function and lymphatic drainage [83]. And as a result of

http://dx.doi.org/10.5772/63962

compression, local hydrostatic pressure increases and superficial venous pressure decreases; thus, the edema dissolves resulting in cutaneous blood flow increase [83]. Other effects of compression therapy are clinical improvement in lipodermatosclerotic skin through lymph propulsion along with the increase in lymph transport and fibrinolysis [4]. Besides the mechanical effect, compression reduces the release of macromolecules into the extravascular space, some of which play role in wound healing [84].

Various types of devices have been used for compression therapy, such as different types of bandages, bandage systems, ready-to-use garments, and several pneumatic devices [31]. It is thought that an external pressure of 35–40 mm Hg at the ankle is necessary to overcome venous hypertension [85]. For acute disease, reducing edema and improving the healing process, inelastic or rigid bandages as well as elastic and multilayered bandages are suggested. The bandage system should have high pressures when the patient walks (working pressure) and low pressure when the patient is on rest (resting pressure). Traditional Unna boot, a moist zinc-impregnated paste bandage, is a prototype of this system [83, 86]. Modified Unna boots (short-stretch bandages) have the same properties. Their stable shape despite the volume changes in leg secondary to edema reduction, unpleasant odor due to wound exudate, and potential development of contact dermatitis are the limiting factors of Unna boots' use [76, 77]. After edema reduces, long-stretch bandages are beneficial as they provide appropriate working pressure and higher resting pressure. Its easy use and providing of frequent dressing changes make the elastic compression bandages practical. Covering the leg by overlapping the bandage between turns will produce a multilayer bandage. Different components of bandages may be applied at each layer. While this application increases the pressure and also makes the final multilayer bandage less elastic and more stiff due to the friction between the surfaces of each bandage [31], intermittent pneumatic compression (IPC) pumps are also used. These devices consist of plastic air chambers, encircling the lower leg. As the air chamber fills to a preset pressure then deflated. With this system, compression of the leg is provided periodically [87].

Although compression therapy is known to be effective in both healing of venous ulcers and prevention of recurrent ulcers, there is still no optimized compression method [31, 88].

6.7. Adjuvant therapies

Systemic pharmacotherapy may be useful as an adjuvant therapy in venous ulcers. Most of the systemic agents used as adjuvant therapy acts in mechanism of one or more points in the pathophysiology of venous leg ulceration.

6.7.1. Pentoxifylline

Pentoxifylline, an antifibrinolytic agent, is thought to promote wound healing as an adjunctive therapy. Pentoxifylline has been shown to play role in microcirculation by promoting leukocyte migration, reducing platelet aggregation and fibrinogen levels, decreasing plasma viscosity, stimulating collagenase production, and blocking the effects of tumor necrosis factor-alpha on fibroblasts [89, 90]. Pentoxifylline may act in venous ulcer healing through the effects of cytokine production [91]. The conventional dose of pentoxifylline in venous leg ulcers is 400 mg three times a day. But recently, it has been proposed that the use of pentoxifylline 800 mg three times a day is more effective in venous ulcer healing. The main side effects reported were gastrointestinal disturbances such as nausea, indigestion, and diarrhea [89, 92, 93]. In studies, pentoxifylline has shown to be an effective adjuvant to compression therapy in venous leg ulcers. According to a Cochrane review, pentoxifylline plus bandaging is more effective than compression plus placebo and pentoxifylline may even be effective in the absence of compression [93].

6.7.2. Aspirin

There is currently insufficient evidence for the effectiveness of aspirin in venous leg ulcers [94]. The use of acetylsalicylic acid as an adjunct for the treatment of venous ulcers has been evaluated in one pilot study and one randomized controlled trial to date. The effect of aspirin in venous ulcers is through its irreversible inhibition of cyclooxygenase, resulting in reduction in thromboxane A2 implicated in platelet aggregation [95].

6.7.3. Split-thickness skin grafting

There are no specific indications for skin grafting of the ulcers of lower extremities [4]. Surgical treatment should only be considered in patients with venous ulcers that do not heal with conservative therapies [96]. Autografts, allografts, or human skin equivalents can be used, with a resulting healing rate of 73% [97]. In venous ulcers, skin grafting can also be followed by additional treatment to accelerate healing. The outcomes of the split-thickness skin grafting in venous ulcers vary in different studies [31]. There is still lack of evidence in the routine use of split-skin thickness skin grafting.

6.7.4. Negative pressure therapy

Negative pressure wound therapy (NPWT) is currently used widely in wound care and is promoted for use on wounds. In this system, a wound dressing is applied to the wound, to which a machine is attached. The negative pressure (or vacuum) that the machine applies sucks any wound and tissue fluid away from the treated area into a canister.

The evidence is insufficient in clinical effectiveness of NPWT in the treatment of leg ulcers. It is thought to be effective in wound healing through providing excess drainage, promoting angiogenesis, and decreasing the bacterial load of the wound [98]. There is some positive evidence that the treatment may reduce time to healing as part of a treatment, tissue granulation, area and volume reduction have also been reported. NPWT is not suggested as a primary treatment for venous leg ulcers [31, 99].

6.7.5. Cellular therapy

In recent years, cellular and/or tissue-derived products (CTPs) such as extracellular matrix (ECM; OASIS®) [100], human skin equivalent (HSE; Apligraf®) [101–103], and living skin equivalent (LSE; Dermagraft®) [104–107] have been explored as alternative therapeutic options.

Studies investigating the effects of CTPs are applied to the wounds that have been stuck in the inflammatory phase. CTPs provide the healing by supplying various biological factors, reducing levels of unnecessary cytokines or enzymes (such as matrix metalloproteinases), and/or forming a temporary ECM (which results in granulation) [108].

Recently, Apligraf, an allogeneic bilayer cellular therapy, has been approved by FDA for use in venous ulcers [31]. Before the application of cellular therapy, appropriate wound bed preparation, including the removal of debris and any necrotic tissue, should be done. The application of the graft is recommended to be done with a period of 1–3 weeks with observations of effectiveness before reapplication is considered. And reapplication is recommended as long as the venous ulcer continues to respond to the therapy [31]. In patients with venous leg ulcers who have failed with standard therapy for 4–6 weeks, cultured allogeneic bilayer skin replacements should be used [31].

Even though cellular treatments are initially more expensive, it may be more effective and less costly in the long term in chronic venous ulcers [109].

6.7.6. Tissue matrices, growth factors, human tissues, or other skin substitutes

In chronic wounds, human tissue (amniotic membrane, cryopreserved skin) or animal tissue (bladder, fetal bovine skin, others) constructs are being used. Growth factors or some other molecules, the tissues contain, may support healing process [110].

Granulocyte macrophage-colony stimulating factor (GMCSF) is a growth factor that has stimulatory effects on keratinocyte proliferation and endothelial cell and fibroblast differentiation [111]. In some studies, both intradermal injections of GM-CSF and topical application of GM-CSF have been shown to be effective in healing rates of venous ulcers [98]. But, injection site and bone pain can limit the intradermal use of GM-CSF [98].

Small intestine submucosa (SIS, Oasis®) is a biomaterial derived from porcine SIS that acts as an extracellular matrix. It is composed of Type I, III, IV, and V collagen, glycosaminogylcans, proteoglycans, proteoglycans, fibronectin, and growth factors [98, 112]. Successful results have only been reported in studies of using porcine small intestinal submucosa in venous leg ulcers [100]. It has been approved by FDA for use in wounds including venous leg ulcers. Use of porcine small intestinal submucosa tissue construct in addition to compression therapy for the treatment of venous leg ulcers is only suggested in patients who did not respond to the standard therapy for 4–6 weeks [31]. It was shown to be well tolerated and nontoxic and did not induce an adverse immunological reaction even in patients given repeated applications.

6.7.7. Therapeutic ultrasound

Ultrasound has been used as a therapeutic tool for nearly 50 years [113]. Recently, ultrasound therapy has been applied for the treatment of chronic wounds in some centers [114]. Although high-frequency ultrasound (HFU) (1–3 MHz) has been shown to promote healing of some injuries [115, 116], it has some disadvantages such as, burns or endothelial injury. However, in some studies low-dose application of ultrasound has been reported to be more successful than high-dose ultrasound in the treatment of skin wounds [117]. Thus, noncontact ultrasound therapy is among the newer modalities. Use of lower frequency (40 kHz) ultrasound in wound management was approved by the FDA in 2004 [118]. Low-frequency ultrasound therapy provides wound healing via the production, vibration, and movement of micron-sized bubbles in the coupling medium and tissue. The healing process improves by the reduced bioburden, increased angiogenesis, stimulated cellular activity, and the removal of necrotic tissues [119]. Additional studies are necessary to determine standardized protocols of therapeutic ultrasound in venous ulcers treatment. Routine use of ultrasound therapy in venous ulcer management is not suggested [31].

6.8. Surgical management

Surgical procedures are often applied when dressings and compression therapies fail in the venous ulcer treatment [76]. There are two approaches in surgical treatment of venous ulcers: ameliorating the cause of the ulcer and treating the ulcer itself by surgical procedures [4].

Superficial venous insufficiency is present in about forty to fifty percent of patients with venous ulcer [2]. Superficial vein surgery, simply comprised of ligation or sclerosis of the long and short saphenous systems, with or without communicating vein ligation or sclerosis, may be useful in patients with superficial venous insufficiency but only when deep veins are competent [120]. Although superficial vein surgery does not affect the success of improvement in venous ulcers, ulcer recurrence has shown to be reduced by the procedure [120]. Subfascial endoscopic perforating vein surgery, a new surgical technique, has proven to be effective in patients with perforator vein insufficiency [8]. In this technique, perforator veins are ligated by an endoscopic camera system through a small incision. This procedure has low complication rates and morbidity [121]. As mentioned above, it has been shown that venous surgery does not seem to improve the healing but delays or reduces the recurrences [76].

Radical excision of the diseased area including the whole ulcer bed, the fibrotic suprafascial tissues, and the abnormal superficial and perforating veins, and flapping this large soft tissue defect have been shown to be successful in a few cases. However, highly invasive character of this procedure limits its application [122].

Skin grafting has proven beneficial to heal large-size recalcitrant ulcers [120]. Contamination with microorganisms and risk of trauma are the main factors that should be kept in mind when grafting for ulcer [123]. Split-thickness skin grafts, punch grafting, and meshed grafts are some of the grafting methods used in venous leg ulcers. While pinched grafts are suitable for small ulcers, meshed grafts are useful for large highly exudative ulcers [4].

6.9. Prevention

In the period that patient has no venous ulcers, it is important to keep in cooperation with and offer some simple lifestyle changes to the patient. Leg elevation is thought to provide venous return, reduce edema, and improve cutaneous circulation [98]. Elevation of the legs above heart level for 30 minutes three or four times a day is a simple and effective method in reducing edema and improving the cutaneous microcirculation in patients with chronic venous insufficiency [87]. Calf muscle pump dysfunction is usually present in venous insufficiency and venous ulcers. Appropriate calf exercise regimes have shown to be useful to improve muscular endurance and may even provide proper functioning of the muscle pump [124]. Even in the first stages of chronic venous disease, starting the effective treatment of symptoms will help for preventing progression to ulcer. The most important step is to persuade the patient, with risk factors or early signs of venous insufficiency, to apply the appropriate compression. It is important to make the patients understand that compression therapy will be a lifelong therapy. The elastic bandages with the appropriate length and strength of compression must be worn daily. Moreover, weight management of obesity, regular exercise programs (with the aim of improving the efficiency of calf muscle pump), and treatment of varicosities (endovenous laser ablation, radiofrequency ablation, and other approaches to repair veins and valves) should be planned. Thrombophilia is increasingly recognized as a major risk factor for DVT, which is the most common identifiable risk factor for the development of chronic venous ulcer. More than 40% of patients with CVU have at least one thrombophilia and chronic venous ulcer patients with post-thrombotic disease are shown to have lower response rates to medical and surgical therapy. Thrombophilia screening is suggested to be performed in patients who have venous ulcer before the age of 50 to stratify the thrombotic risk and start the appropriate prophylactic and therapeutic management. Good nutrition is important in venous ulcer patients as protein deficiency is associated with impaired wound healing. Also smoking affects healing via decreasing the fibroblast proliferation [76]. All these factors together will help to prevent the progression of chronic venous disease to ulceration. Commitment to lifelong exercise programs, weight control, and protection against skin injury is necessary for the prevention of venous leg ulcers [31, 125].

Author details

Aslı Aksu Çerman*, İlknur Kıvanç Altunay and Ezgi Aktaş Karabay

*Address all correspondence to: aksuasli@hotmail.com

Dermatology Department, Sisli Hamidiye Etfal Training and Research Hospital, Istanbul, Turkey

References

[1] Baker SR, Stacey MC, Jopp-McKay AG, et al. Epidemiology of chronic venous ulcers. Br J Surg 1991;78:864–7. doi:10.1002/bjs.1800780729

[2] Nelzen O, Bergquist D, Lindhagen A. Venous and non-venous leg ulcers: clinical history and appearance in a population study. Br J Surg 1994;81:182–7. doi:10.1002/bjs.1800810206

[3] Goldman MP, Fronek A. The Alexander House Group: consensus paper on venous leg ulcer. J Dermatol Surg Oncol 1992;18:592–602. doi:10.1111/j.1524-4725.1992.tb03513.x

[4] Valencia IC, Falabella A, Kirsner R, et al. Chronic venous insufficiency and venous leg ulceration. J Am Acad Dermatol 2001;4:401–21. doi:10.1067/mjd.2001.111633

[5] Callam MJ, Ruckley CV, Harper DR, et al. Chronic ulceration of the leg: extent of the problem and provision of care. Br Med J 1985;290:1855–6.

[6] Callam MJ, Harper DR, Bale JJ, et al. Chronic ulcer of the leg: clinical history. Br Med J 1986;294:1389–91.

[7] Callam MJ. Epidemiology of varicose veins. Br J Surg 1994;81:167–73. doi:10.1002/bjs.1800810204

[8] Etufugh CN, Phillips TJ. Venous ulcers. Clin Dermatol 2007;25:121–30. doi:10.1016/j.clindermatol.2006.09.004

[9] Bergqvist D, Lindholm C, Nelzen O. Chronic leg ulcers: the impact of venous disease. J Vasc Surg 1999;29:752–5. doi:10.1016/S0741-5214(99)70330-7

[10] Ruckley C. Socioeconomic impact of chronic venous insufficiency and leg ulcers. Angiology 1997;46:67–9. doi:10.1177/000331979704800111

[11] Lazarus GS, Cooper DM, Knighton DR, et al. Definitions and guidelines for assessment of wounds and evaluation of healing. Arch Dermatol 1994;130:489–93. doi:10.1001/archderm.1994.01690040093015

[12] Abbade L, Lastoria S. Venous ulcer, epidemiology, physiopathology, diagnosis and treatment. Int J Dermatol 2005;44:449–56. doi:10.1111/j.1365-4632.2004.02456.x

[13] Scott TE, Lamarte WW, Gorin DR, et al. Risk factors for chronic venous insufficiency: a dual case control study. J Vasc Surg 1995;24:703–10. doi:10.1016/S0741-5214(95)70050-1

[14] Alguire PC, Mathes BM. Chronic venous insufficiency and venous ulceration. J Gen Intern Med 1997;12:374–83. doi:10.1046/j.1525-1497.1997.00063.x

[15] Meissner MH. Lower extremity venous anatomy. Semin Intervent Radiol 2005;22:147–56. doi:10.1055/s-2005-921948

[16] Gonsalves CF. Venous leg ulcers. Tech Vasc Interv Radiol 2003;6:132–6. doi:10.1053/S1089-2516(03)00055-6

[17] Browse NL, Burnand KG. The cause of venous ulceration. Lancet 1882;2:243–5. doi:10.1016/S0140-6736(82)90325-7

[18] Falanga V, Kirsner R, Katz MH, et al. Pericapillary fibrin cuffs in venous ulceration: Persistence with treatment and during ulcer healing. J Dermatol Surg Oncol 1992;18:409–13. doi:10.1111/j.1524-4725.1992.tb03694.x

[19] Burnand KG, Whimster I, Naidoo A, et al. Pericapillary fibrin in the ulcer-bearing skin of the lower leg: the cause of lipodermatosclerosis and venous ulceration. Br Med J (Clin Res Ed) 1982;285:1071–2.

[20] Falanga V, Bontempo FA, Eaglstein WH. Protein C and protein S plasma levels in patients with lipodermatosclerosis and venous ulceration. Arch Dermatol 1990;126:1195–7. doi:10.1001/archderm.1990.01670330075010

[21] Falanga V, Kruskal J, Franks JJ. Fibrin and fibrinogen-related antigens in patients with lipodermatosclerosis and venous ulceration. Arch Dermatol 1991;127:75–8.

[22] Paye M, Nusgens BV, Lapiere CM. Factor XIII of blood coagulation modulates collagen biosynthesis by fibroblasts in vitro. Haemostasis 1989;19:274–83.

[23] Dormandy JA, Nash A. Importance of red cell aggregation in venous pathology. Clin Hemorheol 1987;7:119–22.

[24] Thomas PR, Nash Gb, Dormandy JA. White cell accumulation in dependent legs of patients with venous hypertension: a possible mechanism for trophic changes in the skin. Br Med J (Clin Res Ed) 1988;296:1693–5.

[25] Dormandy JA. Pathophysiology of venous ulceration—an update. Angiology 1997;48:71–5. doi:10.1177/000331979704800112

[26] Falanga V, Eaglstein WH. The trap hypothesis of venous ulceration. Lancet 1993;341:1006–8.

[27] Higley HR, Ksander GA, Gerhardt CO, et al. Extravasation of macromolecules and possible trapping of transforming growth factor-β in venous ulceration. Br J Dermatol 1995;132:79–85. doi:10.1111/j.1365-2133.1995.tb08629.x

[28] Maessen-Visch MB, Koedam MI, Hamulyak K, et al. Atrophie blanche. Int J Dermatol 1999;38:161–72. doi:10.1046/j.1365-4362.1999.00581.x

[29] Kirsner RS, Pardes JB, Eaglstein WH, et al. The clinical spectrum of lipodermatosclerosis. J Am Acad Dermatol 1993;28:623–7.

[30] Baldursson B, Sigurgeirsson B, Lindelof B. Venous leg ulcers and squamous cell carcinoma: a large scale epidemiological study. Br J Dermatol 1995;133:571–4. doi: 10.1111/j.1365-2133.1995.tb02707.x

[31] O'Donnell TF Jr, Passman MA, Marston WA, et al. Management of venous leg ulcers: clinical practice guidelines of the Society for Vascular Surgery®and the American Venous Forum. J Vasc Surg 2014;60:3S–59S. doi:10.1016/j.jvs.2014.04.049

[32] McMullin GM, Smith C. An evaluation of Doppler ultrasound and photoplethysmography in the investigation of venous insufficiency. Aust N Z J Surg 1992;62:270–5. doi: 10.1111/j.1445-2197.1992.tb07554.x

[33] Sarin S, Sommerville K, Farrah J, et al. Duplex ultrasonography for assessment of venous valvular function of the lower limb. Br J Surg 1994;81:1591–5. doi:10.1002/bjs.1800811108

[34] Criado E, Farber MA, Marston WA, et al. The role of air plethysmography in the diagnosis of chronic venous insufficiency. J Vasc Surg 1998;27:660–70. doi:10.1016/S0741-5214(98)70231-9

[35] Lurie F, Rooke TW. Evaluation of venous function by indirect noninvasive testing (plethysmography). In: Gloviczki P, editor. Handbook of venous disorders: Guidelines of the American Venous Forum. 3rd ed. London: Hodder Arnold; 2009. p. 156–9. doi:10.1201/b13654-17

[36] Barnes RW. Noninvasive diagnostic assessment of peripheral vascular disease. Circulation 1991;83:120–7.

[37] Porter JM, Moneta GL. International Consensus Committee on Chronic Venous Disease. Reporting standards in venous disease: an update. J Vasc Surg 1995;21:635–45.

[38] Eklöf B, Rutherford RB, Bergan JJ, et al. Revision of the CEAP classification for chronic venous disorders. Consensus statement. J Vasc Surg 2004;40:1248–52. doi:10.1016/j.jvs.2004.09.027

[39] Marston WA, Vasquez MA, Lurie F, et al. Multicenter assessment of the repeatability and reproducibility of the revised venous clinical severity score (rVCSS). J Vasc Surg Venous Lymphat Disord 2013;1:219–24. doi:10.1016/j.jvsv.2012.10.059

[40] Falanga V. Venous ulceration: assessment, classification and management. In: Krasner D, Kane D, editors. Chronic wound care. 2nd ed. Wayne (PA): Health Management Publications; 1997. p. 165–71.

[41] Dissemond J, Körber A, Grabbe S. Differential diagnoses in leg ulcers. J Dtsch Dermatol Ges 2006;4:627–34. doi:10.1111/j.1610-0387.2006.06052.x

[42] Meyer V, Kerk N, Meyer S, et al. Differential diagnosis and therapy of leg ulcers. J Dtsch Dermatol Ges 2011;9:1035–51. doi:10.1111/j.1610-0387.2011.07814.x

[43] Kirsner RS, Vivas AC. Lower-extremity ulcers: diagnosis and management. Br J Dermatol 2015;173:379–90. doi:10.1111/bjd.13953

[44] Fukaya E, Margolis DJ. Approach to diagnosing lower extremity ulcers. Dermatol Therap 2013;26:181–6. doi:10.1111/dth.12054

[45] Goslen JB. Autoimmune ulceration of the leg. Clin Dermatol 1990;3:92–117. doi:10.1016/0738-081X(90)90050-B

[46] Dabiri G, Falanga V. Connective tissue ulcers. J Tissue Viability 2013;22:92–102. doi:10.1016/j.jtv.2013.04.003

[47] Oien RF, Hakansson A, Hansen BU. Leg ulcers in patients with rheumatoid arthritis—a prospective study of aeitology, wound healing, and pain reduction after pinch grafting. Rheumatology (Oxford) 2001;40:816–20. doi:10.1093/rheumatology/40.7.816

[48] Hafner J, Schneider E, Burg G, et al. Management of leg ulcers with rheumatoid arthritis or systemic sclerosis: the importance of concomitant arterial and venous disease. J Vasc Surg 2000;32:322–9. doi:10.1067/mva.2000.106942

[49] Shanmugam VK, Price P, Attinger CE, et al. Lower extremity ulcers in systemic sclerosis: features and response to therapy. Int J Rheumatol 2010:8, article ID 747946, doi: 10.1155/2010/747946

[50] Reddy V, Dziadzio M, Hamdulay S, et al. Lupus and leg ulcers—a diagnostic quandary. Clin Rheumatol 2007;26:1173–5. doi:10.1007/s10067-006-0306-2

[51] Chapnick SL, Merkel PA. Skin ulcers in a patient with Sjögren's syndrome. Arthritis Care Res (Hoboken) 2010;62:1040–6. doi:10.1002/acr.20181

[52] Yamamura K, Takahara M, Masunaga K, et al. Subcutaneous calcification of the lower legs in a patient with mixed connective tissue disease. J Dermatol 2011;38:791–3. doi: 10.1111/j.1346-8138.2010.01177.x

[53] Rozin AP, Braun-Moscovici Y, Bergman R, et al. Recalcitrant leg ulcer due to mixed connective tissue disease. J Med 2006;64:91–4.

[54] Mekkes JR, Loots MAM, Van Der Wal AC, et al. Causes, investigation and treatment of leg ulceration. Br J Dermatol 2003;148:388–401. doi:10.1046/j.1365-2133.2003.05222.x

[55] Harris RJ, Cropley TG. Possible role of hypercoagulability in calciphylaxis: review of the literature. J Am Acad Dermatol 2011;64:405–12. doi:10.1016/j.jaad.2009.12.007

[56] Alguire PC, Mathes BM. Chronic venous insufficiency and venous ulceration. J Gen Intern Med 1997;12:374–83. doi:10.1046/j.1525-1497.1997.00063.x

[57] Philips TJ, Dover JS. Leg ulcers. J Am Acad Dermatol 1991;25:965–87.

[58] Abu-Own A, Scurr JH, Coleridge Smith PD. Effect of leg elevation on the skin microcirculation in chronic venous insufficiency. J Vasc Surg 1994;20:705–10.

[59] Cranley JJ, Krause RJ, Strasser ES. Chronic venous insufficiency of the lower extremity. Surgery 1961;49:48–58.

[60] Falabella AF. Debridement and management of exudative wounds. Dermatol Ther 1999;9:36–43.

[61] Alvarez O, Rozint J, Wiseman D. Moist environment for healing: matching the dressing to the wound. Wounds 1989;1:35–51.

[62] Freidman S, Su WPD. Hydrocolloid occlusive dressing management of leg ulcers. Arch Dermatol 1984;120:1329–31.

[63] Phillips TJ. Successful methods of treating leg ulcers: the tried and true, plus the novel and new. Postgrad Med 1999;105:159–79.

[64] Durham DR, Fortney DZ, Nanney LB. Preliminary evaluation of vibriolysin, a novel proteolytic enzyme composition suitable for the debridement of burn wound eschar. J Burn Care Rehabil 1993;14:544–51.

[65] Falanga V. Occlusive wound dressings: why, when, which? Arch Dermatol 1988;124:544–51.

[66] Sinclair RD, Ryan TJ. Proteolytic enzymes in wound healing: the role of enzymtic debridement. Australas J Dermatol 1994;35:35–41. doi:10.1111/j.1440-0960.1994.tb01799.x

[67] Berger MM. Enzymatic debriding preparations. Ostomy Wound Management 1989;39:61–9.

[68] Falanga V, Carson P, Greenberg A, et al. Topically applied tPA for the treatment of venous ulcers. Dermatol Surg 1996;22:643–4. doi:10.1111/j.1524-4725.1996.tb00611.x

[69] Falanga V. Wound bed preparation and the role of enzymes: a case for multiple actions of the therapeutic agents. Wounds 2002;14:47–57.

[70] Mosher BA, Cuddigan J, Thomas DR, et al. Outcomes of 4 methods of debridement using a decision analysis methodology. Adv Wound Care 1999;12:81–8.

[71] Kennedy KL, Tritch DL. Debridement. In: Krasner D, Kane E, editors. Chronic wound care. 2nd ed. Wayne (PA): Health Management Publications; 1997. p. 227–34.

[72] Donati L, Magliano E, Colonna M, et al. Surgical versus enzymatic debridement. In: Westerhof W, Vanscheidt W, editors. Proteolytic enzymes and wound healing. New York: SpringerVerlag; 1994. p. 38–9. doi:10.1007/978-3-642-78891-8_4

[73] Dunn RM, Fudem GM, Walton RL, et al. Free flap valvular transplantation for refractory venous ulceration. J Vasc Surg 1994;19:525–31.

[74] Weinzwieg N, Schuler J. Free tissue transfer in treatment of the recalcitrant chronic venous ulcer. Ann Plast Surg 1997;38:611–9.

[75] Falanga V. Overview of chronic wounds and recent advances. Dermatol Ther 1999;9:7–17.

[76] Tang JC, Marston WA, Kirsner RS. Wound Healing Society (WHS) venous ulcer treatment guidelines: what's new in five years? Wound Rep Reg 2012;20:619–37. doi: 10.1111/j.1524-475X.2012.00815.x

[77] Gilchrist B, on behalf of the European Tissue Repair Society. Should iodine be reconsidered in wound management? A report of a consensus meeting on the use of iodine in wound care. J Wound Care 1997;6:148–50.

[78] Maessen-Visch MB, van Montfrans C. Wound dressings, does it matter and why? Phlebology 2016;31:63–7. doi:10.1177/0268355516633383

[79] Boateng J, Catanzano O. Advanced therapeutic dressings for effective wound healing- a review. J Pharm Sciences 2015;104:3653–80.

[80] Heyer K, Augustin M, Protz K, et al. Effectiveness of advanced versus conventional wound dressings on healing of chronic wounds: systematic review and meta-analysis. Dermatology 2013;226:172–84. doi:10.1159/000348331

[81] Gottrup F, Apelqvist J, Price P. Outcomes in controlled and comparative studies on non-healing wounds: recommendations to improve the quality of evidence in wound management. J Woundcare 2010;19:239–68. doi:10.12968/jowc.2010.19.6.48471

[82] Erickson CA, Lanza DJ, Karp DL, et al. Healing of venous ulcers in an ambulatory care program: the role of chronic venous insufficiency and patient compliance. J Vasc Surg 1995;22:629–36. doi:10.1016/S0741-5214(95)70051-X

[83] Partsch H. Compression therapy of the legs: a review. J Dermatol Surg Oncol 1991;17:799–808.

[84] Van de Scheur M, Falanga V. Pericapillary fibrin cuffs in venous disease. J Dermatol Surg Oncol 1997;23:955–9. doi:10.1111/j.1524-4725.1997.tb00759.x

[85] Stemmer R, Marescaux J, Furderer C. Compression treatment of the lower extremities, particularly with compression stockings. Dermatologist 1980;31:355–65.

[86] Dickey WJ Jr. Stasis ulcers: the role of compliance in healing. South Med J 1991;84:557–61.

[87] Alguire PC, Mathes BM. Chronic venous insufficiency and venous ulceration. J Gen Intern Med 1997;12:374–83. doi:10.1046/j.1525-1497.1997.00063.x

[88] Moffatt C, Kommala D, Dourdin N, et al. Venous leg ulcers: patient concordance with compression therapy and its impact on healing and prevention of recurrence. Int Wound J 2009;6:386–93. doi:10.1111/j.1742-481X.2009.00634.x

[89] Falanga V, Sabolinski M. A bilayered skin construct (Apligraf) accelerates complete closure of hard-to-heal venous ulcers. Wound Rep Reg 1999;7:201–7.

[90] Bertocchi F, Proserpio P, Lampugnai MG, et al. The effect of pentoxifylline on polymorphonuclear cell adhesion to cultured endothelial cells. In: Mandell GL, Novicl WJ, editors. Pentoxifylline and leukocyte function. Sommerville (NJ): Hoechst Roussel Pharmaceuticals; 1988. p. 68–74.

[91] Zabel P, Wolter DT, Schonharting MM, et al. Oxpentifylline in endotoxaemia. Lancet 1998;2:1474–7. doi:10.1016/S0140-6736(89)92929-2

[92] Falanga V, For the Trental Collaborative Group: Pentoxifylline (Trental) accelerates the healing of venous ulcers in a double blind randomised study. In: Proceedings from the European Tissue Repair Society, Cologne, Germany, Aug 25, 1997.

[93] Jull AB, Arroll B, Parag V, et al. Pentoxifylline for treating venous leg ulcers. Cochrane Database Syst Rev 2012;12:CD001733. doi:10.1002/14651858.CD001733.pub3

[94] de Oliveira Carvalho P, Magolbo NG, De Aquino RF, et al. Oral aspirin for venous leg ulcers. Cochrane Database Syst Rev 2016 Feb 18;2:CD009432. doi: 10.1002/14651858.CD009432.pub2

[95] Cyrus T, Sung S, Zhao L, et al. Effect of low-dose aspirin on vascular inflammation, plaque stability, and atherogenesis in low-density lipoprotein receptor-deficient mice. Circulation 2002;106:1282–7. doi:10.1161/01.CIR.0000027816.54430.96

[96] Serra R, Rizzuto A, Rossi A, et al. Skin grafting for the treatment of chronic leg ulcers—a systematic review in evidence-based medicine. Int Wound J 2016 Mar 4. doi:10.1111/iwj.12575.

[97] Serra R, Buffone G, De Franciscis A, et al. Skin grafting followed by low-molecular-weight heparin long-term therapy in chronic venous leg ulcers. Ann Vasc Surg 2012;26:190–7. doi:10.1016/j.avsg.2011.04.008

[98] Richmond NA, Maderal AD, Vivas AC. Evidence-based management of common chronic lower extremity ulcers. Dermatol Ther 2013;26:187–96. doi:10.1111/dth.12051

[99] Dumville JC, Land L, Evans D, et al. Negative pressure wound therapy for treating leg ulcers. Cochrane Database Syst Rev 2015 Jul 14;7:CD011354. doi: 10.1002/14651858.CD011354.pub2

[100] Mostow EN, Haraway GD, Dalsing M, et al. OASIS Venus Ulcer Study Group. Effectiveness of an extracellular matrix graft (OASIS Wound Matrix) in the treatment of chronic leg ulcers: a randomized clinical trial. J Vasc Surg 2005;41:837–43.

[101] Ehrenreich M, Ruszczak Z. Update on tissue-engineered biological dressings. Tissue Eng 2006;12:2407–24. doi:10.1089/ten.2006.12.2407

[102] Cavorsi J, Vicari F, Wirthlin DJ, et al. Best-practice algorithms for the use of a bilayered living cell therapy (Apligraf) in the treatment of lower-extremity ulcers. Wound Repair Regen 2006;14:102–9. doi:10.1111/j.1743-6109.2006.00098.x

[103] Fivenson D, Scherschun L. Clinical and economic impact of Apligraf for the treatment of nonhealing venous leg ulcers. Int J Dermatol 2003;42:960–5. doi:10.1111/j.1365-4632.2003.02039.x

[104] Purdue GF. Dermagraft-tc pivotal efficacy and safety study. J Burn Care Rehabil 1997;18:13–4.

[105] Marston WA. Dermagraft, a bioengineered human dermal equivalent for the treatment of chronic nonhealing diabetic foot ulcer. Expert Rev Med Devices 2004;1:21–31. doi: 10.1586/17434440.1.1.21

[106] Marston WA, Hanft J, Norwood P, et al. The efficacy and safety of dermagraft in improving the healing of chronic diabetic foot ulcers: results of a prospective randomized trial. Diabetes Care 2003;26:1701–5. doi:10.2337/diacare.26.6.1701

[107] Hart CE, Loewen-Rodriguez A, Lessem J. Dermagraft: use in the treatment of chronic wounds. Adv Wound Care 2011;1:138–41. doi:10.1089/wound.2011.0282

[108] Lazic T, Falanga V. Bioengineered skin constructs and their use in wound healing. Plast Reconstr Surg 2011;127:75–90. doi:10.1097/PRS.0b013e3182009d9f

[109] Carter MJ, Waycaster C, Schaum K, et al. Cost-effectiveness of three adjunct cellular/tissue-derived products used in the management of chronic venous leg ulcers. Value Health 2014;17:801–13. doi:10.1016/j.jval.2014.08.001

[110] Hankin CS, Knispel J, Lopes M, et al. Clinical and cost efficacy of advanced wound care matrices for venous ulcers. J Manag Care Pharm 2012;18:375–84.

[111] Da Costa RM, Ribeiro Jesus FM, Aniceto C, et al. Randomized, double-blind, placebo-controlled, dose-ranging study of granulocyte-macrophage colony stimulating factor in patients with chronic venous leg ulcers. Wound Repair Regen 1999;7:17–25.

[112] Demling RH, Niezgoda JA, Haraway GD, et al. Small intestinal submucosa wound matrix and full-thickness venous ulcers: preliminary results. Wounds 2004;16:18–22.

[113] Hill OR. Ultrasound biophysics: a perspective. Br J Cancer 1982;82:46–51.

[114] Moffatt C, Martin R, Smithdale R. Leg ulcer management. Oxford: Blackwell Publishing Ltd.; 2007.

[115] Cameron MH. Thermal agents: cold and heat, ultrasound, and electrical currents. In: Cameron MH, editor. Physical agents in rehabilitation: from research to practice. St. Louis: WB Saunders; 2003, 2nd ed., p. 133–259.

[116] Busse JW, Bhandari M, Kulkarni AV, et al. The effect of low-intensity pulsed ultrasound therapy on time to fracture healing: a meta-analysis. CMAJ 2002;166:437–41.

[117] Ernst E. Ultrasound for cutaneous wound healing. Phlebology 1995;10:2–4.

[118] Unger PG. Low-frequency, noncontact, nonthermal ultrasound therapy: a review of the literature. Ostomy Wound Manage 2008;54:57–60.

[119] Beheshti A, Shafigh Y, Parsa H, et al. Comparison of high-frequency and MIST ultrasound therapy for the healing of venous leg ulcers. Adv Clin Exp Med 2014;23:969–75. doi:10.17219/acem/37353

[120] Douglas WS, Simpson NB. Guidelines for the management of chronic venous leg ulceration: report of a multidisciplinary workshop. Br J Dermatol 1995;132:446–52. doi: 10.1111/j.1365-2133.1995.tb08681.x

[121] Chong C. Subfascial endoscopic perforating vein surgery (SEPS) for the treatment of venous ulcers. Ostomy Wound Manage 2005;51:26–31.

[122] Weinzwieg N, Schuler J. Free tissue transfer in treatment of the recalcitrant chronic venous ulcer. Ann Plast Surg 1997;38:611–9.

[123] Skouge JW. Techniques for split-thickness skin grafting. J Dermatol Surg Oncol 1987;13:841–9.

[124] Padberg FT, Johnston MV, Sisto SA. Structured exercise improves calf muscle pump function in chronic venous insufficiency: a randomized trial. J Vasc Surg 2004;39:79–87.

[125] Kelechi TJ, Johnson JJ. Chronic venous disease and venous leg ulcers: an evidence-based update. J Vasc Nurs 2015;33:36–46. doi:10.1016/j.jvn.2015.01.003

Chapter 13

Topical Wound Oxygen Versus Conventional Compression Dressings in the Management of Refractory Venous Ulcers

Sherif Sultan, Wael Tawfick, Edel P Kavanagh and Niamh Hynes

Additional information is available at the end of the chapter

http://dx.doi.org/10.5772/63566

Abstract

Topical wound oxygen (TWO_2) proposes an innovative therapy option in the management of refractory non-healing venous ulcers (RVU) that aims to accelerate wound healing. TWO_2 accelerates epithelialisation. This leads to the development of a higher tensile strength collagen, which lessens scarring and the risk of recurrence. Sixty-seven limbs with 67 ulcers were managed using TWO_2 therapy, and 65 limbs with 65 ulcers were managed using conventional compression dressings (CCD). The proportion of ulcers completely healed by 12 weeks was 76% in patients managed with TWO_2, compared to 46% in patients managed with CCD ($p < 0.0001$). The mean reduction in ulcer surface area at 12 weeks was 96% in the TWO_2 therapy group, compared to 61% in patients managed with CCD. The median time to full ulcer healing was 57 days in the TWO_2 group, in contrast to 107 days in patients managed with CCD ($p < 0.0001$). TWO_2 patients had a significantly improved Quality-Adjusted Time Spent Without Symptoms of disease and Toxicity of treatment (Q-TWiST) compared to CCD patients, denoting an improved outcome ($p < 0.0001$). TWO_2 reduces the time needed for RVU healing and is successful in pain alleviation and MRSA elimination. TWO_2 therapy radically degrades recurrence rates. Utilising diffused oxygen raises the capillary partial pressure of oxygen (Po_2) levels at the wound site, stimulating epithelialisation, and granulation of new healthy tissue. Taking the social and individual aspects of chronic venous ulceration into account, the use of TWO_2 can provide an overwhelmingly improved quality of life for long-time sufferers of this debilitating disease.

Keywords: topical wound oxygen, conventional compression dressings, refractory venous ulcers, MRSA, epithelialisation

1. Introduction

Chronic venous ulceration is a common disease. Its prevalence is 1% of the total population, with 20% of venous ulcers presented in octogenarians [1–5]. Refractory venous leg ulceration is a common basis of morbidity [6, 7] and leads to a reduced quality of life [8], especially in the elderly population [4, 5]. It causes a considerable amount of work incapacity, social exclusion and lack of self-esteem [4]. There is a probable underestimation of the true extent of venous leg ulceration in the general population due to its underreporting [7]. Venous ulcers are characterised by a recurring pattern of healing and subsequent 70% recurrence rate at one year [9–14]. Venous ulceration places a huge monetary burden on the healthcare system [15]. The cost of managing venous ulcers accrues to £400 million sterling per year in the UK [16].

Ambulatory venous hypertension is one of the leading causes of chronic reperfusion injury. This in turn provokes venous ulceration with its habitual history of chronicity and recurrence [1]. Over the past 40 years, compression bandaging has been the gold standard form of therapy for treatment of venous ulceration. We have learned that compression will both improve perfusion and enhance healing [2, 17, 18]. Nevertheless, active healthy tissue granulation can take upwards to 3 weeks to cultivate [19]. Therefore, the following question is posed: How can we speed up epithelial coverage in a granulating wound?

1.1. Topical wound oxygen

Topical wound oxygen (TWO_2) proposes an innovative therapy option in the management of refractory non-healing venous ulcers (RVU) that aims to accelerate wound healing. The application of positive pressure oxygen to manage open wounds has been studied extensively and has demonstrated promising clinical results [20–28]. The systemic complications associated with the use of a full-body hyperbaric chamber have been overcome by the application of topical wound pure oxygen at an appropriate cycled pressure to only the specific wound site. This maximizes the beneficial wound healing effects and minimizes the negative systemic side effects [29].

Delivered through a targeted delivery system, a Hyper-Box, TWO_2 accelerates epithelialisation and eliminates MRSA within 72 h. This leads to the development of a higher tensile strength collagen, which lessens scarring and the risk of recurrence [29–32]. Hyperbaric oxygen promotes angiogenesis and increases the expression of angiogenesis-related growth factors [33, 34]. It promotes leukocyte function with enhanced bactericidal activity [35–40]. The intermittent cycled pressure, under which TWO_2 is delivered, stimulates circulation, reduces oedema and provides a sealed humidified environment essential for healing [41].

2. Materials and methods

The aim of this study is to scrutinise the use of TWO_2 when compared to conventional compression dressings (CCD) for managing RVU, with reference to technical and clinical outcomes from our tertiary referral leg ulcer clinic.

A 5-year study of TWO_2 versus CCD for chronic RVU was carried out at our tertiary referral leg ulcer clinic [42, 43]. This parallel group observational comparative study aimed at examining the safety and efficacy of TWO_2 in managing RVU in the short-term (12 weeks), and the mid-term (36 months).

Ethical approval was obtained from the local research ethics committee. Patients with chronic RVU, with an ulcer of more than two years duration, were recruited from the vascular unit. All patients must show no sign of improvement of the ulcer over the past 12 months, despite acceptable compliance with a suitable treatment, provided by community-based leg ulcer clinics. All patients were managed on an intention to treat basis and were given the choice of receiving CCD or TWO_2 therapy. Patients were informed on both CCD and TWO_2 therapies, and the treatment choice was discussed with their primary care physician and local tissue viability nurse. Treatment allocation was based on each patient's choice. All patients signed an informed consent form prior to beginning therapy.

2.1. Technical and clinical endpoints

The end points of this study were the proportion of ulcers healed at 12 weeks and recurrence rates at 36 months. Secondary end-points were time taken for full healing, percentage of reduction in the ulcer size at 12 weeks, methicillin-resistant *Staphylococcus aureus* (MRSA) elimination, pain reduction, recurrence rates and Quality-Adjusted Time Spent Without Symptoms of disease and Toxicity of treatment (Q-TWiST).

2.2. Inclusion criteria

Informed written consent was required from patient's aged ≥ 18 years.

The patients must be treated at a dedicated veins unit with $C_{6,s}$ in the Clinical, Etiological, Anatomical, and Pathophysiological (CEAP) classification [44, 45]. The venous ulcer must have been present for more than 2 years, with no improvement over the past 12 months despite adequate treatment at the veins unit. The patients must also have a normal ankle-brachial index (ABI) with a normal digital pressure.

2.3. Exclusion criteria

Patients who are bedridden, have ischemic or malignant ulcers, or osteomyelitis in the treated limb were primarily excluded. Patients with ischemic diabetic ulcers were excluded; however, it should be noted that diabetes in isolation was not considered an exclusion criterion. A prior study has shown that the AOTI Hyper-Box (AOTI Ltd., Galway, Ireland) is not sufficient in ischemic diabetic ulcers. It may induce iatrogenic deterioration of the affected diabetic limb due to the cyclic pressure of the Hyper-Box [46, 47].

2.4. Statistical analysis

Data was collected and analysed using SPSS 18 software (SPSS Inc., Chicago, IL). An independent sample *t*-test was used for continuous variables, while the Mann-Whitney *U* test was used to compare unpaired, non-parametric data. Categorical proportions were examined using the chi-squared test. Time for healing was examined using Kaplan-Meier with log-rank comparison.

2.5. Quality-Adjusted Time Spent Without Symptoms of disease and Toxicity of treatment (Q-TWiST)

The survival time for patients was divided into three separate phases: the time spent with toxicity of the disease or severe adverse events prior to disease progression known as Toxicity (TOX); the time spent without any symptoms of disease progression or toxicity of treatment known as TWiST; and finally the time spent with progression of the disease known as Progression (PROG). Ulcer recurrence in fully healed ulcers or an increase of size in ulcers that had not fully healed was defined as progression of disease. The Kaplan Meier method was used to determine the mean time spent in each of the TOX, TWiST and PROG periods for each treatment group. Mean Q-TWiST was calculated for each treatment.

2.6. Techniques

The anatomical location and duration of the ulcer, signs of infection, slough, and cellulitis, as well as any other vascular risk factors were observed in each patient. The leg ulcers were swabbed for culture as well as for level of sensitivity. Prior to therapy, a numerical rating scale in regards to pain was used. This was then repeated every three days. To record surface area, maximum length and maximum width of the ulcer, the ulcers were cleaned, debrided and digitally photographed using a Visitrak system (Smith & Nephew Ltd., Hull, United Kingdom). For all patients, ABI with big toe digital pressure measurement and punch biopsy were performed, as well as venous duplex ultrasound scan for full CEAP assessment [44, 45]. Venous Clinical Severity Score was recorded for each patient [48, 49].

2.6.1. TWO_2 therapy

Sixty-seven ulcers were treated with TWO_2 therapy. The limb was placed in the Hyper-Box for twice daily for a duration of 180 min and under pressure of 50 mbar. Oxygen supplied at 10 L/min with continuous humidification. Between each session, wounds were washed and left exposed with no dressings or compression. Wounds were cleaned, debrided and re-measured twice weekly [42, 46, 47].

http://dx.doi.org/10.5772/63566

2.6.2. *Compression therapy*

Sixty-five ulcers were treated with compression therapy. Full compression was performed using Profore ◊ multilayer compression bandage system with underlying non-adherent Profore◊ wound contact layer dressings (Profore◊, Smith & Nephew plc., London, United Kingdom). Dressings were applied by a wound care specialist nurse and changed as required, one to three times per week, depending on the amount of exudates.

Treatment was continued for 12 weeks or until complete healing of the ulcer or whichever can be first. As soon as the ulcer is healed, the leg was fitted with a class 3, closed toe, below knee elastic stocking during the day [50]. Patients were advised to revitalise the skin by soaking the leg with tap water, baby oil or olive oil to prevent itching and dry cracked skin. Patients were followed up at 3 monthly intervals following the end of the therapy. Patients without full healing of their ulcer by 12 weeks were considered failures of treatment. They were managed with CCD and continued to be seen on a weekly basis.

3. Results

Over the course of 5 years at our tertiary referral leg ulcer clinic, 1460 patients were diagnosed of chronic venous ulcers (**Figure 1**). Following application of the inclusion and exclusion criteria, 431 patients were enrolled in this study, but only 148 patients were eligible. One hundred and thirty-two patients consented to join the study, of which 67 limbs with 67 ulcers were treated using TWO_2 therapy, and 65 limbs with 65 ulcers were treated with CCD. Fifty-seven percent of the patients treated with TWO_2 were males ($n = 38$), and 54% of the patients treated with CCD were males ($n = 35$). Risk factors, such as age, gender, the presence of diabetes mellitus, smoking, hypertension and MRSA, were similar, with no statistical significance between each group. There was no significant difference between both the groups in the anatomical distribution of ulcers, size of the ulcers or the duration of the ulcer.

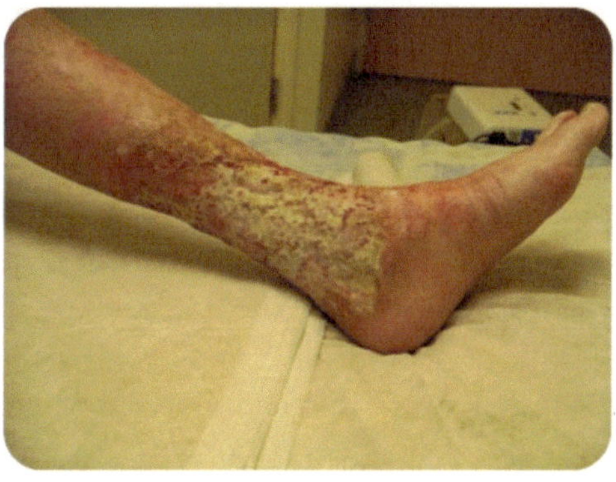

Figure 1. Patient with a chronic venous leg ulcer prior to therapy.

Twenty-four patients (36%) in the TWO_2 group and 19 patients (28%) in the CCD group were MRSA positive. Following treatment, MRSA was eliminated in 11 patients (46%), while zero cases of MRSA were eliminated in the CCD group.

The proportion of ulcers completely healed by 12 weeks was 76% (n = 51/67) in patients managed with TWO_2 compared to 46% (n = 30/65) in patients managed with CCD ($P < 0.0001$). The mean reduction in ulcer surface area at 12 weeks was 96% in the TWO_2 therapy group (**Figure 2**) compared to 61% in patients managed with CCD. The median time to full ulcer healing was 57 days in the TWO_2 group in contrast to 107 days in patients managed with CCD ($P < 0.0001$). Healing time for patients managed with TWO_2 was not affected by the extent of time of the ulcer and its size. In fact, ulcers managed with TWO_2 had a considerably shorter healing time, when compared to CCD ulcers, regardless of duration ($P < 0.0001$) or ulcer size ($P < 0.0001$). TWO_2 patients had a significantly improved Q-TWiST compared to CCD patients, denoting an improved outcome ($p < 0.0001$).

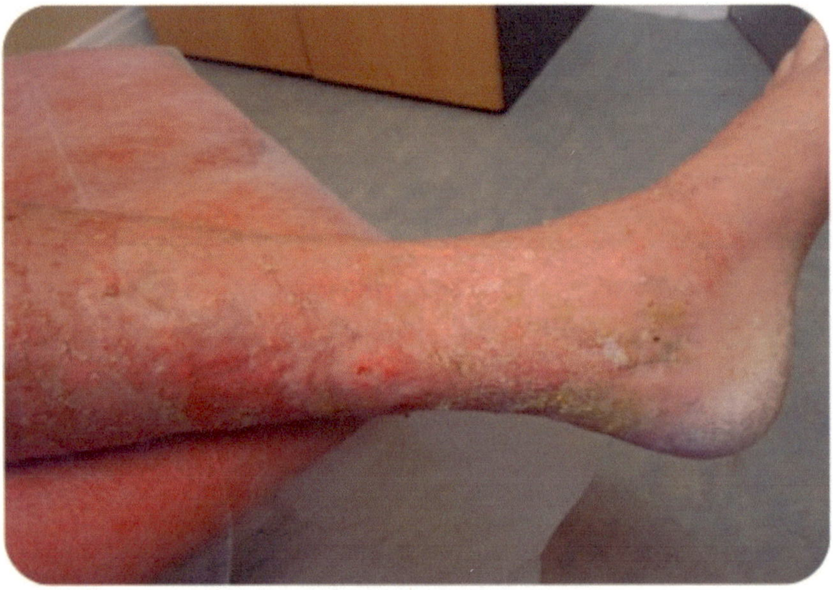

Figure 2. Significant healing and decrease in ulcer surface area post 9 weeks of TWO_2 therapy.

In all, three of the patients managed with TWO_2 were referred to our facility for primary amputation following the failure of other treatment modalities, including skin grafting. These three ulcers fully healed with no need for amputation in any case. After 36 months of follow-up, 14 of the 30 healed CCD ulcers showed recurrence compared to three of the 51 TWO_2-healed ulcers. Two CCD-managed ulcers that had not completely healed showed signs of deterioration and increase in surface area ($P < 0.0001$). All the cases that healed with TWO_2 showed reversed gradient healing phenomena where the ulcer healed from the centre to the periphery. This might be the reason for the absence of scarring and recurrence.

4. Discussion

The socio-economic consequences of management of RVU, merged with high recurrence rates, have encouraged the development of a disruptive technology innovative therapy, such as TWO_2 therapy. Compression therapy within the setup of a leg ulcer clinic is widely recognised as the main modality for managing venous leg ulcers [17, 18, 51, 52]. A previous study mentioned that contemporary dressing materials do not stimulate healing, and expenses are not clinically justified as they have no proven efficacy [19]. After 30 years of research, there is no data to defend using anything other than a simple, inexpensive, low-adherence dressing under multilayer compression [19].

The first publication on the use of TWO_2 was by Fischer in 1969 [20]. Fischer noted that lesions became aseptic and enhanced granulation was witnessed two days after TWO_2. In a prospective randomised study by Heng et al. red granulation tissue was present one week after TWO_2 [27]. Heng noted an absence of clinical scarring and most ulcers healed within 2–16 weeks. Gordillo et al. conducted a study on full-body hyperbaric oxygen (HBO) therapy versus TWO_2. Topical oxygen treatment showed a significant reduction in wound size and was associated with higher vascular endothelial growth factor (VEGF)165 expression in healing wounds [53].

Blackman et al. explored the efficacy of topical oxygen therapy as an adjunctive modality in repairing diabetic ulcers that failed to heal by best practice standard wound care. The healing rate after 12 weeks of topical wound oxygen therapy was 82.4%, and the mean time to complete healing was reduced. Patients also showed very low recurrence rates after 18 months [54].

Results from the Venous ULcer Cost-effectiveness of Antimicrobial dressings (VULCAN) trial showed that it took 101 days to heal 3-cm ulcers, while there was a 1-year recurrence rate of 14% in 86% of small ulcers [55], using silver dressings. These types of dressings are now rarely seen in a standard tertiary vein unit. In our unit, we have abandoned the use of silver dressing in any form as it showed a higher incidence of contacting eczema and an increase in the chronicity of the wounds.

Oxygen plays a major role in the promotion of vascular endothelial cell proliferation, collagen synthesis [56, 57] and infection control [58] by providing a direct microbial growth inhibitory effect [59] and also by activating neutrophils [60]. TWO_2 therapy evades the consequences of a full-body hyperbaric chamber [61], such as grand mal seizures and pulmonary oxygen toxicity [61, 62]. There is also the high associated cost of acquiring and maintaining a chamber to consider.

Utilising diffused oxygen raises the capillary partial pressure of oxygen (Po_2) levels at the wound site, stimulating epithelialisation and granulation of new healthy tissue [29, 32]. Oxygen generates reactive oxygen species at the wound site, acting as signalling substances, which increase the production of VEGF [63, 64]. Repeated treatment therefore accelerates wound closure.

TWO_2 therapy enhances both polymorph nuclear function and bacterial clearance and is fatal to anaerobic bacteria [35–37]. It reduces neutrophil adherence based on hindering the β-2 integrin function [38]. Eleven patients (46%) with MRSA were negative at the end of treatment with TWO_2. This informs us of its effectiveness against MRSA infection in comparison to CCD. TWO_2 therapy supports and strengthens antibiotic distribution for aminoglycosides, cephalosporins, quinilones and amphotericin [39, 40].

While TWO_2 therapy has been available for many years, there is paucity in clinical evidence for its safety and efficacy. Experience from our clinic shows that TWO_2 therapy is effective and valuable in managing RVU. Our course of therapy accomplished enhanced wound healing time, without complications, in a relatively large number of patients. TWO_2 therapy drastically reduced the time required for RVU healing and recurrence rates when compared to CCD. Quality of time spent without symptoms or toxicity of the disease was significantly improved in TWO_2 managed patients compared to CCD patients ($p < 0.0001$).

5. Conclusion

TWO_2 therapy is practical, effective and valuable in managing RVU without the risks associated with full-body hyperbaric chambers. TWO_2 therapy requires no further specialist skills by the primary care physician or local tissue viability nurse. It is therefore readily available for application under most circumstances, even for domiciliary use. The treatment has an extremely low risk of systemic complications when compared to HBO, and single-use devices greatly reduce the possibility of secondary infections.

TWO_2 slashes the time needed for RVU healing and is successful in pain alleviation, MRSA elimination and management. Utilising diffused oxygen raises the capillary partial Po_2 levels at the wound site, stimulating epithelialisation and granulation of new healthy tissue. TWO_2 therapy radically degrades recurrence rates. Taking the social and individual aspects of chronic venous ulceration into account, the use of TWO_2 can provide an overwhelmingly improved quality of life for long-time sufferers of this debilitating disease.

Author details

Sherif Sultan[1,2*], Wael Tawfick[1], Edel P Kavanagh[2] and Niamh Hynes[2]

*Address all correspondence to: sherif.sultan@hse.ie

1 Department of Vascular and Endovascular Surgery, Western Vascular Institute, University College Hospital Galway, Galway, Ireland

2 Department of Vascular and Endovascular Surgery, Galway Clinic, Doughiska, Galway, Ireland

References

[1] Trent JT, Falabella A, Eaglstein WH, Kirsner RS. Venous ulcers: pathophysiology and treatment options. Ostomy/Wound Management. 2005 May;51(5):38–54.

[2] O'Meara S, Cullum NA, Nelson EA. Compression for venous leg ulcers. Cochrane Database Systematic Review. 2009 Jan 21;1:CD000265.

[3] Moffatt CJ, Franks PJ, Doherty DC, Martin R, Blewett R, Ross F. Prevalence of leg ulceration in a London population. QJM. 2004 Jul 1;97(7):431–7.

[4] Graham ID, Harrison MB, Nelson EA, Lorimer K, Fisher A. Prevalence of lower-limb ulceration: a systematic review of prevalence studies. Advances in Skin & Wound Care. 2003 Nov 1;16(6):305–16.

[5] Margolisa DJ, Bilkerb W, Santannab J. Venous leg ulcer: incidence and prevalence in the elderly. Journal of the American Academy of Dermatology. 2002 Mar 31;46(3):381–6.

[6] Anand SC, Dean C, Nettleton R, Praburaj DV. Health-related quality of life tools for venous-ulcerated patients. British Journal of Nursing. 2003 Jan 9;12(1):48–59.

[7] Phillips TJ. Chronic cutaneous ulcers: etiology and epidemiology. Journal of Investigative Dermatology. 1994 Jun 1;102(6):38S–41S.

[8] Persoon A, Heinen MM, Van Der Vleuten CJ, De Rooij MJ, Van De Kerkhof P, Van Achterberg T. Leg ulcers: a review of their impact on daily life. Journal of Clinical Nursing. 2004 Mar 1;13(3):341–54.

[9] Armstrong SA. Compression hosiery. Professional Nurse (London, England). 1997 Apr; 12(7 Suppl):S10–1.

[10] Moffatt CJ, Dorman MC. Recurrence of leg ulcers within a community ulcer service. Journal of Wound Care. 1995 Feb;4(2):57–61.

[11] Monk BE, Sarkany I. Outcome of treatment of venous stasis ulcers. Clinical and Experimental Dermatology. 1982 Jul 1;7(4):397–400.

[12] Lees TA, Lambert D. Prevalence of lower limb ulceration in an urban health district. British Journal of Surgery. 1992 Oct 1;79(10):1032–4.

[13] Callam MJ, Ruckley CV, Harper DR, Dale JJ. Chronic ulceration of the leg: extent of the problem and provision of care. British Medical Journal (Clinical Research ed). 1985 Jun 22;290(6485):1855–6.

[14] Nelzen O, Bergqvist D, Lindhagen A. Venous and non-venous leg ulcers: Clinical history and appearance in a population study. British Journal of Surgery. 1994 Feb 1;81(2):182–7.

[15] Ragnarson Tennvall G, Hjelmgren J. Original research articles—clinical science: annual costs of treatment for venous leg ulcers in Sweden and the United Kingdom. Wound Repair and Regeneration. 2005 Jan 1;13(1):13–8.

[16] Ruckley CV. Socioeconomic impact of chronic venous insufficiency and leg ulcers. Angiology. 1997 Jan 1;48(1):67–9.

[17] Palfreyman SJ, Lochiel R, Michaels JA. A systematic review of compression therapy for venous leg ulcers. Vascular Medicine. 1998 Nov 1;3(4):301–13.

[18] Cullum N, Nelson EA, Fletcher AW, Sheldon TA. Compression for venous leg ulcers. Cochrane Database Syst Rev. 2001;(2):CD000265.

[19] Sultan MJ, McCollum C. Don't waste money when dressing leg ulcers. British Journal of Surgery. 2009 Oct 1;96(10):1099–100.

[20] Fischer B. Topical hyperbaric oxygen treatment of pressure sores and skin ulcers. The Lancet. 1969 Aug 23;294(7617):405–9.

[21] Olejniczak S. Employment of low hyperbaric therapy in management of leg ulcers. Michigan Medicine. 1966 Dec;65(12):1067–8.

[22] Gruber RP, Heitkamp DH, Billy LJ, Amato JJ. Skin permeability to oxygen and hyperbaric oxygen. Archives of Surgery. 1970 Jul 1;101(1):69–70.

[23] Fischer BH. Treatment of ulcers on the legs with hyperbaric oxygen. The Journal of Dermatologic Surgery and Oncology. 1975 Oct 1;1(3):55–8.

[24] Kalliainen LK, Gordillo GM, Schlanger R, Sen CK. Topical oxygen as an adjunct to wound healing: a clinical case series. Pathophysiology. 2003 Jan 31;9(2):81–7.

[25] Edsberg LE, Brogan MS, Jaynes CD, Fries K. Topical hyperbaric oxygen and electrical stimulation: exploring potential synergy. Ostomy/Wound Management. 2002 Nov; 48(11):42–50.

[26] Edsberg LE, Brogan MS, Jaynes CD, Fries K. Reducing epibole using topical hyperbaric oxygen and electrical stimulation. Ostomy/Wound Management. 2002 Apr;48(4):26.

[27] Heng MC, Harker J, Csathy G, Marshall C, Brazier J, Sumampong S, Paterno GE. Angiogenesis in necrotic ulcers treated with hyperbaric oxygen. Ostomy/Wound Management. 2000 Sep;46(9):18–28.

[28] Leslie CA, Sapico FL, Ginunas VJ, Adkins RH. Randomized controlled trial of topical hyperbaric oxygen for treatment of diabetic foot ulcers. Diabetes Care. 1988 Feb 1;11(2): 111–5.

[29] Heng MC. Topical hyperbaric therapy for problem skin wounds. The Journal of Dermatologic Surgery and Oncology. 1993 Aug 1;19(8):784–93.

[30] Prost-Squarcioni C, Fraitag S, Heller M, Boehm N. Functional histology of dermis. Annales de Dermatologie et de Venereologie 2008 Jan; 135(1 Pt 2):1S5–20.

[31] Wirthner R, Balamurugan K, Stiehl DP, Barth S, Spielmann P, Oehme F, Flamme I, Katschinski DM, Wenger RH, Camenisch G. Determination and modulation of prolyl-4-hydroxylase domain oxygen sensor activity. Methods in Enzymology. 2007 Dec 31;435:43–60.

[32] Upson AV. Topical hyperbaric oxygenation in the treatment of recalcitrant open wounds. A clinical report. Physical Therapy. 1986 Sep 1;66(9):1408–12.

[33] Knighton DR, Silver IA, Hunt TK. Regulation of wound-healing angiogenesis-effect of oxygen gradients and inspired oxygen concentration. Surgery. 1981 Aug;90(2):262–70.

[34] Scott G. Topical oxygen alters angiogenesis-related growth factor expression in chronic diabetic foot ulcers. Irish Journal of Medical Science. 2007;176:S2.

[35] Kaufman T, Alexander JW, Nathan P, Brackett KA, MacMillan BG. The microclimate chamber: the effect of continuous topical administration of 96% oxygen and 75% relative humidity on the healing rate of experimental deep burns. Journal of Trauma and Acute Care Surgery. 1983 Sep 1;23(9):806–15.

[36] Park MK, Myers RA, Marzella L. Oxygen tensions and infections: modulation of microbial growth, activity of antimicrobial agents, and immunologic responses. Clinical Infectious Diseases. 1992 Mar 1;14(3):720–40.

[37] Mandell GL. Bactericidal activity of aerobic and anaerobic polymorphonuclear neutrophils. Infection and Immunity. 1974 Feb 1;9(2):337–41.

[38] Thom SR. Effects of hyperoxia on neutrophil adhesion. Undersea & Hyperbaric Medicine. 2004 Apr 1;31(1):123.

[39] Mirhij NJ, Roberts RJ, Myers MG. Effects of hypoxemia upon aminoglycoside serum pharmacokinetics in animals. Antimicrobial Agents and Chemotherapy. 1978 Sep 1;14(3):344–7.

[40] Keck PE, Gottlieb SF, Conley J. Interaction of increased pressures of oxygen and sulfonamides on the in vitro and in vivo growth of pathogenic bacteria. Undersea Biomedical Research. 1980 Jun;7(2):95–106.

[41] Olejniczak S, Zielinski A. Topical oxygen promotes healing of leg ulcers. Medical Times. 1976 Dec;104(12):114–21.

[42] Tawfick W, Sultan S. Does topical wound oxygen (TWO 2) offer an improved outcome over conventional compression dressings (CCD) in the management of refractory venous ulcers (RVU)? A parallel observational comparative study. European Journal of Vascular and Endovascular Surgery. 2009 Jul 31;38(1):125–32.

[43] Tawfick WA, Sultan S. Technical and clinical outcome of topical wound oxygen in comparison to conventional compression dressings in the management of refractory nonhealing venous ulcers. Vascular and Endovascular Surgery. 2012 Dec 5:1538574412467684.

[44] Eklöf B, Rutherford RB, Bergan JJ, Carpentier PH, Gloviczki P, Kistner RL, Meissner MH, Moneta GL, Myers K, Padberg FT, Perrin M. American Venous Forum International Ad Hoc Committee for Revision of the CEAP Classification. Revision of the CEAP classification for chronic venous disorders: consensus statement. Journal of Vascular Surgery. 2004 Dec;40(6):1248–52.

[45] Meissner MH, Gloviczki P, Bergan J, Kistner RL, Morrison N, Pannier F, Pappas PJ, Rabe E, Raju S, Villavicencio JL. Primary chronic venous disorders. Journal of Vascular Surgery. 2007 Dec 31;46(6):S54–67.

[46] Tawfick W, Sultan S. Early results of topical wound oxygen (TWO2) therapy in the management of refractory nonhealing venous ulcers: superior role over conventional compression dressings. Vascular. 2008;16(Suppl 2):S156e7.

[47] Tawfick W, Sultan S. Topical wound oxygen versus conventional compression dressings in the management of refractory venous ulcers: a parallel observational pivotal study. Irish Journal of Medical Science. 2007;176(1):S2.

[48] Meissner MH, Moneta G, Burnand K, Gloviczki P, Lohr JM, Lurie F, Mattos MA, McLafferty RB, Mozes G, Rutherford RB, Padberg F. The hemodynamics and diagnosis of venous disease. Journal of Vascular Surgery. 2007 Dec 31;46(6):S4–24.

[49] Ricci MA, Emmerich J, Callas PW, Rosendaal FR, Stanley AC, Naud S, Vossen C, Bovill EG. Evaluating chronic venous disease with a new venous severity scoring system. Journal of Vascular Surgery. 2003 Nov 30;38(5):909–15.

[50] Nelson EA, Harper DR, Prescott RJ, Gibson B, Brown D, Ruckley CV. Prevention of recurrence of venous ulceration: randomized controlled trial of class 2 and class 3 elastic compression. Journal of Vascular Surgery. 2006 Oct 31;44(4):803–8.

[51] Ghauri AS, Taylor MC, Deacon JE, Whyman MR, Earnshaw JJ, Heather BP, Poskitt KR. Influence of a specialized leg ulcer service on management and outcome. British Journal of Surgery. 2000 Aug 1;87(8):1048–56.

[52] Fletcher A, Cullum N, Sheldon TA. A systematic review of compression treatment for venous leg ulcers. British Medical Journal. 1997 Sep 6;315(7108):576–80.

[53] Gordillo GM, Roy S, Khanna S, Schlanger R, Khandelwal S, Phillips G, Sen CK. Topical oxygen therapy induces vascular endothelial growth factor expression and improves closure of clinically presented chronic wounds. Clinical and Experimental Pharmacology and Physiology. 2008 Aug 1;35(8):957–64.

[54] Blackman E, Moore C, Hyatt J, Railton R, Frye C. Topical wound oxygen therapy in the treatment of severe diabetic foot ulcers: a prospective controlled study. Ostomy/Wound Management. 2010 Jun 1;56(6):24.

[55] Michaels JA, Campbell B, King B, Palfreyman SJ, Shackley P, Stevenson M. Randomized controlled trial and cost-effectiveness analysis of silver-donating antimicrobial dress-

ings for venous leg ulcers (VULCAN trial). British Journal of Surgery. 2009 Oct 1;96(10): 1147–56.

[56] Rodriguez PG, Felix FN, Woodley DT, Shim EK. The role of oxygen in wound healing: a review of the literature. Dermatologic Surgery. 2008 Sep 1;34(9):1159–69.

[57] Schreml S, Szeimies RM, Prantl L, Karrer S, Landthaler M, Babilas P. Oxygen in acute and chronic wound healing. British Journal of Dermatology. 2010 Aug 1;163(2):257–68.

[58] Asano S. Leukocyte. In: Uchiyama T, eds. Miwa Hematology 3rd edn, 292–5, Hakuhodo, Tokyo, 2006.

[59] McAllister TA, Stark JM, Norman JN, Ross RM. Inhibitory effects of hyperbaric oxygen on bacteria and fungi. The Lancet. 1963 Nov 16;282(7316):1040–2.

[60] Hohn DC. Host resistance of infection. In: Hunt TK, ed. Wound healing and wound infection. 264–80, Appleton-Century Crofts, New York, 1980.

[61] Leach RM, Rees PJ, Wilmshurst P. Hyperbaric oxygen therapy. British Medical Journal. 1998 Oct 24;317(7166):1140–3.

[62] Kindwall EP. A history of hyperbaric medicine. Hyperbaric medicine practice. Best Publishing Company, Arizona. 1994:2–16.

[63] Sheikh AY, Gibson JJ, Rollins MD, Hopf HW, Hussain Z, Hunt TK. Effect of hyperoxia on vascular endothelial growth factor levels in a wound model. Archives of Surgery. 2000 Nov 1;135(11):1293–7.

[64] Roy S, Khanna S, Nallu K, Hunt TK, Sen CK. Dermal wound healing is subject to redox control. Molecular Therapy. 2006 Jan 1;13(1):211–20.

Chapter 14

Pressure Ulcers

Jill M. Monfre

Additional information is available at the end of the chapter

http://dx.doi.org/10.5772/63572

Abstract

Pressure ulcers or pressure injuries occur in all health care settings and are considered a quality care indicator. Individuals in every health care setting must routinely be assessed for factors that place them at risk for development of pressure ulcers and have routine skin assessments to assess for the presence of pressure ulcers. If risks for pressure ulcer development or actual pressure ulcers are identified, it is crucial that a prevention and treatment plan be developed and implemented to address the risks and treat the wounds. For a prevention and treatment plan to be comprehensive and effective, it must be evidence based and multidisciplinary. The plan needs to address the risk factors or wound concerns specific to the individual and include education for the providers, caregivers and individuals at risk for pressure ulcer development and/or with pressure ulcers. Expert consensus panels concur that despite evidence-based multidisciplinary comprehensive pressure ulcer prevention plans, there are clinical situations in which pressure ulcers are deemed unavoidable.

Keywords: Pressure, Ulcer, pressure injury, decubitus, bed sore, prevention, treatment

1. Introduction

Pressure ulcers, also referred to as decubitus ulcers, pressure sores or bed sores and recently referred to as pressure injures by the National Pressure Ulcer Advisory Panel (NPUAP) [1], are a common occurrence in all health care settings, including acute care hospitals, long-term care facilities, rehabilitation centers and subacute care centers [2]. Pressure ulcers have a significant impact on patients, families and health care facilities. These wounds can cause pain and suffering to individuals, produce emotional distress for families and significant others, increase the length of a hospital stay and increase the costs to facilities. The incidence of a pressure ulcer can also lead health care providers to feel as though they have failed to deliver quality care to those who have been entrusted to their care [3]. It is important to identify individuals who are at risk for pressure ulcer development or those who have developed a pressure ulcer, in order to implement preventative or treatment measures; these individuals also require close monitoring.

2. Definition

The National Pressure Ulcer Advisory Panel (NPUAP), an organization comprised of leading experts in health care dedicated to the prevention and management of pressure ulcers, during a consensus conference held in the spring of 2016 replaced the term pressure ulcer with pressure injury to more accurately reflect injuries related to pressure in both intact and ulcerated skin [1]. The NPUAP also revised their definition of a pressure injury as *localized damaged to the skin and/or underlying soft tissue usually over a bony prominence or related to a medical or other device. The injury can present as intact skin or an open ulcer and may be painful. The injury occurs as a result of intense and/or prolonged pressure or pressure in combination with shear. The tolerance of soft tissue for pressure and shear may also be affected by microclimate, nutrition, perfusion, comorbidities and condition of the soft tissue* [1]. The European Pressure Ulcer Advisory Panel (EPUAP), also a leading organization of wound care experts, continues to use the term pressure ulcer as well as the definition originally developed in conjunction with the NPUAP, which states a pressure ulcer is a *localized injury to the skin and/or underlying tissue usually over a bony prominence, as a result of pressure, or pressure in combination with shear* [4].

3. Etiology

Pressure ulcers, the term that will be used throughout this chapter, occur across all health care settings with the most common setting for the occurrence of pressure ulcers being acute care hospitals followed by long-term care facilities then equally in occurrence in an individual's home and nursing facilities [5]. Pressure ulcers usually occur on the lower half of the body with two-thirds occurring in the pelvic region such as the sacrum, coccyx or hip areas and one-third occurring on the lower extremities. The occurrence of pressure ulcers on the heels is increasing. **Table 1** indicates bony prominences of the body, the location where pressure ulcers occur most often [6].

Approximately 10% of pressure ulcers are device related [7]. Multiple medical devices or pieces of medical equipment can lead to pressure ulcer development. Items such as endotracheal tubes, feeding tubes, cervical collars, tracheostomy tubes and positive pressure airway masks all have the potential for creating pressure ulcers due to pressure points created by the device. Transfer boards or slide boards place an individual at risk for shear injuries due to sliding over the firm surface.

The most common age group for the incidence of pressure ulcers is the elderly, especially those 70 and older. The occurrence of a pressure ulcer in an elderly individual increases their mortality rate fivefold. In hospital, when a patient has developed a pressure ulcer, mortality increases by 25% in the over 70 age group [5].

Prone position (lying on stomach)

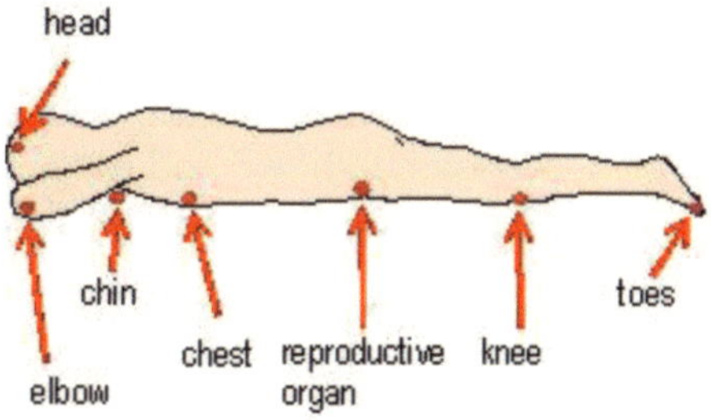

Supine position (lying on back)

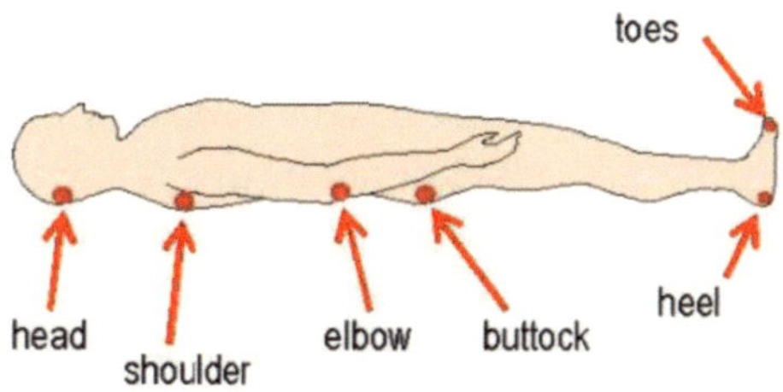

Lateral position (lying on side)

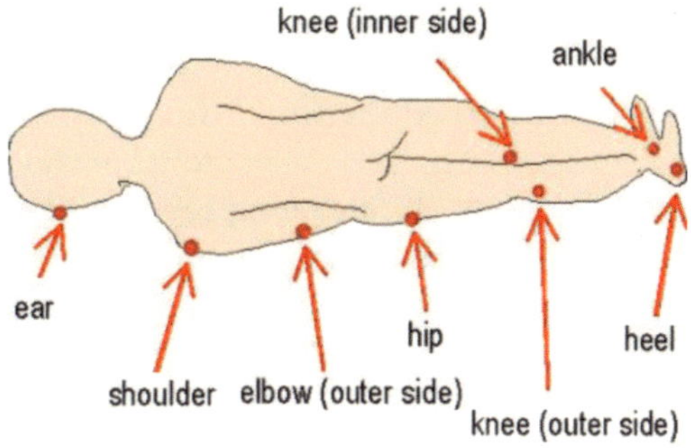

Sitting position

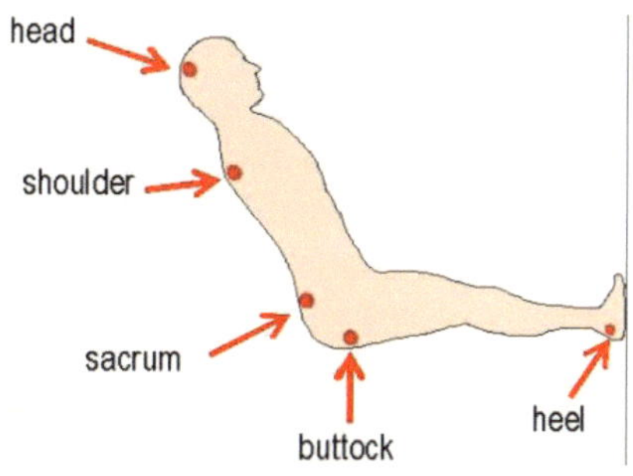

Table 1. Pressure ulcer pressure points.

4. Pathogenesis

The development of a pressure ulcer is not solely dependent upon pressure [8]. Multiple factors that modify the effect of pressure on tissues play a role in the development of pressure ulcers. The tolerance tissues have to external load depends on the duration of the exerted load. High loads can be tolerated for short periods of time, while relatively low loads can be tolerated for longer periods of time. The internal load in the tissues, as a result of the external load, causes cell deformation, occlusion of blood and lymphatic vessels and ischemia. If the internal load could be measured a risk for pressure ulcer, development could potentially be quantified [8].

A pressure ulcer results from sustained compression of soft tissues [5]. This compression occurs most often between a bony prominence and an external surface. Blood flow supplies oxygen and nutrients to the tissues. If pressure is sustained, the blood supply to the tissues is interrupted. When the blood flow is interrupted, oxygen and nutrients are not delivered to the tissues. Without oxygen and nutrients, the tissue will be damaged and eventually die [5].

Not all types of pressure are equally damaging to tissues [9]. Hydrostatic pressure, the pressure exerted by a liquid, as is endured by divers for long periods of time does not result in pressure ulcer formation. Yet localized pressure, as is exerted on the sacrum of a bedbound patient in the supine position for an extended period of time, often causes tissue distortion and blockage of the blood vessels resulting in much more damage. Studies related to localized pressure have found that pressure applied over a bony prominence resulted in more damage to the muscle than to the skin causing the study team to conclude that the muscle is more sensitive to pressure than is the skin or subcutaneous tissue [9].

Further studies identified specific factors associated with the development of a pressure ulcer including; interface pressure, shear, moisture and friction [4]. The NPUAP, after investigating shear and friction which have long been associated with pressure ulcer development, has eliminated friction from its definition of a pressure ulcer the explanation of which will be discussed below [10].

Interface pressure contributes to pressure ulcer development, as it is the pressure that develops between the skin and a surface upon which an individual is sitting or lying. Interface pressure is a measure commonly used to evaluate the effectiveness of a support surface [11]. Pressure mapping measures interface pressures and helps to determine appropriate positioning [8].

Not all localized pressure results in a pressure ulcer. When the pressure of short duration is relieved, blood flow returns to the area. This occurrence is known as reactive hyperemia, blood vessels in the area of pressure dilate in an attempt to overcome the ischemia that occurs with the pressure. Reactive hyperemia is transient and is also described as blanchable erythema—an area that becomes white when pressed with a finger and returns to erythema when the compression is removed [11].

Pressure that is not relieved and is of longer duration leads to further decreased capillary blood flow, occlusion of lymphatic vessels and tissue ischemia. Over a bony prominence, pressure of 20 mmHg can increase to as much as 300 mmHg. If this pressure is sustained, destruction

http://dx.doi.org/10.5772/63572

of deep tissues can occur including destruction of muscle, subcutaneous tissue, dermis and epidermis [11].

When capillaries are occluded metabolic waste begins to accumulate in the surrounding tissues due to the lack of oxygen and nutrients. Capillaries that are damaged become more permeable and leak fluid into the interstitial space-causing edema. Perfusion is slowed through the edematous tissue; therefore, hypoxia worsens. Hypoxia increases cell death that results in an increased metabolic waste released into the surrounding tissues [11]. The ensuing edema further compresses small vessels causing increased edema and ischemia. Local tissue death occurs, which results in a pressure ulcer [7].

Shear is an applied force that causes an opposite yet parallel sliding motion such as when an individual slides in a bed or chair. The individual's skeletal structure slides in one direction yet the skin layer is restrained in the original position secondary to friction forces. In these situations, when shear is involved, multiple studies have found the pressure needed to occlude the blood vessels is much less than in an area where shear force is not involved [5, 8]. Elderly individuals are at higher risk for the effects of shear due to the decreased amount of elastin in their skin which is a normal consequence of aging [5].

Moisture, another factor associated with the development of pressure ulcers, alters the resiliency of the epidermis to external forces [11]. The effects of friction and shear are increased in the presence of moisture. Increased moisture is often associated with incontinence, perspiration or wound exudate [5].

Friction was originally determined to be a causative factor in the development of pressure ulcers after a study by Sidney Dinsdale was published in 1974 [10]. The results of this study showed that significantly less pressure was needed to stimulate the development of a full or partial thickness wound when the pressure was applied in conjunction with friction.

There are several forms of friction as they relate to the development of pressure ulcers. Friction, as a general term, is the rubbing of two body parts together. It is also a force that resists the motion of two bodies and/or material elements sliding against each other. In relation to skin breakdown, the type of friction, that is of concern is dry friction, of which there are two types, namely static and kinetic. Static friction is the force that resists the motion between two bodies when there is no sliding. There are multiple aspects that impact the amount of static friction at the skin surface including an individual's hydration level and what the individual is in contact with, for example bed linen. Moisture is an important factor relative to static friction as humidity and liquid moisture increases the friction and may cause an individual to adhere to a surface. Dynamic friction, also known as kinetic friction, is the force between two bodies relative to one another as they are sliding. Dynamic friction occurs when an individual slides downward in bed or rubs a foot in a shoe causing a blister. Such a blister may be misdiagnosed as a pressure ulcer.

In relation to the Dinsdale study, the type of friction applied during the study was not noted. The results of this study showed that the blood flow to the epidermis in a given area was not significantly different when pressure and friction were applied together and when pressure was applied alone. Investigators concluded that increased susceptibility of lesions with friction was not due to ischemia in the epidermis. Three decades later, it has been hypothesized that the friction used in Dinsdale's study was creating shear strain or deformation in deeper layers of tissue. Current hypothesis is that friction causes mechanically damaging shear strain of superficial tissue cells and tissue damage results directly from excessive deformation not ischemia as previously thought.

Friction is an important factor as it leads to shear stress and strain yet does not alone lead to the development of a pressure ulcer. Friction contributes to the development of a pressure ulcer due to the shear forces it can create. In other words, friction causes the shear forces in the tissue, which can increase the risk of tissue breakdown and lead to the development of a pressure ulcer. Therefore, shear remains in the current NPUAP definition of a pressure ulcer yet friction is eliminated. Including friction would be redundant as friction is now thought to be a cause of shear. Also, eliminating friction may decrease the number of wounds that are misdiagnosed as pressure ulcers when they are caused solely by friction [10].

5. Pressure ulcer stages

Pressure ulcers are classified by the amount of visible tissue loss [4]. Depth of tissue loss is important, as it determines a treatment plan of care and can impact payment. Once a wound is determined to be a pressure ulcer, it is assigned a pressure ulcer-specific stage or category. No other wound utilizes this same staging/categorizing system. A stage or category is assigned after careful and thorough assessment of the pressure ulcer to determine the extent of tissue destruction. To complete this assessment, one must have a competent understanding of the anatomy of the tissue layers involved and of the physiology of pressure ulcer development.

The NPUAP has defined the stages or categories of pressure ulcers as follows (**Table 2**):

EPUAP staging guideline	
Stage I	Nonblanchable erythema—Intact skin with nonblanchable redness of a localized area usually over a bony prominence. Darkly pigmented skin may not have visible blanching; its color may differ from the surrounding area. The area may be painful, firm, soft, warmer or cooler as compared to adjacent tissue. Category I may be difficult to detect in individuals with dark skin tones. May indicate "at-risk" persons.
Stage II	Partial thickness skin loss—partial thickness loss of dermis presenting as a shallow open ulcer with a red pink wound bed, without slough. May also present as an intact or open/ruptured serum-filled or sero-sanguinous-filled blister. Presents as a shiny or dry shallow ulcer without slough or bruising. This category should not be used to describe skin tears, tape burns, incontinence-associated dermatitis, maceration or excoriation
Stage III	Full-thickness skin loss—Full-thickness tissue loss. Subcutaneous fat may be visible but bone, tendon or muscles are not exposed. Slough may be present but does not obscure the depth of tissue loss. May

http://dx.doi.org/10.5772/63572

EPUAP staging guideline	
	include undermining and tunneling. The depth of a category/stage III pressure ulcer varies by anatomical location. The bridge of the nose, ear, occiput and malleolus do not have (adipose) subcutaneous tissue and category/stage III ulcer can be shallow. In contrast, areas of significant adiposity can develop extremely deep category/stage III pressure ulcers. Bone/tendon is not visible or directly palpable.
Stage IV	Full-thickness tissue loss—Full-thickness tissue loss with exposed bone, tendon or muscle. Slough or eschar may be present. Often includes undermining and tunneling. The depth of a category/stage IV pressure ulcer varies by anatomical location. The bridge of the nose, ear, occiput and malleolus do not have (adipose) subcutaneous tissue and these ulcers can be shallow. Category/stage IV ulcers can extend into muscle and/or supporting structures (e.g., fascia, tendon or joint capsule) making osteomyelitis or osteitis likely to occur. Exposed bone/muscle is visible or directly palpable.
Unstageable	Full-thickness skin or tissue loss—depth unknown—Full-thickness tissue loss in which actual depth of the ulcer is completely obscured by slough (yellow, tan, gray, green or brown) and/or eschar (tan, brown or black) in the wound bed. Until enough slough and/or eschar are removed to expose the base of the wound, the true depth cannot be determined, but it will be either a category/stage III or IV. Stable (dry, adherent, intact without erythema or fluctuance) eschar on the heels service as "the body's natural (biological) cover" and should not be removed
Suspected deep tissue injury (sDTI)	SDTI depth unknown—Purple- or maroon-localized area of discolored intact skin or blood-filled blister due to damage of underlying soft tissue from pressure and/or shear. The area may be preceded by tissue that is painful, firm, mushy, boggy, warmer or cooler as compared to adjacent tissue. Deep tissue injury may be difficult to detect in individuals with dark skin tomes. Evolution may include a thin blister over a dark wound bed. The may further evolve and become covered with thin eschar. Evolution may be rapid exposing additional layers of tissue even with optimal treatment.

Table 2. Pressure ulcer staging [4].

An illustration of the pressure ulcer stages/categories is seen in **Table 3** [1].

As pressure ulcers heal, the lost muscle, subcutaneous fat or dermis are not replaced with like tissue before they re-epithelialize [12]. A pressure ulcer fills in with scar tissue, which is composed primarily of endothelial cells, fibroblasts, collagen and extracellular matrix. Therefore, a stage-III pressure ulcer, for example, cannot, as the wound heals, become a stage-II pressure ulcer and progress on to a stage-I pressure ulcer because the term stage I would not accurately reflect the structures that are now present under the newly re-epithelialized tissue. Referring to a healing stage-III pressure ulcer as a stage II, then a stage-I pressure ulcer is known as reverse staging or down staging and is not acceptable. The stage needs to reflect the scar tissue that has developed. Therefore, the stage for this healing pressure ulcer is "healing stage-III pressure ulcer" and when the pressure ulcer has healed, the stage is a "healed stage-III pressure ulcer," indicating the pressure ulcer is now filled with granulation or scar tissue and resurfaced with epithelium [12].

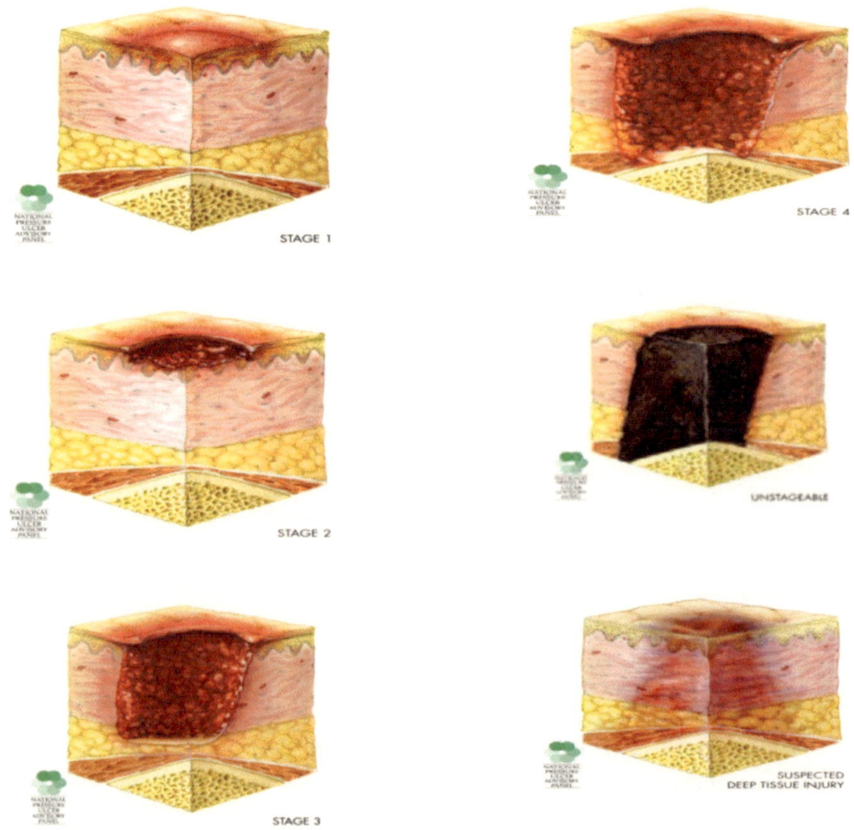

Table 3. Pressure ulcer injury/ulcer stages/categories.

Mucosal pressure injuries are *pressure injuries found on mucous membranes with a history of a medical device in use at the location of the ulcer* [1]. A mucous membrane is the moist lining of a body cavity, such as the gastrointestinal tract, nasal passages, urinary tract and vaginal canal, that communicates with the exterior. When pressure is applied to a mucous membrane, ischemia can result that can lead to a pressure ulcer. Mucous membranes are vulnerable to pressure especially related to medical devices such as oxygen tubing, feeding tubes, urinary catheters and fecal containment devices [13].

The anatomy of mucous membranes impacts the staging or categorizing of a mucous membrane pressure injury [13]. There are two types of mucous membrane tissue; nonkeratinized stratified squamous epithelium and an underlying connective tissue layer, the lamina propria. These layers are similar to the epidermis and dermis and are connected via rete pegs. At the interface of the two layers is a basal laminal layer. The epithelial layer is continuously renewed through migration of lower layers of epithelium to the surface. The epithelium of the mucosa, although is not keratinized like the epithelium of the skin. The lamina propria generally contains blood vessels, elastin and collagen fibers [13].

http://dx.doi.org/10.5772/63572

Injured mucosa heals similarly as skin with the exception of scar formation [13]. There is an increasing evidence that the fibroblasts in mucosa resembles fetal fibroblasts. Most mucosal injuries heal without scar formation [13].

The staging or categorizing of pressure ulcers that is used for the skin cannot be used to stage mucosal pressure injuries [13]. Nonblanchable erythema cannot be seen in mucous membranes, as superficial tissue losses of the nonkeratinized epithelium are so shallow they cannot be differentiated from deeper, full thickness injuries. The coagulum seen on a mucous membrane pressure injury resembles slough yet it is actually soft blood clot. Muscle is seldom seen in a mucous membrane pressure injury and bone is not present in these tissues. Therefore, pressure injuries located on a mucous membrane are referred to as mucous membrane pressure injuries [13].

6. Pressure ulcer prevention

There are several factors that have been associated with the development of pressure ulcers. Many of these factors affect an individual's ability to withstand episodes of pressure and shear as well as decrease the length of time or amount of pressure necessary to cause tissue damage. Risk factors that can lead to pressure ulcer development include age, immobility, nutritional deficiencies, skin moisture and incontinence, vasopressor use, chronic diseases such as diabetes or stroke, smoking, behavioral issues leading to noncompliance, poor general health and sensory loss [14, 15]. No single factor can explain all pressure ulcers rather it is a complex interaction among factors which increases the probability of pressure ulcer development

Braden scale	Norton scale	Waterlow scale	Jackson Cubbin scale
Sensory perception	Physical condition	Sex	Age
Moisture	Mental status	Age	Weight
Activity	Activity	Appetite	Skin condition
Mobility	Mobility	Nurses' visual assessment of skin	Mental status
Nutrition status	Continence	condition	Mobility
Friction/shear		Mobility	Nutrition
		Continence	Respiration
		Factors contributing to tissue Malnutrition	Continence
		Neurologic deficits	Hygiene
		Major surgery or trauma	Hemodynamic status
		Medication	

Table 4. Pressure ulcer risk assessment tools.

Prevention begins with identifying those individuals at risk for pressure ulcer development. A pressure ulcer risk assessment instrument that has been validated for use in the specific age group should be utilized. In the Unites States, the most common adult risk assessment instruments are The Braden and Norton scales that have been tested for validity in predicting pressure ulcer development risk [7, 16]. In Britain, the most common scales are the Braden and the Waterlow. The Jackson Cubbin Scale is specific to European critical care (**Table 4**).

These scales will identify specific factors related to assessment categories that place an individual at risk for pressure ulcer development. Once specific factors are identified, a prevention plan to address those factors can be implemented to reduce or eliminate the risk of pressure ulcer development [3, 16]. With the implementation of an evidence-based pressure ulcer prevention plan, pressure reduction can occur which will preserve the microcirculation and prevent the development of pressure ulcers [17]. A pressure ulcer prevention plan is multifaceted. Factors related to prevention and discussed further in treatment, as these factors are also included in a treatment plan, include; mobility, moisture and continence care, nutrition and hydration, support surfaces, documentation and education. No single intervention has been found that will consistently, reliably and completely reduce pressure ulcer development. Pressure ulcer prevention involves multiple interventions and a multidisciplinary team to affect the identified factors and reduce the risk of pressure ulcer development.

7. Pressure ulcer treatment

The treatment of pressure ulcers is based on the physiology of wound healing. Wound healing is a complex process that changes with the health status of the individual [17]. A health care provider needs to have a basic knowledge of the phases of wound healing including; hemostasis, inflammation, proliferation and maturation. Once a provider understands wound healing, one has a significant piece of the knowledge necessary to develop a pressure ulcer treatment plan [18].

7.1. Phases of wound healing

The first phase of wound healing is hemostasis. Briefly, in this phase, damaged blood vessels are sealed when platelets form a stable clot to seal the blood vessel. The platelets also stimulate the clotting cascade through the production of thrombin that initiates the production of fibrin. The fibrin mesh ultimately strengthens the platelet aggregate into a hemostatic plug. Hemostasis occurs within minutes of injury unless the injured individual has underlying clotting disorders [18].

In the second phase of wound healing, the inflammation phase, the erythema, swelling and warmth that occur are often associated with pain. This phase of wound healing usually lasts up to 4 days after injury. During this phase, neutrophils or PMN's (polymorphonucleocytes) and plasma are leaked from the blood vessels into the surrounding tissue. These factors clean debris from the surrounding tissue and provide the first line of defence against infection. Macrophages are also active in the second phase of wound healing acting to destroy bacteria and secreting growth factors which direct the third phase of wound healing.

Chronic wounds, wounds that take longer than 12 weeks to heal, often remain in the inflammatory stage longer than occurs with acute wounds. Cellular and molecular abnormalities within a wound bed prevent progression through the stages of healing [19]. Chronic wounds contain elevated inflammatory cytokines and proteases. Chronic wounds do not respond to growth factors in the same manner in which acute wounds do. Specifically related to pressure ulcers, the volume of exudate is often times increased in chronic wounds. Secondary to infection, the exudate may be more purulent. If protein levels are low, the exudate may appear thinner [19]. Chronic wounds often have inadequate blood supply that also contributes to delayed healing and the formation of unhealthy granulation tissue.

The third phase of wound healing, the proliferation phase, begins approximately 4 days after injury and usually lasts until day 21 postinjury. The activity during this phase is replacement of dermal tissue and possibly subdermal tissue and contraction of the wound. Fibroblasts secrete collagen, which is the framework upon which new dermal regeneration, can occur. Angiogenesis, development of new capillaries, also occurs during this phase of wound healing. Keratinocytes differentiate to form the protective outer layer.

In the final phase of wound healing, maturation, remodeling of the dermal layer occurs to produce greater tensile strength. The cells that are involved in this process are fibroblasts. This process can take up to 2 years to complete [18].

7.2. Principles of wound healing

In addition to knowledge of wound healing, a provider must also be aware of the principles of wound treatment and intervention. For a wound to progress to healing, the wound bed must be well vascularized, free of devitalized tissue, free of infection and moist. Continual evaluation of a wound is necessary as the wound progresses through the stages of wound healing.

7.3. Dressings

No one dressing is appropriate for all wounds. There are multiple factors that will affect the dressing selected for a particular wound **Table 5**.

Knowledge of the properties of available wound dressings and an understanding that a treatment plan may need to change as the wound progresses through the stages of healing is vital. Wounds that do not advance through the process of healing in a reasonable or expected time frame must be assessed for issues that have not been previously identified or wound changes that have occurred and the treatment plan re-evaluated **Table 6**.

The principles in selecting dressings for pressure ulcer treatment include eliminate dead space, control exudate, prevent bacterial overgrowth, ensure proper moisture balance, cost-efficiency, and manageability for the individual, caregiver and providers.

Several adjuvant therapies/advanced dressings have been used to treat pressure ulcers. These therapies include (a) platelet-derived growth factor (PDGF) applied to the wound bed, which will stimulate the growth of cells involved in wound healing and granulation tissue formation; (b) negative pressure wound therapy (NPWT), which utilizes subatmospheric pressure applied to a wound via a sealed dressing to promote wound healing, the applied suction removes drainage and increases blood flow to the wound; and (c) hyperbaric oxygen therapy, delivered in multiple modes—total body, body part or mask—exposes the body to 100% oxygen at a higher pressure than normally experienced, this therapy provides oxygen necessary to stimulate wound healing and combats infection by enhancing leukocyte and macrophage activity [20]. PDGR and hyperbaric oxygen, although supported for use, have less support than does NPWT in studies conducted on individuals with pressure ulcers [20].

Wound depth	Partial thickness Full thickness
Wound description	Necrotic Slough Granulating Epithelializing
Wound characteristics	Dry Moist Heavily exudating Malodorous Excessively painful Difficult to dress
Bacterial description	Colonized Infected

Table 5. Wound description.

Alginate	Highly absorbent, useful for wounds with copious exudate. Alginate rope is particularly useful to pack exudate cavities or tracts
Hydrofiber	Absorbent dressing used for exudative wounds
Debriding agents	Useful for necrotic wounds, often used as an adjunct to surgical debridement
Foam	Useful for clean granulating wounds with minimal exudate
Hydrocolloid	Useful for dry necrotic wounds, wounds with minimal exudate or clean granulating wounds
Hydrogel	Useful for dry, sloughy, necrotic wounds
Transparent film	Useful for clean, dry wounds with minimal exudate, protect high friction areas
Negative pressure wound therapy	Conforms to the wound bed by suction and stimulates wound contraction while removing exudate

Table 6. Dressings [17].

There is limited evidence, although moderate strength, indicating support for the use of radiant heat dressings to improve pressure ulcer healing. Radiant heat dressings are noncontact dressings attached to a heating element. These dressings provide warmth to the wound and have been found to increase capillary blood flow to the area and thus increase wound healing. Also with limited yet moderate strength of evidence is the use of electrical stimulation, which provides a direct electrical current through the wound bed using electrodes on the surface of the wound. One hour daily session has been shown to be most effective. Caution has been noted not to use electrical stimulation on individuals with cancer as the treatment could stimulate the cancerous cells. The American College of Physicians specifically notes electrical stimulation in its guidelines [15].

http://dx.doi.org/10.5772/63572

7.4. Treatment plan

Prior to the development of a comprehensive pressure ulcer treatment plan, consideration should be given to an individual's psychological, behavioral and cognitive status. The individual's goals and prognosis need to be determined as well as the resources an individual has available, both financially and as caregivers.

A multidisciplinary team is needed to develop a comprehensive pressure ulcer prevention and treatment plan, as numerous factors are addressed. The team may include the individual's primary care provider, a wound care specialist, nurses or medical assistants who will provide wound care or education, social workers who will assist the individual and family members with resources and emotional concerns, a physical therapist who will provide assistance with mobility therapy and any other necessary consultants.

Within the plan, the following needs may need to be addressed.

Debridement of necrotic tissue within an acute wound may be necessary to be able to completely assess the wound. Necrotic tissue may obscure underlying fluid collections that need to be identified. Necrotic tissue also promotes bacterial growth that impairs wound healing and therefore should be debrided [17]. However, debridement is not recommended for stable dry eschar on heel wounds with no edema, erythema or fluctuance. Debridement can be achieved by multiple methods including sharp debridement, mechanical, enzymatic or autolytic debridement. Most sharp debridement can be completed at bedside, yet if more extensive sharp debridement is needed it may need to be performed in an operating room [17].

Mobilization of an individual is an important component to a pressure ulcer treatment plan. Since, by definition, a pressure ulcer is caused, in part, by pressure, if an individual begins to mobilize pressure will be relieved individuals who cannot ambulate redistributing pressure on a support surface needs to be investigated.

Moisture management, controlling incontinence and excess perspiration by wicking moisture away from the skin, will impact the effect of moisture. Managing moisture will increase the ability of the epidermis to return to its original state after being exposed to pressure. Shear and friction also will not be as detrimental to the skin when moisture is not allowed to be in contact with the skin for prolonged periods of time.

Nutrition studies indicated weak evidence that nutritional interventions provide benefits in the prevention or treatment of pressure ulcers [15]. A guideline presented by the American College of Physicians in 2015 cited moderate quality evidence supporting protein supplements in treating pressure ulcers. A Cochrane review in 2014 concluded that there is no evidence to support nutritional interventions, including protein, provide any benefits in preventing or treating pressure ulcers. A study regarding vitamin C supplements concluded that there was no change in wound healing. No results were noted related to zinc due to insufficient evidence. Although, evidence supports that providing adequate nutrition is important. Oral nutrition is preferred, yet if not possible; provide nutrition by the most appropriate route.

Oxygenation and perfusion must be ensured. A primary reason for inadequate tissue oxygenation is vasoconstriction as a result of sympathetic over activity. Blood volume deficit, pain and hypothermia are common causes of sympathetic overactivity for which the end result could be increased risk for pressure ulcer development.

Infection is usually determined clinically [15]. All open wounds contain some degree of bacteria. Healing is most often not impaired until bacteria reach a high colony count. If a wound culture needed, evidence indicates the Levine technique should be used. This technique involves rotating a swab over a 1 cm^2 patch of wound with enough pressure to express fluid from the wound for 5 s. A tissue or bone biopsy is the preferred method of identification of osteomyelitis, although biopsies of this nature are not always feasible. Magnetic resonance imaging (MRI) and nuclear medicine tests are more sensitive and specific than conventional plain radiography in identifying osteomyelitis. When bone is exposed in a pressure ulcer, osteomyelitis is often presumed.

An individual with increasing pain may be exhibiting a sign of a wound infection. Other signs of an acute wound infection include erythema around the ulcer's edges, induration, warmth and purulent drainage, no progression toward healing for 2 weeks, friable granulation tissue, foul odor, new necrotic tissue or lack of even spread of granulation tissue across the base of the wound. An individual may also exhibit systemic symptoms of a wound infection including fever, delirium and confusion [15].

Repositioning is replacing the term turning. The aim of repositioning individuals at risk for pressure ulcer development is to relieve pressure and/or redistribute pressure. It has been found that a slight change in position can be adequate to aid in relieving pressure. A turn of 30°, as previously encouraged for an individual in bed, for pressure relief, is not always needed to relieve pressure from bony prominences.

There is no research to support repositioning individuals every 2 h will aid in preventing the development of pressure ulcers; this recommendation is based on expert opinion [15]. The frequency of repositioning will, in part, be determined by an individual's tissue tolerance or the ability of both the individual's skin and its underlying structures to withstand pressure without an adverse effect.

As a provider or caregiver, when an individual at risk for pressure ulcer development is in bed, avoid positions with the head of the bed elevated to the point in which excess pressure and shear are applied to the sacrum and coccyx. This is most often any point beyond 30°.

In the seated position, the greatest exposure to pressure is to the ischial tuberosities. The area of the ischial tuberosities is relatively small; therefore, the pressure will be high. Without pressure relief, a pressure ulcer will develop quickly.

If a patient has a reddened area as a result of a previous episode of pressure loading, it is not advisable to position the individual on the same body surface. The reddened area indicates the body has not recovered from the previous position on the body surface and continues to require relief from the pressure load.

If heels are left in contact with a surface for a prolonged period of time, it is not unusual for heel pressure ulcers to develop due to the significant volume of bony structure in relation to the soft tissue in the heel. For the protection of the heels or treatment of heel, pressure ulcers

http://dx.doi.org/10.5772/63572

assure that heels are elevated off any surface. Heels should be elevated so as to distribute the weight of the leg along the calf without putting pressure on the Achilles tendon. To avoid obstruction of the popliteal vein, which begins behind the knee, which may lead to a deep vein thrombosis, care must be taken to not hyperextend the knee.

Physical conditions of certain populations require additional care in positioning. These populations include those with spinal cord injuries, those that are insensate, older adults, individuals that have sustained hip fractures or those that do not maintain a healthy lifestyle.

Support surface use has been validated in studies for the prevention of pressure ulcers in high-risk individuals and for the treatment of individuals with pressure ulcers. A support surface reduces pressure by spreading the tissue load over a larger area, thus decreasing the load over bony prominences. A support surface also manages the microclimate including moisture and temperature.

Support surface selection is based on mobility, comfort and circumstances of care. In a home setting, consideration is given to the structure of the home including width of doors, power supply and available ventilation for heat from the motor as these factors relate to the support surface to be utilized. If a spouse or significant, other will share the bed consideration should be given to his or her comfort also.

Regular foam does not distribute patient weight uniformly and may worsen or cause pressure ulcers. A higher specification foam mattress is more effective in preventing pressure ulcers

When an individual is placed on a low-air loss, surface consideration must be given to the linens and pads used on the surface. Linens and pads should not be of materials that will block the air flow.

An issue that can negatively impact an individual at risk for pressure ulcer development or with a pressure ulcer that is related to any support surface is bottoming out. Bottoming out occurs when an individual's pelvic region or buttocks sink down and the support surface no longer provides adequate redistribution of pressure. An assessment for bottoming out can be performed with a hand check. Place a hand, palm side up under the support surface directly below the individual's buttocks region. If the individual can feel your hand or if less than an inch of support material is evident, the individual has bottomed out and the surface should be replaced [16].

Physician consults are generally part of a comprehensive treatment plan for individuals with pressure ulcers. Specialists may be consulted to debride wounds or with more complex wounds to perform flap procedures. Infectious disease physicians may be consulted to provide input or to monitor infected wounds especially if osteomyelitis is suspected or confirmed.

Education of providers, caregivers and individuals with pressure ulcers is a vital component to any prevention or treatment plan. Without adequate education, failure of a plan is probable. Education of providers should include how to complete a comprehensive skin and wound assessment as well as documentation of the assessments. Providers also require education on the facilities process for wound care treatment, including the principles of wound care and the products available on the wound care formulary.

Caregivers or the individual with a pressure ulcer need to be educated on the cause of the pressure ulcer, the contributing factors, prevention measures, proper nutrition, appropriate wound treatment and appropriate times to contact a provider. Education should include materials in a format understandable for the caregivers and individuals. For individuals with chronic conditions, such as spinal cord injuries, there are often times formal education programs in rehabilitation centers. It is also common to request a caregiver to receive education in the hospital prior to a patient being discharged. Education is crucial to an effective prevention and treatment plan.

8. Unavoidable pressure ulcers

In 2014, the NPUAP hosted a multidisciplinary international conference to explore the issue of unavoidable pressure ulcers. This conference brought experts together to explore, within the context of organ systems, the issue of unavoidable pressure ulcers [14]. At a previous conference in 2010, also hosted by the NPUAP, an unavoidable PU was defined *as one that may occur even though providers have evaluated the individual's clinical condition and PU risk factors have been evaluated and defined and interventions have been implemented that are consistent with individual needs, goals and recognized standards of practice.*

It was agreed upon by those in attendance at the 2014 conference that unavoidable pressure ulcers do occur. This conference also established consensus on risk factors that have in some situations been shown to increase the likelihood of the development of unavoidable pressure ulcers. In summary, the organ systems which were identified that may in some situations contribute to the development of unavoidable pressure ulcers included; (a) impaired tissue oxygenation/cardiopulmonary dysfunction—an individual cannot be repositioned due to the potential for a fatal event related to hemodynamic status, (b) hypovolemia—an individual is hemodynamically unstable which often leads to an inability to reposition an individual, (c) body edema/anasarca–leads to decrease pressure-loading tolerance and increased risk of pressure ulcer development, (d) peripheral vascular disease, lower extremity arterial and venous disease—compromised circulation that contributes to ischemia which leaves tissues more vulnerable to pressure ulcer development. Within this category, other subcategories were identified including chronic kidney disease, whereas the change in tissue tolerance may increase the likelihood of pressure ulcer development, hepatic injury which results in hypoalbuminemia that leads to edema and anasarca, sensory impairment, skin issues related to extremes in age, multiorgan dysfunction syndrome, critical status and burns all which leave patients prone to pressure ulcer development, (e) body habitus—obesity compromises an individual's ability to prevent shear injury during movement, pressure ulcer development related to moisture due to increased diaphoresis and inability to redistribute pressure over bony prominences and (f) immobility—associated with vascular congestion, dependent edema, compromised lung aeration, decreased red blood cell mass, dyspnea and activity tolerance leading to increased risk for unavoidable pressure ulcer development. The consensus panel also agreed that further research is necessary to examine the issue of unavoidable pressure ulcers [21].

http://dx.doi.org/10.5772/63572

9. Summary

A pressure ulcer rate is considered a quality care indicator in most health care settings and being an international health care concern. Most pressure ulcers are preventable. With a thorough assessment, including an assessment of an individual's skin and an assessment of pressure ulcer development risk, a comprehensive prevention and treatment plan can be developed and implemented to enhance positive outcomes.

Author details

Jill M. Monfre

Address all correspondence to: jmonfre@uwhealth.org

University Hospital, University of Wisconsin, Madison, Wisconsin, USA

References

[1] National Pressure Ulcer Advisory Panel. NPUAP Pressure Injury Stages [Internet]. April 13, 2016. Available from: http://www.npuap.org/resources/educational-and-clinical-resources/npuap-pressure-injury [Accessed: April 27, 2016]

[2] Lyder C. H. Pressure ulcer prevention and management. JAMA. 2003;289(2):223–226.

[3] Satekova L., Ziakova K. Validity of pressure ulcer risk assessment scales: review. Central European Journal of Nursing and Midwifery. 2014;5(2):85–92.

[4] National Pressure Ulcer Advisory Panel. NPUAP Pressure Ulcer Stages/Categories [Internet]. 2014. Available from: http://www.npuap.org/resources/educational-and-clinical-resources [Accessed: February 18, 2016]

[5] Grey J. E., Enoch S., Harding K. G. ABC of wound healing: pressure ulcers. BMJ. 2006;332(25):472–475.

[6] Images of Imgarcade. [Internet]. April 2015, Available from: http://www.Imgarcade.com [accessed February 13, 2016]

[7] Cooper K. L. Evidence-based prevention of pressure ulcers in the intensive care unit. Critical Care Nurse. 2013;33(6):57–66.

[8] Reenalda J., Jannink M., Nederhand M., Ijzerman M. Clinical use of interface pressure to predict pressure ulcer development: a systematic review. Assistive Technology. 2009;21:76–85.

[9] Loerakker, S. Aetiology of pressure ulcers [thesis]. Eindhoven, Netherlands: Eindhoven University of Technology; 2007. 24 p.

[10] National Pressure Ulcer Advisory Panel. Friction Induced Skin Injuries-Are They Pressure Ulcers? A National Pressure Ulcer Advisory Panel White Paper [Internet]. November 20, 2012. Available from: http://NPUAP.org [Accessed: February 14, 2016]

[11] Pieper B. Mechanical forces: pressure, shear and friction. In: Ruth A. Bryant, editor. Acute & Chronic Wound Nursing Management. 2nd ed. St. Louis: Mosby; 2000. pp. 221–264.

[12] National Pressure Ulcer Advisory Panel. The Facts about Reverse Staging in 2000. The NPUAP Position Statement [Internet]. 2000. Available from: http://www.NPUAP.org [Accessed: February 26, 2016]

[13] National Pressure Ulcer Advisory Panel. Mucosal Pressure Ulcers [Internet]. August 2008. Available from: http://www.NPUAP.org [Accessed: February 23, 2016]

[14] Edsberg L. E., Langemo D., Baharestani M. M., Posthauer M. E., Goldberg M. Unavoidable pressure injury. J Wound Ostomy Continence Nurs. 2014;41(4):313–334.

[15] Raetz J., Wick K. Common questions about pressure ulcers. American Family Physician. 2015;92(10):888–894.

[16] Ratliff C. R. Pressure ulcer prevention. Advance for NP's and PA's. 2016;18(6):24–29.

[17] Bluestein D., Javaheri A. Pressure ulcers: prevention, evaluation, and management. American Family Physician. 2008;78(10):1186–1194.

[18] The Canadian Association of Wound Care. The Basic Principles of Wound Healing [Internet]. Available from: http://cawc.nwt [Accessed: February 24, 2016]

[19] Ousey, K. Chronic wounds-an overview. Journal of Community Nursing 2009;23(7):20–24.

[20] National Pressure Ulcer Advisory Panel, European Pressure Ulcer Advisory Panel, PAN Pacific Pressure Ulcer Injury Alliance, editors, London England. Prevention and Treatment of Pressure Ulcers: Clinical Practice Guideline. 2nd ed. Australia: Cambridge Media; 2014. 308 p.

[21] Black J. M., Edsberg L., Baharestani M. M., Langemo D., Goldberg M., McNichol L., Cuddigan J. Pressure ulcers: avoidable or unavoidable? results of the national pressure ulcer advisory panel consensus conference. Ostomy Wound Management. 2011;57(2): 24–36.

Section 3

Current Deeds and Future Challenges in Wound Therapy

Chapter 15

Surgical Management of Wounds

Peter Mekhail, Shuchi Chaturvedi and
Shailesh Chaturvedi

Additional information is available at the end of the chapter

http://dx.doi.org/10.5772/64536

Abstract

In surgical speciality, understanding of the wound healing is absolutely necessary. There are different kinds of wounds that require treatment which is most appropriate to them. In this chapter, we have discussed treatment for different types of wounds in four main types according to WHO Classification. Pros and cons of different types of materials used for cleaning and dressing are discussed. Dressing materials are discussed in detail. We have described the process of wound healing. There are various factors that influence wound healing and we have specifically described how they differ in primary and secondary wound healing. Usage of various kinds of dressing materials and their mechanism of action is described in detail. We have specifically highlighted the role of community nurses and tissue viability nurses. Since the availability and the recognition of tissue viability nurses, the cost of wound treatment has come down considerably and it is also very popular with the patients. Vacuum-assisted closure (VAC) therapy is very helpful in large wounds that are producing a lot of exudates. The VAC pulls the skin edges together and removes the exudate. Other adjunctive therapies are also mentioned but they are not available in most hospitals and therefore detailed descriptions are not provided.

Keywords: wound, closer, techniques, infection, surgical

1. Introduction

Wound management is considered one of the main pillars of patients' care at all levels of health service. The financial burden on the health service and the community in relation to wound management are due to prolonged stay, the cost of different materials required for wound care, delayed discharge, loss of earnings, continuous input and follow up at primary care level. No reliable data are available for the cost of treating the wound which do not close with primary intention. A report by Lewis et al. [1] has carried out a comprehensive review of the literature and has found that the cost of dressings and other material alone could be as high as £37 million per year in England. Data for primary care are easily available as they purchase on Form 10 but the data for secondary care are difficult to find as most hospitals buy directly from manufacturers at specially negotiated price, therefore factoring this in is quite difficult and no reliable study has been found on literature search. If patient stays in hospital the cost of stay in hospital could be as high as £400–500 per day depending upon the geographic location of hospital. Additionally, the cost of staffing, local or general anaesthetic, has to be factored in as well.

Significant developments have taken place with regards to wound management over the course of the years. Thanks to the evolving technology, better understanding of the healing process and relevant contributing factors we are now able to address the problem in a timely, cost-effective and efficient manner. It is a developing area and therefore the means of management will only improve with time.

2. Understanding tissue healing

Understanding tissue healing is fundamental in wound management. Such a complex physiological process is proven to be dependent on multiple inter-related factors [2].

Wound healing can be defined as the process by which the body restores and replaces function to damaged tissues [3]. Following tissue trauma, healing can be initiated through one of the two mechanisms:

1. Regeneration, which means replacement of damaged tissue by an identical type of tissue. This process is only confined to a few types of cells, for example epithelial, liver and nerve cells [2].

2. Repair, where damaged tissues are replaced by connective tissue to form a scar. This mechanism occurs in vast majority of cases [2].

3. Stages of wound healing

In general terms, the wound healing process can be divided into four stages with some potential overlap between the stages. Identification and recognition of the wound stage enables appropriate treatment objectives for that particular stage. When treating, practitioner at times may fail to establish correct treatment objectives due to failure to correctly recognise the healing stage of that particular wound.

3.1. Stage 1 (vascular response)

Tissue trauma leads to activation of coagulation cascade resulting in formation of a fibrin mesh to fill the gap within the tissue. It usually lasts up to 3 days [3].

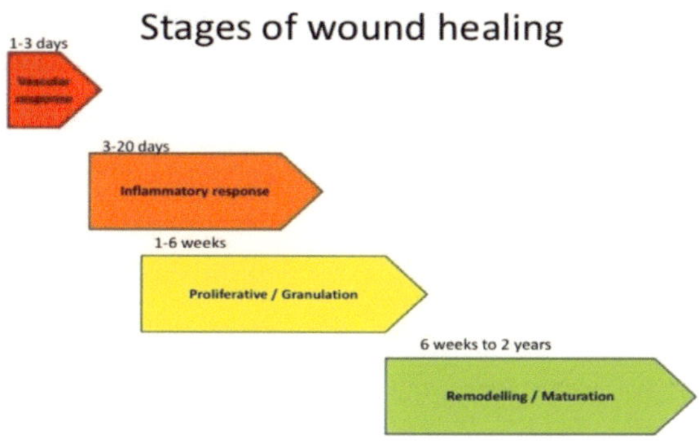

Scheme 1. Stages of Wound healing.

3.2. Stage 2 (inflammatory response)

At this stage, vasodilatation and increased permeability of the adjacent blood vessels are noted. This is the result of inflammatory mediators like histamine and prostaglandins released by mast cells. Clinically, this is characterised by redness, swelling, localised heat, pain and functional limitation. Clinical presentation at this stage might be confused with wound infection, as hyperaemia occurs in the first 3 weeks of healing.

Increased capillary permeability at this phase leads to exudates production containing essential growth factors, nutrients and enzymes mandatory for wound healing in addition to their anti-microbial characteristics [4].

Immuno-compromised patients might not be able to produce appropriate inflammatory response resulting in failure of activation of normal healing process [5].

3.3. Stage 3 (proliferative/granulation phase)

New connective tissue starts to fill the wound and a decrease of the wound size is noted. This occurs as a result of epithelialisation, wound contraction and granulation [2]. Collagen and other extra-cellular materials form scaffolding on which the new capillaries grow (angiogenesis) to form connective tissue. The process is referred to as granulation formation [2]. Angiogenesis is promoted by material produced by macrophages including transforming growth factor (TGF) and tumour necrosis factor (TNF) [6].

Fibroblast contraction that takes place during this stage is responsible for wound contraction and hence reducing wound size. This is considered to be a crucial part of a large and open wound healing [7].

Growth factor	Abbreviation	Main origins	Effects
Epidermal growth factor	EGF	Activated macrophages	Keratinocyte and fibroblast mitogen Keratinocyte migration Granulation tissue formation
Transforming growth factor-α	TGF-α	Activated macrophages T-lymphocytes Keratinocytes	Hepatocyte and epithelial cell proliferation Expression of anti-microbial peptides Expression of chemotactic cytokines
Hepatocyte growth factor	HGF	Mesenchymal cells	Epithelial and endothelial cell proliferation Hepatocyte motility
Vascular endothelial growth factor	VEGF	Mesenchymal cells	Vascular permeability Endothelial cell proliferation
Platelet-derived growth factor	PDGF	Platelets Macrophages Endothelial cells Smooth muscle cells Keratinocytes	Granulocyte, macrophage, fibroblast and smooth muscle cell chemotaxis Granulocyte, macrophage and fibroblast activation Fibroblast, endothelial cell and smooth muscle cell proliferation Matrix metalloproteinase, fibronectin and hyaluronan production Angiogenesis Wound remodelling Integrin expression regulation
Fibroblast growth factors 1 and 2	FGF-1, -2	Macrophages Mast cells T-lymphocytes Endothelial cells Fibroblasts	Fibroblast chemotaxis Fibroblast and keratinocyte proliferation Keratinocyte migration Angiogenesis Wound contraction Matrix (collagen fibres) deposition
Transforming growth factor-β	TGF-β	Platelets T-lymphocytes Macrophages Endothelial cells Keratinocytes Smooth muscle cells Fibroblasts	Granulocyte, macrophage, lymphocyte, fibroblast and smooth muscle cell chemotaxis TIMP synthesis Angiogenesis Fibroplasia Matrix metalloproteinase production inhibition Keratinocyte proliferation
Keratinocyte growth factor	KGF	Keratinocytes	Keratinocyte migron and differentiation

Table 1. Various growth factors involved in wound healing [10].

During the final phase of proliferation, re-epithelialisation takes place across the wound surface. This process will be delayed until the wound bed is filled with granulation tissue in cases of wound healing with secondary intention [2].

3.4. Stage 4 (remodelling/maturation phase)

This is the fourth and final stage of wound healing and it might extend up to 2 years from the time of tissue trauma. During this stage, the raised and reddish scar becomes more flat, smooth and lighter in colour. This relates to a reduction in the blood supply. Mature scars are hairless, avascular and do not contain sweat or sebaceous glands.

Collagen fibres are reorganised to maximise tensile strength, a process called remodelling and it is stimulated by macrophages [8].

Hypertrophic scar and keloid formation are two known abnormalities associated with this stage. While the former takes place after initial repair, the latter occurs sometime after healing is completed and continues to grow afterwards [9]. Keloid formation occurs 10 times more commonly in the Black Afro-Caribbean population in comparison to Caucasian population [9] **Table 1**.

4. Wound classification

Surgical wounds are commonly classified according to the degree of contamination and breaching of the aerodigestive tract epithelium into four categories:

A. Clean

Uncontaminated wounds without breaching of the respiratory, gastrointestinal (GI) or genitourinary (GU) tract. Examples include mastectomy, neck dissection, thyroid surgery and hernia surgery. These wounds are commonly managed with primary closure.

B. Clean-contaminated

Gastrointestinal, respiratory or Genitourinary tracts are entered in a controlled fashion. Usually no gross contamination or spillage should happen if proper precautions, i.e. minimising spillage, protecting the wound edges, etc., are taken. Examples of these types of wounds include cholecystectomy, Whipple operation, elective colonic or gastric surgery.

C. Contaminated

Any gross spillage of GI tract contents or major breach in the sterile technique either as causative agent or accidental can lead to contamination of wound. Perforated appendicitis, bile spillage, diverticular perforation or penetrating wounds come within this category. Although primary closure is still feasible in these wounds, thorough washout with copious amount of saline to remove as much contaminating agent, i.e. faeces or pus, as possible and prophylactic intra-operative antibiotics are advisable. Most randomised controlled trials (RCTs) prove the reduction in major sepsis though minor wound infection may still occur. In cases of gross contamination of abdominal cavity with faecal matter and when one is not sure of complete removal of contaminating agent it is better to leave the abdomen open and covered with wet packs for 48 hours and then re-checking the abdomen under general anaesthetic by removing the pack. If the abdominal cavity looks clean and there is no dead tissue or bowel then the closure can be attempted. These wounds are best closed in one layer with whole thickness sutures with either nylon or prolene as tension sutures.

D. Dirty wounds

This refers to old traumatic wounds with necrotic tissue, ongoing infection or perforation and presence of known organisms in the wound prior to intervention. Primary closure is not advisable and debridement is essential. Examples include abscesses, perforated bowel and faecal peritonitis. In cases of gross contamination of abdominal cavity with faecal matter and when one is not sure of complete removal of contaminating agent it is better to leave the abdomen open and covered with wet packs for 48 hours and then re-checking the abdomen under general anaesthetic by removing the pack. If the abdominal cavity looks clean and there is no dead tissue or bowel then the closure can be attempted. These wounds are best closed in one layer with whole thickness suture with either nylon or prolene as tension sutures.

Techniques of wound closure:

A. Closure by primary intention

In this technique, approximation of wound edges and deeper tissue layers is meticulously carried out with appropriate sutures in layers. Skin is approximated by sub-cuticular sutures or staples. Sterstrips™ are used to relieve tension on suture line and to give more aesthetically pleasing and functional scar. Elimination of dead space minimises new tissue formation, and careful epidermal alignment minimises scar formation [11, 12].

B. Closure by secondary intention

This is considered an adequate alternative to primary intention closure, particularly in cases where major tissue loss or gross contamination is expected. It might include closure of deeper facial planes while leaving the skin open [13].

5. Factors affecting wound healing [14]

The World Health Organisation (WHO) considers wound healing a multi-factorial process and each factor contributes to the healing process either directly or indirectly.

A. Patient-related factors

a. Age

b. Nutritional status

c. Underlining co-morbidity including diabetes, anaemia and compromised immunity

http://dx.doi.org/10.5772/64536

d. Patients' physiological status, for instance, multi-organ dysfunction, inotropic/vasopressor support

B. Wound-related factors

a. Type of organ or tissue

b. Extent/severity of injury

c. Nature of injury, e.g. clean laceration versus crushing injury

d. Wound contamination

e. Time lapse between the injury and initiation of treatment

C. Local factors related to the surgical technique itself

a. Appropriate haemostasis to ensure viable and well vascularised wound edges is a necessity but at the same time there should be no continuous oozing

b. Decision to perform (or not to perform) wound debridement as part of the surgical wound management does affect the final outcome

c. Timing of closure can be as important as any of the above factors in determining the fate of the wound

6. Surgical approaches to wound management [14]

There are certain golden surgical principles that must be followed in order to achieve adequate wound management.

6.1. For primary repair

A. Primary closure requires clean, well approximated and tension free suturing technique.

B. Infection and delayed healing are almost inevitable when primary closure of contaminated wound takes place without proper debridement or washout.

C. Various suturing techniques mean each technique is ideal for certain types of wounds. For example, while a subcuticular skin suture is considered to be an excellent option of good alignment for the wound edges, it is not the best haemostatic technique and in wounds with oozing edges or expected oozing a continuous mattress suture might be a better option in those cases where oozing is expected.

D. Choosing the correct suture material is vital in ensuring a desirable outcome. In general, a monofilament stitch carries less risk of infection in comparison to braided (multifilament) stitches [15]. Correct tensile strength of the material used is essential in maintaining the integrity of the wound until the healing is complete [15].

E. Size of sutures and interval between stitches should be proportional to the thickness of approximated tissues.

F. Deep wounds should be closed in layers whenever possible.

G. Timing of suture removal is determined by site and vascularity. For example, while skin stitches on the face can be removed as early as in 3 days, abdominal closure, usually, necessitate keeping suture material for up to 7–10 days.

H. Some operations that leave quite a large raw area may require drains as the chances of haematoma formation are high. The most common example is mastectomy. In these cases use of human fibrin glue spray reduces the drainage and also Seroma formation is reduced to a significant degree [16]. The product ARTISS is produced by Baxter Ltd. It contains 5% fibrin and 95% prothrombin and comes loaded in syringe. The product must be connected to a pressurised air source and before using the temperature of fluid must be at 25°C. This solution is good where one may need adjusting the flaps as it takes roughly 3 minutes for it to work [16]. If immediate fixation of the surfaces is required, Tessil (Baxter) is a good product [17]. This contains 95% fibrin and 5% prothrombin and adheres immediately. This is very useful in thoracotomy where it is sprayed straight to the chest wall and pleura [17].

For delayed primary closure:

A. Delayed primary closure is a good alternative in clean contaminated wounds and whenever washout is required. Wounds can be left open with saline-soaked sterile gauze and then patient should be taken back to the theatre, the gauze is removed and if wound looks clean and free of contaminant, sutures can be applied after 48 hours.

6.2. For healing with secondary intention

A. Promote healing with secondary intention after performing surgical debridement.

B. Surgical debridement includes washout of wound edges with antiseptic solutions, thorough washout with copious amounts of saline, excising dead and necrotic tissue down to healthy bleeding edges and gentle tissue handling to minimise iatrogenic tissue trauma.

7. Post-operative wound care

Regardless of the nature of the wound, healing mechanism or the type of closure, the aims of post-operative wound care remain the same. The main goal is to promote fast, complication-free healing with the best possible functional and aesthetic outcome [18]. Special consideration is given to wound healing with primary intention. As there is minimal tensile strength at the wound edges due to lack of remodelling collagen fibres, additional support in the form of sutures, tapes or staples is usually required until epithelisation takes place [19].

8. Guidance for reducing post-operative surgical site infection (SSI) [20]

A. Dressings and wound cleaning

a. Aim not to disturb the wound in the first 48 hours as this can damage the new delicate layer of epithelium. If necessary, use sterile saline for cleaning wound during this period and not to rub the surface.

b. Aseptic non-touch technique is mandatory for changing/removing dressings.

c. Advise patients that they can have a shower 48 hours post-operatively as by this time the top layer of epithelium has formed and the wound becomes water tight.

d. Early referral to tissue viability services is preferable in cases of wounds healing by secondary intention.

B. Anti-microbial treatment

a. Consider giving antibiotics whenever SSI (cellulites) is suspected.

b. Antibiotic choice should be broad spectrum initially then spectrum should be narrowed to target specific organisms once the culture and sensitivity report is available [21].

C. Further debridement

a. If debridement becomes necessary, surgical debridement in the theatre is always preferred in grossly contaminated wounds.

b. Avoid gauze dressings as when gauze is removed it damages granulation tissue which sticks to it. Though in certain superficial pussy wounds this method is still used and statistically no difference has been found in the healing time in comparison to more costly dressings.

c. Some non-healing wound with lot of dead tissue can be treated with sterile Green Bottle Larvae (*Lucilia sericata*) which destroy the necrotic tissue with enzyme and then ingest it. Larvae are applied directly to the wound and then held in place with an occlusive dressing. These can be applied to wound infected with MRSA (Methecillin Resistant Staphylococcus Aureus) as the larvae digest the bacteria as well and reduce the chance of continued infection. It is stipulated that the enzyme also produces growth of granulation tissue, however, some patients may find having larvae on their body unacceptable and if left too long the enzyme produced may destroy the keratinised epithelium [2].

d. Different types of special dressings can be applied to absorb the exudates and let the wound heal quicker and with less pain when changing the dressing. There are numerous dressings available for this kind of wounds and are described in the next section.

e. Cleaning the wound with hydrojets and by putting the patient in whirlpool has also been tried and found helpful in cleaning grossly contaminated wounds or quite large wounds. If wound is small and irrigation is required to remove exudates and debris that might interfere with wound healing, gentle irrigation with a syringe filled with saline or sterile water is preferred [3, 22].

f. Irrigation of wounds with antiseptic solution has been tried with hypochloride (*Eusol*) solution, Aserbane™ and hydrogen peroxide as caustic agents have been tried but there are no reliable data available to prove their efficacy [3]·

D. Structured wound care approach

a. Using flowcharts and a structured approach with clear guidance is essential to ensure continuity within the team.

b. Continuous education about recent updates in wound care.

E. Methods to avoid

a. Topical antibiotics in wounds healing by primary intention.

b. Moist cotton gauze or mercury-based antiseptic solutions.

F. Post-operative wound complications: The most common and significant post-operative wound complications are wound infection and wound dehiscence. Once suspected, active management should start and this includes swabs for culture and sensitivities, followed by empirical antibiotics administration in the first instance [21]. Debridement in some cases might be necessary to promote wound healing.

9. Dressings

a. The ideal dressing should carry certain characteristics to assist wound healing. It must maintain some moisture at the wound site, act as a barrier against fluid or bacterial contamination, potentially remove excess exudates that might lead to wound maceration and finally it should be adherent to skin but removed with no/minimal trauma [24]. Tegaderm™ and Opsite™ dressings are two such dressings. These are water resistant and allow patient to have a wash next day if the patients wish so.

b. Wound which are producing lot of debris and discharge need cleaning with aseptic technique. There are a number of different materials available, some of the commonly used ones are described below.

- Hydrocolloid dressings. These contain sodium carboxymethylcellulose which is combined to elastomers and applied to a carrier, usually polyurethane foam. The hydrocolloid absorbs the exudates and becomes gel and when dressing is removed the whole lot lifts off without disturbing the granulation tissue. Common ones are Granuflex™, Comfeel Plus™, Aquacel™ and DuoDerm Extra Thin™.

- Polysaccharide beads. This comes in powder form and swells when it comes in contact with fluid or exudates. This can be left in place for a few days and then removed with gentle wash with saline. It is available as Debrisan (Pharmacia Ltd) and Iodosorb (Perstrop).

http://dx.doi.org/10.5772/64536

- Alginates. These are made from the sodium salts of algenic acid. Alginic acid is produced from seaweed. When exposed to fluid it is activated and forms a gel and absorbs the exudates. It comes in different size and shape as flat squares and ribbons. It is very commonly used in UK. Flat square and ribbons are manufactured by many pharmaceuticals. Kaltostat (Convatec) is the most widely used in our institute.
- Foam dressing. These are made from polyurethane or silicon which absorbs liquid by capillary action. They can be applied to wound as a filler for the cavities. Dressings can be removed every couple of days and the foam can be washed and cut to size for re-application. Lyofoam (Seton) and Silastic (Dow Corning Ltd) are common examples.
- Silver impregnated dressings. These dressings also come as squares or ribbon. They are made of alginate, carboxymethylcellulose and silver impregnated nylon fibres. Silver is used for its anti-microbial action and at the same time the alginate absorbs the exudate to form gel. It is quite effective for the superficial wounds infected with gram positive bacteria and as ribbon for the cavities after surgery for pilonidal sinuses. Most common one is Silver-cel (Systagenix). Aquacel™ is also available with silver.
- Iodine containing dressings. These are gauze dressings impregnated with iodine which is usually good for quite superficial wounds. Iodine acts as antiseptic. Inadine (Systagenix) is readily available. The only problem with this dressing is that it sticks to the granulation tissue, so have to soak the wound in saline for 5 minutes before removing the dressing.
- Allograft and Xenograft for challenging skin loss situations [22, 23]

Skin is considered the largest organ of the human body representing about 16% of the total body weight. Skin loss is commonly encountered in problems such as burns or de-gloving injuries. The skin plays a vital role in terms of immunity, protection and thermoregulation of the human body. Consequently, skin loss can be associated with significant morbidities and even mortalities. Over decades, Research has been carried out to provide biologic skin substitutes that can take the skin function and can be readily available. Cadaveric and porcine grafts have been used for decades as a biologic skin substitutes. When cadaveric grafts are used, they are called allograft as they are originated from the same species. On the contrary, porcine grafts are called xenografts because they are taken from one species and transplanted on to another one.

10. Role of district nurses for wound management

While the journey of wound management starts at the acute hospital, a major part of it takes place in the community. District nurses and practice nurses in the community play a role in wound care. District nurse care is usually provided to patients who cannot physically attend their general practice for various reasons. Once the patients' condition enables them to move freely outside their homes, they are strongly advised to consult the practice nurses in the general practice and this allows appropriate resource allocation and provides a good service for the people who really need it. Moreover, it promotes recovery of the relatively fitter patient population.

11. Tissue viability services [25]

The concept of tissue viability nurses is relatively new though the idea originated in the 1980s. It covers all aspects of skin and soft tissue wounds. Although surgical wound management is a major part of their role, it is not their sole field of expertise. They also cover various soft tissue-related areas such as pressure sores and chronic leg ulceration. In addition to their bedside role, they provide education to the entire healthcare team. Across the UK, they are also working on preventing common hospital-related skin problems like pressure sores, thereby saving costs in the long term. Their role extends into the community where they provide support to district and practice nurses and help them to choose the correct dressing material and other essential tools for wound healing. The Tissue Viability Society has been established since 2014 and it is considered an excellent forum to discuss all new techniques and materials used for wound healing [26].

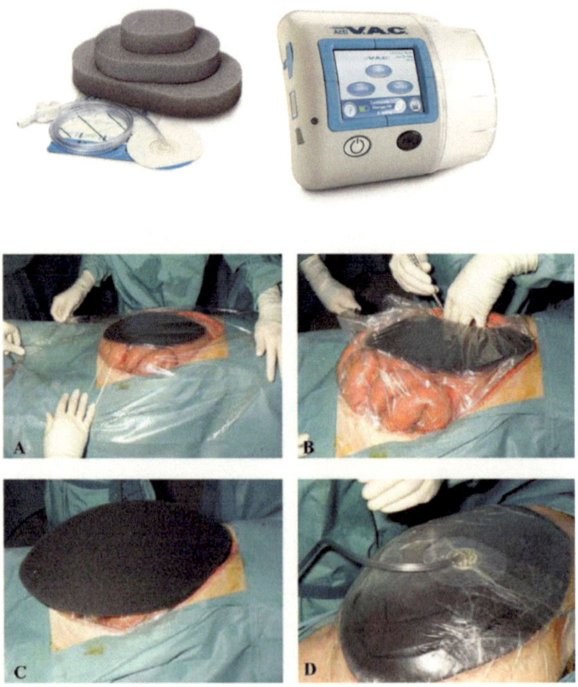

Figure 1. Prospective evaluation of vacuum-assisted closure in abdominal compartment syndrome and severe abdominal sepsis, *J Am Coll Surg*. 2007; **205**: 586–592 (Courtesy of KCI medical).

http://dx.doi.org/10.5772/64536

11.1. Vacuum-assisted closure (VAC) therapy and its role in wound healing

VAC therapy is a simple but effective method of promoting rapid healing. It is currently considered to be an effective means of managing large complex acute and chronic wounds (**Figures 1** and **2**) [27].

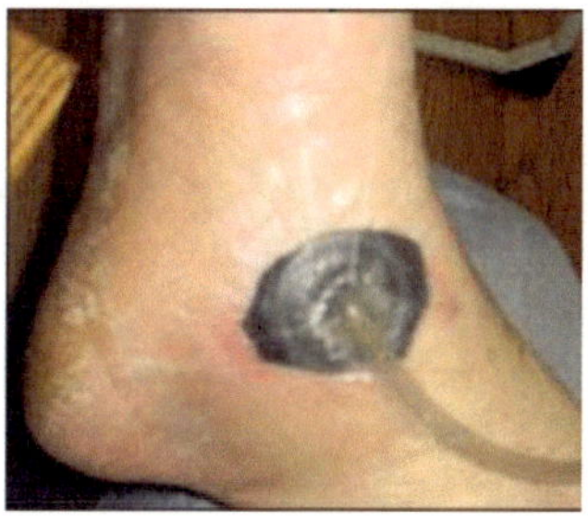

Figure 2. Vacuum dressing or small oozing wound (Courtesy of WWW.REHABPUB.COM).

VAC is an active wound therapy that was first described in 1997 by Morykwas and Argenta [28]. The system applies negative pressure to the wound bed via an open-cell polyurethane foam dressing [28]. The foam will be in direct contact with the wound and connects to a canister via a suction tube. An effective airtight seal is mandatory for the system to function.

Treatment objectives

A. Removal of excessive exudate and promoting a moist rather than wet environment for wound healing [27].

B. Increase angiogenesis which promotes granulation formation [28].

C. Ability to promote healing in complex wounds and wounds that fail to heal with the conventional methods [27, 28].

Wounds that can be treated with VAC therapy [29]

A. Pressure ulcers

B. Diabetic foot ulcers

C. Trauma wounds with tissue loss

D. Burns

E. Leg ulcers

F. Skin grafts

G. Surgical wound dehiscence

Contraindications and precautions [29]

A. Known or suspected malignant wounds

B. Gastrointestinal fistulation

C. Untreated osteomyelitis

D. Direct exposure of large blood vessels due to risk of bleeding

E. Thick/necrotic eschar.

11.2. Adjunctive measurements contributing to wound management

1. Ultrasound waves, electrotherapy or laser therapy. These adjuncts have always been thought to contribute towards better wound management. In a recent RCT, Cullum et al. concluded that there is lack of sufficient reliable evidence to draw conclusions about the contribution of laser therapy, therapeutic ultrasound, electrotherapy and electromagnetic therapy to chronic wound healing [30].

2. Hyperbaric oxygen therapy. Tissue hypoxia is one of the characteristics of chronic wounds. Therefore, means of increasing O_2supply to tissues could potentially improve chronic wound healing. In a recent Cochrane review of 12 randomised trials, it was concluded that hyperbaric O_2 therapy can improve the chance of healing of diabetic foot ulcers only on short term but not on long term bases [31]. It can also reduce the size of wounds caused by chronic venous insufficiency but it was found to have no effect in wounds/ulcers caused by arterial insufficiency [31].

12. Conclusion

After reading this chapter the reader would have full understanding of types of wounds (WHO Classification) and how to treat them. We have described in details how to deal with different types of wound from clean surgical wound to heavily contaminated wounds. Closure of wounds by primary intention when the wound is clean and debridement and then leaving the wound to heal by secondary intention with or without secondary closure with sutures as deemed necessary. Different types of dressings are described in details with pros and cons of each one of them. Role of all personnel involved in treating the wound is defined. More specific types of method, i.e. laser therapy, ultrasound, hyperbaric oxygen and compression used for treating the wound are enumerated but not described in details as there is not enough evidence available.

Acknowledgements

We would like to express our sincere thanks to Dr Jaina Chauhan and Miss Janaki Solanki for poof reading the article and making linguistic changes where necessary. We would also like to acknowledge the help provided by Miss Shona Stewart in co-ordinating the project.

http://dx.doi.org/10.5772/64536

Author details

Peter Mekhail[1], Shuchi Chaturvedi[2] and Shailesh Chaturvedi[3*]

*Address all correspondence to: s.chaturvedi@nhs.net

1 Aberdeen Royal Infirmary, Aberdeen, UK

2 Kings College London, London, UK

3 Department of General Surgery, Aberdeen Royal Infirmary, Aberdeen, UK

References

[1] Lewis R, Whiting P, ter Riet G, O'Meara S, Glanville J. A rapid and systemic review of the clinical effectiveness and cost effectiveness of debriding agents in treating surgical wounds healing by secondary intention. Health Technol Assess. 2001:5 (14):3–4,26–29,35–39,59–61.

[2] M. Flanagan. The physiology of wound management. Journal of Wound Care. June, Vol 9, No 6, 2000:209–300

[3] Tortora, G.J., Grabowski, S.R. *Principles of Anatomy and Physiology* (8th edn). New York: Harper Collins College Publications, 1996.

[4] Hutchinson, J.J. Prevalence of wound infection under occlusive dressings: a collective survey of reported research. *Wounds* 1989; 1: 123–133.

[5] Baxter, C.R. Immunologic reactions in chronic wounds. *Am J Surgery* 1994; 167: S: 12S–14S.

[6] Nathan, C.F. Secretory products of macrophages. *J Clin Investigation* 1987; 79: 319–326.

[7] Brown, G.L. Acceleration of tensile strength of incisions treated with EGF and TGF. *Annals of Surgery* 1988; 208: 788–794.

[8] Diegelmann, R. et al. The role of macrophages in wound repair: a review. *Plastic Reconstructive Surgery* 1991; 68: 107–113.

[9] Eisenbeiss, W., Peter, P.W., Bakhtiari, C. et al. Hypertrophic scars and keloids. *J Wound Care* 1998; 7: 5, 255–257.

[10] Mitchell, Richard Sheppard; Kumar, Vinay; Abbas, Abdul K;Faust, Nelson (2007). Robins Basic Pathology. Philadelphia: Saunders. ISBN 1-4160-2973-7. 8th Edition.

[11] Kanzler MH, Gorsulowsky DC, Swanson NA. Basic mechanisms in the healing cutaneous wound. *J Dermatol Surg Oncol*. 1986 Nov. 12(11):1156–64.

[12] Singer AJ, Clark RA. Cutaneous wound healing. *N Engl J Med*. 1999 Sep 2. 341(10): 738–46.

[13] Diwan R, Tromovitch TA, Glogau RG, Stegman SJ. Secondary intention healing. The primary approach for management of selected wounds. *Arch Otolaryngol Head Neck Surg*. 1989 Oct. 115(10):1248–9.

[14] Best practice guidelines in disaster situations. WHO/EHT/CPR 2005, formatted 2009.Chapter 9:9–11

[15] Mohan H. Kudur , Sathish B. Pai, H. Sripathi, Smitha Prabhu. Sutures and suturing techniques in skin closure .Indian J Dermatol Venereol Leprol. July-August 2009. Vol 75. Issue 4:425–433.

[16] Benevento R, Santoriello A, Pellino G, Sciaudone G, Candilio G, De Fatico GS, Selvaggi F; EBSQ Colo, Canonico S. The effects of low-thrombin fibrin sealant on wound serous drainage, seroma formation and length of postoperative stay in patients undergoing axillary node dissection for breast cancer. A randomized controlled trial. Int J Surg. 2014 Nov;12(11):1210–5.

[17] Sierra D, Fibrin sealant adhesive systesm: a review of their chemistry, material properties and clinical applications. *J Biomat App* 1993;7:309–352.

[18] Singer AJ, Dagum AB. Current management of acute cutaneous wounds. NEJM 2008;359:1037–46.

[19] Yao K, Bae L, Yew WP. Post-operative wound management. Aust Fam Physician. 2013 Dec;42(12):867–70.

[20] Mark Collier et al. National Institute for Health and Care Excellence. Prevention and treatment of surgical site infections. Available at publications.nice.org.uk/ surgical-site-infection-cg74. Published 2008.

[21] Singhal H, Kaur K, Zammit C. Medscape reference: wound infection treatment and management. Available at emedicine.medscape.com/ article/188988,; Updated Dec. 2015; Section2:2–3.

[22] Benjamin C Wood et al. Skin Grafts and Biologic Skin Substitutes. Available at emedicine.medscape.com/article/1295109-overview; Updated March 2015; Section 3: 3

[23] Ennis WJ, Valdes W, Salzman S, Fishman D, Meneses P. Trauma and wound care. In: Morison MJ, Ovington LG, Wilkie K, editors. Chronic wound care. A problem-based learning approach. London: Mosby Elsevier Limited; 2004. p. 291–307.

[24] Ruszczak Z, Schwartz RA, Joss-Wichman E, Wichman R, Zalewska A. Medscape reference: surgical dressings. Available at emedicine.medscape.com/article/1127868-overview#showall; Section 6–7.

[25] Fanja Pagnamenta. Tissue viability The role of the tissue viability nurse. Wound Essentials 2014, Vol 9 No 2.(65–67).

[26] Tissue Viability Society (2014) Available at: http://tvs.org.uk.

[27] Joseph E, Hamori CA, Bergman S, et al. A prospective randomised trial of vaccum-assisted closure versus standard therapy of chronic nonhealing wounds. Wounds2000; 3:60–7.

[28] Morykwas MJ, Argenta LC, Shelton-Brown EI, et al. Vacuum-assisted closure: a new method for wound control and treatment: animal studies and basic foundation. Ann Plast Surg1997;38:553–62.

[29] Baxter Helena, Ballard Kate. Vacuum Assisted Closure. Nursing Times 2001;Vol 97(35): 51–53.

[30] Cullum N, Nelson EA, Flemming K, Sheldon T. Systematic reviews of wound care management: (5) beds; (6) compression; (7) laser therapy, therapeutic ultrasound, electrotherapy and electromagnetic therapy. Health Technol Assess: 2001:Vol 5(9):161–163.

[31] Kranke P, Bennett MH, Martyn-St James M, Schnabel A, Debus SE, Weibel S. Hyperbaric oxygen therapy for chronic wounds. Cochrane Database of Systematic Reviews 2015, Issue 6. Art. No.: CD004123. DOI: 10.1002/14651858.CD004123.pub4

Chapter 16

Physical Modalities in the Management of Wound(s)

Amir Feily, Fatemeh Moeineddin and
Shadi Mehraban

Additional information is available at the end of the chapter

http://dx.doi.org/10.5772/64340

Abstract

Wound is caused by disruption of the integrity of body skin as a result of environmental or medical factors. Managing chronic and refractory wounds is a significant dilemma physicians are facing. Large varieties of treatment modalities have been used to enhance wound healing among which were different medicines, surgical procedures, physical therapy, hyperbaric oxygen therapy, and physical modalities such as laser and shockwave. In this chapter, the authors discuss physical modalities that are most used in the management of wound healing with a focus on lasers, shockwaves, photodynamic therapy, UVB therapy, and lights and describe some important experimental and clinical trials that have been done in this regard with an attempt to explain their mechanisms.

Keywords: wound healing, low-level lasers, shockwave, photodynamic therapy, phototherapy, CO_2 laser

1. Introduction

Wound is caused by disruption of the integrity of body skin as a result of environmental or medical factors. Managing chronic and refractory wounds represents a significant dilemma that physicians are facing. Wound healing is a complex cascade of events that restores skin integrity by replacing damaged cells and tissues which consists of four phases: hemostasis, inflammation, proliferation, and remodeling. In the first phase, hemostatic changes result in a reduced blood flow and clot formation. Activated platelets as well as the injury itself attract inflammatory agents, neutrophils, and predominantly macrophages, which clear the apoptotic cells. By releasing growth factors, these leukocytes trigger proliferation of fibroblasts, epithelial and endothelial cells in the trauma site forming the granulation tissue. Turnover of collagen from type III to I restores skin integrity in the remodeling phase. Various factors can influence the quality of wound healing including nutrition, vitamin deficiencies, smoking, sex hormones, oxygenation, age, stress, diabetes, alcoholism, and medications such as glucocorticoid steroids, chemotherapeutic agents, and nonsteroidal antiinflammatory drugs [1].

Large varieties of treatment modalities have been used to enhance wound healing such as different medicines, surgical procedures, physical therapy, hyperbaric oxygen therapy, and physical modalities such as laser and shockwave. Some substances like honey have also proved to be beneficial in wound healing as a result of antiinflammatory and antibacterial features [2]. The ideal physical therapy modality is chosen based on the patient's factors, type of wound, previous therapies, and clinician's preference.

Electrical stimulation is another method of physical therapy used for accelerating wound healing. Electrotherapy works by stimulating cell migration, cell proliferation rate, and growth factor secretion via creating an electrical current. The anode attracts macrophages, neutrophils, and keratinocytes. The cathode attracts activated neutrophils, fibroblasts, myofibroblasts, and endothelial cells [3].

Low-level laser therapy (LLLT) is also a novel approach for treating wounds. Greatest benefits have been achieved through wavelengths of 632–1000 nm. The mechanism of action of LLLT is defined through wound contraction which accelerates the wound healing process [4].

Pulsed radiofrequency energy also promotes chronic wound healing by contracting the wound [5]. It has minimum side effects as well as the advantage of reducing wound pain.

Light-emitting diode (LED) has somewhat similar effects as light amplification by stimulated emission of radiation (LASER) in expediting the process of wound healing by increasing fibroblasts and collagens and decreasing inflammatory cells in the trauma site [6].

Shockwaves have also proved to be beneficial in overcoming chronic and intractable wounds such as diabetic ones with minimal adverse effects and long-lasting results. The mechanism through which they work remains unknown; however, several factors are considered to be effective in this procedure including stimulation of microcirculation and metabolism, reduction of inflammatory cells, release of growth factors, and stimulation of stem cells [7].

Photodynamic therapy (PDT) has also proved to be effective in wound healing. However, it seems to display best results when used in conjunction with lasers [8].

The effect of ultraviolet therapy on wound healing seems not promising and may even delay the process as it has shown to affect focal adhesion dynamics [9]. On the other hand, there are studies which suggest that ultraviolet C can be beneficial in expediting wound healing with antibacterial effects [10].

In this chapter, the authors tend to discuss physical modalities that are most used in the management of wound healing with a focus on lasers, shockwaves, photodynamic therapy, UVB therapy, and lights.

http://dx.doi.org/10.5772/64340

2. Low-level laser and wound healing

In the recent years, it has been shown that the laser therapy had the potential to improve wound healing and reduce pain and inflammation [11].

The main indications of low-reactive-level laser therapy (LLLT) are reduction of pain and inflammation. It amplifies tissue repair, enhances regeneration of different nerves and tissues, and prevents tissue injury in situations where it is likely to occur [12, 13].

Low-reactive-level laser therapy (LLLT) enhances the activation of intracellular or extracellular chromophores and the initiation of cellular signaling by exposing cells or tissue to low levels of red and near infrared (NIR) light [11]. The biological effects of LLLT are decreased inflammatory cells, increased fibroblast reproduction and angiogenesis, and stimulation of granulation tissue and augmented collagen synthesis [14].

LLLT assumes the use of photons at a nonthermal irradiation to alter biological activity. LLLT is composed of two sources: coherent light and noncoherent light sources (lasers) consisting of filtered lamps or light-emitting diodes (LED) or, on occasion, a combination of both [13, 14].

The reason of the term "low level" is the use of low-power contents compared to the other forms of laser therapy such as cutting, ablation, and thermally coagulating tissue.

The mechanism of LLLT on wound healing is not yet fully understood nevertheless it appears that LLLT has a wide area of effects at all the levels of molecular, cellular, and tissue ingredients. The main biological mechanism behind the effects of LLLT is proposed to be absorption of red and NIR light by mitochondrial components, in particular cytochrome c oxidase (CCO) which is concluded in the respiratory chain located within the mitochondria [15–17], and also in the plasma membrane of cells. Accordingly, a chain of events and various process carries out in the mitochondria [18] leading to wound healing.

Although LLLT is now used as a portable minimally invasive, easy-to-use, and cost-effective modality to promote wound healing, it is also employed for treatment of diabetic lower extremity ulcer. However, it remains controversial in this therapy for two reasons. First, there are uncertainties about the basic molecular and cellular mechanisms responsible for appropriate biological effects on the affected tissue. Second, there are significant variations in terms of parameters measuring: wavelength, irradiation or power density, pulse structure, coherence, polarization, energy, fluence, irradiation time, contact versus noncontact application, and repetition regimen. Lower level parameters can result in lower impact of the treatment and higher ones can lead to tissue injury [12, 14].

Inappropriate choice of light source and dosage can be the cause of negative results of many of the published studies on LLLT. In addition, eventual mismatch of the patient's skin to the application of LLLT were described, such as: improper preparation and oily debris that can interfere with the influence of the light source, and cause failure to account for skin pigmentation [19]. Unsuitable maintenance of the LLLT devices can reduce its efficiency and interfere with clinical results as well. It is important to notice that there is an optimal dose of light for any particular issues [14].

Nevertheless, many systematic reviews point that LLLT is an effective therapeutic modality on wound healing and diabetic foot ulcer recovery [20], but additional clinical studies must be performed in order to find out the best parameters of wavelength, dosage, and methodology and especially appropriate treatment protocol.

3. Relative contraindications/precautions

3.1. Relative contraindications

3.1.1. Cancer

Do not use LLLT over any known malignant lesions unless: for pain relief during the terminal stages of the illness, and for cancer therapy side effects (e.g., oral mucositis, radiation dermatitis, etc.).

3.1.2. Pregnancy

There is no evidence of harm to an unborn baby; however, there are no safety tests either, so for medico legal reasons it is recommended to not treat directly over the developing fetus.

3.1.3. Thyroid

Although relatively low intensity is far less likely to trigger any adverse events when treating that region of the neck, we suggest not applying lasers directly over the thyroid.

4. Photodynamic therapy and wound healing

Photodynamic therapy (PDT) as a photochemistry process can kill cancer cells, inactivate infected pathogens, and demolish target tissue. In PDT process, one special material called photosensitizer or nontoxic dyes absorbs visible light and produces excited singlet state such as singlet oxygen and hydroxyl radicals that are able to attack to target cells [21]. Administration of photosensitizer either topically or systemically in combination with irradiation appropriate wavelength laser is a promising treatment modality in wound healing especially for chronic pressure and decubitus wounds frequently encountered in diabetic and disable patients. The healing of chronic wounds and venous stasis ulcers of the leg is compromised by infection, yet PDT has an antimicrobial action [22]. Bacterial burden in chronic ulcer decreases by treatment with infrared radiation. A radiation via endogenous protoporphyrin (and/or protoporphyrin IX [PpIX] of bacteria) is virtually similar to a mild PDT [23]. It appears that PDT with suitable PS together with suitable laser parameters represents effective treatment modalities in promoting wound healing. PSs associates with three main groups of agents: azine dyes, macrocyclic dyes, and metallated derivatives [24–27]. An extensive range of PSs from different groups including azines, porphyrins, phthalocyanines, and chlorophyll derivatives have been described in eradication of many pathogens such as a variety of bacteria, parasites, viruses, and fungi [22].

Several types of first- and second-generation PSs have been used at minimal doses with laser irradiation performed at wavelengths ranging from 630 to 690 nm, and showed that PDT of acute wounds can lead to an improvement of healing outcomes. Interestingly in one study, the healing of skin flaps after being subjected to ischemia was impaired by PDT treatment, although only one PS (Photofrin) was tested. Further animal model and human wound studies are required to find the main process of enhancement of reepithelization and granulation tissue formation with PDT.

In photodynamic therapy, irradiation of cells with low dosage or small energy may incite proliferation. In using PDT clinically, it is essential to use the suitable doses of both the PS and the activating light source in order to achieve cell death for cancer therapy, or regeneration for wound healing [23]. The newest generations of PSs allowing a faster clearance time of normal tissues are more selective for tumor cells. Although PDT may be nontraumatic but in comparison with nature of lower laser therapy it is almost always traumatic and can cause burns, swelling, pain, and scarring in nearby normal tissue [28].

4.1. Contraindication

Cutaneous hypersensitivity, porphyria, known allergies to porphyrins.

Both Aminolevulinic acid (ALA) and Methyl aminolevulinate (MAL) are in FDA pregnancy category C; reproduction studies have not been performed on animals.

Photodynamic therapy is not approved for use in children.

5. Phototherapy (UV irradiation) and wound healing

New contemporary research shows that controlled UV exposure might have some eventual benefit in wound healing and cutaneous homeostasis. The effectiveness of UV energy in enhancing biological changes depends on the chosen irradiation parameters, with maximal effective wavelength and lowest irradiation level [29]. The main mechanism of phototherapy is related to the depth of penetration. UVA, for example, has the longest wavelength and penetrates to the upper part of dermis in human skin, and UVB only penetrates down to the basal layer; however, UVC only reaches the upper part of the epidermis [30].

UV has bactericidal effect and its radiation to the skin can increase blood flow, producing erythema and epidermal hyperplasia [31]. The induced erythema via vasodilatation and inflammatory response represents the first phase of healing. In addition, UV light irradiation increases cellular proliferation in the stratum corneum [32], which can be a protective mechanism against further sunlight damage.

Although UV protection and antisolars are commonly advised during and after wound healing, it is possible that UV also affects the melanocyte redistribution and prevents the normal cutaneous response to injury [33].

It has been shown that UVC light *per se* could stimulate wound healing. UVC light enhances fibronectin and growth factors release leading to increase healing cascade and wound contraction [34, 35]. UV can promote endothelial cell proliferation [36] and augment epidermal thickness and reepithelialization or desquamation of the leading edge of periulcer epidermal cells [31].

UVC (200–280 nm) has a significant antimicrobial effect and can be used as efficient bactericide agent for treatment of acute wound infections and killing pathogens without undesirable injury to host tissue. UVB (280–315 nm) irradiation to the wound has wound healing stimulating effect and extracorporeal UVB irradiation of blood adds immune system stimulating effects too. Although UVA (315–400 nm) has specific effects on cell biologic events, it has not yet been extensively applied to wound treatment [31].

An interesting study compared the efficacy of phototherapy on wound healing in rats under the normal and high-fat diets and revealed increased wound healing by regulating oxidative stress in rats with metabolic disorders under a high-fat diet [37]. The efficacy of UV therapy on pressure ulcer is not clear due to eventual bias and limited number of trials available for consideration. Further research is recommended to determine possible benefit or drawbacks of this treatment [38].

While low level laser (or light) and photodynamic therapy both have considerable applications in wound care, but penetration of UV light into tissues and its efficacy is restricted. UVC and UVB can damage DNA in host cells and chronic exposure to UV can be carcinogenic. Accordingly, additional study of cellular signaling that occurs after UV exposure of tissue is needed to better indicate the risk and benefits of UV irradiation in wound healing.

5.1. Contraindication of phototherapy

- Childhood
- Pregnancy and breastfeeding (PUVA)
- Immobility or inability to stand unassisted for 10 min or longer
- Very fair skin (skin type 1 and 2, especially PUVA)
- Past excessive exposure to natural sun light or phototherapy
- Immunosuppressive medication
- Photosensitizing creams or medications
- Past skin cancer, especially melanoma [39]

http://dx.doi.org/10.5772/64340

6. Shock wave and wound healing

Although hearing extracorporal shock wave brings the treatment of urinary stones in the mind [40–43] but it also has some benefits in the treatment of acute and chronic wounds [44]. Shock waves are biphasic high-energy acoustic waves that can be produced by electrohydraulics. Although the exact mechanisms of shock wave therapy are not entirely elucidated, it may harbor eventual immunomedulatory effects, acting by transient micromechanical forces in altering various biologic activities. Shock wave therapy increased expression of macromolecules in wound healing such as VEGF, proliferating cell nuclear antigen, and endothelial nitric oxide synthesis. Because of the considerable experience in using shock wave in the treatment of urolithiasis and other conditions in humans, it appears to be a safe technology. The clinical effect of this technology in various wound types and the particular mechanisms of action are now beginning to be understood. Shock waves may also stimulate sensory nerve fibers and decrease pain. Clinical studies of shock wave therapy in wound healing suggest that many factors such as wound cause, size, and duration may impact response to shock wave therapy. However, the actual administration of shock wave therapy in current clinical studies varies in type (unfocused versus focused). Primary studies suggest that unfocused shock wave therapy is more effective than focused one in the treatment of superficial soft tissue defects yet, without direct comparison between unfocused and focused shock wave therapy in clinical trials to date [33]. Importantly, additional basic science studies along with randomized controlled trials will be necessary to determine the optimal shock wave therapy settings. Currently, the U.S. Food and Drug Administration has approved devices that administer shock wave therapy for the treatment of plantar fasciitis and lateral epicondylitis. Application of such devices for treatment of acute and chronic wounds has not been approved yet. We look forward to future innovation in this field to find out the accurate mechanisms of action and optimal treatment of specific wound types.

6.1. Contraindications

6.1.1. Absolute

Lungs: Treatments must not be performed across or directed to the lungs and heart.

Eyes: Tissue of the eye could be adversely affected by shock wave.

Brain: The destructive forces seen at transitions could damage and destroy brain matter.

Major blood vessels: Both the major blood vessels in the neck and thigh should be avoided to prevent damage and potential catastrophic bleeding.

Major nerves: Superficial major nerves like the brachial plexus, ulna/radial nerve should not be treated directly (treatment around these areas is acceptable just not directly to the nerve).

Open wounds/postsurgical wounds with or without stabilization (glue, stitches, steristrips): Shock wave damages tissues and local circulation. This could lead to degradation of the wound, further bleeding, and delayed healing.

Implanted devices or hormones.

Epiphysis: Open growth plates could potentially be damaged by shock wave either by using settings that create more growth and close them too quickly or by using settings that delay growth.

6.1.2. Relative

Genitals; pregnancy; clotting disorders/anticoagulants; joint replacements, certain settings have been used to loosen previously implanted joints ready for a new implant; infection; and cancer.

Corticosteroid injection: Generally people recommend waiting 1 month before application [45].

7. CO_2 laser and wound healing

There are some anecdotal reports of CO_2 laser and wound healing. In an interesting case series two pediatric patients with chronic wounds within scars showed rapid healing with a single-pass treatment by fractionated carbon dioxide (CO_2) laser [46]. In another case series done by Phillips et al., CO_2 laser was used in the treatment of posttraumatic slow healing wounds in three elderly patients. In their report each wound was healed by 60% or greater within 3 weeks [47]. In an interesting article reepithelialization and accelerated wound healing within 4 weeks was reported in one recessive dystrophic epidermolysis bullosa (RDEB) patient with CO_2 laser without blistering or other adverse effects [48]. Although there are no considerable reports of the efficacy of fractional carbon dioxide laser on wound healing, it seems that it has a promising effect on chronic wound without remarkable complications.

7.1. Contraindication

Isotretinoin use within the previous 6 months, active cutaneous bacterial or viral infection in the area to be treated, history of keloid formation or hypertrophic scarring, ongoing ultraviolet exposure, prior radiation therapy to treatment area, collagen vascular disease, chemical peel, and dermabrasion [49].

8. Conclusion

Managing chronic and refractory wounds represents a significant dilemma that physicians are facing and needs invention of new treatment modalities. Wide ranges of the above physical modalities have been introduced and used in wound-healing treatment with different efficacies, but most of them, to some extent, are strange for patients and physicians. Although additional clinical studies must be performed in order to find out the best modalities and the best parameters of wavelength, dosage, and methodology, and especially appropriate treatment protocols, we think these modalities need more attention to be paid and should be kept in mind for treating persistent ulcers.

Author details

Amir Feily[1*], Fatemeh Moeineddin[1] and Shadi Mehraban[2]

*Address all correspondence to: dr.feily@yahoo.com

1 Skin and Stem Cell Research Center, Tehran University of Medical Sciences, Tehran, Iran

2 Jahrom University of Medical Sciences, Jahrom, Iran

References

[1] Guo S, Dipietro LA. Factors affecting wound healing. J Dent Res. 2010 Mar;89(3):219–229.

[2] Pazyar N, Yaghoobi R, Rafiee E, Mehrabian A, Feily A. Skin wound healing and phytomedicine: a review. Skin Pharmacol Physiol. 2014;27(6):303–310.

[3] Walter C, Chua MD. Advanced wound care modalities for the treatment of pressure ulcers. PVA Summit. 2011; 2011:35–37.

[4] Hopkins JT, McLoda TA, Seegmiller JG, David Baxter G. Low-level laser therapy facilitates superficial wound healing in humans: a triple-blind, Sham-controlled study. J Athl Train. 2004 Jul–Sep; 39(3):223–229.

[5] Li Q, Kao H, Matros E, Peng C, Murphy GF, Guo L. Pulsed radiofrequency energy accelerates wound healing in diabetic mice. Plast Reconstr Surg. 2011 Jun;127(6):2255–2262.

[6] de Abreu Chaves ME, de Araújo AR, Piancastelli ACC, Pinotti M. Effects of low-power light therapy on wound healing: LASER×LED. An Bras Dermatol. 2014 Jul–Aug; 89(4): 616–623.

[7] Kuo YR, Wang CT, Wang FS, Chiang YC, Wang CJ. Extracorporeal shock-wave therapy enhanced wound healing via increasing topical blood perfusion and tissue regeneration in a rat model of STZ-induced diabetes. Wound Repair Regen. 2009 Jul–Aug; 17(4): 522–530.

[8] Jayasree RS, Gupta AK, Rathinam K, Mohanan PV, Mohanty M. The influence of photodynamic therapy on the wound healing process in rats. J Biomater Appl. 2001 Jan;15(3):176–186.

[9] Liu H, Yue J, Lei Q, Gou X, Chen SY, He YY, Wu X. Ultraviolet B inhibits skin wound healing by affecting focal adhesion dynamics. Photochem Photobiol. 2015 Jul–Aug; 91(4):909–916.

[10] Thai TP, Houghton PE, Campbell KE, Woodbury MG. Ultraviolet light C in the treatment of chronic wounds with MRSA: a case study. Ostomy Wound Manage. 2002 Nov;48(11):52–60.

[11] Kushibiki T, Hirasawa T, Okawa S, Ishihara M. Low reactive level laser therapy for mesenchymal stromal cells therapies. Stem Cells Int. 2015;2015:974864.

[12] Chung H, Dai T, Sharma SK, Huang YY, Carroll JD, Hamblin MR. The nuts and bolts of low-level laser (light) therapy. Ann Biomed Eng. 2012 Feb;40(2):516–533.

[13] Gupta A, Avci P, Sadasivam M, et al. Shining light on nanotechnology to help repair and regeneration. Biotechnol Adv. Biotechnol Adv. 2013 Sep–Oct;31(5):607–631.

[14] Avci P, Gupta A, Sadasivam M, Vecchio D, Pam Z, Pam N, Hamblin MR. Low-level laser (light) therapy (LLLT) in skin: stimulating, healing, restoring. Semin Cutan Med Surg. 2013 Mar;32(1):41–52.

[15] Karu TI, Kolyakov SF. Exact action spectra for cellular responses relevant to phototherapy. Photomed Laser Surg. 2005 Aug;23(4):355–361.

[16] Greco M, Guida G, Perlino E, Marra E, Quagliariello E. Increase in RNA and protein synthesis by mitochondria irradiated with helium-neon laser. Biochem Biophys Res Commun. 1989 Sep 29;163(3):1428–1434.

[17] Karu TI, Pyatibrat LV, Kalendo GS. Photobiological modulation of cell attachment via cytochrome c oxidase. Photochem Photobiol Sci. 2004 Feb;3(2):211–216.

[18] Oron U. Light therapy and stem cells: a therapeutic intervention of the future? Interven Cardiol. 2011;3(6):627–629.

[19] Posten W, Wrone DA, Dover JS, Arndt KA, Silapunt S, Alam M. Low-level laser therapy for wound healing: mechanism and efficacy. Dermatol Surg. 2005 Mar;31(3):334–340.

[20] Tchanque-Fossuo CN, Ho D, Dahle SE, Koo E, Li CS, Rivkah Isseroff R, Jagdeo J. A systematic review of low-level light therapy for treatment of diabetic foot ulcer. Wound Repair Regen. 2016; 24:418–26.

[21] Silva ZS Jr, Bussadori SK, Fernandes KP, Huang YY, Hamblin MR. Animal models for photodynamic therapy (PDT). Biosci Rep. 2015; 28;35(6), pii:e00265.

[22] O'Riordan K, Akilov OE, Hasan T. The potential for photodynamic therapy in the treatment of localized infections. Photodiagnosis Photodyn. Ther. 2005;2:247–262.

[23] Peplow PV, Chung TY, Baxter GD. Photodynamic modulation of wound healing: a review of human and animal studies. Photomed Laser Surg. 2012 Mar;30(3):118–148.

[24] Malik Z, Hanania J, Nitzan Y. Bactericidal effects of photoactivated porphyrins – an alternative approach to antimicrobial drugs. J Photochem Photobiol B. 1990 May;5(3–4):281–293.

[25] Wainwright M. Photodynamic antimicrobial chemotherapy (PACT). J Antimicrob Chemother. 1998;42:13–28.

[26] Ali H, van Lier JE. Metal complexes as photo and radio-sensitizers. Chem Rev. 1999;99:2379–2450.

[27] Josefsen LB, Boyle RW. Photodynamic therapy and the development of metal-based photosensitisers. Met Based Drugs. 2008;2008:276109.

[28] Vrouenraets MB, Visser GW, Snow GB, van Dongen GA. Basic principles, applications in oncology and improved selectivity of photodynamic therapy. Anticancer Res. 2003 Jan–Feb;23(1B):505–522.

[29] Nussbaum EL, Biemann I, Mustard B. Comparison of ultrasound/ultraviolet-C and laser for treatment of pressure ulcers in patients with spinal cord injury. Phys Ther. 1994;74:812.

[30] Ennis WJ, Lee C, Meneses P. A biochemical approach to wound healing through the use of modalities. Clin Dermatol. 2007;25:63.

[31] Gupta A, Avci P, Dai T, Huang YY, Hamblin MR. Ultraviolet radiation in wound care: sterilization and stimulation. Adv Wound Care (New Rochelle). 2013 Oct;2(8):422–437.

[32] Sauder DN, Stanulis-Praeger BM, Gilchrest BA. Autocrine growth stimulation of human keratinocytes by epidermal cell-derived thymocyte-activating factor: implications for skin aging. Arch Dermatol Res.1988;280:71.

[33] Rennekampff HO, Busche MN, Knobloch K, Tenenhaus M. Is UV radiation beneficial in postburn wound healing? Med Hypotheses. 2010;75:436.

[34] Morykwas M, Marks M. Effects of ultraviolet light on fibroblast fibronectin production and lattice contraction. Wounds. 1998;10:111.

[35] James LC, Moore AM, Wheeler LA, Murphy GM, Dowd PM, Greaves MW. Transforming growth factor alpha: in vivo release by normal human skin following UV irradiation and abrasion. Skin Pharmacol.1991;4:61.

[36] Eaglstein WH, Weinstein GD. Prostaglandin and DNA synthesis in human skin: possible relationship to ultraviolet light effects. J Invest Dermatol. 1975;64:386.

[37] Leite SN, Leite MN, Caetano GF, Ovidio PP, Jordão Júnior AA, Frade MA. Phototherapy improves wound healing in rats subjected to high-fat diet. Lasers Med Sci. 2015 Jul; 30(5):1481–1488.

[38] Chen C, Hou WH, Chan ES, Yeh ML, Lo HL. Phototherapy for treating pressure ulcers. Cochrane Database Syst Rev. 2014 Jul 11;7:CD009224.

[39] Schaden W, Fischer A, Sailler A. Extracorporeal shock wave therapy of nonunion or delayed osseous union. Clin Orthop Relat Res. 2001;387:90–94.

[40] Contrandication of phototherapy. http://www.dermnetnz.org/doctors/scaly-rashes/phototherapy.html#contra. Accessed at 7 May, 2016.

[41] Wang CJ, Liu HC, Fu TH. The effects of extracorporeal shockwave on acute high-energy long bone fractures of the lower extremity. Arch Orthop Trauma Surg. 2007;127:137–142.

[42] Wang CJ, Chen HS, Chen CE, Yang KD. Treatment of nonunions of long bone fractures with shock waves. Clin Orthop Relat Res. 2001;387:95–101.

[43] Elster EA, Stojadinovic A, Forsberg J, Shawen S, Andersen RC, Schaden W. Extracorporeal shock wave therapy for nonunion of the tibia. J Orthop Trauma 2010;24:133–141.

[44] Qureshi AA, Ross KM, Ogawa R, Orgill DP. Shock wave therapy in wound healing. Plast Reconstr Surg. 2011;128:721e-7e.

[45] Contrandication of shock wave therapy. http://www.shockwavetherapy.education/index.php/theory/contraindications. Accessed at 7 May, 2016.

[46] Krakowski AC, Diaz L, Admani S, Uebelhoer NS, Shumaker PR. Healing of chronic wounds with adjunctive ablative fractional laser resurfacing in two pediatric patients. Lasers Surg Med. 2016 Feb;48(2):166–169.

[47] Phillips TJ, Morton LM, Uebelhoer NS, Dover JS. Ablative fractional carbon dioxide laser in the treatment of chronic, posttraumatic, lower-extremity ulcers in elderly patients. JAMA Dermatol. 2015 Aug;151(8):868–871.

[48] Krakowski AC, Ghasri P. Case report: rapidly healing epidermolysis bullosa wound after ablative fractional resurfacing. Pediatrics. 2015 Jan;135(1):e207-10.

[49] Krupa Shankar DS, Chakravarthi M, Shilpakar R. Carbon dioxide laser guidelines. J Cutan Aesthet Surg. 2009 Jul–Dec;2(2):72–80.

Chapter 17

Antimicrobial Dressings for Improving Wound Healing

Omar Sarheed, Asif Ahmed, Douha Shouqair and
Joshua Boateng

Additional information is available at the end of the chapter

http://dx.doi.org/10.5772/63961

Abstract

Wound healing occurs by a series of interrelated molecular events which work together to restore tissue integrity and cellular function. These physiological events occur smoothly in normal healthy individual and/or under normal conditions. However, in certain cases, these molecular events are retarded resulting in hard-to-heal or chronic wounds arising from several factors such as poor venous return, underlying physiological or metabolic conditions such as diabetes as well as external factors such as poor nutrition. In most cases, such wounds are infected and infection also presents as another complicating phenomenon which triggers inflammatory reactions, therefore delaying wound healing. There has therefore been recent interests and significant efforts in preventing and actively treating wound infections by directly targeting infection causative agents through direct application of antimicrobial agents either alone or loaded into dressings (medicated). These have the advantage of overcoming challenges such as poor circulation in diabetic and leg ulcers when administered systemically and also require lower amounts to be applied compared to that required via oral or iv administration. This chapter will review and evaluate various antimicrobial agents used to target infected wounds, the means of delivery, and current state of the art, including commercially available dressings. Data sources will include mainly peer-reviewed literature, clinical trials and reports, patents as well as government reports where available.

Keywords: antimicrobial, bioburden, dressings, infection, wounds, wound healing, bacterial resistance

1. Introduction

A wound may be defined as a disruption to the physiological arrangement of the skin cells and a disturbance to its function in connecting and protecting underlying tissues and organs. It may be primary caused by accidental cut, tear, scratch, pressure, extreme temperatures, chemicals, and electrical current, or secondary to surgical intervention or disease (i.e., diabetes, ulcers, or carcinomas) [1]. It ranges from superficial (affecting the epidermis) to partial-thickness (affecting both epidermis and parts of the dermis) and full-thickness (including subcutaneous fat and bones) wounds [2]. Wound healing is a physiological process, by which the living body repairs tissue damages, restores its anatomical integrity, and regains the functionality of the injured parts. A wound can be closed by primary intention or left to heal by secondary intention, and in both ways the healing process occurs through a series of overlapping events and is influenced by a number of intrinsic and extrinsic factors [3].

1.1. Acute wounds

Acute wounds can heal within a limited amount of time, usually show no complications, and are characterized by the loss of skin integrity (injury) that occurs suddenly. The injured tissue heals in a predictable manner where platelets, keratinocytes, immune surveillance cells, microvascular cells, and fibroblasts play major roles in the restoration of tissue integrity [4]. These wounds are either surgical or traumatic [5].

1.2. Chronic wounds

Chronic wounds are wounds that do not heal within normal period and are associated with predisposing factors that weaken the integrity of dermal and epidermal tissues. Those factors either disrupt the balance between wound bioburden and the patient's immune system or impair the wound healing cycle. In terms of duration, if the wound fails to heal or shows no sign of recovery within 12 weeks, it is considered a chronic wound. Predisposing factors may affect the tissue perfusion causing chronic wounds such as vascular ulcers, associated with metabolic disorders such as diabetes causing diabetic foot ulcers [6]. They can be identified by criteria such as delayed healing and friable granulation tissue, prolonged inflammatory phase, persistent infection, and presence of resistant microorganisms [7–10].

1.3. Wound healing

The repair (wound healing) process involves four overlapping biochemical, physiological, and molecular phases.

I. Hemostasis

> This stage is characterized by microvascular injury and release of blood components at the wound site. Platelets come into contact with and adhere to the wall of the injured blood vessels. This adherence activates the platelets to release cytokines, growth factors, and numerous pro-inflammatory mediators, resulting in platelet aggregation and triggering the intrinsic and extrinsic coagulation path-

http://dx.doi.org/10.5772/63961

ways to form a fibrin clot which limits further blood loss. Growth factors produced by the platelets initiate the healing cascade [11, 12].

II. Inflammatory phase

The inflammatory phase starts at the same time as hemostasis sometime between a few minutes after injury up to 24 h and lasts for about 3 days. Aggregated platelets store vasoactive amines such as prostaglandins and histamine while other amines from granules released by mast cells, in response to injury, result in increased microvascular permeability and vasodilation, leading to exudation of fluid into the extravascular space [13]. This allows the migration of monocytes and protein-rich exudate into the wound and surrounding tissue, resulting in edema. These are typical signs of the inflammation process, and patients start complaining about pain at the site of injury within 24 h.

III. Proliferative phase

This phase commences after the inflammatory phase wanes. The remaining inflammatory cells produce growth factors to initiate angiogenesis, which is important to keep adequate blood supply within the wound bed [14]. Newly formed blood vessels will contribute to granulation tissue (composed of collagen and extracellular matrix) formation and provide the required nutrients.

IV. Maturation phase

This commences when the wound is superficially sealed. It involves the re-epithelialization and remodeling of newly formed tissues in the proliferative phase and restoration of epidermal integrity [15]. It also involves transferring collagen III to collagen I.

1.4. Factors affecting wound healing

Multiple factors affect wound healing and lead to the impairment of healing classified into local and systemic factors [16].

1.4.1. Oxygenation

Oxygen is crucial to wound healing and for resistance to infection, and used for cellular energy production by adenosine triphosphate [17]. It acts on different levels of wound healing by inducing angiogenesis, keratinocytes differentiation, migration, re-epithelialization, fibroblast proliferation, and collagen synthesis, and promotes wound contraction [18]. When injury occurs, temporary hypoxia and oxygen are useful to trigger wound healing by inducing the production of cytokines and growth factors from macrophages, keratinocytes, and fibroblasts [16]. Chronic wounds are generally hypoxic with oxygen tissue tension of 5–20 mm Hg compared to normal levels of 30–50 mm Hg [19]. Factors predisposing chronic wounds such as advancing age and diabetes can induce poor oxygenation through impaired vascular flow. Interventional revascularization therapies have been used to reverse hypoxic conditions in diabetic foot ulcers [20]. However, it has also been reported that such procedures can cause adverse effects to diabetic patients [21]. Recently, some topical foam dressings containing dissolved oxygen were developed to increase oxygen perfusion into the chronic wound area [22]. Results showed that dissolved oxygen from topical foam dressing penetrates into skin layers compared to topical gaseous oxygen.

1.4.2. Wound bioburden and infection

1.4.2.1. Bioburden

The intact skin acts to control the microbial population on the skin surface itself [23]. Once the integrity is lost through injury, the subcutaneous tissue becomes exposed, providing an environment for colonization and growth of microbes. However, this does not necessarily lead to an infection as there is a balance between the wound bioburden and the immune system [24].

1.4.2.2. Wound infection

Skin microflora is present to about 10^5 colonies without any clinical problems [25]. However, if the balance is disrupted, microorganisms will proliferate and start a microbiological chain of events by invading tissues resulting in an inflammatory response which may lead to tissue damage and delayed healing [7]. Once it causes damage to the host tissue, infection will arise. One of the consequences of infection is the prolonged inflammation due to prolonged elevation of pro-inflammatory cytokines, which causes the wound to enter the chronic stage and fail to heal within the expected 8–12 weeks [26]. This prolonged inflammation is also associated with increased levels of matrix metalloproteases which are capable of degrading the extracellular matrix which is the key component of proliferative phase of wound healing [9]. This increase in protease levels happens at the expense of the naturally occurring protease inhibitor levels that are decreased. From a microbiological perspective, wound infection is described as the presence of replicating microorganisms at the wound site overwhelming the host's immune system. It delays wound healing due to the release of toxins and exhibits active signs and symptoms of infections.

1.4.2.3. Common bacterial species present in chronic wounds

Generally, most infected wounds are polymicrobial and are commonly contaminated by pathogens found in the immediate environment, the endogenous microbes living in the mucous membranes, and the microflora on adjacent skin. Bacteria are the main cause of wound infection among other microorganisms present in the skin, though other microorganisms such as fungi have been implicated in certain mixed infections. In the initial stages of chronic wound formation, Gram-positive organisms such as *Staphylococcus aureus* and *Escherichia coli* are predominant [9]. In the later stages, Gram-negative *Pseudomonas* species are common and tend to invade deeper layers in the wound causing significant tissue damage [27]. Other aerobes implicated include *Staphylococci* and *Streptococci* species as well as anaerobic bacteria and are estimated in 50% of chronic wounds [28, 29].

1.4.3. Chronic wounds and biofilm

Biofilm is defined as "a microbially derived sessile community characterized by cells that are irreversibly attached to a substratum or interface or to each other, are embedded in a secreted matrix of extracellular polymeric substances (EPSs), and exhibit an altered phenotype with respect to growth rate and gene transcription" [30]. Firstly, conditioning film forms and is composed of proteins and polysaccharide molecules adsorbed onto the solid surface. This makes the surface ready to receive the first cells of the insipient biofilm. Secondly, bacteria will start to approach and attach onto the surface by forces such as van der Waals forces and the negative electrostatic charges of bacterial surface [31]. The attached bacteria become encased in a polymeric matrix called extracellular polymeric substance (EPS). This bacterial attachment induces a phenomenon called quorum sensing, which is responsible for "the regulation of gene expression in response to fluctuations in cell population density" [32]. This causes the bacteria within biofilm to alter their phenotypes resulting in the production of more virulent factors in response to signals from other bacteria within biofilm. These factors with barrier made from EPS contribute to the increased resistance to antibiotics. It has been suggested that EPS can interact with antibiotics spontaneously thereby preventing them reaching the bacteria to exert their antimicrobial activity [33]. The biofilm also protects the bacteria from host defenses by the covering of glycocalyx while bacteria secrete products within the film which makes phagocytic penetration poor [34].

This understanding is of great importance for intervention modalities in chronic wounds especially the use of antimicrobial wound dressing. For example macrolides can have inhibitory effect on the film formation or induce phagocytic invasion into biofilms [35]. Furthermore, in clinical wound management, it is always essential to promptly clean the wound and remove necrotic tissue and foreign material (e.g. bacteria and biofilms) from areas around the wound to improve the chances of enhanced wound healing, and this is known as debridement [1]. This is important because the presence of necrotic tissue increases the risk of infection and sepsis, which prolongs the inflammatory phase. Several approaches are employed including surgical removal, wound irrigation (e.g. saline and antiseptics such as chlorhexidine), autolytic rehydration using hydrogel dressings, applying enzymes such as collagenases or streptokinase preparations as well as using maggots to selectively dissolve necrotic and infected tissue (including biofilms) without destroying healthy or newly formed tissue [1].

2. Wound dressings

Wound dressings can maintain a moist environment in the wound which helps in proliferation and migration of fibroblast and keratinocytes. Moisture in the wound serves as a transporter for enzymes, growth factors, and hormones, thus inducing cell growth. Moist wound dressings promote collagen synthesis and decrease scar formation [36] which help wounds to heal faster [37]. Modern moist wound dressings can be classified depending on their materials (synthetic and natural polymers) and physical forms (hydrogels, hydrocolloids, films, and wafers).

Hydrogels consist of hydrated polymers which make them hydrophilic in nature. Water content is higher than 95%, and as a result they cannot absorb much exudate and cause maceration. But, this dressing is very useful in dry wound which can maintain moisture within wounds [36]. A Cochrane Review [38] of hydrogel dressings for healing diabetic foot ulcers suggests that hydrogel dressings are more effective than basic wound contact dressing. Hydrogels have advantages of autolytic debridement of slough and necrotic tissue and do not support bacterial growth [39, 40]. Hydrocolloid dressings are occlusive and can absorb wound exudate into the matrix to help improve healing. It can work for a sustained period of time, thus reducing the frequency of dressing changes. It also assists autolysis of necrotic materials [40]. Due to its extra absorbent nature, it is widely used in the treatment of cavity wounds [41]. A Cochrane Review [42] reported that any type of hydrocolloid and other dressings have no difference in efficacy. Foam dressings are highly absorptive, protective, and comfortable to the body surface. They promote thermal insulation, angiogenesis, and autolysis [43]. Film dressings are adhesive, transparent, durable, comfortable, and cost effective. Due to their transparency, the wound bed can be monitored without removing the dressing. However, films are suitable for superficial pressure wounds. The disadvantage of film dressing is maceration of wound exudate [36]. Lyophilized wafers are one of the most recent moist dressings proposed for wound care. Due to their highly porous nature, they can absorb high amounts of exudate rapidly which improves wound healing. Wafers can carry both antibacterial and anti-inflammatory drugs at the same time which give dual effects of inhibiting bacteria and reducing inflammation [44]. Wafers have good adhesion and diffusion properties [45] while Labovitiadi et al. [46] reported that wafers are a compatible delivery system for both insoluble and soluble antimicrobial drugs that exhibit better antimicrobial activity.

3. Antimicrobial wound dressings

3.1. Need for antimicrobial wound dressing

The major need for antimicrobial dressing is drug resistance to bacteria. Zubair et al. [47] isolated bacteria from diabetic foot ulcer patients and their resistance to different classes of drugs with the penicillins showing highest susceptibility to resistance followed by cephalosporins (54%), quinolones and fluoroquinolones (52.8%), aminoglycosides (38.5%), beta lactams (32.2%), and carbapenems (18.4%). Further, most chronic wound sufferers such as older patients and diabetics with leg and foot ulcers suffer from complications of poor circulation at the lower extremities, which makes oral and IV antibiotics ineffective. In addition, topical dressings are able to avoid the adverse effects of systemic administration (oral and IV) of high antibiotic doses including nausea, vomiting, diarrhea, allergic reactions, leukocyturia, insomnia, headache, and vaginosis, when only small doses above the minimum inhibitory concentration are required at the infected wound site. Finally, production costs of most dressings are less than those of IV or oral products.

3.2. Advanced medicated antimicrobial wound dressings

Antimicrobial dressings can be broadly classified into two groups as antiseptic or antibiotic dressings. Antiseptic dressings have broad spectrum activity which can kill or inhibit bacteria, fungus, protozoa, viruses, and prions [48]; however, some antiseptic dressings often show dose-dependent cytotoxicity to the host cells including keratinocytes, fibroblasts, and leukocytes [49, 50]. The concentration of povidone iodine greater than 0.004 and 0.05% is completely toxic to keratinocytes and fibroblasts, respectively [51]. Cadexomer iodine is reported to be nontoxic to fibroblasts *in vitro* at concentrations of up to 0.45% [52]. Chlorhexidine also shows dose-dependent toxicity to fibroblasts at concentrations between 0.2 and 0.001% [53, 54]. Moreover, silver-impregnated dressings have been reported to be more cytotoxic to epidermal keratinocytes and dermal fibroblasts than honey-based dressings [55]. On the other hand,

Dressing type	Polymers	Drug	Reference
Pads	Bovine serum albumin	Ciprofloxacin	[58]
Nanofibers patch	PVA/sodium alginate	Ciprofloxacin	[59]
Hydrogel	Polyethylene glycol	Ciprofloxacin	[60]
Sponges	Alginate/chitosan	Ciprofloxacin	[61]
Films	Chitosan/gelatin	Ciprofloxacin	[62]
Nanofibers	PVA/regenerated silk fibroin	Ciprofloxacin	[63]
Nanofiber mats	Polyurethane/dextran	Ciprofloxacin	[64]
Nanofiber mats	PVA/poly(vinyl acetate)	Ciprofloxacin	[65]
Films	Poly (2-hydroxymethacrylate)	Ciprofloxacin	[66]
Films	PVA/aminophenylboronic acid	Ciprofloxacin	[67]
Collagen dressing	Collagen	Ciprofloxacin	[68]
Hydrogels	Keratin	Ciprofloxacin	[69]
Films	Sodium carboxymethyl cellulose/gelatin	Ciprofloxacin	[70]
Scaffolds	Chitosan/polyethylene glycol	Ciprofloxacin	[71]
Hydrogel films	Carboxymethyl chitin	Chlorhexidine gluconate	[72]
Gel	Chitosan	Ofloxacin	[73]
Wafers and films	Polyox/carrageenan	Streptomycin	[74–76]
Films	PVA/sodium alginate	Clindamycin and nitrofurazone	[77, 78]
Films	PVA/dextran	Gentamicin	[79]
Scaffolds	Collagen	Doxycycline	[80]
Microspheres	Gelatin	Doxycycline	[81]
Microspheres	Chitosan	Levofloxacin	[82]
Nanofibrous scaffolds	Chitosan/poly(e-caprolactone)	Levofloxacin	[82]
Hydrogels	Polyvinylalcohol	Nitric oxide	[83]
Hydrogels	poly(2-hydroxyethyl methacrylate)	Nitric oxide	[84]
Hydrogels	*S*-Nitrosothiol	Nitric acid	[85]

Table 1. Summary of antibiotic dressings reported in the literature.

antibiotic dressings (**Table 1**) are nontoxic and can work effectively on the target sites without damaging host tissues [49]. The ideal antimicrobial dressing should have broad spectrum activity against all major microorganisms, be nonallergic and nontoxic to host cells, have the ability to drain exudate and maintain a moist wound environment, should release drugs rapidly in a sustained manner, should reduce malodor, and be cost effective [56, 57].

3.3. Silver-based dressings

Silver is a natural broad spectrum antibiotic, and its dressings have not yet shown any bacterial resistance. Silver exists in different forms such as silver oxide, silver nitrate, silver sulfate, silver salt, silver zeolite, silver sulfadiazine (SSD), and silver nanoparticles (AgNPs). Before the eighteenth century, silver nitrate was used for leg ulcers, epilepsy, acne, and venereal infections [86]. Currently different forms of silver are widely used in acute wound (burns, partial-thickness burns, freshly grafted burns, second-degree burns, surgical/traumatic wounds, colorectal surgical wounds, pilonidal sinus, and donor site), and chronic wound (pressure ulcers, leg ulcers, and diabetic foot ulcers) healing [87].

3.3.1. Antimicrobial activity of silver dressings

Antimicrobial activity of silver dressings depends on the amount and rate of silver release and its toxicity to bacterial, fungal, and algal cells. Silver works by interacting with thiol groups present in bacterial cells thus stop their respiration process. In the case of *E. coli*, silver prevents phosphate uptake and catalysation of disulfide bonds with silver tending to change the nature of protein structure in *E. coli*. The degenerative changes in cytosolic protein cause cell death [86, 88]. Feng et al. [89] reported antibacterial mechanism of action of silver ions on *E. coli* and *S. aureus* and showed that silver ions penetrate into bacterial cells and condense DNA molecules which inhibit their replication capabilities leading to cell death. Matsumura et al. [90] introduced two bactericidal mechanism actions of silver zeolite on *E. coli*. Firstly, silver ions released from silver zeolite come into contact with cells and penetrate into cells, altering the cellular functions that cause cell death. Secondly, silver ions inhibit respiration process through the generation of reactive oxygen molecules. Silver zeolite has also been reported against oral microorganisms (*Streptococcus mutans, Lactobacillus casei, Candida albicans, and S. aureus*) [91].

Silver nanoparticles show the most efficient antimicrobial activity amongst all forms of silver. The bactericidal effects of AgNPs depend on the size, shape, surface characteristics, and their dose [88, 92–101]. It has been reported that 75 $\mu g\ ml^{-1}$ of AgNPs having 1–100 nm particle size inhibits all bacterial strains (specifically, *E. coli, Vibrio cholerae, Salmonella typhi, and Pseudomonas aeruginosa)*. It has also been reported nanoparticles having particle size ~1–10 nm have higher affinity of attaching to the surface of the cell membrane as compared to larger nanoparticles. Because of this nature, AgNPs can attach to the larger surface area of bacterial cell membrane and cause native membrane porations which cause cell damage [92]. Ivask et al. [93] examined toxicity of silver nanoparticles to bacteria (*E. coli*), yeast (*Saccharomyces cerevisiae*), algae (*Pseudokirchneriella subcapitata*), crustacean (*Daphnia magna*), and mammalian cells (murine fibroblast) according to their particle sizes ranging from 10 to 80 nm. They confirmed that the smaller-sized nanoparticles showed highly toxic effect. The review of Rai et al. [88] and Rizzello

http://dx.doi.org/10.5772/63961

et al. [92] explained that truncated triangular nanoparticles are the strongest biocidal active products compared to spherical- and rod-shaped nanoparticles. 1 μg of truncated triangular nanoparticles shows greater activity than 12.5 μg of spherical-shaped nanoparticles and 50–100 μg of rod-shaped nanoparticles due to the enhancement of electrostatic interaction with bacterial cells (**Table 2**).

Dressing type	Brand name	Silver form
Contact layer dressings	Restore contact layer	Silver sulfate
	Acticoat Flex 3; Acticoat Flex 7	Elemental silver
	KerraContact Ag	Silver salt
	SilverDerm 7	Ionic silver
	Silverlon Wound & Burn Contact Dressings	Ionic silver
	Therabond 3D with Silvertrak™ Technology	Silver
Foams	RTD	Silver zirconium phosphate
	Acticoat Moisture Control	Elemental silver
	Allevyn Ag	Silver sulfadiazine
	Aquacel Ag	Ionic silver
	Biatain Ag Adhesive	Silver
	HydraFoam/Ag	Silver
	MediPlus Comfort Border Foam Ag+	Silver
	Mepilex Ag	Silver
	Optifoam Ag Adhesive	Ionic silver
	PolyMem MAX Silver Non-Adhesive Dressing	Silver
	Silverlon Negative Pressure	Ionic silver
	UrgoCell Silver/Cellosorb Ag	Silver salts
	V.A.C GranuFoam Silver	Silver
	Silverlon Acute Burn Glove	Silver
	Silvercel	Elemental silver
Fibers/clothes/mats /pads/others	Tegaderm Ag Mesh Dressing	Silver sulfate
	Absorbent Dermanet Ag+ Border	Silver
	Acticoat	Elemental silver
	Allevyn Ag Non-Adhesive	Silver sulfadiazine
	Durafiber Ag	Ionic silver
	Exsalt SD7	Silver

Dressing type	Brand name	Silver form
	Gentell Calcium Alginate Ag	Silver
	Silverlon Calcium Alginate	Silver
	Simpurity Silver Alginate Pads	Silver particles
	Urgotul SSD	Silver sulfadiazine
	Vliwaktiv Ag	Silver
	Acticoat 7	Elemental silver
	Arglaes film	Silver
Films/meshes	Avance	Silver
	Acticoat Absorbent	Elemental silver
	Algicell Ag	Silver
Alginate based	Algidex Ag	Ionic silver
	Biatain Alginate Ag	Silver
	CalciCare	Silver zirconium
	DermaGinate/Ag	Silver
	Dermanet Ag+	Silver
	Maxorb ES Ag+	Silver
	Maxorb Extra Ag+	Silver zirconium phosphate
	McKesson Calcium Alginate with Antimicrobial Silver	Silver
	Opticell Ag+	Ionic silver
	Restore Calcium Alginate Dressing with Silver	Ionic silver
	Sofsorb Ag	Silver
	Sorbalgon Ag	Ionic silver
	Suprasorb A + Ag Calcium Alginate	Silver
	Askina Calgitrol Ag	Silver alginate
	Invacare Silver Alginate	Silver sodium hydrogen zirconium phosphate
	Melgisorb Ag	Silver
	SeaSorb Ag	Ionic silver
	Silvasorb	Ionic silver
	Sorbsan Silver	Silver Sorbsan
	Algidex Ag	Ionic silver
	Urgotul SSD/S.Ag	Silver sulfadiazine

http://dx.doi.org/10.5772/63961

Dressing type	Brand name	Silver form
Gauze	Aquacel Ag	Ionic silver
	Arglaes Powder	Silver
Hydrofiber	Cardinal Health Hydrogel +Ag	Silver
Powder	DermaSyn/Ag	Ionic silver
Hydrogel	Elta Silver Gel	Silver
	ExcelGinate Ag	Silver
	Gentell Hydrogel Ag	Silver sulfadiazine
	SilvaSorb Antimicrobial Silver Dressing	Ionic silver
	Silver-Sept Silver Antimicrobial Skin & Wound Gel	Silver
	SilverMed Amorphous Hydrogel	Silver
	Silverseal	Silver
	SilvrSTAT Gel	Silver nanoparticles
	Viniferamine Hydrogel Ag	Silver
	Silverseal	Silver oxide
	Silver-Sept Antimicrobial Gel	Silver salt
	DermaCol Ag Collagen Matrix	Silver
	Puracol Plus Ag+ MicroScaffold Collagen	Silver
Collagen based	SilvaKollagen Gel	Silver
	Silverlon Adhesive Strips	Silver
	Contreet Hydrocolloid	Silver
Adhesive strips	Silverseal Hydrocolloid	Silver
Hydrocolloid	SilverMed Antimicrobial Wound Cleanser	Silver microparticles

Table 2. List of selected commercially available antimicrobial silver-containing dressings [22, 102, 103].

3.3.2. Silver dressings in wound healing

AgNPs (~11 to ~12 nm) containing gelatin fiber mats were prepared by electrospinning process and inhibited major microorganisms present in wounds [104]. Lin et al. [105] compared silver-containing carbon-activated fibers with commercially available silver-containing dressings and showed the silver-containing carbon-activated fibers to exhibit antibacterial activity and biocompatibility and promoting granulation and collagen deposition. A novel chitosan–hyaluronic acid composite with nanosilver was reported as a potential antimicrobial wound healing dressing for diabetic foot ulcers possessing high porosity, swelling, water uptake abilities, and biodegradable and potential blood clotting ability. The authors proved the inhibitory effects on *S. aureus, E. coli,* MRSA, *P. aeruginosa,* and *Klebsiella pneumoniae* [106].

In a related study, chitosan incorporated with polyphosphate and AgNPs was studied. The polyphosphate acts as a procoagulant which boosts blood clotting, platelet adhesion, and thrombin generation [107]. A similar scaffold dressing was developed by incorporating silver nanoparticles with chitin and showed antibacterial and blood clotting activity [108]. In another study, AgNPs containing hydrogel without any cytotoxicity but with antibacterial activity were reported [109]. Various inorganic forms of silver including silver zeolite, silver zirconium phosphate silicate, and silver zirconium phosphate demonstrate antimicrobial activity against oral microorganisms [91]. Pant et al. [110] stated AgNPs containing nylon-6 nanofibers prepared by one-step electrospinning process could be an effective antimicrobial wound dressing to kill both Gram-negative *E. coli* and Gram-positive *S. aureus*. Archana et al. [111] evaluated chitosan-blended polyvinyl pyrrolidone (PVP)–nano silver oxide (CPS) as an effective wound dressing *in vitro* and *in vivo*.

Lansdown et al. [112] investigated two forms of silver-containing dressings (Contreet foam and Contreet hydrocolloid) and found these promoted healing in chronic venous leg ulcers and diabetic foot ulcers. Polyvinylpyrolidone and alginate-based hydrogel-containing nanosilver has been functionally evaluated for efficient fluid handling capacity and strong antimicrobial activity against all major microorganisms such as *Pseudomonas, Staphylococcus, Escherichia, and Candida* [113]. Jodar et al. [114] demonstrated silver sulfadiazine-impregnated hydrogel for antimicrobial topical application for wound healing. Silver sulfadiazine (SSD)-impregnated hydrogel was prepared by polyvinyl alcohol (PVA) and dextran blending. Boateng et al. [115] formulated an ideal lyophilized wafer dressing composed of alginate and gelatin containing silver sulfadiazine for wound healing and showed the controlled release of SSD over 7 h and expected to diminish microbial load in the wound area. A novel SSD-loaded bilayer chitosan membrane was prepared with sustained release of silver which inhibits the growth of *P. aeruginosa and S. aureus* [116]. Shanmugasundaram et al. [117] formulated SSD-impregnated collagen-based scaffold with strong antibacterial activity *in vitro*. Ammons et al. [118] formulated dressings by combining commercial silver dressings (Acticoat™ Absorbent, Aquacel® Ag, and Tegaderm™Ag) with lactoferrin and xylitol and demonstrated greater efficacy against MRSA and *P. aeruginosa*.

There are several clinical studies with silver-containing dressings in the treatment of infected wounds to enhance wound healing, and the reader is referred to these [119–125].

3.4. Iodine and other antiseptics

Iodine is an old agent used in the treatment of chronic wounds and was used by soldiers during wars. The antibacterial activity of iodine was first investigated by Davaine in 1880 [126]. Iodine penetrates into the cell wall of microorganisms and damages the cell membrane by blocking hydrogen bond. This phenomenon alters the structure and function of cell proteins and enzymes, leading to cell death [127]. Iodine is active against a broad spectrum of microorganisms including *S. aureus, E. coli, Pseudomonas, Streptococcus, Salmonella, Candida, Enterobacter, Klebsiella, Clostridium, Corynebacterium, and Mycobacterium* [126]. Iodine dressings can be found in two preparations as povidone iodine and cadexomer iodine, and the various commercial formulations are summarized in **Table 3**.

http://dx.doi.org/10.5772/63961

Polyhexamethylene biguanide (PHMB) is an another antiseptic and widely used as antimicrobial dressing in wound healing. PHMB is known to be effective against *E. coli. S. aureus* and *S. epidermidis*. PHMB also works like iodine as it attaches to the bacterial cells and disrupts cell membrane resulting in leakage of potassium ions and cytosolic components that lead to cell death [128]. A study by Eberlein et al. [129] confirmed that PHMB containing biocellulose wound dressings were more effective than silver-containing dressing in retarding microbial loads present in locally infected wounds. Loke et al. [130] developed a two-layer dressing with sustained release of chlorhexidine which showed activity against *S. aureus* and *P. aeruginosa in vitro*.

Dressing type	Product name	Antiseptic
Pad	Iodoflex 0.9% Cadexomer Iodine Pad	Cadexomer iodine
Foam	IodoFoam	Iodine
Fibers	**Inadine**	Povidone iodine
Colloidal ointment base	Braunovidon ointment/ointment gauze	Povidone
Hydrogel dressing	Iodozym	Iodine
Liposome hydrogel	Repithel	Povidone
Foam	Kerlix AMD	PHMB
Sponges	Telfa AMD	PHMB
Foam	Kendall AMD	PHMB
Gauzes sponges	Curity AMD Antimicrobial Gauze Sponges	PHMB

Table 3. List of other commercially available antiseptics [36, 127].

3.5. Honey dressings

Honey has been used as wound dressing over centuries [131]. Honey has been reported in several clinical studies for treating chronic diabetic foot ulcers [132–135] and has antimicrobial and anti-inflammatory activity [136–138]. It is reported that honey can inhibit around 60 species of bacteria including *Alcaligenes faecalis, Citrobacter freundii, E. coli, Enterobacter aerogenes, Klebsiella pneumoniae, Mycobacterium phlei, Salmonella california, Salmonella enteritidis, Salmonella typhimurium, Shigella sonnei, S. aureus, and Staphylococcus epidermidis* [139]. In addition, it is reported Manuka honey and Cameroonian honey have an effect on *Pseudomonas aeruginosa*, methicillin-resistant *S. aureus* (MRSA), and vancomycin-resistant *Enterococcus* species [137, 140]. The antimicrobial properties of honey are ascribed to its low pH, hygroscopic nature, and peroxide-containing compounds [141]. The rich contents of sugar in honey generate high osmotic pressure and present an unsuitable environment to bacterial growth and cell proliferation [139]. Van den Berg et al. [142] investigated the anti-inflammatory properties of different types of honey *in vitro* by testing reactive oxygen species (ROS) inhibition capability and found American buckwheat honey exhibits high ROS inhibition ability. Many clinical studies have been performed on the basis of the antimicrobial effect of honey [143–145]. Clinical studies and bioactivity demonstrate the efficiency of honey in wound healing, maintaining a moist environment, promoting drainage of wound exudate and autolytic debridement [144]. It has been reported in minimizing malodour and scar formation of the wound [145] as well as angiogenic activity [146].

Sasikala et al. [147] developed a chitosan-based film dressing loaded with Manuka honey. They identified chitosan–lactic acid with 6% honey showed ideal dressing properties in terms of water vapor transmission rate, water absorption, tensile strength, elongation, and antibacterial activity against *E. coli* and *S. aureus.* **Table 4** summarizes the commercially available honey-based dressings currently sold on the market.

Dressing type	Product Name	Honey type
Hydrocolloid	MediHoney	Leptospermum honey
Alginate-based	MediHoney	Leptospermum honey
Fibers	MANUKAhd	Manuka honey
Pure honey	Surgihoney	Bioengineered honey
Foam	Ligasano	Honeycomb
Pure honey	MGO Manuka Honey	Manuka honey
Sterile Manuka honey	ManukaFill	Manuka honey
Honey-impregnated gauze	Manuka IG	Manuka honey
Sheets, ribbon, gel	TheraHoney	Manuka honey
Knitted viscose mesh dressing, pure honey	Activon	Manuka honey
Alginate ribbon and dressing	Algivon	Manuka honey
Composite, foam/silicone dressings	Actilite	Manuka honey
Nonadherent gauze fibers	MelDra	Buckwheat honey

Table 4. List of selected commercially available honey dressings used in wound healing [22, 148, 149].

3.6. Polymer-based antimicrobial dressings

Natural and synthetic polymers are widely used in acute and chronic wound healing due to their biodegradability, biocompatibility, and wound exudate handling capacity. However, some polymers themselves have an antimicrobial activity [150]. The combination of polymers and antimicrobial drugs provides effective dressings to improve wound healing. Biazar et al.

http://dx.doi.org/10.5772/63961

[151] evaluated a synthetic polymer-based hydrogel dressing that exhibits biocompatible and antimicrobials activity. In another study, synthetic polyvinyl alcohol was blended with calcium alginate to produce nano fiber matrix by electrospinning technique. *In vitro* antibacterial test showed the rate of inhibition of *S. aureus* depends on the concentration of calcium alginate [152]. Chitosan is a cationic polymer whose positive charge interacts with a negative charge of the microbial cell membrane, resulting in disruption and agglutination [153]. Carboxymethyl chitosan has been reported as a broad spectrum antibiofilm agent which can prevent biofilm formation for *E. coli and S. aureus* by 81.6 and 74.6%, respectively [154].

4. Summary

In this chapter, wound healing processes and types of dressings incorporating antimicrobial agents have been briefly discussed. Antimicrobials loaded into dressings for direct application to infected wound sites are becoming more popular worldwide in terms of safety, efficacy, cost effective, and convenience. The key antimicrobial agents ranging from antiseptics such as iodine, metals such as silver, antibiotics such as cephalosporins and aminoglycosides as well as natural products such as honey have been covered. In addition, the driving forces behind the developing of advanced therapeutic dressings have been reviewed. Furthermore, this review has demonstrated different and wide range of antimicrobial-loaded dressings, and a few clinical studies and commercially available antimicrobial dressings have been highlighted. Given the wide range of scientific studies and commercial products publicly available, it is evident that more evidence-based clinical trials are required to select appropriate dressings for the patients. It is also important to note the interdisciplinary fields (including formulation technology, biopharmaceutics, microbiology, materials and polymer chemistry and molecular biology) required for developing an effective antimicrobial dressing able to treat infection and also contribute towards enhanced wound healing.

Author details

Omar Sarheed[1*], Asif Ahmed[2], Douha Shouqair[1] and Joshua Boateng[2*]

*Address all correspondence to: sarheed@rakmhsu.ac.ae and j.s.boateng@gre.ac.uk

1 RAK College of Pharmaceutical Sciences, RAK Medical and Health Sciences University, Ras Al Khaiamah, United Arab Emirates

2 Department of Pharmaceutical, Chemical and Environmental Sciences, Faculty of Engineering and Science, University of Greenwich, Kent, UK

References

[1] Boateng JS, Matthews KH, Stevens HN, Eccleston GM. Wound healing dressings and drug delivery systems: a review. J Pharm Sci. 2008;97(8):2892–2923.

[2] Flanagan M. Wound care. Assessment criteria. Nurs Times. 1994;90(35):76–88.

[3] Hutchinson J. The Wound Programme. Centre for Medical Education: Dundee; 1992.

[4] Singer AJ, Clark RA. 1999. Cutaneous wound healing. N Engl J Med. 1999;341:738–746.

[5] Gottrup F, Melling A, Hollander DA. An overview of surgical site infections: aetiology, incidence and risk factors. EWMA J. 2005;5(2):11–15.

[6] Alavi A, Sibbald RG, Phillips TJ, Miller OF, Margolis DJ, Marston W, Woo K, Romanelli M, Kirsner RS. What's new: management of venous leg ulcers: approach to venous leg ulcers. J Am Acad Dermatol. 2016;74(4):627–640.

[7] Moffatt C. Identifying criteria for wound infection. EWMA Position document: 1–5 [Internet]. 2005. http://ewma.org/fileadmin/user_upload/EWMA/pdf/Position_Documents/2005__Wound_Infection_/English_pos_doc_final.pdf. [Accessed 17 Mar 2016].

[8] Eming SA, Krieg T, Davidson JM. Inflammation in wound repair: molecular and cellular mechanisms. J Invest Dermatol. 2007;127(3):514–525.

[9] Edwards R, Harding KG. Bacteria and wound healing. Curr Opin Infect Dis. 2004;17:91–96.

[10] Wolcott RD, Rhoads DD, Dowd SE. Biofilms and chronic wound inflammation. J Wound Care. 2008;17(8):333–341.

[11] Weyrich AS, Zimmerman GA. Platelets: signaling cells in the immune continuum. Trends Immunol. 2004;25(9):489–495.

[12] Reinke JM, Sorg H. Wound repair and regeneration. Eur Surg Res. 2012;49(1):35–43.

[13] Singer AJ, Clark RA. Cutaneous wound healing. N Engl J Med. 1999;341:738–746.

[14] Li J, Zhang YP, Kirsner RS. Angiogenesis in wound repair: angiogenic growth factors and the extracellular matrix. Microsc Res Tech. 2003;60(1):107–114.

[15] Steed, DL. The role of growth factors in wound healing. Surg Clin North Am. 1997;77(3): 575–586.

[16] Guo S, Dipietro LA. Factors affecting wound healing. J Dent Res. 2010;89(3): 219–229.

[17] Gottrup F. Oxygen in wound healing and infection. World J Surg. 2004;28(3):312–315.

[18] Rodriguez PG, Felix FN, Woodley DT, Shim EK. The role of oxygen in wound healing: a review of the literature. Dermatol Surg. 2008;34(9):1159–1169.

[19] Tandara AA, Mustoe TA. Oxygen in wound healing—ore than a nutrient. World J Surg. 2004;28(3):294–300.

[20] Faries PL, Teodorescu VJ, Morrissey NJ, Hollier LH, Marin ML. The role of surgical revascularization in the management of diabetic foot wounds. Am J Surg. 2004;187(5):S34–S37.

[21] Smith SC, Faxon D, Cascio W, Schaff H, Gardner T, Jacobs A, et al. Prevention conference VI: diabetes and cardiovascular disease: writing group VI: revascularization in diabetic patients. In: Proceeding of the American Heart Association; 18–20 January 2001; Circulation. 2002;105(18). p. 165–169.

[22] Boateng JS, Catanzano O. Advanced therapeutic dressings for effective wound healing —a review. J Pharm Sci. 2015;104(11):3653–3680.

[23] Bowler PG, Duerden BI, Armstrong DG. Wound microbiology and associated approaches to wound management. Clin Microbiol Rev. 2011;14 (2):244–269.

[24] Sue E. Gardner, Rita A. Frantz. Wound bioburden and infection-related complications in diabetic foot ulcers. Biol Res Nurs. 2008;10(1): 44–53.

[25] Noble WC. Ecology and Host Resistance in Relation to Skin Disease. 5th ed. New York: McGraw-Hill; 1999. p. 184–191.

[26] Menke NB, Ward KR, Witten TM, Bonchev DG, Diegelmann RF. Impaired wound healing. Clin Dermatol. 2007;25(1):19–25.

[27] Dow G, Browne A, Sibbald RG. Infection in chronic wounds: controversies in diagnosis and treatment. Ostomy Wound Manage. 1999;45(8):23–7, 29–40; quiz 41–2.

[28] Sun Y, Smith E, Wolcott R, Dowd SE. Propagation of anaerobic bacteria within an aerobic multi-species chronic wound biofilm model. J Wound Care. 2009;18(10):426–431.

[29] Stephens P, Wall IB, Wilson MJ, Hill KE, Davies CE, Hill CM, Harding KG, Thomas DW. Anaerobic cocci populating the deep tissues of chronic wounds impair cellular wound healing responses in vitro. Br J Dermatol. 2003;148(3):456–66.

[30] Donlan RM1, Costerton JW. Biofilms: survival mechanisms of clinically relevant microorganisms. Clin Microbiol Rev. 2002;15(2):167–193.

[31] Garrett TR, Bhakoo M, Zhang Z. Bacterial adhesion and biofilms on surfaces. Prog Natl Sci. 2008;18(9):1049–1056.

[32] Miller MB, Bassler BL. Quorum sensing in bacteria. Annu Rev Microbiol. 2001;55:165–199.

[33] Song C, Sun XF, Xing SF, Xia PF, Shi YJ, Wang SG. Characterization of the interactions between tetracycline antibiotics and microbial extracellular polymeric

substances with spectroscopic approaches. Environ Sci Pollut Res Int. 2014;21(3): 1786–1795.

[34] Costerton JW, Stewart PS, Greenberg EP. Bacterial biofilms: a common cause of persistent infections. Science. 1999;284(5418):1318–1322.

[35] Yamasaki O, Akiyama H, Toi Y, Arata J. A combination of roxithromycin and imipenem as an antimicrobial strategy against biofilms formed by *Staphylococcus aureus*. J Antimicrob Chemother. 2001;48(4):573–577.

[36] Moura LI, Dias AM, Carvalho E, de Sousa HC. Recent advances on the development of wound dressings for diabetic foot ulcer treatment—a review. Acta Biomater. 2013;9(7):7093–7114.

[37] Harding KG, Jones V, Price P. Topical treatment: which dressing to choose. Diabetes Metab Res Rev. 2000;16: S47–S50.

[38] Dumville JC, O'Meara S, Deshpande S, Speak K. Hydrogel dressings for healing diabetic foot ulcers. Cochrane Database Syst Rev. 2011;9:CD009101.

[39] Fonder M., Lazarus G, Cowan D, Aronson-Cook B, Kohli A, Mamelak A. Treating the chronic wound: a practical approach to the care of nonhealing wounds and wound care dressings. J Am Acad Dermatol. 2008;58(2):185–206.

[40] Hilton JR, Williams DT, Beuker B, Miller DR, Harding KG. Wound dressings in diabetic foot disease. Clin Infect Dis. 2004;39(Suppl 2):S100–S103.

[41] Lloyd LL, Kennedy JF, Methacanon P, Paterson M, Knill CJ. Carbohydrate polymers as wound management aids. Carbohydr Polym. 1998;37(3):315–322.

[42] Dumville JC, Deshpande S, O'Meara S, Speak K. Hydrocolloid dressings for healing diabetic foot ulcers. Cochrane Database Syst Rev. 2013; 8:CD009099.

[43] Skórkowska-Telichowska K, Czemplik M, Kulma A, Szopa J. The local treatment and available dressings designed for chronic wounds. J Am Acad Dermatol. 2013;68(4):117–126.

[44] Pawar HV, Boateng JS, Ayensu I, Tetteh J. Multifunctional medicated lyophilised wafer dressing for effective chronic wound healing. J Pharm Sci. 2014;103(6):1720–1733.

[45] Boateng JS, Pawar HV, Tetteh J. Evaluation of in vitro wound adhesion characteristics of composite film and wafer based dressings using texture analysis and FTIR spectroscopy: a chemometrics factor analysis approach. RSC Adv. 2015;5(129): 107064–107075.

[46] Labovitiadi O, Lamb AJ, Matthews KH. In vitro efficacy of antimicrobial wafers against methicillin-resistant *Staphylococcus aureus*. Ther Deliv. 2012; 3(4):443–55.

[47] Zubair M, Malik A, Ahmad J. Clinico-microbiological study and antimicrobial drug resistance profile of diabetic foot infections in North India. Foot (Edinburgh, Scotland). 2011;21(1):6–14.

[48] Gethin G. Role of topical antimicrobials in wound management. J Wound Care. 2009;Nov:4–8.

[49] Lipsky BA, Hoey C. Topical antimicrobial therapy for treating chronic wounds. Clin Infect Dis. 2009;49(10):1541–1549.

[50] Drosou A, Falabella A, Kirsner RS. Antiseptics on wounds: an area of controversy. Wounds Compend Clin Res Pract. 2003;15(5):149–166.

[51] Burks RI. Povidone-iodine solution in wound treatment. Phys Ther. 1998;78(2):212–218.

[52] Zhou LH, Nahm WK, Badiavas E, Yufit T, Falanga V. Slow release iodine preparation and wound healing: in vitro effects consistent with lack of in vivo toxicity in human chronic wounds. Br J Dermatol. 2002;146(3):365–374.

[53] Mirhadi H, Azar MR, Abbaszadegan A, Geramizadeh B, Torabi S, Rahsaz M. Cytotoxicity of chlorhexidine-hydrogen peroxide combination in different concentrations on cultured human periodontal ligament fibroblasts. Dent Res J. 2014;11(6):645–648.

[54] Severyns AM, Lejeune A, Rocoux G, Lejeune G. Non-toxic antiseptic irrigation with chlorhexidine in experimental revascularization in the rat. J Hosp Infect. 1991;17(3): 197–206.

[55] Du Toit, DF, Page BJ. An in vitro evaluation of the cell toxicity of honey and silver dressings. J Wound Care. 2009;18:383–389.

[56] Vowden K, Vowden K, Carville K. Antimicrobials made easy. Wounds Int. 2011;2(1):1–6.

[57] Cutting K. Wound dressings: 21st century performance requirements. J Wound Care. 2010;19(Suppl 1):4–9.

[58] Phoudee W, Wattanakaroon W. Development of protein-based hydrogel wound dressing impregnated with bioactive compounds. Nat Sci. 2015;49(1):92–102.

[59] Kataria K, Gupta A, Rath G, Mathur RB, Dhakate SR. In vivo wound healing performance of drug loaded electrospun composite nanofibers transdermal patch. J Pharm Sci. 2014;469(1):102–110.

[60] Shi Y, Truong V, Kulkarni K, Qu Y, Simon G, Boyd R. Light-triggered release of ciprofloxacin from an in situ forming click hydrogel for antibacterial wound dressings. J Mater Chem B. 2015;3(45):8771–8774.

[61] Öztürk E, Ağalar C, Keçeci K, Denkba E. Preparation and characterization of ciprofloxacin-loaded alginate/chitosan sponge as a wound dressing material. J Appl Polym Sci. 2006;101(3):1602–1609.

[62] Hima Bindu, TVL, Vidyavathi M, Kavitha K, Sastry T P, Kumar RVS. Preparation and evaluation of chitosan-gelatin composite films for wound healing activity. Trends Biomater Artif Organs. 2010;24(3):122–130.

[63] El-Shanshory A, Chen W, Mei M. Preparation of antibacterial electrospun PVA/regenerated silk fibroin nanofibrous composite containing ciprofloxacin hydrochloride as a wound dressing. J Donghua Univ. 2014;31(5):566–571.

[64] Unnithan AR, Barakat NA, Pichiah PB, Gnanasekaran G, Nirmala R, Cha YS, Jung CH, El-Newehy M, Kim HY. Wound-dressing materials with antibacterial activity from electrospun polyurethane–dextran nanofiber mats containing ciprofloxacin HCl. Carbohydr Polym. 2012;90(4):1786–1793.

[65] Jannesari M, Varshosaz J, Morshed M, Zamani M. Composite poly(vinyl alcohol)/poly(vinyl acetate) electrospun nanofibrous mats as a novel wound dressing matrix for controlled release of drugs. Int J Nanomed. 2011;6:993–1003.

[66] Tsou TL, Tang ST, Huang YC, Wu JR., Young JJ, Wang HJ. Poly(2-hydroxyethyl methacrylate) wound dressing containing ciprofloxacin and its drug release studies. J Mater Sci Mater Med. 2005;16(2):95–100.

[67] Manju S, Antony M, Sreenivasan K. Synthesis and evaluation of a hydrogel that binds glucose and releases ciprofloxacin. J Mater Sci. 2010;45(15):4006–4012.

[68] Puoci F, Piangiolino C, Givigliano F, Parisi OI, Cassano R, Trombino S, Curcio M. Ciprofloxacin–collagen conjugate in the wound healing treatment. J Funct Biomater. 2012;3(2):361–371.

[69] Roy DC, Tomblyn S, Burmeister DM, Wrice NL, Becerra SC, Burnett LR., Saul J. Ciprofloxacin-loaded keratin hydrogels prevent infection and support healing in a porcine full-thickness excisional wound. Adv Wound Care. 2015;4(8):457–468.

[70] Okoye EI, Okolie TA. Development and in vitro characterization of ciprofloxacin loaded polymeric films for wound dressing. Int J Health Allied Sci. 2015;4(4):234–42.

[71] Sinha M, Banik RM, Haldar C, Maiti P. Development of ciprofloxacin hydrochloride loaded poly(ethylene glycol)/chitosan scaffold as wound dressing. J Porous Mater. 2013;20:799–807.

[72] Loke WK, Lau SK, Yong LL, Khor E, Sum CK. Wound dressing with sustained antimicrobial capability. J Biomed Mater Res. 2000;53(1):8–17.

[73] Kota S, Jahangir M, Ahmed M, Kazmi I, Bhavani P, Muheem A, Saleem M. Development and evaluation of ofloxacin topical gel containing wound healing modifiers from natural sources. Sch Res Library. 2015;7(10):226–233.

[74] Boateng JS, Pawar HV, Tetteh J. Polyox and carrageenan based composite film dressing containing anti-microbial and anti-inflammatory drugs for effective wound healing. Int J Pharm. 2013;1–2(441):181–191.

[75] Pawar HV, Boateng JS, Ayensu I, Tetteh, J. Multifunctional medicated lyophilised wafer dressing for effective chronic wound healing. J Pharm Sci. 2014;103(6):1720–1733.

[76] Pawar HV, Tetteh J, Boateng JS. Preparation, optimisation and characterisation of novel wound healing film dressings loaded with streptomycin and diclofenac. Colloid Surf B: Biointerfaces. 2013;102:102–110.

[77] Kim JO, Choi JY, Park JK, Kim JH, Jin SG, Chang SW, Li DX. Development of clindamycin-loaded wound dressing with polyvinyl alcohol and sodium alginate. Biol Pharm Bull. 2008;December(31):2277–2282.

[78] Kim JO, Park JK, Kim JH, Jin SG, Yong CS, Li DX, Choi JY. Development of polyvinyl alcohol–sodium alginate gel-matrix-based wound dressing system containing nitrofurazone. Int J Pharm. 2008;1–2(359): 79–86.

[79] Hwang MR, Kim JO, Lee JH, Kim YI, Kim JH, Chang SW, Jin SG. Gentamicin-loaded wound dressing with polyvinyl alcohol/dextran hydrogel: gel characterization and in vivo healing evaluation. AAPS PharmSciTech. 2010;11(3):1092–103.

[80] Adhirajan N, Shanmugasundaram N, Shanmuganathan S, Babu M. Collagen-based wound dressing for doxycycline delivery: in-vivo evaluation in an infected excisional wound model in rats. J Pharm Pharmacol. 2009; 61(12):1617–23.

[81] Adhirajan N, Shanmugasundaram N, Shanmuganathan S, Babu M. Functionally modified gelatin microspheres impregnated collagen scaffold as novel wound dressing to attenuate the proteases and bacterial growth. Eur J Pharm Sci. 2009;36(2–3):235–245.

[82] Guan J, Dong LZ, Huang SJ, Jing ML. Characterization of wound dressing with microspheres containing levofloxacin. In: Proceedings of the International Conference on Information Technology and Scientific Management; 20 December 2010; Tianjin, China: 2010;1–2. p. 344–348.

[83] Bohl MKS, Leibovich SJ, Belem P, West JL, Poole WLA. Effects of nitric oxide releasing poly(vinyl alcohol) hydrogel dressings on dermal wound healing in diabetic mice. Wound Repair Regen. 2002;10(5):286–294.

[84] Halpenny GM, Steinhardt RC, Okialda KA, Mascharak, PK. Characterization of pHEMA-based hydrogels that exhibit light-induced bactericidal effect via release of NO. J Mater Sci Mater Med. 2009;20(11):2353–2360.

[85] Li Y, Lee PI. Controlled nitric oxide delivery platform based on *S*-nitrosothiol conjugated interpolymer complexes for diabetic wound healing. Mol Pharm. 2010;7(1):254–266.

[86] Lansdown AB. Silver. I: its antibacterial properties and mechanism of action. J Wound Care. 2002;11(4):125–130.

[87] Leaper D. Appropriate use of silver dressings in wounds: international consensus document. Int Wound J. 2012;9(5):461–464.

[88] Rai M, Yadav A, Gade A. Silver nanoparticles as a new generation of antimicrobials. Biotechnol Adv. 2009;27(1):76–83.

[89] Feng QL, Wu J, Chen GQ, Cui FZ, Kim TN, Kim JO. A mechanistic study of the antibacterial effect of silver ions on *Escherichia coli* and *Staphylococcus aureus*. J Biomed Mater. 2000;52(4):662–668.

[90] Matsumura Y, Yoshikata K, Kunisaki SI, Tsuchido T. Mode of bactericidal action of silver zeolite and its comparison with that of silver nitrate. Appl Environ Microbiol. 2003;69(7):4278–4281.

[91] Saengmee-anupharb S, Srikhirin T, Thaweboon B, Thaweboon S, Amornsakchai T, Dechkunakorn S, Suddhasthira T. Antimicrobial effects of silver zeolite, silver zirconium phosphate silicate and silver zirconium phosphate against oral microorganisms. Asian Pac J Trop Biomed. 2013;3(1):47–52.

[92] Rizzello L, Pompa PP. Nanosilver-based antibacterial drugs and devices: mechanisms, methodological drawbacks, and guidelines. Chem Soc Rev. 2014;43(5):1501–18.

[93] Ivask A, Kurvet I, Kasemets K, Blinova I, Aruoja V, Suppi S, Vija H. Size-dependent toxicity of silver nanoparticles to bacteria, yeast, algae, crustaceans and mammalian cells in vitro. PLoS One. 2014;9(7):e1–14.

[94] Sondi I, Salopek-Sondi B. Silver nanoparticles as antimicrobial agent: a case study on *E. coli* as a model for Gram-negative bacteria. J Colloid Interface Sci. 2004;275(1):177–182.

[95] Shrivastava S, Bera T, Roy A, Singh G, Ramachandrarao P, Dash D. Characterization of enhanced antibacterial effects of novel silver nanoparticles. Nanotechnology. 2010;18(22):1–9.

[96] Kazachenko A, Legler A, Per'yanova O, Vstavskaya Y. Synthesis and antimicrobial activity of silver complexes with histidine and tryptophan. Pharm Chem J. 2000;34(5): 257–258.

[97] Baker C, Pradhan A, Pakstis L, Pochan DJ, Shah SI. Synthesis and antibacterial properties of silver nanoparticles. J Nanosci Nanotechnol. 2005;5(2):244–249.

[98] Morones JR, Elechiguerra JL, Camacho A, Holt K, Kouri JB, Ram JT, Yacaman MJ. The bactericidal effect of silver nanoparticles. Nanotechnology. 2005;16(10):2346–53.

[99] Panacek A, Kvítek L, Prucek R, Kolar M, Vecerova R., Pizúrova N, Sharma VK. Silver colloid nanoparticles: synthesis, characterization, and their antibacterial activity. J Phys Chem B. 2006;110(33):16248–16253.

[100] Kim JS, Kuk E, Yu KN, Kim JH, Park SJ, Lee HJ, Kim SH. Antimicrobial effects of silver nanoparticles. Nanomed Nanotechnol Biol Med. 2007;3(1):95–101.

[101] Gade AK, Bonde P, Ingle AP, Marcato PD, Durán N, Rai MK. Exploitation of *Aspergillus niger* for synthesis of silver nanoparticles. J Biobased Mater Bioenergy. 2008;2(3):1–5.

[102] Lindsay S. Silver white paper—everything you ever wanted to know about the use of silver in wound therapy [Internet]. 2011. http://www.systagenix.co.uk/cms/uploads/1458_Silver_WhitePaperA4_LP3_060.pdf. [Accessed 10 Mar 2016].

[103] Wound Source [Internet]. http://www.woundsource.com/product-category/dressings/antimicrobial-dressings. [Accessed 10 Mar 2016].

[104] Rujitanaroj PO, Pimpha N, Supaphol P. Wound-dressing materials with antibacterial activity from electrospun gelatin fiber mats containing silver nanoparticles. Polymer. 2008;49(21):4723–4732.

[105] Lin YH, Hsu WS, Chung WY, Ko TH, Lin JH. Evaluation of various silver-containing dressing on infected excision wound healing study. J Mater Sci Mater Med. 2014;25(5): 1375–1386.

[106] Anisha BS, Biswas R, Chennazhi KP, Jayakumar R. Chitosan–hyaluronic acid/nano silver composite sponges for drug resistant bacteria infected diabetic wounds. Int J Biol Macromol. 2013;62:310–320.

[107] Ong SY, Wu J, Moochhala SM, Tan MH, Lu J. Development of a chitosan-based wound dressing with improved hemostatic and antimicrobial properties. Biomaterials. 2008;29(32):4323–4332.

[108] Madhumathi K, Sudheesh Kumar PT, Abhilash S, Sreeja V, Tamura H, Manzoor K, Nair SV. Development of novel chitin/nanosilver composite scaffolds for wound dressing applications. J Mater Sci Mater Med. 2010;21(2):807–813.

[109] Boonkaew B, Suwanpreuksa P, Cuttle L, Barber PM, Supaphol P. Hydrogels containing silver nanoparticles for burn wounds show antimicrobial activity without cytotoxicity. J Appl Polym Sci. 2014;131(9):40215.

[110] Pant B, Pant HR, Pandeya DR, Panthi G, Nam KT, Hong ST, Kim CS. Characterization and antibacterial properties of Ag NPs loaded nylon-6 nanocomposite prepared by one-step electrospinning process. Colloid Surf A: Physicochem Eng Aspects. 2012;395:94–99.

[111] Archana D, Singh BK, Dutta J, Dutta PK. Chitosan-PVP-nano silver oxide wound dressing: in vitro and in vivo evaluation. Int J Biol Macromol. 2015;73(1):49–57.

[112] Lansdown BG, Jensen K, Jensen MQ. Contreet foam and contreet hydrocolloid: an insight into two new silver-containing dressings. J Wound Care. 2003;12(6):205–210.

[113] Singh R., Singh D. Radiation synthesis of PVP/alginate hydrogel containing nanosilver as wound dressing. J Mater Sci Mater Med. 2012;23(11):2649–2658.

[114] Jodar KSP, Balcão VM, Chaud MV, Tubino M, Yoshida VMH, Oliveira JM, Vila MMDC. Development and characterization of a hydrogel containing silver sulfadiazine for antimicrobial topical applications. J Pharm Sci. 2015;104(7):2241–2254.

[115] Boateng JS, Burgos AR, Okeke O, Pawar H. Composite alginate and gelatin based bio-polymeric wafers containing silver sulfadiazine for wound healing. Int J Biol Macromol. 2015;79:63–71.

[116] Mi FL, Wu YB, Shyu SS, Schoung JY, Huang YB, Tsai YH, Hao JY. Control of wound infections using a bilayer chitosan wound dressing with sustainable antibiotic delivery. J Biomed Mater Res. 2002;59(3):438–449.

[117] Shanmugasundaram N, Sundaraseelan J, Uma S, Selvaraj D, Babu M. Design and delivery of silver sulfadiazine from alginate microspheres-impregnated collagen scaffold. J Biomed Mater Res B: Appl Biomater. 2006;77(2):378–388.

[118] Ammons M, Ward L, James G. Anti-biofilm efficacy of a lactoferrin/xylitol wound hydrogel used in combination with silver wound dressings. Int Wound J. 2011;8(3):268–273.

[119] Rayman G, Rayman A, Baker NR, Jurgeviciene N, Dargis V, Sulcaite R., Pantelejeva O. Sustained silver-releasing dressing in the treatment of diabetic foot ulcers. Br J Nurs (Mark Allen Publishing). 2005;14(2):109–114.

[120] Jude EB, Apelqvist J, Spraul M, Martini J, Jones G, Harding K, Benbow S. Prospective randomized controlled study of Hydrofiber® dressing containing ionic silver or calcium alginate dressings in non-ischaemic diabetic foot ulcers. Diabet Med. 2007;24(3):280–288.

[121] Gago M, Garcia F, Gaztelu V, Verdu J, Lopez P, Nolasco A. A comparison of three silver-containing dressings in the treatment of infected, chronic wounds. Wound Res. 2008;20(10):273–278.

[122] Hiro ME, Pierpont YN, Ko F, Wright TE, Robson MC, Payne WG. Comparative evaluation of silver-containing antimicrobial dressings on in vitro and in vivo processes of wound healing. Eplasty. 2012;12:48.

[123] Thomas S, McCubbin P. A comparison of the antimicrobial effects of four silver-containing dressings on three organisms. J Wound Care. 2003;12(3):101–107.

[124] Thomas S, McCubbin P. An in vitro analysis of the antimicrobial properties of 10 silver-containing dressings. J Wound Care. 2003;12(8):305–308.

[125] Gaisford S, Beezer AE, Bishop AH, Walker M, Parsons D. An in vitro method for the quantitative determination of the antimicrobial efficacy of silver-containing wound dressings. Int J Pharm. 2009;1–2(366):111–116.

[126] Sunil KP, Raja BP, Jagadish RG, Uttam A. Povidone iodine—revisited. Indian J Dent Adv. 2011;3(3):617–620.

[127] Sibbald R, Leaper D, Queen D. Iodine made easy. Wounds Int. 2011;2(2):1–6.

[128] Gilliver S. PHMB: a well-tolerated antiseptic with no reported toxic effects. J Wound Care. 2009; Active Health Care Suppl:9–14.

[129] Eberlein T, Haemmerle G, Signer M, Gruber MU, Traber J, Mittlboeck M, Abel M. Comparison of PHMB-containing dressing and silver dressings in patients with critically colonised or locally infected wounds. J Wound Care. 2012;21(1):13–19.

[130] Loke WK, Lau SK, Yong LL, Khor E, Sum CK. Wound dressing with sustained anti-microbial capability. J Biomed Mater Res. 2000;53(1):8–17.

[131] Forrest RD. Early history of wound treatment. J R Soc Med. 1982;75(3):198–205.

[132] Hammouri S. The role of honey in the management of diabetic foot ulcers. JRMS. 2004;11(2):20–22.

[133] Schumacher HH. Use of medical honey in patients with chronic venous leg ulcers after split-skin grafting. J Wound Care. 2004;13(10):451–452.

[134] Molan P, Betts J. Using honey to heal diabetic foot ulcers. Adv Skin Wound Care. 2008;21(7):313–316.

[135] Mclennan ASV, Henshaw FR, Twigg SM. What's the buzz: bee products and their potential value in diabetic wound healing. J Diabet Foot Complic. 2014;6(2):24–39.

[136] Boateng JS, Diunase K. Comparing the antibacterial and functional properties of Cameroonian and Manuka honeys for potential wound healing—have we come full cycle in dealing with antibiotic resistance? Molecules. 2015;20(9):16068–16084.

[137] Subrahmanyam M. A prospective randomised clinical and histological study of superficial burn wound healing with honey and silver sulfadiazine. Burns J Int Soc Burn Inj. 1998;24(2):157–161.

[138] Cooper RA, Halas E, Molan, PC. The efficacy of honey in inhibiting strains of Pseudo-monas aeruginosa from infected burns. J Burn Care Rehabil. 2002;23(6):366–370.

[139] Aggad H, Guemour D. Honey antibacterial activity. Med Aromat Plants. 2014;2(3):1–2.

[140] Song JJ, Salcido R. Use of honey in wound care: an update. Adv Skin Wound Care. 2011;24(1):40–4; quiz 45–6.

[141] Karayil S, Deshpande SD, Koppikar GV. Effect of honey on multidrug resistant organisms and its synergistic action with three common antibiotics. J Postgrad Med. 1998;44(4):93–96.

[142] Van den Berg AJ, Van den Worm E, Van Ufford HC, Halkes SB, Hoekstra MJ, Beukelman CJ. An in vitro examination of the antioxidant and anti–inflammatory properties of buckwheat honey. J Wound Care. 2008;17(4):172–174, 176–178.

[143] Gethin G, Cowman S. Bacteriological changes in sloughy venous leg ulcers treated with Manuka honey or hydrogel: an RCT. J Wound Care. 2008;17(6):241–244, 246–247.

[144] Molan P, Betts J. Clinical usage of honey as a wound dressing: an update. J Wound Care. 2004; 13(9):353–356.

[145] Alam F, Islam M, Gan S, Khalil M. Honey: a potential therapeutic agent for managing diabetic wounds. Evidence Based Complement Altern Med. 2014; 2014:Article ID 169130

[146] Rossiter K, Cooper AJ, Voegeli D, Lwaleed BA. Honey promotes angiogeneic activity in the rat aortic ring assay. J Wound Care. 2010;19(10):440, 442–446.

[147] Sasikala L, Durai B, Rathinamoorthy R. Manuka honey loaded chitosan hydrogel films for wound dressing applications. Int J PharmTech Res. 2013;5(4):1774–1785.

[148] Halstead F, Webber M, Rauf M, Burt R, Dryden M, Oppenheim B. In vitro activity of an engineered honey, medical-grade honeys, and antimicrobial wound dressings against biofilm-producing clinical bacterial isolates. J Wound Care. 2016;25(2):93–102.

[149] Molan PC. The evidence and the rationale for the use of honey as a wound dressing. Wound Practice Res. 2011;19(4):204–220.

[150] Mogosanu GD, Grumezescu AM. Natural and synthetic polymers for wounds and burns dressing. Int J Pharm. 2014;463(2):127–136.

[151] Biazar E, Roveimiab Z, Shahhosseini G, Khataminezhad M, Zafari M, Majdi A. Biocompatibility evaluation of a new hydrogel dressing based on polyvinylpyrrolidone/polyethylene glycol. J Biomed Biotechnol. 2012; 2012:Article ID 343989.

[152] Tarun K, Gobi N. Calcium alginate/PVA blended nano fibre matrix for wound dressing. Indian J Fibre Textile Res. 2012;37(2):127–132.

[153] Dai T, Tanaka M, Huang YY, Hamblin MR. Chitosan preparations for wounds and burns: antimicrobial and wound-healing effects. Exp Rev Anti-infect Ther. 2011;9(7): 857–879.

[154] Tan Y, Han F, Ma S, Yu W. Carboxymethyl chitosan prevents formation of broad-spectrum biofilm. Carbohydr Polym. 2011;84(4):1365–1370.

Chapter 18

The Need for Increased Attention to Low-Level Laser Therapy as Treatment for Wounds and Ulcers

Mohammad Bayat

Additional information is available at the end of the chapter

http://dx.doi.org/10.5772/64339

Abstract

Light amplification by stimulated emission of radiation (lasers) is a device that typically generates electromagnetic radiation of uniform wavelength, phase, and polarization. The term low-level laser therapy (LLLT) is broadly defined as the therapeutic benefit of lasers. This review aims to discuss the positive effects of LLLT on skin wounds, diabetic foot ulcers, and burn healing. Different LLLT protocols have been widely used as treatment for these conditions to accelerate tissue regenerative processes. We have classified eligible papers in the fields of skin wounds, ulcers, and burns into in vivo and in vitro experimental studies and clinical trials that evaluated the use of LLLT as treatments that promote healing. An electronic search of scientific peer reviewed papers was conducted in the PubMed database. Our search has shown that the use of LLLT in biology and medicine is growing rapidly, and advancements in LLLT research dramatically improved the clinicians' ability to safely and effectively treat wounds and ulcers. There is increased clinical use of laser for wound and ulcer treatment. Several recent studies have confirmed the potential beneficial effects of LLLT for wound healing.

Keywords: low-level laser therapy, skin wound, diabetic foot ulcer, burn

1. Introduction

The term low-level laser therapy (LLLT) is broadly defined as the therapeutic benefit of lasers. After Professor Mester from Hungary first revealed the therapeutic importance of lasers, different wavelengths of continuous wave (CW) LLLT have been shown to promote healing in skin from healthy humans and animals, as well as a number of experimental pathological cases. Different LLLT protocols have been widely used in numerous medical situations with the intent to accelerate the regenerative processes of tissues.

In this review, the author characterized eligible papers into in vivo and in vitro experimental studies and clinical trials that evaluated the use of LLLT on skin wounds for promotion of healing. The author conducted an electronic search of scientific peer reviewed papers in the PubMed database of English language studies published from 2004 to 2016 with the keyword "low-level laser therapy." As inclusion criteria, the author chose articles with availability of access to the full text. This review intended to show the positive effects of LLLT on healing of skin wounds, diabetic foot ulcers, and burns. Initially, the author introduced wounds, ulcers, and burns and showed their importance. Next, a number of important related papers in the field were reported.

2. Definition

Devices that provide light amplification by stimulated emission of radiation (LASERS) typically generate electromagnetic radiation of a uniform wavelength, phase, and polarization. In 1960, Theodore Maiman has originally described a ruby laser. A laser is described as a source of light or radiation energy [1].

3. History

The term "LLLT" is broadly applied to the therapeutic effects of lasers; other terms, such as low power laser therapy, laser biomodulation, laser bioactivation, laser biostimulation, laser irradiation, and laser photostimulation, may be substituted for LLLT. In this review, the author have chosen the term LLLT photostimulation because of the observed stimulatory effects of the laser beam and photochemical nature of its interaction with biological systems. LLLT is a special type of laser that influences biologic systems through nonthermal means [2]. The use of LLLT as a therapeutic modality has originated from Eastern Europe approximately 50 years ago [2]. In 1967, Professor Mester, an employee of Semmelweis University in Budapest, Hungary, observed that applying laser light to the shaven backs of mice could cause more rapid regrowth of hair compared to unshaven mice [3]. He reported that the helium-neon (He-Ne) laser had the capability to promote wound healing in mice [4]. Professor Mester applied these findings to humans when he used lasers to treat patients with nonhealing skin ulcers [5, 6]. The clinical applications of LLLT have become the leading edge of clinical research in several countries, such as the former USSR, Japan, Canada, Australia, United Kingdom, China, and several Scandinavian countries. The history, origin, and development of various lasers are well authorized [2]. The clinical application of laser photobiostimulation is growing rapidly. Several review articles that explain the clinical applications of LLLT have been published [2]. LLLT is currently considered not only as a therapeutic procedure primarily used for relief of inflammation, edema, and chronic joint disorders; escalate healing of the wounds, deeper tissues, and nerves; but also as a treatment for neurological disorders and pain [7].

4. Objective

LLLT exposes tissues and cells to low levels of red and near infrared (NIR) and IR light. This treatment is introduced to as "low level" because of usage of light at lower energy densities in comparison to other types of laser therapy such as cutting, ablation, and thermal coagulation of tissue. LLLT is also defined as "cold laser" therapy because of the lower power densities used compared to those needed to produce tissue heating [7]. LLLT is currently used to treat a wide variety of diseases in which a large number of laser parameters such as the energy density, wavelength, pulse structure, power density, and timing of the applied light must be chosen for each treatment. A less than optimal choice of parameters can lead to not only reduced effectiveness of the treatment but also result in negative therapeutic outcomes. Thus, numerous published results on LLLT include negative findings simply because of an inappropriate choice of light source and dosage. This choice is particularly important because of the optimal dose of light needed for any particular application; doses higher or lower than this optimal value may have no therapeutic effect. LLLT is defined by a biphasic dose response: lower doses of light are often more advantageous than high doses [7]. This review aims to discuss the positive effects of LLLT on healing diabetic wounds and burns. Low-level laser energy density (J/cm^2) calculation: power (W) × duration of laser radiation (s)/laser beam surface area (cm^2).

5. Wound healing

Wound healing, which is a normal physiological process, takes places in four particular phases: hemostasis, inflammation, proliferation, and remodeling. For a successful healing process, all four phases must follow in the appropriate sequence and time. Numerous factors can put adverse effects on different phases of this process, resulting in an inappropriate wound healing process. The most important factors that influence healing of the cutaneous wound and the potential cellular and/or molecular mechanisms involved consist of local and systemic factors. Local factors include oxygenation, infections, foreign bodies, and venous sufficiency, whereas systemic factors comprise age and gender, sex hormones, stress, diseases, such as diabetes mellitus (DM), keloids, fibrosis, hereditary healing disorders, jaundice, uremia, obesity, medications (glucocorticoid steroids, nonsteroidal anti-inflammatory drugs), chemotherapy, alcoholism, and smoking, as well as immunocompromised conditions (cancer, radiation therapy, AIDS, and nutrition). A better understanding of the effects of these factors on the wound healing process may lead to therapeutics that accelerate wound healing and resolve impaired wounds. However, the influences of these factors are not mutually exclusive. One or multiple factors may play a role in any of the individual phases by contributing to the overall outcome of the healing process [8].

6. Diabetic wound healing in animals and patients (diabetic foot ulcers (DFU))

DM is the general name for a heterogeneous group of metabolic disorder characterized by high blood glucose levels that result from defects in insulin secretion and/or action [9]. The percentage of the population diagnosed with DM continues to increase. A study projects that as many as one in three US adults may have DM by the year 2050 if current trends continue. The expense of DM in the United States, at more than $174 billion per year in 2007, is anticipated to become an increasingly large financial burden in the future [10].

DFUs are a common problem among individuals with DM. These ulcers are among the most serious complications of DM that may result in amputation and mortality [11]. The prevalence of DFU in people with DM vary from 4% to 10% with a lifetime incidence as high as 25% [12]. Treatment of diabetic foot is extremely hard because these wounds are delineated by delayed healing; often result in chronic wound [13]. It has been reported that the 5-year mortality leading to lower extremity amputations may be as high as 68% [14]. Therefore, successful treatment of diabetic ulcers is a field of huge importance [15].

Many elements considered to be sources for the lack of healing in diabetic wounds involve peripheral neuropathy, the presence of an impaired immune system, peripheral microvascular disease, glycation of hemoglobin that leads to inadequate oxygen delivery to tissues, alterations in the red blood cell membrane [13] due to glycation, interchange in the proportion of type III to type I collagen in the skin [16], impaired biomechanical properties of the diabetic skin [17], impaired proliferation of skin fibroblasts [18], and impaired L-lactate production [19]. The diabetic wound is a disorder of the wound healing process, especially in the inflammatory and proliferative phases [13], pathologic angiogenesis [20], and a significant diminishing of the tensile strength of wound repair, detected in studies on diabetic animal models [21].

According to a review of the literature, numerous in vitro and in vivo studies, as well as clinical trials have reported positive effects of LLLT on the wound healing process both in animals and human patients.

7. Literature review

Dahmardehei et al. have stated that significant numbers of patients in burn centers are diabetics. The healing process in these patients is more difficult due to complications attributed to diabetes. Despite the fact that the gold standard treatment for a grade 3 burn ulcer patient is split-thickness skin grafting (STSG), however in diabetic patients, the rate of graft rejection and organ amputation is high due to impaired tissue perfusion. Previous studies show that LLLT accelerates fibroblast proliferation, increases collagen synthesis and tissue perfusion, and accelerates wound healing. Dahmardehei et al. have recommended a new therapeutic method for improving the healing process with better prognosis for these patients. Their study enrolled type II diabetes patients with 13, grade 3 burn ulcers considered candidates for amputation.

In these patients, the grade 3 burn ulcers were treated by a 650 nm red laser light at 2 J/cm^2 for the bed of the ulcer and an 810 nm infrared laser light at 6 J/cm^2 for the margins, along with intravenous LLLT with a 660 nm red light, before and after STSG. The results showed complete healing for all patients considered candidates for amputation [22]. Góralczyk et al. reported that that chronic hyperglycemia was the source of endothelial activation. On the other hand, the inflammatory process in DM has been associated with the secretion of inflammatory cytokines by endothelial cells, such as tumor necrosis factor-alpha (TNF-α) and interleukin 6 (IL-6). Góralczyk et al. evaluated the effects of 635 and 830 nm wavelength LLL irradiation on the secretion of inflammatory factors (TNF-α and IL-6) in an endothelial cell culture-human umbilical vein endothelial cell (HUVEC) line under hyperglycemic conditions. Adverse effects of hyperglycemia on vascular endothelial cells might be recovered by the action of LLLT, especially at a wavelength of 830 nm. LLLT decreased TNF-α concentration in the supernatant and improved cell proliferation [23]. Lau et al. carried out a study to investigate the biophotonic effect of irradiance on collagen production in a rat model of a diabetic wound. The skin's tensile strength was a parameter to characterize the wound. The rat models received intravenous injections of streptozotocin (STZ) to induce diabetes. Skin-breaking strength was measured. The experimental animals were treated with an 808 nm diode laser at two power densities of 0.1 and 0.5 W/cm^2. The tensile strength was optimized after treatment with a high-power diode laser. The photostimulation effect was shown by the accelerated healing process and enhanced tensile strength of the wound. Lau et al. concluded that LLLT facilitated collagen production in diabetic wound healing [24]. Sharifian et al. assessed the influence of pulsed wave (PW) LLLT on healing of the diabetic wound in diabetic (STZ-D) rats. They divided rats into two groups: nondiabetic and diabetic. They induced type I DM in the diabetic rat group through injection of STZ. The rats were submitted to two full-thickness skin incisions on the dorsal region of each one. One month after the injection of STZ, wounds of the nondiabetic and diabetic rats were subjected to a pulsed, infrared 890 nm wavelength laser with an 80 Hz frequency and 0.2 J/cm^2 energy density for each wound point. PW LLLT significantly accelerated the numbers of macrophages, fibroblasts, and blood vessel sections in comparison with the corresponding control groups. Semiquantitative analysis of basic fibroblast growth factor (bFGF) gene expression indicated significant increase in gene expression in both nondiabetic and diabetic rats following LLLT [25]. Houreld reported that due to advancements in laser technology, irradiation of diabetic wounds with low-intensity laser irradiation (LILI) or phototherapy has vastly accelerated wound healing. At the correct laser parameters, LILI increased migration, viability, and proliferation of diabetic cells in vitro. A stimulatory effect on the mitochondria that resulted in increased adenosine triphosphate (ATP) was observed. In addition, LILI also showed anti-inflammatory and protective effects on these cells. In light of the continual threat of diabetic foot, infection, and amputation, new better therapies and the developing of wound healing research deserves better prioritization [26]. Esmaeelinejad and Bayat evaluated the effects of LLLT on human skin fibroblasts (HSFs) cultured in high glucose concentration and physiological glucose condition media. Release of IL-6 and bFGF was evaluated by enzyme-linked immunosorbent assay (ELISA). Statistical analysis demonstrated that certain previously mentioned laser doses (energy densities) promoted the release of IL-6 in HSFs which were cultured in high glucose concentration medium in comparison with nonirradiated HSFs cultured in the same medium. LLLT with 2 J/cm^2 energy density enhanced secretin of bFGF and IL-6 from fibroblast cultured in media mentioned above (hyperglycemic condition media). When HSFs were cultured in physiologic glucose concentration medium during laser irradiation, LLLT more effectively released IL-6 and bFGF [27]. In a single case study, Dixit et al. outlined the possible effect of LLLT on delayed wound healing and pain in a diabetic patient with chronic dehiscent sternotomy. After irradiation, they observed proliferation of healthy granulation tissue with decreased scores from the pressure ulcer scale of healing for sternal According to the results, LLLT could be a new potential treatment for chronic sternal dehiscence following coronary artery bypass graft, as it reinforced wound healing with an early closure of the wound deficit [28]. Fathabadie et al. conducted a study on the influence of PW LLLT on mast cells in wounds of nondiabetic and diabetic rats. The induction of type I DM and LLLT protocol was the same as Sharifian et al.'s study [25]. They assessed mast cell numbers and degranulation in all subgroups at 4, 7, and 15 days after infliction of the wounds. According to the paired *t*-test, there were significantly more total numbers of laser-treated mast cells compared to the placebos in the nondiabetic and diabetic groups. They observed significantly more granulated mast cells compared with degranulated mast cells for all laser-treated mast and placebo mast cells in the nondiabetic and diabetic groups [29]. Aparecida Da Silva et al. performed a study not only to determine if LLLT restored the balance between mRNA expression of matrix metalloproteinases (MMP)-2 and MMP-9 but also to determine the ratio between collagen types I and III during the diabetic wounds healing. The diabetes model was induced efficiently by STZ as demonstrated through increased levels of blood glucose. A diode laser (50 mW, 660 nm, 4 J/cm^2, 80 s) was administered once after scare induction. After LLLT, the rats were euthanized. The scarred areas were collected for MMP-2 and MMP-9 mRNA and histological analyses (inflammation and types I and III collagen). The results determined that scare significantly increased MMP-2 and MMP-9 expressions in untreated diabetic rats compared to nondiabetic rats. LLLT significantly reduced MMP-2 and MMP-9 expressions compared with untreated diabetic rats. Aparecida Da Silva et al. concluded that LLLT altered the expression of MMP-9, stimulated collagen production, and increased the total percentage of collagen type III in diabetic animals [30]. Esmaeelinejad et al. evaluated the effects of LLLT on HSFs cultured in high glucose concentration medium. HSFs were cultured either in physiologic glucose (5.5 mM/l) or high glucose (11.1 and 15 mM/l) media. LLLT was performed with a He-Ne laser unit at energy densities of 0.5, 1, and 2 J/cm^2. The viability and proliferation rate of these cells were determined by MTT assay. The results indicate that LLLT stimulate the viability and proliferation rate of HSFs, which were cultured in physiologic glucose medium compared to their control cultures. LLLT had stimulatory effects on the proliferation rate of HSFs cultured in high glucose concentrations compared with their control cultures. Esmaeelinejad et al. announced that HSFs originally cultured for 2 weeks in high glucose concentration attended to culture in physiologic glucose during laser irradiation increase cell viability and proliferation. Therefore, LLLT had a stimulatory effect on these HSFs [31]. Dadpay et al. studied the effect of LLLT in experimentally induced diabetic rats. They generated two full thickness skin incisions on the dorsal regions of each rat. The healthy (nondiabetic) groups received a pulsed-infrared 890 nm laser with an 80 Hz frequency and 0.03 J/cm^2 for each wound point in the first group and 0.2 J/cm^2

in the second group. Laser-treated diabetic wounds of the animals subjected to the same pulsed-infrared laser treatments as the second group for each wound point. Laser irradiation with 0.03 J/cm^2 significantly diminished the maximum load for wound repair in healthy rats. Laser irradiation with 0.2 J/cm^2 significantly escalated the maximum load in wounds from the healthy control and diabetic groups [32]. Peplow et al. have used a 660 nm laser diode in genetic diabetic mice to promote the healing process of wounds covered with a Tegaderm™ HP dressing that causes delayed contraction (splinted wounds). Possibly, the stimulation of healing could be due to the potential diabetes-modifying properties of laser light. Nonwounded diabetic mice and wounded diabetic mice was subjected to the 660 nm laser to at the same dose and location. They measured body weight and water intake of the mice. The left flank in the experimental group received 660 nm and 100 mW of irradiation 20 s/day for 7 days. There were no significant differences in body weight and water intake over 22 days between mice in the experimental and control groups. On day 14, the mean blood plasma glucose level did not significantly differ between the two groups. There was no glycated hemoglobin A1c detected in the samples. Peplow et al. concluded that irradiation of the left flank in diabetic mice with the 660 nm laser system did not have a significant hypoglycemic effect. The laser-stimulated healing of wounds in diabetic mice resulted from cellular and biochemical changes to the immediate wound environment [33]. Jahangiri et al. studied the effects of combined 670 and 810 nm diode lasers on diabetic wound healing parameters in rats. Two intervention (laser) groups underwent LLLT using 670 nm diode laser (500 mW, 10 J, 48 s) in the wound context and 810 nm diode laser (250 mW, 12 J, 50 s) to the wound margins. Never could they find statistically significant differences between the diabetic and nondiabetic groups in the wound area, percentage of open wound area, and wound healing rate by the repeated measurements. After 7 days of LLLT in the nondiabetic group, urine excretion significantly increased compared with the control group. Jahangiri et al. showed that no significant difference existed between the LLLT and control groups. The increased urine volume in nondiabetic rats after LLLT was an incidental observation that deserved future study [34]. Mirzaei et al. examined the impact of LLLT on cellular changes in organ culture and cell culture of skin from STZ-D rats. Type I DM was induced in rats by STZ. Fibroblasts extruded from the samples were proliferated in vitro and another set of samples were cultured as the organ culture. The researchers used an He-Ne laser. They administered 0.9–4 J/cm^2 energy densities four times to each organ and cell culture. The organ cultures were analyzed by light and transmission electron microscopy. Cell proliferation was evaluated by the MTT assay. Statistically, 4 J/cm^2 irradiation significantly increased the fibroblast numbers compared with the sham-exposed cultures [35].

8. Skin burn healing

Burn injuries are common traumatic injuries that cause considerable mortality and morbidity. Additionally, they are among the most expensive traumatic injuries due to the extended hospitalization and rehabilitation, as well as costly wound and scar treatments [36]. Annually in the United States, 1.25 million burn patients are treated. Of these, at least 50,000 require hospitalization [36]. Burn wounds generate special interest due to the large numbers of burn cases encountered. These wounds can generate a destructive effect functionally and cosmetically, which necessitates the search for a more efficient cure [37]. LLLT has beneficial effects on burn healing.

9. Literature review

Khoshvaghti et al. studied the effects of LLLT on mast cells in a third-degree burn rat model. Rats from all groups each received third-degree burns at three different locations. The first burn site on group I rats subjected to 890 nm pulsed laser, with 0.924 J/cm^2 energy density. 0.2% nitrofurazone cream was administrated for treatment of the second burn site on both groups of rats. They evaluated mast cell degranulation and numbers at each burn site on each group of rats. Analysis of variance on day 4 showed significantly lower total numbers of mast cells in the laser-treated burn sites compared with the other burn sites in both groups of rats. On day 8, the total numbers of mast cells were significantly lower at the laser-treated burn sites compared with the other burn sites. On day 13, there were significantly lower numbers of types I and II mast cells at the laser-treated burn sites compared with the other burn sites. Khoshvaghti et al. [38] concluded that LLLT significantly declined total numbers of mast cells through the proliferation and remodeling phases of healing in a rat model of third-degree burn. Ezzati et al. investigated the influence of PW LLLT on healing of a deep second-degree burn model in rats. In their study, two groups of laser-treated burns were treated by a 3000 Hz pulsed infrared diode laser that had 2.3 or 11.7 J/cm^2 energy densities, respectively. Treatment response was assessed both microbiologically and macroscopically. The incidence of *Staphylococcus aureus* diminished significantly in group 3 in comparison to group 1 on day 28. Analysis of variance showed that the 11.7 J/cm^2 LLLT significantly increased the wound closure rate at 2 and 3 weeks after infliction of the burn when compared with placebo burns. Independent sample *t*-tests demonstrated that LLLT with 11.7 J/cm^2 significantly enhance the wound closure rate though 4 weeks after infliction of the burn in comparison to the control burns. Ezzati et al. concluded that pulsed LLLT with 11.7 J/cm^2/890 nm of a deep second-degree burn model in rats significantly escalated the rate of wound closure compared with the control burns [39]. Ezzati et al. studied the influence of PW LLLT on the healing process of a third-degree burn in a rat model. They treated two groups of rats with a 3000 Hz-pulsed infrared diode laser that had 2.3 or 11.7 J/cm^2 energy densities and evaluated the response to treatment both microbiologically and macroscopically. They indicated that the incidence of *Staphylococcus epidermidis*, Lactobacillus, and Diphtheria diminished significantly in the laser-treated groups compared to the other groups by the chi-square test. The independent sample *t*-test illustrated that LLLT with 11.7 J/cm^2 energy density significantly escalated the wound-closure rate at 3 and 4 weeks after infliction of the burn compared with the control burns [40]. Vasheghani et al. evaluated 80 Hz pulsed infrared diode LLLT for third-degree burn healing in rats. The laser-treated burns were exposed to an 80 Hz pulsed 890 nm infrared diode laser at 0.396 J/cm^2, three times per week. Burn wounds were clinically examined. There were a significantly higher number of laser-treated burns that closed compared to the controls. The paired Student's *t*-test indicated that the wound closure rate of laser-treated burns was significantly longer than the control burns. Chi-square tests showed no significant difference between each microorganism (*Staphylococcus epidermis, S. aureus*, and *Pseudomonas aeruginosa*). Vasheghani et al. concluded that LLLT with an 80 Hz pulsed infrared diode laser accelerated third-degree burn healing in rats [41]. Bayat et al. studied the effects of LLLT on mast cell number during the inflammation, proliferation, and remodeling phases of the wound healing process of experimental burns. In the two laser-treated groups, burned areas were subjected to the LLLT with a He-Ne laser at energy densities of 38.2 or 76.4 J/cm^2. They observed that on day 7 in the first laser group, there were significantly more total numbers of mast cells compared with the other groups. On day 16 in the nitrofurazone-treated group, the total number of mast cells was significantly higher compared with the control, first laser, and normal groups [42]. In another study, Vashghani et al. investigated the effect of LLLT administered with a He-Ne laser on mast cell number and degranulation in rats with second-degree burns. All rats received deeply inflicted second-degree burns. In the two laser-treated groups, the burns received daily LLLT, with energy densities of 1.2 or 2.4 J/cm^2. In the fifth group, the burns were treated topically with daily administration of 0.2% nitrofurazone cream. Vashghani et al. concluded that administration of LLLT for deep second-degree cutaneous burns in rats not only significantly enhanced the number of intact mast cells during the inflammatory and proliferative phases of healing but also diminished the total number of mast cells during the remodeling phase [43]. In another study, Bayat et al. researched the effects of LL He-Ne LT on burn healing. The two laser treated groups, underwent daily treatment with LL He-Ne LT at energy densities of 1.2 or 2.4 J/cm^2. The response to treatment was assessed histologically and microbiologically. Analysis of variance demonstrated significantly greater mean blood vessel sections in the 1.2 J/cm^2 laser group compared with the other groups. Compared with the nitrofurazone-treated group, the mean depth of new epidermis in the 2.4 J/cm^2 laser group on day 16 was significantly lower. *P. aeruginosa* and *S. aureus* grew in more than 50% of samples obtained from control group, however these bacteria did not grow in the samples from the 2.4 J/cm^2 laser group. Bayat et al. concluded that LL He-Ne LT stimulated the destruction of *S. aureus* and *P. aeruginosa* in rats with third-degree burns. However, the histological evaluation demonstrated that LL He-Ne LT not only made a significant escalation in the mean blood vessel sections on day 7 after infliction of the third degree burns but also reduced the mean of the depth of new epidermis on day 16 after infliction of these burns in rats [44]. Bayat et al. studied the effects of two different doses of LLLT on healing deep second-degree burns. They inflicted a deep second-degree burn in each rat. The control group burns remained untreated. The two laser treated group burns were irradiated daily with LL He-Ne LT with energy densities of 1.2 or 2.4 J/cm^2. The response to treatments was assessed histologically and microbiologically. *S. epidermidis* was found in the 70% of the rats' wounds in the laser-treated groups in comparison to 100% of rats in the control group. Despite the fact that they found *S. aureus* in 40% of the rat wounds which were treated by nitrofurazone, they did not find this bacterium in the wounds of the laser treated and control groups. Bayat et al. determined that LLLT of deep second-degree burns made significant reduction in the number of macrophages and depth of the new epidermis.

Moreover, this treatment diminished the incidence of *S. epidermidis* and *S. aureus* [45]. It seems that special LLLT protocols have potential antimicrobial activity.

10. Cellular and tissue mechanisms of LLLT

It appears that LLLT not only has a great range of effects at the molecular, cellular, and tissue levels and also its specific modes of action may vary among different applications. Within the cell, there is strong evidence to suggest that LLLT causes the mitochondria [46] to enhance ATP production [27, 31], modification of reactive oxygen species (ROS), and induce transcription factors [47].

LLLT also enhances the proliferation, maturation, and motility of fibroblasts, and increases the production of bFGF [48]. When a chromophore absorbs a photon of light (laser) in the treated cells, an electron in the chromophore has the potential to become excited and move from low-energy orbit to a higher energy orbit [49]. The system can then use this stored energy to achieve various cellular tasks. There are several pieces of data that suggest that a mitochondria chromophore is as the initial LLLT target. Radiation of tissue with light makes mitochondrial products such as ATP, nicotinamide adenine dinucleotide (NADH), proteins, and RNA, as well as a reciprocal augmentation in oxygen consumption to increase. Various in vitro experiments have showed that cellular respiration is upregulated when mitochondria are subjected to a He-Ne laser or other forms of illumination [50]. The relevant chromophore can be detected by matching the action spectra for the biological response to light in the NIR range to the absorption spectra of the four membrane-bound complexes identified in mitochondria. This procedure demonstrates that complex IV or cytochrome *c* oxidase (CCO) is the essential chromophore in the cellular response to LLLT. CCO that consists of two copper and two heme-iron centers (components of the respiratory electron transport chain) is a large transmembrane protein complex [51]. The high-energy electrons are passed from electron carriers through a series of transmembrane complexes (such as CCO) to the final electron acceptor which makes a proton gradient used to produce ATP. Therefore, the administration of light directly affects ATP production by influencing one of the transmembrane complexes in the chain. Especially, LLLT increases ATP production and electron transport [52].

11. Contraindications and precautions

11.1. Contraindications

Direct irradiation of the eyes, within 4–6 months after radiotherapy, hemorrhaging region, locally to the endocrine glands [53].

11.2. Precautions

Epilepsy, fever, malignancy, to the low back or abdomen during pregnancy or menstruation, embryo or fetus, over the gonads, epiphyseal lines in children confused or disoriented patient, area of decreased sensation, infected tissue, sympathetic ganglia, vagus nerves, or cardiac region in patients with heart disease [53].

12. Conclusion

The effects of LLLT depend on the physiological state of the target cells, type of laser, radiation wavelength, energy density, and number of laser sessions. The biostimulation efficiency of LLLT is also dependent on the delivered energy density, which appears to be restricted to a very narrow therapeutic window. Compared with CW LLLT devices, PW LLLT devices provide more laser parameters. By investigating different values of these parameters, research models can be more effectively studied in these devices (PWLLLT) in comparison with CW LLLT devices, with the purpose of achieving better outcomes [54]. There were different LLLT protocols for different tissues. Clinical applications of LLLT have significantly impacted medicine and attracted the interest of clinicians, the public, and the media. The use of LLLT in biological applications and medicine is growing rapidly; advances in LLLT research have dramatically improved the clinician's ability to safely and effectively treat various medical conditions. According to several studies if the general condition of patients (such as blood glucose level, hydration, Na level, etc.) is controlled, LLLT can be useful for the treatment of diabetic foot ulcer. Nevertheless, additional research is required to elucidate the exact mechanism of laser photostimulations action at the cellular and molecular levels. Standardized treatment parameters of LLLT should be followed. Efforts should be made to evaluate precise dosimetry for skin wounds, DFUs, and burns.

Author details

Mohammad Bayat

Address all correspondence to: bayat_m@yahoo.com

Cellular and Molecular Biology Research Center, and Department of Biology and Anatomical Sciences, School of Medicine, Shahid Beheshti University of Medical Sciences, Tehran, Iran

References

[1] Farivar S, Malekshahabi T, Shiari R. Biological effects of low level laser therapy. J Lasers Med Sci. 2014;5:58–62.

[2] Reddy GK. Photobiological basis and clinical role of low-intensity lasers in biology and medicine. J Clin Laser Med Surg. 2004;22:141–50. doi: 10.1089/104454704774076208.

[3] Mester E, Szende B, Gartner P. The effect of laser beams on the growth of hair in mice. Radiobiol Radiother. 1968;9:621–6.

[4] Mester E, Spiry T, Szende B, Tota JG. Effect of laser rays on wound healing. Am J Surg. 1971;122:532–5. doi: 10.1016/0002-9610(71)90482-X.

[5] Mester E, Nagylucskay S, Doklen A, Tisza S. Laser stimulation of wound healing. Acta Chir Acad Sci Hung. 1976;17(1):49–55.

[6] Mester E, Szende B, Spiry T, Scher A. Stimulation of wound healing by laser rays. Acta Chir Acad Sci Hung. 1972;13:315–24.

[7] Chung H, Dai T, Sharma SK, Huang YY, Carroll JD, Hamblin MR. The nuts and bolts of low-level laser (light) therapy. Ann Biomed Eng. 2012;40:516–33. doi: 10.1007/s10439-011-0454-7.

[8] Guo S, Dipietro LA. Factors affecting wound healing. J Dent Res. 2010;89(3):219–29.

[9] Couch R, Jetha M, Dryden DM, Hooton N, Liang Y, Durec T, et al. Diabetes education for children with type 1 diabetes mellitus and their families. Evid Rep/Technol Assess. 2008;(166):1–144.

[10] Boyle JP, Thompson TJ, Gregg EW, Barker LE, Williamson DF. Projection of the year 2050 burden of diabetes in the US adult population: dynamic modeling of incidence, mortality, and prediabetes prevalence. Popul Health Metrics. 2010;8:1. doi: 10.1186/1478-7954-8-29.

[11] Noble-Bell G, Forbes A. A systematic review of the effectiveness of negative pressure wound therapy in the management of diabetes foot ulcers. Int Wound J. 2008;5:233–42. doi: 10.1111/j.1742-481X.2008.00430.x.

[12] Singh N, Armstrong DG, Lipsky BA. Preventing foot ulcers in patients with diabetes. JAMA. 2005;293(2):217–28. doi: 10.1001/jama.293.2.217.

[13] Breitbart AS, Laser J, Parrett B, Porti D, Grant RT, Grande DA, et al. Accelerated diabetic wound healing using cultured dermal fibroblasts retrovirally transduced with the platelet-derived growth factor B gene. Ann Plastic Surg. 2003;51:409–14. doi: 10.1097/01.SAP.0000084461.83554.71.

[14] Reiber GE, Boyko EJ, Smith DG. Lower extremity foot ulcers and amputations in diabetes. In Aubert R, editor. Diabetes in America. Diane Publishing Co. National Institutes of Health, USA; 1995. p. 409–27.

[15] Kawalec J, Pfennigwerth T, Hetherington V, Logan J, Penfield V, Flauto J, et al. A review of lasers in healing diabetic ulcers. Foot. 2004;14:68–71. doi: 10.1016/j.foot.2003.11.001.

[16] Kern P, Moczar M, Robert L. Biosynthesis of skin collagens in normal and diabetic mice. Biochem J. 1979;182:337–45. doi: 10.1042/bj1820337.

[17] Bermudez DM, Herdrich BJ, Xu J, Lind R, Beason DP, Mitchell ME, et al. Impaired biomechanical properties of diabetic skin: implications in pathogenesis of diabetic wound complications. Am J Pathol. 2011;178:2215–23. doi: 10.1016/j.ajpath.2011.01.015.

[18] Loots MA, Lamme EN, Mekkes JR, Bos JD, Middelkoop E. Cultured fibroblasts from chronic diabetic wounds on the lower extremity (non-insulin-dependent diabetes mellitus) show disturbed proliferation. Arch Dermatol Res. 1999;291(2–3):93–9.

[19] Hehenberger K, Hansson A, Heilborn JD, Abdel-Halim SM, Östensson CG, Brismar K. Impaired proliferation and increased l-lactate production of dermal fibroblasts in the GK-rat, a spontaneous model of non-insulin dependent diabetes mellitus. Wound Repair Regener. 1999;7:65–71. doi: 10.1007/s004030050389.

[20] Francis-Goforth KN, Harken AH, Saba JD. Normalization of diabetic wound healing. Surgery. 2010;147:446–9. doi: 10.1016/j.surg.2009.04.038.

[21] Kwon DS, Gao X, Liu YB, Dulchavsky DS, Danyluk AL, Bansal M, et al. Treatment with bone marrow-derived stromal cells accelerates wound healing in diabetic rats. Int Wound J. 2008;5:453–63. doi: 10.1111/j.1742-481X.2007.00408.x.

[22] Dahmardehei M, Kazemikhoo N, Vaghardoost R, Mokmeli S, Momeni M, Nilforoushzadeh MA, et al. Effects of low level laser therapy on the prognosis of split-thickness skin graft in type 3 burn of diabetic patients: a case series. Lasers Med Sci. 2016 31:497–502. doi: 10.1007/s10103-016-1896-9.

[23] Góralczyk K, Szymańska J, Szot K, Fisz J, Rość D. Low-level laser irradiation effect on endothelial cells under conditions of hyperglycemia. Lasers Med Sci. 2016:1–7.

[24] Lau PS, Bidin N, Krishnan G, Nassir Z, Bahktiar H. Biophotonic effect of diode laser irradiance on tensile strength of diabetic rats. J Cosmet Laser Ther. 2015;17:86–9.

[25] Sharifian Z, Bayat M, Alidoust M, Farahani RM, Bayat M, Rezaie F, et al. Histological and gene expression analysis of the effects of pulsed low-level laser therapy on wound healing of streptozotocin-induced diabetic rats. Lasers Med Sci. 2014;29:1227–35. doi: 10.1007/s10103-013-1500-5.

[26] Houreld NN. Shedding light on a new treatment for diabetic wound healing: a review on phototherapy. Scientific World J. 2014;2014. doi: 10.1155/2014/398412.

[27] Esmaeelinejad M, Bayat M. Effect of low-level laser therapy on the release of interleukin-6 and basic fibroblast growth factor from cultured human skin fibroblasts in normal and high glucose mediums. J Cosmet Laser Ther. 2013;15:310–7. doi: 10.3109/14764172.2013.803366.

[28] Dixit S, Maiya A, Umakanth S, Borkar S. Photobiomodulation of surgical wound dehiscence in a diabetic individual by low-level laser therapy following median sternotomy. Indian J Palliat Care. 2013;19:71. doi: 10.4103/0973-1075.110242.

[29] Fathabadie FF, Bayat M, Amini A, Bayat M, Rezaie F. Effects of pulsed infra-red low level-laser irradiation on mast cells number and degranulation in open skin wound

healing of healthy and streptozotocin-induced diabetic rats. J Cosmet Laser Ther. 2013;15:294–304. doi: 10.3109/14764172.2013.764435.

[30] Aparecida Da Silva A, Leal-Junior ECP, Alves ACA, Rambo CS, Dos Santos SA, Vieira RP, et al. Wound-healing effects of low-level laser therapy in diabetic rats involve the modulation of MMP-2 and MMP-9 and the redistribution of collagen types I and III. J Cosmet Laser Ther. 2013;15:210–6. doi: 10.3109/14764172.2012.761345.

[31] Esmaeelinejad M, Bayat M, Darbandi H, Bayat M, Mosaffa N. The effects of low-level laser irradiation on cellular viability and proliferation of human skin fibroblasts cultured in high glucose mediums. Lasers Med Sci. 2014;29:121–9. doi: 10.1007/s10103-013-1289-2.

[32] Dadpay M, Sharifian Z, Bayat M, Bayat M, Dabbagh A. Effects of pulsed infra-red low level-laser irradiation on open skin wound healing of healthy and streptozotocin-induced diabetic rats by biomechanical evaluation. J Photochem Photobiol B: Biol. 2012;111:1–8. doi: 10.1007/s10103-013-1289-2.

[33] Peplow PV, Chung TY, Baxter GD. Laser photostimulation (660 nm) of wound healing in diabetic mice is not brought about by ameliorating diabetes. Lasers Surg Med. 2012;44:26–9. doi: 10.1002/lsm.21133. Epub 2011 Nov 22.

[34] Jahangiri Noudeh Y, Shabani M, Vatankhah N, Hashemian SJ, Akbari K. A combination of 670 nm and 810 nm diode lasers for wound healing acceleration in diabetic rats. Photomed Laser Surg. 2010;28(5):621–7.

[35] Mirzaei M, Bayat M, Mosafa N, Mohsenifar Z, Piryaei A, Farokhi B, et al. Effect of low-level laser therapy on skin fibroblasts of streptozotocin-diabetic rats. Photomed Laser Surg. 2007;25:519–25. doi: 10.1089/pho.2009.2634.

[36] Gamelli RL. Cost-utility analysis applied to the treatment of burn patients in a specialized center—invited critique. Arch Surg. 2007;142:57. doi: 10.1001/archsurg.142.1.50.

[37] Ghieh F, Jurjus R, Ibrahim A, Geagea AG, Daouk H, El Baba B, et al. The use of stem cells in burn wound healing: a review. Biomed Res Int. 2015;684084:7. doi: 10.1155/2015/684084.

[38] Khoshvaghti A, Zibamanzarmofrad M, Bayat M. Effect of low-level treatment with an 80-Hz pulsed infrared diode laser on mast-cell numbers and degranulation in a rat model of third-degree burn. Photomed Laser Surg. 2011;29:597–604. doi: 10.1089/pho.2010.2783.

[39] Ezzati A, Bayat M, Khoshvaghti A. Low-level laser therapy with a pulsed infrared laser accelerates second-degree burn healing in rat: a clinical and microbiologic study. Photomed Laser Surg. 2010;28:603–11. doi: 10.1089/pho.2009.2544.

[40] Ezzati A, Bayat M, Taheri S, Mohsenifar Z. Low-level laser therapy with pulsed infrared laser accelerates third-degree burn healing process in rats. J Rehabil Res Dev. 2009;46:543. doi: 10.1089/pho.2009.2544.

[41] Vasheghani MM, Bayat M, Dadpay M, Habibie M, Rezaei F. Low-level laser therapy using 80-Hz pulsed infrared diode laser accelerates third-degree burn healing in rat. Photomed Laser Surg. 2009;27:959–64. doi: 10.1089/pho.2008.2366.

[42] Bayat M, Vasheghani MM, Razavie N, Jalili MR. Effects of low-level laser therapy on mast cell number and degranulation in third-degree burns of rats. J Rehabil Res Dev. 2008;45:931.

[43] Vasheghani MM, Bayat M, Rezaei F, Bayat A, Karimipour M. Effect of low-level laser therapy on mast cells in second-degree burns in rats. Photomed Laser Surg. 2008;26:1–5. doi: 10.1089/pho.2007.2103.

[44] Bayat M, Vasheghani MM, Razavi N. Effect of low-level helium–neon laser therapy on the healing of third-degree burns in rats. J Photochem Photobiol B: Biol. 2006;83:87–93. doi: 10.1016/j.jphotobiol.2005.12.009.

[45] Bayat M, Vasheghani MM, Razavi N, Taheri S, Rakhshan M. Effect of low-level laser therapy on the healing of second-degree burns in rats: a histological and microbiological study. J Photochem Photobiol B: Biol. 2005;78:171–7. doi: 10.1016/j.jphotobiol.2004.08.012.

[46] Greco M, Guida G, Perlino E, Marra E, Quagliariello E. Increase in RNA and protein synthesis by mitochondria irradiated with helium-neon laser. Biochem Biophys Res Commun. 1989;163:1428–34. doi: 10.1016/0006-291X(89)91138-8.

[47] Karu T. Primary and secondary mechanisms of action of visible to near-IR radiation on cells. J Photochem Photobiol B: Biol. 1999;49:1–17. doi: 10.1016/S1011-1344(98)00219-X.

[48] Chen AC, Arany PR, Huang Y-Y, Tomkinson EM, Sharma SK, Kharkwal GB, et al. Low-level laser therapy activates NF-kB via generation of reactive oxygen species in mouse embryonic fibroblasts. PLoS One. 2011;6:e22453. doi: 10.1371/journal.pone.0022453.

[49] Karu TI. Photobiological fundamentals of low-power laser therapy. Quant Electron. IEEE J. 1987;23:1703–17. doi: 10.1109/JQE.1987.1073236.

[50] Karu T, Afanas' eva N. Cytochrome *c* oxidase as the primary photoacceptor upon laser exposure of cultured cells to visible and near IR-range light. Dokl Akad Nauk/[Rossiiskaia akademii nauk]. 1995;342:693–5.

[51] Fuller S, Capaldi R, Henderson R. Structure of cytochrome *c* oxidase in deoxycholate-derived two-dimensional crystals. J Mol Biol. 1979;134(2):305–27.

[52] Karu T, Pyatibrat L, Kalendo G. Irradiation with He-Ne laser increases ATP level in cells cultivated in vitro. J Photochem Photobiol B: Biol. 1995;27(3):219–23. doi:10.1016/1011-1344:07078-3.

[53] Cameron MH. Physical agents in rehabilitation: from research to practice. Elsevier Health Sciences; St Louis, Missouri, USA; 2012.

[54] Bayat M. The necessity for increased attention to pulsed low-level laser therapy. Photomed Laser Surg. 2014;32:427–8. doi: 10.1089/pho.2014.9858.

Chapter 19

The Use of Amniotic Membrane in the Management of Complex Chronic Wounds

Gregorio Castellanos, Ángel Bernabé-García,
Carmen García Insausti, Antonio Piñero,
José M. Moraleda and Francisco J. Nicolás

Additional information is available at the end of the chapter

http://dx.doi.org/10.5772/64491

Abstract

Chronic wounds do not follow the usual wound healing process; instead, they are stuck in the inflammatory or proliferative phase. This is particularly evident in large, massive wounds with considerable tissue loss, which become senescent and do not epithelialize. In these wounds, we need to remove all the factors that prevent or delay normal wound healing. After that, soft tissue granulation is stimulated by local negative pressure therapy. Lastly, after the granulation is completed, the epithelialization process must be activated. Although a plethora of wound dressings and devices are available, chronic wounds persist as a unresolved medical concern. We have been using frozen amniotic membrane (AM) to treat this type of wounds with good results. Our studies have shown that AM is able to induce epithelialization in large wounds that were unable to epithelialize. AM induces several signaling pathways involved in cell migration and/or proliferation. Among those, we can highlight the mitogen-activated protein kinase (MAPK) and Jun N-terminal kinase (JNK) signaling pathways. Additionally, AM is able to selectively antagonise the anti-proliferative effect of TGFß by modifying its genetic program on keratinocytes. The combined effect of AM on keratinocytes, promoting cell proliferation/migration and antagonising TGFß-effect, is the perfect combination allowing chronic wounds to progress into epithelialization.

Keywords: soft-tissue chronic wounds, amniotic membrane, TGF-β, epithelialization

1. Introduction

The evolution of knowledge about the biology of wound healing makes it possible to predict the sequence and prognosis of the events that occur in this complex process. However, there are wounds in which healing can be either prolonged over time or not fully achieved [1, 2].

Therefore, The keys to providing adequate and efficient treatment involve identifying, as soon as possible, the combination of either internal or external factors that contribute to the complexity of the wound and affect the healing process, and to detect at an early stage when it is likely that a wound would be slow or difficult to heal.

The actions undertaken should be aimed at reducing the aspects that lead to complexity, including factors related to the patient, the wound, relationships with healthcare personnel, and available resources. Only by assessing and understanding the interaction between these factors and their effect on healing will it be possible to develop efficient and appropriate strategies for improving results. Similarly, certain characteristics of the wound, such as its anatomical location, time duration, size, depth, and the state of the wound bed, are correlated with adequate healing [3–5].

The presence of necrotic tissue, crusts, slough, or foreign bodies in the wound bed, which are all obstacles for wound assessment, can lead to a delay in healing, and they can also be a focus of infection. Therefore, it is important to provide frequent, extensive, and efficient debridement until healthy tissue is found [6]. There are other situations that can have an influence and cause healing to fail, such as ischemia. Poor perfusion deprives tissue of an efficient oxygen and metabolic exchange, and causes an increase in vascular permeability, leukocyte retention, synthesis and the liberation of oxygen free radicals and proteolytic enzymes [7]. Inflammation in chronic wounds brings about a prolongation in healing time, resulting in an exacerbated inflammatory reaction, which in turn causes the hyperproduction of pro-inflammatory cytokines and proteolytic enzymes. This activity is combined with a decrease in the secretion of metalloproteinase tissue inhibitors, and it intensifies as the wound bed pH alters. As a consequence, we find that in the wound bed there is a sustained inflammation with matrix degradation, a limited bioavailability of growth factors and intense fibroblast aging, all of which reduce tissue repair, cell proliferation, and angiogenesis [8, 9].

In the same way, chronic wounds are characterized by the presence of one or more bacterial strains, with antibiotic-resistant microorganisms, and the presence of biofilms within which the bacteria are protected against the action of the silver-based antimicrobials [10–13].

The initial response to treatment is indicative of the viability of the tissue and its capacity to heal. When a patient's wound does not heal in the planned period of time using conventional treatment, it is essential to reassess the patient and modify the therapeutic guidelines [14, 15].

Thus, tissue wound healing usually follows a predictable sequence, although in some cases, it is prolonged over time or it is never achieved. The wound healing process is the result of a complex interaction between the patient and wound factors, the treatment adopted, and the skills and knowledge of healthcare professionals. Only by carrying out a detailed initial

http://dx.doi.org/10.5772/64491

assessment and repeated treatment assessment will it be possible to identify the factors that contribute to the complexity of the wound and to assess its potential state. The challenge for professionals is to utilize the most efficient therapeutic strategies at the right time and in the most cost-effective way, in order to reduce the complex nature of wounds, to treat the symptoms, and whenever possible, to achieve wound healing.

2. How should chronic and complex soft-tissue wounds be managed?

2.1. Management and treatment strategies

Chronic and complex soft-tissue wounds usually involve difficult healing, which means that they require an appropriate management-treatment strategy using a comprehensive and dynamic approach, applying new therapies to confront this old problem: wound healing [16]. In order to carry out this comprehensive approach, we should take into account the complex nature of the wound and its healing, its relationship with psychosocial factors and delays in wound healing, together with the economic cost for the patient, family, community, and the healthcare system. The steps to follow in order to achieve this approach should take into account the complete assessment of the patient, the control of causal factors, general healthcare, and the preparation of the wound bed.

2.2. Preparation of the wound bed

The preparation of the wound bed is an essential and dynamic process that provides an appropriate framework for a structured approach to wound management. This notion stresses a comprehensive and systematic approach with the aim of assessing and eliminating barriers to the normal wound healing process. It develops the appropriate treatment strategies to be directed at the patient in general and for treating the underlying condition causing the wound. Its objective is to create an optimum healing setting, a well-vascularized wound, with a stable and balanced bed in terms of exudate production, aimed at reducing scar healing time and facilitating the efficiency of other therapeutic measures. The wound bed should be prepared in each phase of the wound healing process following an agreed-upon procedure.

The "Tissue, Inflammation-infection, Moisture, Edge" (T.I.M.E.) scheme, proposed by the European Wound Management Association (EWMA), is based on the research of the International Wound Bed Preparation Advisory Board (IWBPAB), which established an algorithm through the development of the acronym T.I.M.E., whose objective is to describe the characteristics of chronic wounds during wound bed preparation. Following on from this, the concept was updated by placing emphasis on the treatment of the cause of the wound and general patient factors during treatment, before dealing with local wound factors. This algorithm consists of four components that cover the different physiopathological alterations present in chronic wounds: the management and conditioning of non-viable tissue, the monitoring of inflammation and infection, the disequilibrium of moisture due to excess exudate, and the stimulation and progression of the wound edges. So we can see that the T.I.M.E. framework involves the overall strategies that can be applied to the management of different kinds of wound with the aim of maximizing the ability to heal wounds [16–18] (**Figure 1**).

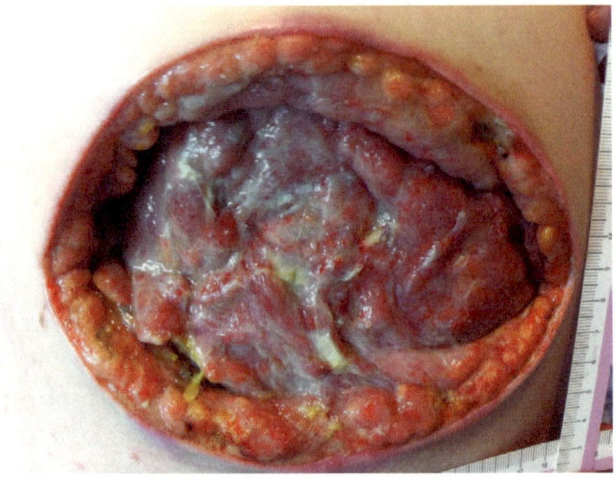

Figure 1. Complex and traumatic soft-tissue wound. Management and treatment of wound bed.

Wound treatment is initiated with a hydrodynamic washing using 0.9% saline solution at room temperature, with a 1–4 kg/cm effective washing pressure, without any damage being caused (a 20-ml syringe, with a 0.9-mm-diameter catheter), and the surrounding area is washed with a soapy antiseptic solution consisting of chlorhexidine digluconate.

For the monitoring of the non-viable tissues (necrotic tissue, crust, slough, and foreign bodies), episodic or continuous debridement is carried out until healthy tissue is found. It can be surgical, using tangential hydrodissection (Versajet™Plus, Smith & Nephew, London, United Kingdom); enzymatic, applying exogenous enzymes locally (collagenase, fibrolysine, trypsin, or chymotrypsin); chemical (cadexomer iodine); autolytic (due to the conjunction of three factors: hydration of the bed, fibrinolysis and the action of the endogenous enzymes on the devitalized tissue); or osmotic (hyperosmotic solutions). On occasions, an instillation therapy can also be used (VeraFlo™, KCI, Acelity LPI, San Antonio, TX) either in deep wounds with a viscous exudate or in uncontrolled infections on prosthetic materials, in order to eliminate the biofilm, reduce the pain, and reactivate healing. A noninvasive treatment option, for the debridement of chronic wounds, is low-frequency guided ultrasound [3].

In the management of the bacterial load (a contaminated or colonized lesion, with critical or infected colonization), foci of local and/or systemic infection have to be removed, which is why it is necessary to clean and debride the wound; take a wound culture; monitor the wound proteases; and use topical antimicrobials (silver, cadexomer iodine), systemic antibiotics according to the antibiogram data, anti-inflammatory drugs, and protease inhibitors if required.

It is important to monitor the exudate and achieve the equilibrium in the moisture, given that a dry wound makes it difficult for cell migration and exudate encourages infection and macerates the perilesional skin area. We should be aware that scarring is faster with wounds in an optimally moist environment in which the physiological and atmospheric conditions of the wound bed are maintained, thus fostering basal keratinocyte migration. A moist environment also prevents cell desiccation, encourages cell migration, promotes angiogenesis, stimulates collagen synthesis, and facilitates intercellular communication. A moist wound environment preserves a slightly acid pH and a low oxygen tension on the surface of the wound [18–20].

Thus, the edges of the wound do not advance because there are keratinocytes that do not migrate, senescent cells, and alterations in the extracellular matrix secondary to the disequilibrium in protease activity.

2.3. Clinical protocols

The preparation of the wound bed requires specific management protocols, which can be grouped into three sections following the T.I.M.E. procedure:

- Nonsurgical debridement with moisture monitoring and dressing every 48 h (**Table 1**).
- Local infection with moisture monitoring and dressing every 72 h (**Table 2**).
- A granulation phase with moisture monitoring and dressing every 72 h (**Table 3**).

Protocol 1: (T/M= Tissue and moisture) **-Non-viable tissue and moisture monitoring** **-Non-surgical debridement** **-Dressing every 48 h**			
-Type of wound	-Necrotic tissue -Low exudate	-Sloughy tissue -Moderate exudate	-Infected sloughy tissue -High exudate
-Debridement	-Collagenase + hydrogel	-Collagenase	-Cadexomer iodine + alginate
-Moist dressing	-Hydrocellular with acrylic adhesive or silicone adhesive	-Hydrocellular with acrylic adhesive or silicone adhesive	-Hydrocellular with acrylic adhesive or silicone adhesive

Table 1. Preparing the wound bed: management protocol (T/M).

Protocol 2: (I/M = Infection and moisture) **-Infection and moisture monitoring** **-Wounds with local infection** **-Dressing every 72 h**			
-Type of wound	-Infection -Low exudate	-Infection -Moderate exudate	-Infection -High exudate
-Decrease in bacterial load	-Nanocrystalline silver or -Silver-impregnated activated carbon+ hydrogel	-Nanocrystalline silver or -Silver-impregnated activated carbon	-Nanocrystalline silver or -Silver-impregnated activated carbon + alginate
-Moist dressing	-Hydrocellular with acrylic adhesive or silicone adhesive	-Hydrocellular with acrylic adhesive or silicone adhesive	-Hydrocellular with acrylic adhesive or silicone adhesive

Table 2. Preparing the wound bed: management protocol (I/M).

Protocol 3: (E/M = Edges and moisture) **-Epithelialization of edges and moisture monitoring** **-Wounds in the granulation phase** **-Dressing every 72 h**		
-Type of wound	-Granulation tissue -Low or moderate exudate	-Granulation tissue -High exudate
-Granulation	-Collagen with silver protease modulator matrix or -Powder collagen	-Collagen with silver protease modulator matrix or -Powder collagen + alginate
-Moist dressing	-Hydrocellular with acrylic adhesive or silicone adhesive	-Hydrocellular with acrylic adhesive or silicone adhesive

Table 3. Preparing the wound bed: management protocol (E/M).

After finalizing the preparation of the wound bed, the wound remains open ready for its closure by secondary intention with granulation tissue and the re-establishment of the epidermis. At this point, the surgeon comes across two new problems: how to granulate the wound, and afterwards, how to epithelialize it.

2.4. Wound granulation using negative topical pressure therapy

For the granulation, we use a noninvasive topical negative pressure wound therapy (NPWT) (**Figure 2**), using aspirated drainage to eliminate the secretions, facilitate the closure and prevent complications. Its scientific fundamentals and physiopathology are based on the application of mechanical stress on the tissues, by creating a negative pressure on the surface of the wound [21]. The effect of the macrotension on the tissues is carried out using a sponge dressing (polyurethane-polyvinyl alcohol), with open pores, that contract under the negative pressure, bringing the edges closer together [22], eliminating the exudate, the non-viable tissue, and the soluble wound healing inhibitors (cytokines and matrix metalloproteinases) [23]. Other effects are a reduction in the edema, an increase in neutrophils and monocytes on the bacterial load and an improvement in local perfusion [24]. The effect of microtension, at the cell level, triggers cell stretching, which increases fibroblasts, the formation and division of new cells and the rapid growth of granulation tissue [25], the migration of fibroblasts to the area of the wound (displacing new cells to its surface), the formation of new blood vessels [26], and the formation of granulation tissue through mitosis stimulation. In this way, moist healing of the wound helps wound debridement (**Figure 3**).

The NPWT is contraindicated when either the wound has not been well explored, it has necrotic tissue with eschar or it has weakened blood vessels due to irradiation or suture. Also, NPWT is contraindicated in case of intestinal anastomosis, exposed nerves, the presence of tumors or untreated osteomyelitis. Equally, it is not advisable for either enterocutaneous or enteroatmospheric fistulas. Finally, active bleeding wounds and/or patients treated with anticoagulants are not suitable for NPWT treatment.

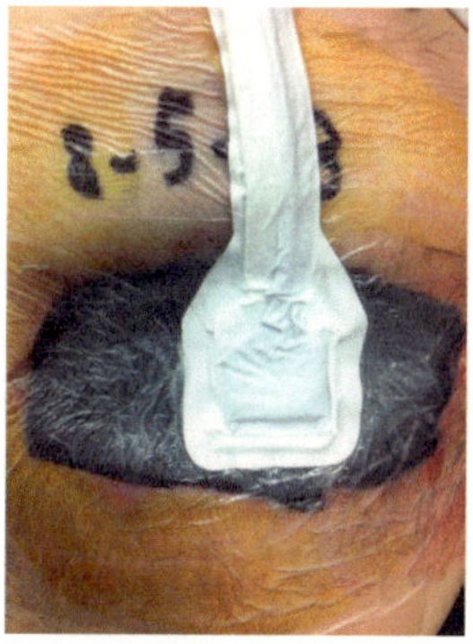

Figure 2. Complex and traumatic soft-tissue wound. Treatment with TNP therapy.

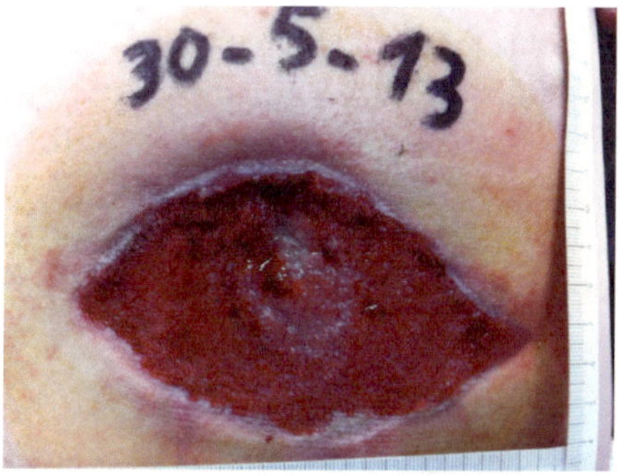

Figure 3. Complex and traumatic soft-tissue wound. Completed granulation after TNP therapy.

2.5. Epithelialization of the chronic and complex soft-tissue wounds

A large variety of wound coverings and procedures have become available over the past two decades, including several types of synthetic dressings and allo-skin or auto-skin substitutes, although their cost is too high for routine clinical practice [27, 28]. New technologies involving growth factors and bioengineered tissues are relatively new and have produced relatively good results; however, they are quite expensive.

2.6. Amniotic membrane and wound healing

Amniotic membrane (AM), the innermost layer of the placenta, has a fetal origin and can easily be separated from the placenta by blunt dissection. AM, due to its special structure, biological properties and immunological characteristics, is a tissue of particular interest as a biological dressing. AM exhibits low immunogenicity and well-documented reepithelialization effects. Moreover, AM shows anti-inflammatory, antifibrotic, antimicrobial, analgesic and nontumorigenic properties. This diversity of its effects is related to its capacity to synthesize and release biologically active molecules including cytokines and signaling factors such as tumor necrosis factor (TNF)-α, transforming growth factor (TGF)-α, TGF-β, basic fibroblast growth factor (b-FGF), epidermal growth factor (EGF), keratinocyte growth factor (KGF), hepatic growth factor (HGF), interleukin-4 (IL-4), IL-6, IL-8, natural inhibitors of metalloproteases, β-defensins, and prostaglandins among others [29–31]. Moreover, AM is a biomaterial that can be easily obtained, processed, and transported. On the other hand, AM may function as a substrate where cells can easily proliferate and differentiate [32]. When compared to skin transplantation, AM treatment offers considerable advantages. Its application does not produce rejection because it has low immunogenicity and does not induce uncontrolled proliferation [33]. All these effects are related to its capacity for the production and release of biologically active substances (see above).

AM has been applied in medicine for more than 100 years. In 1910, Davis [34] reported a comprehensive review of 550 cases of skin transplantation to various types of burns and wounds using natural AM obtained from labor and delivery at the Johns Hopkins University. In 1913, Sabella [35] and Stern [36] separately reported on the use of preserved AM in skin grafting for burns and ulcers. Since then, there have been several reports of the uses of AM in the treatment of wounds of different etiologies and other applications: first, in the reconstructive surgery of different tissues and organs including the mouth, tongue, nasal mucosa, larynx, eardrum, vestibule, bladder, urethra, vagina, and tendons [37–43]; second, as a peritoneum substitute in reconstruction procedures of pelvic exenteration surgery; third, in adherence prevention in the abdomen and pelvic surgery; and finally, as a covering of onphaloceles and the like [34–37, 44].

In ophthalmology, the use of AM was reported for the first time in 1940 by De Rötth, who used fresh fetal membranes, namely amnion and chorion, at the ocular surface as a biological dressing in the management of conjunctival alterations [45]. Later, Sorsby et al. [46] used preserved AM as a temporary coating in the treatment of acute caustic ocular lesions. Even though the results were favorable, its use was abandoned for almost four decades. In 1995, with the reconstitution assays of rabbit corneas with limbic disorder using human preserved AM, by Kim and Tseng [47], there was a renewed widespread interest in the use of AM in ophthalmology. Several publications appeared related to the efficacy of the AM in various ocular surface conditions and in diseases like epidermolysis bullosa [44, 48, 49]. Nowadays, AM is a resource widely used in ophthalmology [49–51] and to a lesser degree in the treatment of wounds, burns lesions, and chronic ulcers of the legs [48, 52–54] and in other surgical and nonsurgical procedures [38–43, 55–59].

3. Using AM in chronic wound healing

Once granulation of the wound is finalized, the process of epithelialization by using AM can be initiated. The source of AM for wound healing is donated placenta. AM has been used for wound healing either as intact AM without epithelium removal or as denuded AM, without the epithelium, [60, 61]. In some cases, AM was used fresh, and in others AM was preserved. Nowadays, it is known that the use of fresh AM is not practical for clinical use [62]. Methods

http://dx.doi.org/10.5772/64491

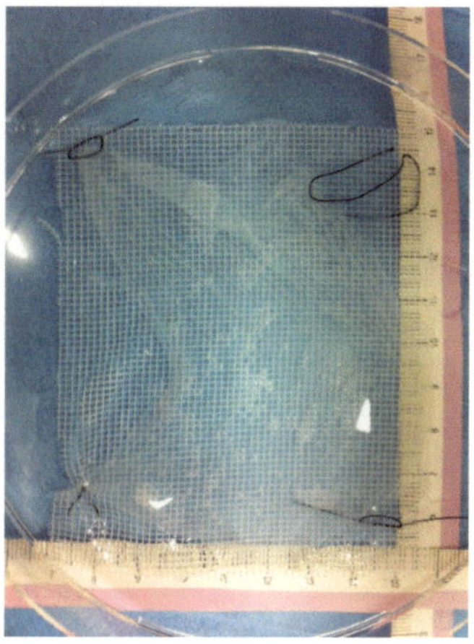

Figure 4. Amniotic membrane fixed to sterile petrolatum gauze (Tulgrasum®) ready for its application.

to remove the epithelium or preserve AM are very diverse and exceed the scope of this chapter. In our case, the placenta is obtained from an uncomplicated elective cesarean of a healthy mother, excluding patients with positive human immunodeficiency virus (HIV), hepatitis B virus (HBV), and hepatitis C virus (HCV) serology. Using an aseptic technique, AM is separated from the subjacent chorion by blunt dissection and stored in saline solution or phosphate buffered saline with antibiotics (cotrimoxazol, tobramycin, vancomycin, and amphotericin B). In this solution, AM is taken to the clean room [55]. Then, its processing, under sterile conditions, is carried out in a type II vertical laminar flow cabinet (HEPA filter). Then it is cut up into fragments measuring 10 × 10cm, which are then placed on a sterile scaffold of sterile petrolatum gauze (Tulgrasum®) and fixed with silk points at their ends (**Figure 4**). Finally, individual fragments are introduced into a bag with cryopreservative solution to freeze them in liquid nitrogen. These fragments cannot be used in the clinical practice until 3 months have passed, when there is a certainty that their donor has not been seroconverted to HIV, HBV, or HCV. After its defrosting in a 37°C bath, they are taken back to the surgical area and are applied on the wounds of the selected patient [55] (**Figures 5** and **6**).

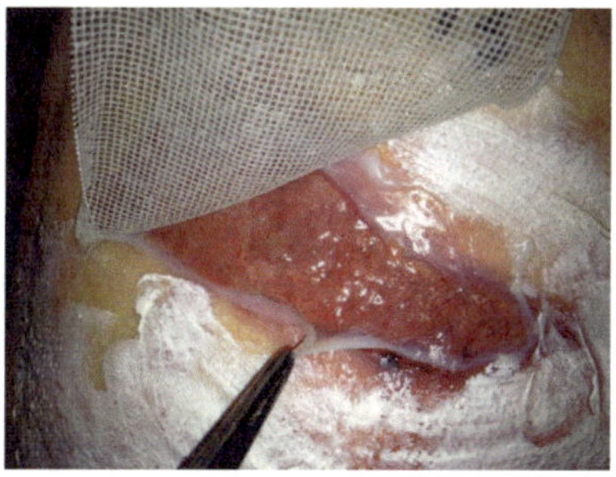

Figure 5. Complex and traumatic soft-tissue wound. Application of the amniotic membrane.

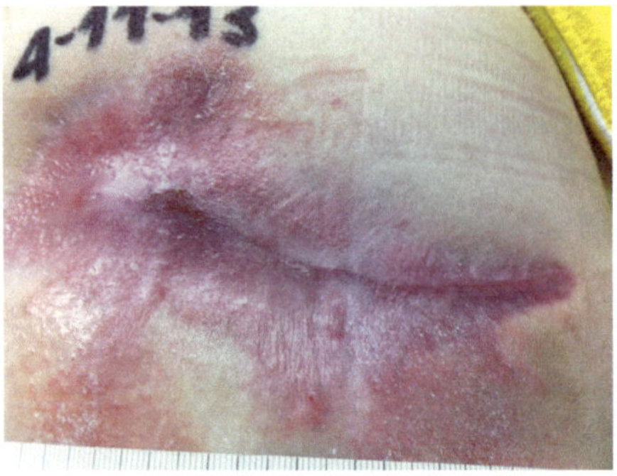

Figure 6. Complex and traumatic soft-tissue wound. Complete epithelialization after amniotic membrane treatment.

3.1. Molecular mechanisms underlying AM-induced skin reepithelialization

The molecular mechanisms underlying AM-induced skin reepithelialization are largely unknown. AM might have a wound healing effect by improving keratinocyte migration from the wound edge and stimulating its differentiation, thereby generating an intact epithelium [63]. Niknejad et al. [64] reflected that the stimulatory effect on epithelialization from the wound bed and/or the wound edge is facilitated by growth factors and progenitor cells released by AM. In addition, it has been described that the preservation of the integrity of the basement membrane and stromal matrix increases the healing potency of AM and is crucial in promoting a fast reepithelialization [65].

Insausti et al. [55] had previously worked on HaCaT cells, a spontaneously immortalized human keratinocyte cell line, as a model to comprehend the molecular consequences of AM application on human wounds [66]. This research showed that HaCaT cells exhibited different molecular reactions upon stimulation with AM that were attributed to the effects of soluble AM-released factors on HaCaT cells [55]. The application of AM to keratinocytes induced the activation of the phosphorylation of ERK1/2, JNK1/2, and p38 [55]. Also, AM-conditioned medium induced similar responses, suggesting a trans-effect of AM on the triggering of these events. Additionally, the authors reported that HaCaT cells stimulated with AM showed an increased expression of *c-JUN*. Members of the AP1 family had been involved in keratinocyte migration and the wound healing process [67–70]. AM induced the phosphorylation of Jun N-terminal kinase (JNK)1 and two kinases in HaCaT cells [55]; JNK1 is a positive regulator of c-JUN, contributing to its phosphorylation and stabilization [71, 72]. Finally, the expression of c-Jun in the wounds treated with AM was very strong, and particularly evident at the basal epithelium near the leading edge and at the dermal leading edge or keratinocyte tongue, indicating that c-Jun expression might be an important event for epithelialization occurring at the AM-stimulated wound borders [55].

3.2. Chronic wound healing, AM, and TGF-β

Wound fluid derived from chronic venous leg ulcers is rich in pro-inflammatory cytokines such as TNF-α, interleukin-1β (IL-1β), and TGF-β1 [73]. In addition, the quantities of these cytokines drop as the chronic wound commences to heal, denoting a strong correlation between non-healing wounds and an increased level of pro-inflammatory cytokines [74]. TGF-β has a critical role in regulating multiple cellular responses that occur in all phases of wound healing [75]. Of the many cytokines shown to influence the wound healing process, TGF-β has the broadest spectrum of action because it affects the behavior of a wide variety of cell types and mediates a diverse range of cellular functions [76]. Platelets are thought to be the primary source of TGF-β at the wound site; also, activation of latent TGF-β occurs immediately after wounding [75]. The TGF-β signaling pathway is considered as a promising target for the treatment of many pathological skin conditions including chronic non-healing wounds [75]. Keratinocytes, fibroblasts, and monocytes are among the targeted cells in the TGF-β management of the wound [76]. Monocytes/macrophages and fibroblasts then contribute to autocrine-perpetuated high concentrations of TGF-β at the wound site [76].

TGF-β exerts its effect on cells by increasing the phosphorylation of members of the receptor activated (R-)Smad family (Smad2 and 3). Additionally, non-Smad pathways are also activated, including the extracellular-signal-regulated kinase (ERK), JNK, and p38 mitogen-activated protein (MAP) kinase pathways, the tyrosine kinase Src, and phosphatidylinositol 3-kinase (PI3K) [77, 78]. Once receptor-induced phosphorylation has taken place, R-Smads form complexes with the common-mediator (Co-) Smad4, which are translocated to the nucleus [79] where they, in cooperation with other transcription factors, co-activators, and corepressors, regulate the transcription of specific genes [80].

The effects of TGF-β on full-thickness wound reepithelialization have been studied in a transgenic mouse. The study in the ear mouse model suggests that TGF-β has an inhibitory effect on epithelialization when the wound involves all the layers of the skin [81]. Also, the overexpression of TGF-β, at the epidermis level, causes a decrease in reepithelialization [82, 83]. Abolishing part of the TGF-β signaling pathway has been suggested as a way to improve wound healing, so abolishing part of the TGF-β-stimulated Smad pathways may enhance wound healing and benefit the effect of TGF-β signaling over matrix synthesis by fibroblasts, for instance [76]. TGF-β causes the growth arrest of epithelial cells. The mechanisms, which differ somewhat between different cell types, involve the inhibition of the expression of the transcription factor Myc and members of the Id family, and the transcriptional induction of the cell cycle inhibitors *CDKN2B* (*p15*) and *CDKN1A* (*p21*) [84].

In order to further unravel the molecular mechanism by which AM may contribute to the epithelialization and wound border proliferation in chronic post-traumatic wounds, Alcaraz et al. [85] analyzed the association between TGF-β signaling and AM regulation in wound healing using keratinocytes. Strikingly, AM was capable of attenuating the TGF-β-induced phosphorylation of Smad2 and Smad3 in HaCaT cells. Both the strength and duration of TGF-β signaling, expressed as sustained phosphorylation of Smads, are essential to achieve proper cell responses to TGF-β; the impossibility to do so produces a loss of the cell cycle arrest in response to TGF-β [86]. AM attenuates TGF-β-induced Smad2 and Smad3 phosphorylation and hence attenuates *CDKN2B (p15)* and *CDKN1A (p21)* expression [85], which has been connected to cell cycle regulation [86]. Therefore, the presence of AM counteracts the cell cycle arrest induced by TGF-β on keratinocytes, releasing them from the restrain imposed by TGFß [85]. The effect of AM on TGF-β-regulated genes is not indiscriminate, and not all genes are affected by the presence of AM. Interestingly, genes that positively participate in wound healing such as *SNAI-2* and *PAI-1* were synergistically up-regulated by the presence of AM and TGF-β [85]. Finally, the expression of c-Jun was maximal when both TGF-β and AM were present in either HaCaT or primary keratinocyte cells [85].

It has been suggested that AM might exert its wound healing effect by increasing keratinocyte migration speed from the wound edge [63]. Growth factors and progenitor cells released by AM [64] are supposed to mediate the epithelialization stimulatory effect. AM induces cell migration in a wound healing assay in keratinocytes and mesenchymal cells [85]. Furthermore, in keratinocytes, inhibition of cell proliferation with mitomycin C, affected the migrating properties of AM. In the same study, the use of JNK1 inhibitors prevented AM-induced cell migration in both cell types. Moreover, a closer inspection of the margins of the scratch wound healing assays showed a high expression of c-JUN in the AM-stimulated cells engaged in the migratory wave. The AM-induced high expression of c-JUN at the wound border was prevented by inhibitors SP600125 and PD98059, which is consistent with the fact that AM induces the activation of a signaling cascade that produces the phosphorylation of ERK1/2 and JNK1/2. A local increase of c-JUN was observed in the patient wound border when the wound had been treated with AM. This is coherent with the AM effect on cell migration. In fact, in the examination of patient wound borders a few days after AM application, a clear proliferation/migration was observed [85]. This correlates well with the robust expression of c-Jun at the wound border, which is particularly robust at the *stratum basale* of the epidermis that overlaps the keratinocyte tongue, the area where the migration of keratinocytes happens to epithelialize the wound [85]. Additionally, in that investigation, the authors revealed that the application of AM promotes healing in chronic wounds by refashioning the TGF-β-induced genetic program, stimulating keratinocyte migration and proliferation [85]. Additionally, there might be a synergy of AM and TGF-β signaling for the resolution of chronic wounds [85, 87]. Thus, stimulation of keratinocytes with both AM and TGF-β was synergistic when compared to both stimulus being added separately [85]. Moreover, the treatment of cells with TGF-β signaling inhibitors hampered the effect of AM, indicating that both AM and TGF-β signaling positively contribute to cell migration [87]. The down-regulation of Smad3 has been suggested as a possible way of improving wound healing [76]. In this sense, the effect of R-Smads, Smad2 or 3, seems to be different given that the overexpression of Smad2 increased AM-induced cell migration while the overexpression of Smad3 prevented it [87]. Notably, the ability of keratinocytes to sense TGF-β through Smad3 prevents the cell proliferation of keratinocytes and consequently prevents wound healing resolution when the levels of TGF-β are high [88].

Presently, in order to evaluate the effect of AM on chronic post-traumatic wounds, a clinical trial is being conducted in our hospital, with exceptional results. The TGF-β-stimulated Smad pathway has also been involved in the production of fibrosis and inflammation in response to TGF-β. Thus, interfering with TGF-β signaling may be a good way of interfering with fibrosis and improving the evolution of wound healing [76]. In different experimental models, the application of AM is able to ameliorate fibrosis [89–92]. Currently, we are exploring whether the application of AM is able to reduce fibrosis and inflammation in chronic wounds.

http://dx.doi.org/10.5772/64491

4. Summary

To summarize, AM is a biological dressing that stimulates proper epithelialization in chronic wounds. It has several advantages; among them, it is economical, easy to obtain, and in endless supply. Additionally, AM can be cryopreserved at a low temperature while preserving all its biological functions. Finally, it can be used as a treatment in the outpatient clinic, which reduces costs even more. Thus, AM must be taken into account as a consolidated treatment option for chronic wounds.

Acknowledgements

We would like to thank other members of the different laboratories who contribute in our daily task of increasing our knowledge of AM and chronic wound healing. Ana M García, María D. López and Mónica Rodríguez working in the clean room and providing AM. Paola Romencín, José E. Millán, David García and Noemi Marín, working on AM and animal models, and Miguel Blanquer, working in the cell therapy group. Antonia Alcaraz, Catalina Ruiz-Cañada, Ania Mrowiec, Eva M. García, and Sergio Liarte working on molecular aspects of AM and wound healing using cell models. This work was supported by a grant from the Fundación Séneca de la Región de Murcia and a grant from the Instituto de Salud Carlos III, Fondo de Investigaciones Sanitarias. Plan Estatal I+D+i and the Instituto de Salud Carlos III-Subdirección General de Evaluación y Fomento de la Investigación (Grant no.: PI13/00794) http://www.isciii.es/Fondos FEDER (ERDF funds) http://ec.europa.eu/regional_policy/es/funding/erdf/. We are indebted to the Hospital Clínico Universitario Virgen de la Arrixaca for strongly supporting this research.

Author details

Gregorio Castellanos[1], Ángel Bernabé-García[2], Carmen García Insausti[3], Antonio Piñero[1], José M. Moraleda[3] and Francisco J. Nicolás[2*]

*Address all correspondence to: Franciscoj.nicolas2@carm.es

1 Surgery Service, Virgen de la Arrixaca University Clinical Hospital, El Palmar, Murcia, Spain

2 Molecular Oncology and TGFβ, Research Unit, Virgen de la Arrixaca University Hospital, El Palmar, Murcia, Spain

3 Cell Therapy Unit, Virgen de la Arrixaca University Clinical Hospital, El Palmar, Murcia, Spain

References

[1] Troxler M, Vowden K, Vowden P. Integrating adjunctive therapy into practice: the importance of recognising 'hard-to-heal' wounds. World Wide Wounds (online) 2006; available from URL: http://www.worldwidewounds.com/2006/december/Troxler/Integrating-Adjunctive-Therapy-Into-Practice.html.

[2] Falanga V, Saap LJ, Ozonoff A. Wound bed score and its correlation with healing of chronic wounds. Dermatol Ther. 2006;19(6):383–90.

[3] Doerler M, Reich-Schupke S, Altmeyer P, Stucker M. Impact on wound healing and efficacy of various leg ulcer debridement techniques. J Dtsch Dermatol Ges. 2012;10(9): 624–32.

[4] Margolis DJ, Berlin JA, Strom BL. Risk factors associated with the failure of a venous leg ulcer to heal. Arch Dermatol. 1999;135(8):920–6.

[5] Henderson EA. The potential effect of fibroblast senescence on wound healing and the chronic wound environment. J Wound Care. 2006;15(7):315–8.

[6] Steed DL. Clinical evaluation of recombinant human platelet-derived growth factor for the treatment of lower extremity diabetic ulcers. Diabetic Ulcer Study Group. J Vasc Surg. 1995;21(1):71–8; discussion 9–81.

[7] Mogford J., Mustoe T. Experimental models of wound healing.In: Falanga V., editor. Cutaneous Wound Healing. London: Martin Dunitz Ltd.; 2001. p. 109–22.

[8] Medina A, Scott PG, Ghahary A, Tredget EE. Pathophysiology of chronic nonhealing wounds. J Burn Care Rehabil. 2005;26(4):306–19.

[9] Shukla VK, Shukla D, Tiwary SK, Agrawal S, Rastogi A. Evaluation of pH measurement as a method of wound assessment. J Wound Care. 2007;16(7):291–4.

[10] Bowler PG, Duerden BI, Armstrong DG. Wound microbiology and associated approaches to wound management. Clin Microbiol Rev. 2001;14(2):244–69.

[11] Ngo Q, Vickery K, Deva AK. PR21 Role of Bacterial Biofilms in Chronic Wounds. ANZ Journal of Surgery. 2007;77:A66.

[12] Percival SL, Bowler PG, Dolman J. Antimicrobial activity of silver-containing dressings on wound microorganisms using an in vitro biofilm model. Int Wound J. 2007;4(2):186–91.

[13] Bjarnsholt T, Kirketerp-Moller K, Kristiansen S, Phipps R, Nielsen AK, Jensen PO, et al. Silver against Pseudomonas aeruginosa biofilms. APMIS. 2007;115(8):921–8.

[14] Attinger CE, Janis JE, Steinberg J, Schwartz J, Al-Attar A, Couch K. Clinical approach to wounds: débridement and wound bed preparation including the use of dressings and wound-healing adjuvants. Plast Reconstr Surg. 2006;117(7 Suppl):72S–109S.

[15] Baharestani M, de Leon J, Mendez-Eastman S, et al. Consensus statement: a practical guide for managing pressure ulcers with negative pressure wound therapy utilizing vacuum-assisted closure-understanding the treatment algorithm. Adv Skin Wound Care. 2008(21(Suppl 1)):1–20.

[16] EWMA, editor. Position Document: Wound Bed Preparation in Practice. (EWMA). London: MEP Ltd.; 2004.

[17] Falanga V. Classifications for wound bed preparation and stimulation of chronic wounds. Wound Repair Regen. 2000;8(5):347–52.

[18] Sibbald RG, Williamson D, Orsted HL, Campbell K, Keast D, Krasner D, et al. Preparing the wound bed--debridement, bacterial balance, and moisture balance. Ostomy Wound Manage. 2000;46(11):14–22, 4–8, 30–5; quiz 6–7.

[19] Falanga V. Wound bed preparation: science applied to practice. In: (EWMA). EWMA, editor. Position Document: Wound Bed Preparation in Practice. London: MEP Ltd.; 2004. p. 2–5.

[20] Halim AS, Khoo TL, Saad AZ. Wound bed preparation from a clinical perspective. Indian J Plast Surg. 2012;45(2):193–202.

[21] Morykwas MJ, Argenta LC, Shelton-Brown EI, McGuirt W. Vacuum-assisted closure: a new method for wound control and treatment: animal studies and basic foundation. Ann Plast Surg. 1997;38(6):553–62.

[22] Banwell PE, Musgrave M. Topical negative pressure therapy: mechanisms and indications. Int Wound J. 2004;1(2):95–106.

[23] Stechmiller JK, Kilpadi DV, Childress B, Schultz GS. Effect of vacuum-assisted closure therapy on the expression of cytokines and proteases in wound fluid of adults with pressure ulcers. Wound Repair Regen. 2006;14(3):371–4.

[24] Timmers MS, Le Cessie S, Banwell P, Jukema GN. The effects of varying degrees of pressure delivered by negative-pressure wound therapy on skin perfusion. Ann Plast Surg. 2005;55(6):665–71.

[25] Saxena V, Hwang CW, Huang S, Eichbaum Q, Ingber D, Orgill DP. Vacuum-assisted closure: microdeformations of wounds and cell proliferation. Plast Reconstr Surg. 2004;114(5):1086–96; discussion 97–8.

[26] Greene AK, Puder M, Roy R, Arsenault D, Kwei S, Moses MA, et al. Microdeformational wound therapy: effects on angiogenesis and matrix metalloproteinases in chronic wounds of 3 debilitated patients. Ann Plast Surg. 2006;56(4):418–22.

[27] Greaves NS, Iqbal SA, Baguneid M, Bayat A. The role of skin substitutes in the management of chronic cutaneous wounds. Wound Repair Regen. 2013;21(2):194–210.

[28] Lorenz HP, Longaker M. Wounds: biology, pathology, and management. Essential practice of surgery. New York: Springer; 2003. p. 77–88.

[29] Yang L, Shirakata Y, Shudou M, Dai X, Tokumaru S, Hirakawa S, et al. New skin-equivalent model from de-epithelialized amnion membrane. Cell Tissue Res. 2006;326(1):69–77.

[30] Parolini O, Soncini M. Human placenta: a source of progenitor/stem cells? J Reproduktionsmed Endokrinol. 2006;3(2):117–126.

[31] Parolini O, Alviano F, Bagnara GP, Bilic G, Buhring HJ, Evangelista M, et al. Concise review: isolation and characterization of cells from human term placenta: outcome of the first International Workshop on Placenta Derived Stem Cells. Stem Cells. 2008;26(2): 300–11.

[32] Miki T, Strom SC. Amnion-derived pluripotent/multipotent stem cells. Stem Cell Rev. 2006;2(2):133–42.

[33] Insausti CL, Blanquer M, Bleda P, Iniesta P, Majado MJ, Castellanos G, et al. The amniotic membrane as a source of stem cells. Histol Histopathol. 2010;25(1):91–8.

[34] Davis JS. A method of splinting skin grafts. Skin transplantation. 1910; 21:44.

[35] Sabella N. Use of fetal membranes in skin grafting. Med Records NY. 1913;83:478–80.

[36] Stern M. The grafting of preserved amniotic membrane to burned and ulcerated surfaces, substituing skin grafts: a preliminary report. J Am Med Assoc. 1913;60(13): 973–4.

[37] Ganatra MA. Amniotic membrane in surgery. J Pak Med Assoc. 2003;53(1):29–32.

[38] Tolhurst DE, van der Helm TW. The treatment of vaginal atresia. Surg Gynecol Obstet. 1991;172(5):407–14.

[39] Georgy M, Aziz N. Vaginoplasty using amnion graft: new surgical technique using the laparoscopic transillumination light. J Obstet Gynecol. 1996;16(4):262–4.

[40] Morton KE, Dewhurst CJ. Human amnion in the treatment of vaginal malformations. Br J Obstet Gynaecol. 1986;93(1):50–4.

[41] Fishman IJ, Flores FN, Scott FB, Spjut HJ, Morrow B. Use of fresh placental membranes for bladder reconstruction. J Urol. 1987;138(5):1291–4.

[42] Brandt FT, Albuquerque CD, Lorenzato FR. Female urethral reconstruction with amnion grafts. Int J Surg Investig. 2000;1(5):409–14.

[43] Zohar Y, Talmi YP, Finkelstein Y, Shvili Y, Sadov R, Laurian N. Use of human amniotic membrane in otolaryngologic practice. Laryngoscope. 1987;97(8 Pt 1):978–80.

[44] Trelford JD, Trelford-Sauder M. The amnion in surgery, past and present. Am J Obstet Gynecol. 1979;134(7):833–45.

[45] de Rötth A. Plastic repair of conjunctival defects with fetal membranes. Arch Ophthalmol. 1940;23(3):522–5.

[46] Sorsby A, Symons HM. Amniotic membrane grafts in caustic burns of the eye: (burns of the second degree). Br J Ophthalmol. 1946;30(6):337–45.

[47] Kim JC, Tseng SC. Transplantation of preserved human amniotic membrane for surface reconstruction in severely damaged rabbit corneas. Cornea. 1995;14(5):473-84.

[48] Mermet I, Pottier N, Sainthillier JM, Malugani C, Cairey-Remonnay S, Maddens S, et al. Use of amniotic membrane transplantation in the treatment of venous leg ulcers. Wound Repair Regen. 2007;15(4):459–64.

[49] Gomes JA, Romano A, Santos MS, Dua HS. Amniotic membrane use in ophthalmology. Curr Opin Ophthalmol. 2005;16(4):233–40.

[50] Dua HS, Gomes JAP, King AJ, Maharajan VS. The amniotic membrane in ophthalmology. Surv Ophthalmol. 2004;49(1):51–77.

[51] Baradaran-Rafii A, Aghayan HR, Arjmand B, Javadi MA. Amniotic membrane transplantation. Iranian J Ophthalmic Res. 2007;2(1):58–75.

[52] Colocho G, Graham WP, Iii, Greene AE, Matheson DW, Lynch D. Human amniotic membrane as a physiologic wound dressing. Arch Surg. 1974;109(3):370–3.

[53] Singh R, Chouhan US, Purohit S, Gupta P, Kumar P, Kumar A, et al. Radiation processed amniotic membranes in the treatment of non-healing ulcers of different etiologies. Cell Tissue Bank. 2004;5(2):129–34.

[54] Hasegawa T, Mizoguchi M, Haruna K, Mizuno Y, Muramatsu S, Suga Y, et al. Amnia for intractable skin ulcers with recessive dystrophic epidermolysis bullosa: report of three cases. J Dermatol. 2007;34(5):328–32.

[55] Insausti CL, Alcaraz A, Garcia-Vizcaino EM, Mrowiec A, Lopez-Martinez MC, Blanquer M, et al. Amniotic membrane induces epithelialization in massive posttraumatic wounds. Wound Repair Regen. 2010;18(4):368–77.

[56] Sangwan VS, Matalia HP, Vemuganti GK, Fatima A, Ifthekar G, Singh S, et al. Clinical outcome of autologous cultivated limbal epithelium transplantation. Indian J Ophthalmol. 2006;54(1):29–34.

[57] Díaz-Prado S, Rendal-Vázquez ME, Muiños-López E, Hermida-Gómez T, Rodríguez-Cabarcos M, Fuentes-Boquete I, et al. Potential use of the human amniotic membrane as a scaffold in human articular cartilage repair. Cell Tissue Bank. 2010;11(2):183–95.

[58] Yeager AM, Singer HS, Buck JR, Matalon R, Brennan S, O'Toole SO, et al. A therapeutic trial of amniotic epithelial cell implantation in patients with lysosomal storage diseases. Am J Med Genet. 1985;22(2):347–55.

[59] Redondo P, Giménez de Azcarate A, Marqués L, García-Guzman M, Andreu E, Prósper F. Amniotic membrane as a scaffold for melanocyte transplantation in patients with stable vitiligo. Dermatol Res Pract. 2011;2011:6.

[60] Akle C, McColl I, Dean M, Adinolfi M, Brown S, Fensom AH, et al. Transplantation of amniotic epithelial membranes in patients with mucopolysaccharidoses. Exp Clin Immunogenet. 1985;2(1):43–8.

[61] Wilshaw SP, Kearney JN, Fisher J, Ingham E. Production of an acellular amniotic membrane matrix for use in tissue engineering. Tissue Eng. 2006;12(8):2117–29.

[62] Zelen CM, Snyder RJ, Serena TE, Li WW. The use of human amnion/chorion membrane in the clinical setting for lower extremity repair: a review. Clin Podiatr Med Surg. 2015;32(1):135–46.

[63] Lee SH, Tseng SC. Amniotic membrane transplantation for persistent epithelial defects with ulceration. Am J Ophthalmol. 1997;123(3):303–12.

[64] Niknejad H, Peirovi H, Jorjani M, Ahmadiani A, Ghanavi J, Seifalian AM. Properties of the amniotic membrane for potential use in tissue engineering. Eur Cell Mater. 2008;15:88–99.

[65] Kubo M, Sonoda Y, Muramatsu R, Usui M. Immunogenicity of human amniotic membrane in experimental xenotransplantation. Invest Ophthalmol Vis Sci. 2001;42(7): 1539–46.

[66] Boukamp P, Petrussevska RT, Breitkreutz D, Hornung J, Markham A, Fusenig NE. Normal keratinization in a spontaneously immortalized aneuploid human keratinocyte cell line. J Cell Biol. 1988;106(3):761–71.

[67] Angel P, Szabowski A, Schorpp-Kistner M. Function and regulation of AP-1 subunits in skin physiology and pathology. Oncogene. 2001;20(19):2413–23.

[68] Yates S, Rayner TE. Transcription factor activation in response to cutaneous injury: role of AP-1 in reepithelialization. Wound Repair Regen. 2002;10(1):5–15.

[69] Gangnuss S, Cowin AJ, Daehn IS, Hatzirodos N, Rothnagel JA, Varelias A, et al. Regulation of MAPK activation, AP-1 transcription factor expression and keratinocyte differentiation in wounded fetal skin. J Invest Dermatol. 2004;122(3):791–804.

[70] Li G, Gustafson-Brown C, Hanks SK, Nason K, Arbeit JM, Pogliano K, et al. c-Jun is essential for organization of the epidermal leading edge. Dev Cell. 2003;4(6):865–77.

[71] Ronai Z. JNKing Revealed. Mol Cell. 2004;15(6):843–4.

[72] Sabapathy K, Hochedlinger K, Nam SY, Bauer A, Karin M, Wagner EF. Distinct roles for JNK1 and JNK2 in regulating JNK activity and c-Jun-dependent cell proliferation. Mol Cell. 2004;15(5):713–25.

[73] Harris IR, Yee KC, Walters CE, Cunliffe WJ, Kearney JN, Wood EJ, et al. Cytokine and protease levels in healing and non-healing chronic venous leg ulcers. Exp Dermatol. 1995;4(6):342–9.

[74] Trengove NJ, Bielefeldt-Ohmann H, Stacey MC. Mitogenic activity and cytokine levels in non-healing and healing chronic leg ulcers. Wound Repair Regen. 2000;8(1):13–25.

[75] Finnson KW, McLean S, Di Guglielmo GM, Philip A. Dynamics of transforming growth factor beta signaling in wound healing and scarring. Advances Wound Care. 2013;2(5): 195–214.

[76] Ashcroft GS, Roberts AB. Loss of Smad3 modulates wound healing. Cytokine Growth Factor Rev. 2000;11(1–2):125–31.

[77] Moustakas A, Heldin CH. Non-Smad TGF-beta signals. J Cell Sci. 2005;118(Pt 16):3573–84.

[78] Mu Y, Gudey SK, Landstrom M. Non-Smad signaling pathways. Cell Tissue Res. 2012;347(1):11–20.

[79] Pierreux CE, Nicolas FJ, Hill CS. Transforming growth factor beta-independent shuttling of Smad4 between the cytoplasm and nucleus. Mol Cell Biol. 2000;20(23): 9041–54.

[80] Heldin CH, Moustakas A. Role of Smads in TGFbeta signaling. Cell Tissue Res. 2012;347(1):21–36.

[81] Tredget EB, Demare J, Chandran G, Tredget EE, Yang L, Ghahary A. Transforming growth factor-beta and its effect on reepithelialization of partial-thickness ear wounds in transgenic mice. Wound Repair Regen. 2005;13(1):61–7.

[82] Chan T, Ghahary A, Demare J, Yang L, Iwashina T, Scott PG, et al. Development, characterization, and wound healing of the keratin 14 promoted transforming growth factor-beta1 transgenic mouse. Wound Repair Regen. 2002;10(3):177–87.

[83] Yang L, Chan T, Demare J, Iwashina T, Ghahary A, Scott PG, et al. Healing of burn wounds in transgenic mice overexpressing transforming growth factor-beta 1 in the epidermis. Am J Pathol. 2001;159(6):2147–57.

[84] Heldin CH, Landstrom M, Moustakas A. Mechanism of TGF-beta signaling to growth arrest, apoptosis, and epithelial-mesenchymal transition. Curr Opin Cell Biol. 2009;21(2):166–76.

[85] Alcaraz A, Mrowiec A, Insausti CL, Bernabe-Garcia A, Garcia-Vizcaino EM, Lopez-Martinez MC, et al. Amniotic membrane modifies the genetic program induced by TGFss, stimulating keratinocyte proliferation and migration in chronic wounds. PLoS One. 2015;10(8):e0135324.

[86] Nicolas FJ, Hill CS. Attenuation of the TGF-beta-Smad signaling pathway in pancreatic tumor cells confers resistance to TGF-beta-induced growth arrest. Oncogene. 2003;22(24):3698–711.

[87] Ruiz-Canada C, Bernabé-García A, Angosto D, Castellanos G, Insausti CL, Moraleda JM, et al. Amniotic membrane stimulates migration by modulating TFG-β signaling. (In press).

[88] Ashcroft GS, Yang X, Glick AB, Weinstein M, Letterio JL, Mizel DE, et al. Mice lacking Smad3 show accelerated wound healing and an impaired local inflammatory response. Nat Cell Biol. 1999;1(5):260–6.

[89] Hodge A, Lourensz D, Vaghjiani V, Nguyen H, Tchongue J, Wang B, et al. Soluble factors derived from human amniotic epithelial cells suppress collagen production in human hepatic stellate cells. Cytotherapy. 2014;16(8):1132–44.

[90] Cargnoni A, Gibelli L, Tosini A, Signoroni PB, Nassuato C, Arienti D, et al. Transplantation of allogeneic and xenogeneic placenta-derived cells reduces bleomycin-induced lung fibrosis. Cell Transplant. 2009;18(4):405–22.

[91] Cargnoni A, Piccinelli EC, Ressel L, Rossi D, Magatti M, Toschi I, et al. Conditioned medium from amniotic membrane-derived cells prevents lung fibrosis and preserves blood gas exchanges in bleomycin-injured mice-specificity of the effects and insights into possible mechanisms. Cytotherapy. 2014;16(1):17–32.

[92] Cargnoni A, Ressel L, Rossi D, Poli A, Arienti D, Lombardi G, et al. Conditioned medium from amniotic mesenchymal tissue cells reduces progression of bleomycin-induced lung fibrosis. Cytotherapy. 2012;14(2):153–61.

Chapter 20

Progress and Perspectives in the Management of Wound Infections

Federica Paladini, Mauro Pollini,
Alessandro Sannino and Luigi Ambrosio

Additional information is available at the end of the chapter

http://dx.doi.org/10.5772/64280

Abstract

The progress in nanotechnology and the medical application of novel generations of nanomaterials have opened new horizons in the definition of non-conventional approaches against multiple diseases. Biomaterials coated with antimicrobial metal nanoparticles, along with the topical applications of zinc, silver or copper-based formulations have demonstrated huge potential in prevention from infections associated with implantable medical devices and in biofilm eradication. In wound healing, in particular, the increasing healthcare costs and the antibiotic resistance demonstrated by several microorganisms have encouraged researchers and companies in the development of innovative wound dressings with antibacterial properties and capability to promote and enhance the healing process. Supported by scientific evidence, many formulations have been proposed and a large number of works involves the use of hybrid metal nanoparticles/polymer products, which have demonstrated encouraging results both *in vitro* and *in vivo*. In this chapter, recent progress in the development of novel wound dressings based on antibacterial metal nanoparticles is presented, along with the most interesting results achieved by the authors, mainly devoted to the application of silver nanocoatings in wound management.

Keywords: infection, antibacterial, wound dressings, metal nanoparticles

1. Introduction

The Wound Healing Society has defined the wound as the result of 'disruption of normal anatomic structure and function'. A wound can be also described as a defect or break in the skin, which results from physical or thermal damage, or from medical and physiological conditions [1]. The wound healing is a dynamic process consisting of four continuous and precisely programmed phases, namely haemostasis, inflammation, proliferation and remodelling. Multiple factors, such as infections, stress, diabetes, smoking and obesity, can lead to impaired wound healing by interfering with one or more of these phases [2]. Once injured, the skin loses many of the protective defence mechanism of the intact skin and is colonized by the microorganisms on its surface. According to the replication status of the microorganisms, a wound can be classified as contaminated, colonized, locally infected and/or with spreading invasive infection [3]. The main bacterial mode of living in an infected wound is biofilm, which can be defined as a confluent community of adherent bacteria characterized by high cell densities and encased in an extracellular polymeric matrix that acts as physical barrier for biological and pharmaceutical antimicrobials [4, 5]. The presence of bacterial biofilm is associated with impaired epithelialization and granulation tissue formation and promotes a low-grade inflammatory response that interferes with wound healing [6]. The biofilm matrix plays an important role in the increased antibiotic resistance and has an enormous impact on medicine in terms of both therapeutic options and costs. Biofilm has been estimated to be associated with 65% of nosocomial infections, and the treatment costs associated with biofilm infection and chronic wounds have been estimated to be more than 1 billion USD annually in the United States [4, 7].

The increasing resistance of bacteria to antibiotics represents a huge concern, so that the World Health Organization recently has described the problem as 'so serious that it threatens the achievements of modern medicine' [8, 9]. Moreover, the large number of wound dressings and the limited guidelines available have induced an undesirable inconsistency in wound-care practice [10]. The local treatment of wounds is crucial for preventing infections, controlling exudates and providing the moist environment necessary for wound healing. At this purpose, efforts have been made by many research groups in the development of bioactive dressings, which can play an active role in wound protection and healing, and/or are able to release biomolecules and antimicrobials for prevention and treatment of wound infections [8, 11, 12]. A strategy for the treatment of infected wounds with increased resistance to traditional antibiotic therapy is the use of specific antibacterial agents immobilized on the surface of a material, thus providing a wide spectrum of activity in terms of bacterial toxicity and destructuration of the bacterial biofilm matrix [13].

This chapter aims to provide the reader with an overview of the most promising routes to develop advanced biomaterials with antimicrobial properties for the management of wound infections through nanotechnology approaches. The new generation and application of nanomaterials with novel properties are one of the century's key technology developments, which offer extraordinary opportunities in the pharmaceutical and medical field [14]. The great potential of nanometals such as zinc, copper and silver in wound dressing formulations and their use as antimicrobial agent in wound infections will be presented, along with the most recent efforts and results achieved by several research group in the definition of effective strategies for prevention of wound infection and for enhanced wound healing. Moreover, the most relevant results obtained by the authors of this chapter in the field of silver-based antibacterial treatments for wound-healing application will be presented and discussed.

2. Wound infections

The skin represents a complex and effective barrier between the organism and the environment, preventing invasion of pathogens, chemical and physical insults and unregulated loss of water and solutes [15]. From a microbiological point of view, the primary function of normal and intact skin is to control the microbial populations that live on the skin surface and to prevent the underlying tissues from invasion and colonization by potential pathogens [16]. A wound, which represents the loss of skin integrity and following exposure of subcutaneous tissue, provides a moist, warm and nutritious environment for microbial colonization and proliferation. The abundance and diversity of microorganisms in any wound depend on different factors such as wound type, depth, location and quality, the level of tissue perfusion and the antimicrobial efficacy of the host immune response [16]. As all open wounds lack the protective covering of skin, microorganisms from endogenous or exogenous sources can be introduced onto the wound surface and can lead to colonization [17, 18]. Colonization is defined as the presence of proliferating bacteria on the surface of a wound, without a noticeable host response and without clinical signs and symptoms. Differently, wound infection depends on the pathogenicity of the microorganisms and on the immune competency of the host, and it is characterized by the presence of the clinical signs of infection such as erythema, pain, tenderness, heat, oedema, cellulites and abscess or pus [19, 20]. Within an infected wound, the main bacterial mode of living is a biofilm [4]. Bacterial biofilm consists of a complex microenvironment of single or mixed bacterial species encased within an extracellular polymeric substance (EPS) produced by bacteria. The moist, adhesive and proteinaceous wound surface represents the ideal environment for biofilm development [21]. If microbes attach to the wound surface and proliferate, the biofilm begins to develop and, when it is well established, it exhibits resistance to the host immune system and antimicrobials. At this stage, the biofilm is considered mature and difficult to eradicate, thus requiring specialized management practices and increasing the risk of non-healing and clinically infected wound (i.e. showing signs of inflammation or purulence) [17]. Biofilm infections compromise wound closure and contribute to wound chronicity. Persistent infections may arrest the growth of the repairing tissue and significantly [22] impairing the key healing processes such as the inflammatory immune response, granulation tissue formation and epithelialization. Although a moist environment is necessary for optimal wound healing, poor moisture/exudate control within a wound environment promotes the development of biofilm. Consequently, moisture balance is essential to optimize the wound environment for healing and minimize the opportunity for biofilms to develop [23–25]. Preventing biofilm is fundamental for faster and more effective treatment of chronic wounds [17]. However, despite the evidence for the presence of biofilm in wounds, research studies are required to detect biofilm and to determine the exact role played by multispecies biofilms in terms of delayed wound-healing process [26]. Different biofilms can be identified within a wound environment, such as aggregates of cells dispersed within the wound exudate, in slough or on necrotic tissue or on the wound dressing [27]. The microbial community presents multiple difficulties for clinicians in attempting to heal a chronic wound. Biofilms are resistant to many biocides, antibiotics and wound-care products. So, managing biofilm often involves its physical removal from the wound surface with sharp or surgical debridement [28].

The control of biofilm is a key part of chronic wound management, but the use of antiseptic dressings for preventing and managing biofilm and infection still needs further research involving well-designed, randomized controlled trials [29]. The concept of a bacterial contamination, colonization and biofilm-related infection is now widely accepted in wound care, and the recognition of the biofilm and the evolution of topical antiseptics to control bioburden in wounds are considered strictly related to the concept of TIME (tissue, infection/inflammation, moisture balance and edge of wound) and to its relation with the current best practice [30]. In healthcare, infections lead to longer hospital stays for patients, specifically wound dressings and increased hospital costs [12]. Also worsened by an ageing population and the incidence of diabetes and obesity, the huge economic and social impact of wounds requires higher level of attention and resources to understand biological mechanisms underlying cutaneous wound complications [31].

Infections of the dermis, including burns, surgical site infections and non-healing diabetic foot ulcers affect over a million people. Individuals with diabetes represent a particularly vulnerable category because many of them develop foot ulceration during the course of their disease and undergo amputation. In addition to diabetics, several other groups of immune-compromised patient populations are plagued by slow-healing and non-healing wounds, such as trauma and burn victims, cancer patients and pressure ulcers in the elderly [32]. The incidence, morbidity, mortality and costs associated with non-healing of chronic skin wounds are dramatic. Chronic wounds cost millions of dollars annually in the healthcare industry of the United States, and biofilm significantly contributes many billions of dollars to the global cost of chronic wounds because of its role in delaying the wound-healing process and extending the inflammatory phase of repair [19, 33–35].

Along with the direct medical costs borne by the hospital or insurer, also indirect costs including lost patient productivity and diminished functional status should be considered [36]. The control of bioburden is recognized as an important aspect of wound management, which requires new solutions against microbes and their biofilms. Octenidine dihydrochloride and polyhexanide are effective and tolerated antiseptics used in wound management today, but antiseptics alone may not be able to achieve wound healing without addressing other factors such as the general health of patients or the wound's physical environment [37, 38]. Next generation of wound treatment strategies for non-healing chronic wounds can be achieved by adopting a biofilm-based management approach to wound care, in order to kill and prevent reattachment of microorganisms [26].

3. The antibacterial activities of metals

The antibiotic resistance of microorganisms determines serious complications like infection, and delayed wound healing and great concerns are related to the numbers and types of residing microorganisms and the ability of the host's immune system to control their proliferation [39–41]. Along with the emergence of microorganisms' resistance to multiple antibiotics, the increased healthcare costs and the huge social and economic impact of wound care have increased attention towards the biological mechanisms underlying cutaneous wound complications and have encouraged the researchers towards the development of new bactericide agents [31, 42]. The new frontier in clinical medicine and disease burden is represented by the medical applications of nanotechnology. Antimicrobial nanoparticles (NPs) offer an effective approach against numerous microorganisms where conventional antimicrobial agents fail [43, 44] and, compared with micron-sized particulate matter, have greater potential to enter cells and be more biologically active due to their small size and large surface area [X3]. Endowing ordinary products with new functionalities, consumer products containing engineered nanoparticles, are growing tremendously, and the global nanotechnology industry is becoming a major economic force of the twenty-first century [45, 46]. Some natural antibacterial materials such as zinc, silver and copper possess great antibacterial properties at nanometric size and their way of interaction with bacteria provides unique bactericidal mechanisms [43, 47].

Zinc is a transitional metal known since ancient time and widely distributed in the human environment. Today, many zinc-containing products are available for topical application in wound management due to the demonstrated improved re-epithelialization, reduced inflammation and bacterial growth. [48, 49]. ZnO has demonstrated to possess both antibacterial and anti-inflammatory properties and to accelerate the healing of both acute and chronic wounds. ZnO-NPs have exhibited antimicrobial capability and effectiveness against Gram-positive and Gram-negative bacteria, including pathogens such as *Escherichia coli, Salmonella, Listeria monocytogenes* and *Staphylococcus aureus* [49]. Several mechanisms have been reported for the antibacterial activity of ZnO-NPs. Some of them involve the interaction with membrane lipids and structure, leading to loss of membrane integrity, malfunction, and finally to bacterial death. ZnO-NPs may also penetrate into bacterial cells, thus resulting in the production of toxic oxygen radicals, which damage DNA, cell membranes or cell proteins [50–52]. The direct interaction between ZnO nanoparticles and cell surfaces affects the permeability of membranes and results in the inhibition of cell growth and cell death. Recent studies have also shown that these nanoparticles have selective toxicity to bacteria but exhibit minimal effects on human cells, thus suggesting their potential as nanomedicine-based antimicrobial agents [53, 54].

The bactericidal effect of metal nanoparticles has been attributed to their small size and high surface to volume ratio, and it is not merely due to the release of metal ions in solutions [55]. Copper ions released subsequently may bind with bacterial DNA molecules and disrupt biochemical processes inside bacterial cells. The exact mechanism behind bactericidal effect of copper nanoparticles is not fully elucidated; however, Cu-NPs were found to cause multiple toxic effects such as generation of reactive oxygen species, lipid peroxidation, protein oxidation and DNA degradation in *E. coli* [47, 56]. Although the potential use of copper-based nanomaterials in wound healing has recently emerged and also supported by the hypothesis that copper ions regulate the activity and expression of proteins involved in the wound repair process, however, the synthesis of stable metallic Cu-NPs still remains a challenge because of the rapid oxidation to $Cu2^{+}$ ions in air or aqueous media [47, 57].

In combination with silver, copper nanoparticles may give rise to more complete bactericidal effect against a mixed bacterial population [56]. The broad-spectrum antimicrobial activity of silver has been demonstrated against a wide range of microorganisms, including methicillin resistant bacteria, fungi and viruses [58]. Although the exact antimicrobial mechanism still represents a debated topic, many theories on the action of silver nanoparticles on microbes have been proposed. One of them involves the anchorage and penetration of the nanoparticles into the bacterial cell wall, which cause structural changes in the cell membrane such as permeability and respiration [59–62]. *E. coli* cells treated with silver nanoparticles appear damaged and show the formation of 'pits' in the cell wall of the bacteria, where the silver nanoparticles accumulate [59, 63]. Another antibacterial mechanism involves the release of silver ions and their interaction with the enzymes of the respiratory chain, the cell membrane and the DNA. The binding of silver to the membrane can inhibit the passage of nutrients through the membrane, interfering with normal concentration gradients between the cell and the surrounding environment, so leading to cell death [64, 65]. The formation of free radicals has also the ability to damage the cell membrane and makes it porous, thus causing the death of bacteria [66].

Nanosilver products safety data available in EPA's formal incident reporting database indicates that nanosilver products are safe. Silver nanoparticles can be easily incorporated into matrix materials and have demonstrated a great potential in applications of huge interest in nanotechnology [66]. When incorporated into wound treatment systems, silver nanoparticles can provide clinically relevance in the development of ideal environment for rapid and effective healing. These systems may significantly reduce the time required for the homeostatic equilibrium, while reducing the risk of complications and improving the physical appearance of the scar [67]. Silver nanoparticles induce rapid healing and improved cosmetic appearance in a dose-dependent manner and exert positive effects through their antimicrobial properties, reduction in wound inflammation and modulation of fibrogenic cytokines [68].

4. Metal nanoantimicrobials for wound dressing applications

Wound healing still represents a clinical challenge, which requires efficient wound management strategies [69]. Indeed, a crucial component of wound care is the choice of dressing. Many modern wound dressings have been developed to promote wound healing, such as dressings designed to absorb exudate, to provide an ideal moisture balance at the wound surface, to prevent maceration of surrounding tissue and infections and to reduce the bacterial load [70, 71]. Biomaterials, such as chitosan, alginate and collagen, play an important role as wound dressing materials by accelerating the healing of wounds and also because they can embed many nanoparticles for the development of metal nanoparticles-based wound dressings [69, 72]. Hydrogel-based wound dressings provide a cooling sensation and a moisture environment [73]. Several systems based on the combination of hydrogel and metal nanoparticles, such as zinc, copper and silver, have been recently proposed by many authors, aiming to develop wound dressings with antibacterial and enhanced wound-healing properties. For example, an alginate hydrogel/zinc oxide nanoparticles composite bandage was developed by Mohandas *et al.* using a freeze-drying method. The results obtained demonstrated controlled degradation profile and faster blood clotting ability, along with excellent antimicrobial activity against different microorganisms such as *Escherichia coli, Staphylococcus aureus, Candida albicans* and methicillin resistant *S. aureus* (MRSA) [74]. β-chitin hydrogel/nZnO composite bandages with interconnected micro-porous structure were also obtained by freeze-drying technique and proposed for infected wounds with large volume of exudate. Indeed, the wounds treated with the composite bandages promoted the healing and the re-epithelialization, enhanced collagen deposition and showed reduced number of bacterial colonies [75]. Other formulations involving the use of chitin hydrogel/nano ZnO composite bandages were proposed by Kumar *et al.* for burn, diabetic and chronic wound defects, because of the enhanced swelling, blood clotting and antibacterial properties achieved [76]. Kumar *et al.* have also developed a flexible and microporous chitosan hydrogel/nano zinc oxide composite bandages by incorporating the zinc oxide nanoparticles into chitosan hydrogel. *In vivo* wound-healing evaluations proved the enhanced healing ability of the materials without causing toxicity to cells [73]. Chitosan and copper nanoparticles co-introduced into an ointment preparation were investigated by Rakhmetova *et al.* and their combination at certain ratio of components, concentrations and physicochemical characteristics enhanced the antibacterial and wound-healing properties of the individual components [77]. Babushkina *et al.* demonstrated the efficacy of local application of a suspension of copper and zinc nanoparticles and of a drug based on chitosan and copper/zinc on bacterial contaminated purulent wound in rats [78]. Copper (II) cross-linked alginate hydrogels with body fluid absorption ability and haemostatic properties were developed and suggested by Klinkajon and Supaphol for the treatment of exudation/bleeding wounds and burns [79].

Among the recent trends against burn infections involving the use of noble metal antimicrobials, the most prevalent is represented by silver [80]. For nearly 50 years, silver-containing compounds have been the mainstay of burn wound care and silver sulfadiazine (SSD) has been the standard topical antimicrobial for burn wounds for decades [64, 81].

Silver has been used as an antimicrobial agent for a long time in the form of metal silver and silver sulfadiazine ointments [41], and today, there is scientific evidence supporting the use of silver-based wound dressings highlighting antimicrobial efficacy on biofilms within the *in vitro* and *in vivo* environments [40]. A number of wound dressings developed using silver have been approved by the US Food and Drug Administration (FDA) [82]. In addition to antimicrobial activity, silver dressings may modulate or reduce wound pain and limit the frequency of changes [83]. While topical silver creams and solutions require frequent application, the dressings can control the release of silver to the wound and require to be changed with less frequency [84]. Nanocrystalline silver dressings are considered as the gold standard in the conservative treatment of wounds and burns. It has been demonstrated that nanosilver has both anti-inflammatory effects and improves wound healing [85]. The healing response studied by Chowdhury *et al.* in laparotomy wounds after application of silver nanoparticles determined increased collagen expression from dermal fibroblasts, improved wound healing and reduced microbial load [86]. Rigo *et al.* have observed that the application of Ag NP-based dressing for prolonged time does not affect the proliferation of fibroblasts and keratinocytes, leading to the restoration of the organized skin structure in previously unhealed parts of the wound [87]. Polyvinyl alcohol (PVA) hydrogels loaded with a controlled concentration of silver could combine the hydrogel property of keeping a moisturized environment, thus stimulating healing, with the effect of silver of inhibiting or killing the bacteria [88]. PVA-Ag NPs mats, fabricated by Nguyen *et al.* from a suspension of PVA and Ag NPs after microwave irradiation, possess high tensile stress and anti-bacterial activities at the same time and were proposed as a promoter of wound healing [89].

Hydrogels with polyvinyl pyrrolidone (PVP) and alginate were synthesized by Singh *et al.*, and silver nanoparticles were incorporated in hydrogel network using gamma radiation. The hydrogel-containing nanosilver demonstrated strong antimicrobial effect and complete inhibition of microbial growth, absorption capacity, moisture permeability and the ability to prevent fluid accumulation in exudating wound [90]. Chitosan-PVP-nanosilver oxide wound dressings showed excellent results such as good swelling capability, good antibacterial activity and also transparency of the film, which helps to regularly monitor the condition of wound without removing it from the wound site [81]. The silver nanocrystalline chitosan dressing described by Lu *et al.* significantly increased the rate of wound healing and was associated with silver levels in blood and tissues well below those associated with the silver sulfadiazine dressing ($p < 0.01$) [91]. Silver released in a moist wound surface environment significantly increases the rate of re-epithelialization compared to a standard antibiotic solution, as demonstrated by Demling *et al.* [92].

The application of both silver dressings and antibiotic therapy can have a synergistic effect in improving wound healing, since the interaction of silver released from the dressings significantly increases the susceptibility of bacterial cells within biofilms to antibiotics. Moreover, the reduction of the silver particle size to nanoscale level provides better penetration and accumulation of silver within biofilms, thus contributing to the effectiveness of the silver based product [93]. As silver is the most widely used substance to obtain antimicrobial effects, different formulations involving the use of silver-containing solution or silver nanoparticles have been developed. Among the most widespread antimicrobial dressings, silver foam dressings and silver alginate dressings are applied to exuding wounds and demonstrate improved performances than the traditional gauze dressings [94]. Silver alginate wound dressings have demonstrated beneficial effects on wound healing, in terms of wound exudates levels and prevention from wound infections [95–97]. Silver alginate dressings are particularly known for the prolonged antimicrobial efficacy, which indicates sustained availability of ionic silver and suggests the necessity of reduced dressings changes [98]. Excellent and sustainable controllability of Ag^+ release were obtained by the AgNP-bacterial cellulose hybrid nanostructure developed by Wu *et al.*, which offered promising results for antimicrobial wound dressing through the addition of silver nanoparticles. Indeed, bacterial cellulose has attracted great attention as novel wound dressing material, but it has no antimicrobial activity [99]. The silver nanoparticle/bacterial cellulose gel membranes developed by Wu *et al.* demonstrated *in vivo* excellent healing effects in a second-degree rat wound model and were proposed as promising antimicrobial wound dressing with good biocompatibility to promote scald wound healing [100].

The use of cellulose/nanosilver sponge materials was strongly encouraged in case of serious wound infection and *in vivo* tests confirmed accelerate infected wound healing and absorbing capacity for wound exudate [101]. Other examples of composite scaffolds are biocomposite films containing alginate and sago starch impregnated with silver nanoparticles [102], chitin/nanosilver composite scaffolds and electrospun mats doped with nanosilver, zinc oxide, etc., as degradable and non-degradable polymers [103, 104]. For example, polymeric nanofilm-containing silver nanoparticles exhibit antimicrobial activity at loadings and release rates of silver lower than conventional dressings. When placed on a moist wound, the PVA dissolves and the silver-loaded nanofilm results immobilized on the wound bed, thus allowing the normal and complete wound closure by re-epithelialization [104]. A general overview of some relevant techniques adopted to incorporate nanometals into hydrogel network for wound dressing production is reported in **Table 1**.

Nanomaterial	Description of the technique	References
Zinc oxide (ZnO)	Hydrogel/zinc oxide nanoparticles (nZnO) composite wound dressings developed by freeze-dry method from the mixture of nZnO and alginate or chitosan hydrogels.	[73–76]
Copper oxide (CuO)	Cu^{2+} cross-linked alginate hydrogels by a two-step cross-linking technique. (i) Preparation of solid alginate films through solvent-casting method from soft gels of alginate solutions lightly cross-linked using a Cu^{2+} sulphate solution; (ii) further cross-linking of the films in Cu^{2+} sulphate solution using a dipping method.	[79]
Silver nanoparticles	Silver nanoparticles incorporated in hydrogels network using microwave/electro-spinning, gamma radiation, self-assembling. Composite sponges and films obtained by freeze drying and solvent casting.	[89–91, 101, 102]

Table 1. Overview of some relevant techniques for production of nanometal-based antimicrobial wound dressings.

The widespread use of silver-based dressings in surgery is promising, inexpensive and well tolerated. The placement of silver-nylon dressings over incision sites in colorectal, neurological, spinal, cardiovascular and orthopaedic procedures at the time of primary closure has been described by Abboud *et al.* as effective in reducing surgical site infection rates [105]. Commercial dressings impregnated by immersion in solutions of AgNPs using different concentrations of silver from 125 to 1000 ppm demonstrated anti-biofilm efficacy against *Pseudomonas aeruginosa* [70]. Conventional cotton gauzes were modified by Sannino *et al.* through the deposition of silver-based nanocoatings obtained by a patented photo-assisted deposition process, which allows the silver treatment of natural and synthetic materials for different applications [106–108]. Particularly, the technology adopted involves the preparation of a silver-based solution, and then the deposition of the silver solution onto the surface of the material through spray coating or dip coating and the following exposure of the wet material to ultraviolet light, in order to induce the photo-chemical deposition of silver nanoparticles on the surface of the product. Indeed, the synthesis and deposition of the silver nanoparticles occur simultaneously onto the surface of the material because the photo-reduction reaction induced by UV irradiation determines the conversion from the silver precursor to metal silver nanoparticles. The silver coatings deposited are characterized by a strong adhesion to the substrate, good antimicrobial capability and biocompatibility and low silver release [109]. Cotton gauzes treated with low amounts of silver have demonstrated good antimicrobial activity against different bacterial strains and fungi, and the good antibacterial properties were further confirmed in simulated working conditions such as after incubation in artificial exudate inoculated with bacteria [110]. **Figure 1** reports the agar diffusion test performed on untreated gauze and gauze treated with silver by adopting the technology described using *Staphylococcus aureus* as tester microorganism.

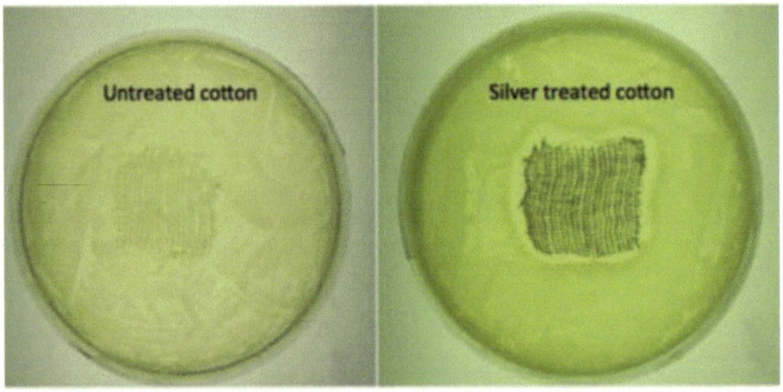

Figure 1. Agar diffusion tests on untreated gauze and cotton gauze treated by photo-reduction technology.

Description of the product	Application	References
Polyester textile mesh impregnated with hydrocolloid particles, vaseline and silver sulphate.	Low to moderate exuding acute and chronic wound at risk of infection.	[112, 113]
Sodium carboxymethylcellulose hydrofibres combined with ionic silver.	Acute and chronic wounds at risk of infection, with moderate and abundant exudate.	[112, 113]
Flexible polyethylene cloth coated with nanocrystalline Ag particles.	Infected ulcers, surgical wounds and burns.	[87, 112]
Silver nylon cloth/activated charcoal.	Most type of chronic wounds and infected wounds and ulcers.	[112, 114]

Table 2. Examples of commercial silver-containing dressings.

Although the impregnating silver solution was prepared by using a percentage of silver lower than 0.5 wt/v%, the antibacterial test clearly demonstrated that the presence of the silver coating successfully inhibited the bacterial growth beneath and around the sample, thus indicating a good potential of product as antibacterial wound dressing. Also flax substrates have been treated with silver by adopting the same technology and the microbiological activity was still confirmed after industrial washing, thus suggesting the excellent stability of the coating on the surface of the textile material [111, 112]. In order to provide flax substrates with a moist environment and antibacterial capability at same time, Paladini *et al.* has developed a wound dressing biomaterial based on silver-doped self-assembling di-phenylalanine hydrogels. These peptide-based hydrogels have some similarities to the extracellular matrix due to their high hydration and nanofibrous architecture, which make them suitable for wound dressing applications where the wound environment needs to be controlled to prevent microbial invasion and to favour tissue regeneration [113]. Along with research efforts, in recent years, many silver-based wound dressings have been marketed for medical problems such as wide-body burns, sepsis in traumatic wounds and chronic diabetic ulcers [114, 115]. Some examples are collected in **Table 2**.

5. Conclusion and future perspectives

Nanotechnology is gaining huge impetus in the present century due to the drastic changes of chemical, physical and optical properties of metals at nanoscale size [84]. The cutting-edge combination of nanotechnology with medicine offers unprecedented opportunities to revolutionize currently available macro-scale therapeutics. Nanoparticles-based delivery systems can be highly beneficial to improve the therapeutic power of biological and synthetic molecules [90]. Due to the knowledge of cellular and molecular processes underlying wound healing, the new therapeutic approaches act directly on cellular and subcellular events during the healing process [90].

In recent years, metal nanoparticles/polymer composites have created lot of attraction due to their wide range of applications [41]. The interest in broad-spectrum antimicrobial agents is particularly increasing for medicated wound dressings, in order to control colonization of wounds by opportunistic pathogens. Medicated wound dressings have demonstrated efficacy *in vitro* against planktonic microorganisms; however, *in vivo* bacteria are organized in biofilms, which is more challenging to control and eradicate [116]. Silver nanoparticles, in particular, have been identified as potent antimicrobial agent and are being evaluated in different medical applications ranging from silver based dressings to silver coated medical devices [117]. Silver in ionized form or nanoparticles exhibits excellent antimicrobial and antifungal properties and efficacy in preventing biofilm formation by pathogenic bacteria. Silver-based wound dressings are widely used in clinical practice and show promising results in healing of contaminated wounds [118].

Despite its recognized importance, there have not been systemic studies that probe the targeting efficiency of nanoparticles nor international standards on their toxicology and biocompatibility [119]. Despite their promise, further studies are needed to elucidate the pharmacokinetics of nanoparticles and potential for *in vivo* toxicity. However, to date, studies have found limited toxicity without evidence of systemic absorption [120].

Author details

Federica Paladini[1*#], Mauro Pollini[1,2#], Alessandro Sannino[1,2] and Luigi Ambrosio[3]

*Address all correspondence to: federica.paladini@unisalento.it

1 Department of Engineering for Innovation, University of Salento, Lecce, Italy

2 Silvertech Ltd, Via per Monteroni, Lecce, Italy

3 Department of Chemical Sciences & Materials Technology, National Research Council of Italy, Rome, Italy

#these authors contributed equally to this work

References

[1] Boateng JS, Matthews KH, Stevens HN, Eccleston GM. Wound healing dressings and drug delivery systems: a review. J. Pharm. Sci. 2008;97:2892–2923. doi:10.1002/jps.21210

[2] Guo S, Di Pietro LA. Factors affecting wound healing. J. Dent. Res. 2010;89:219–229. doi:10.1177/0022034509359125

[3] Edwards R, Harding KG. Bacteria and wound healing. Curr. Opin. Infect. Dis. 2004;17:91–96. doi:10.1097/01.qco.0000124361.27345.d4

[4] Thet NT, Alves DR, Bean JE, Booth S, Nzakizwanayo J, Young AE, Jones BV, Jenkins AT. Prototype development of the intelligent hydrogel wound dressing and its efficacy in the detection of model pathogenic wound biofilms. ACS Appl. Mater. Interfaces. 2015. doi:10.1021/acsami.5b07372

[5] Schierle CF, De la Garza M, Mustoe TA, Galiano RD. Staphylococcal biofilms impair wound healing by delaying reepithelialization in a murine cutaneous wound model. Wound Repair Regen. 2009;17:354–359. doi:10.1111/j.1524-475X.2009.00489.x

[6] Metcalf DG, Bowler PG. Biofilm delays wound healing: a review of the evidence. Burns Trauma. 2013;1:5–12. doi:10.4103/2321-3868.113329

[7] Mah TF, O'Toole GA. Mechanisms of biofilm resistance to antimicrobial agents. Trends Microbiol. 2001;9:34–39. doi:10.1016/S0966-842X(00)01913-2

[8] Straccia MC, d'Ayala GG, Romano I, Oliva A, Laurienzo P. Alginate hydrogels coated with chitosan for wound dressing. Mar. Drugs. 2015;13:2890–2908. doi:10.3390/md13052890

[9] World Health Organisation. Antimicrobial Resistance: Global Report on Surveillance. Geneva, Switzerland: WHO Press; 2014.

[10] Ubbink DT, Brölmann FE, Go PM, Vermeulen H. Evidence-based care of acute wounds: a perspective. Adv. Wound Care (New Rochelle). 2015;4:286–294. doi:10.1089/wound.2014.0592

[11] Eming SA, Krieg T, Davidson, JM. Inflammation in wound repair: molecular and cellular mechanisms. J. Investig. Dermatol. 2007;127:514–525. doi:10.1038/sj.jid.5700701

[12] Finnegan S, Percival SL. EDTA: an antimicrobial and antibiofilm agent for use in wound care. Adv. Wound Care (New Rochelle). 2015;4:415–421. doi:10.1089/wound.2014.0577

[13] Marcano A, Ba O, Thebault P, Crétois R, Marais S, Duncan AC. Elucidation of innovative antibiofilm materials. Colloids Surf. B Biointerfaces. 2015;136:56–63. doi:10.1016/j.colsurfb.2015.08.007

[14] Landsiedel R, Ma-Hock L, Kroll A, Hahn D, Schnekenburger J, Wiench K, Wohlleben W. Testing metal-oxide nanomaterials for human safety. Adv. Mater. 2010;22:2601–2627. doi:10.1002/adma.200902658

[15] Proksch E, Brandner JM, Jensen JM. The skin: an indispensable barrier. Exp. Dermatol. 2008;17:1063–1072. doi:10.1111/j.1600-0625.2008.00786.x

[16] Bowler PG, Duerden BI, Armstrong DG. Wound microbiology and associated approaches to wound management. Clin. Microbiol. Rev. 2001;14:244–269. doi:10.1128/CMR.14.2.244-269.2001

[17] Percival SL, McCarty SM, Lipsky B. Biofilms and wounds: an overview of the evidence. Adv. Wound Care (New Rochelle). 2015;4:373–381. doi:10.1089/wound.2014.0557

[18] Kwei J, Halstead FD, Dretzke J, Oppenheim BA, Moiemen NS. Protocol for a systematic review of quantitative burn wound microbiology in the management of burns patients. Syst. Rev. 2015;4:150. doi:10.1186/s13643-015-0137-9

[19] Zhao G, Usui ML, Lippman SI, James GA, Stewart PS, Fleckman P, Olerud JE. Biofilms and inflammation in chronic wounds. Adv. Wound Care (New Rochelle). 2013;2:389–399. doi:10.1089/wound.2012.0381

[20] Bessa LJ, Fazii P, Di Giulio M, Cellini L. Bacterial isolates from infected wounds and their antibiotic susceptibility pattern: some remarks about wound infection. Int. Wound J. 2015;12:47–52. doi:10.1111/iwj.12049

[21] Hill KE, Malic S, McKee R, Rennison T, Harding KG, Williams DW, Thomas DW. An *in vitro* model of chronic wound biofilms to test wound dressings and assess antimicrobial susceptibilities. J. Antimicrob. Chemother. 2010;65:1195–1206. doi:10.1093/jac/dkq105

[22] Ganesh K, Sinha M, Mathew-Steiner SS, Das A, Roy S, Sen CK. Chronic wound biofilm model. Adv. Wound Care (New Rochelle). 2015;4:382–388. doi:10.1089/wound.2014.0587

[23] Seth AK, Geringer MR, Hong SJ, Leung KP, Mustoe TA, Galiano RD. *In vivo* modeling of bio- film-infected wounds: a review. J. Surg. Res. 2012;178:330–338. doi:10.1016/j.jss. 2012.06.048

[24] Seth AK, Geringer MR, Gurjala AN, Hong SJ, Galiano RD, Leung KP, Mustoe TA. Treatment of *Pseudomonas aeruginosa* biofilm-infected wounds with clinical wound care strategies: a quantitative study using an *in vivo* rabbit ear model. Plast. Reconst. Surg. 2012;129:262–274. doi:10.1097/PRS.0b013e31823aeb3b

[25] Hurlow J, Couch K, Laforet K, Bolton L, Metcalf D, Bowler P. Clinical biofilms: a challenging frontier in wound care. Adv. Wound Care (New Rochelle). 2015;4:295–301. doi:10.1089/wound.2014.0567

[26] Percival SL, Hill KE, Williams DW, Hooper SJ, Thomas DW, Costerton JW. A review of the scientific evidence for biofilms in wounds. Wound Repair Regen. 2012;20:647–657. doi:10.1111/j.1524-475X.2012.00836.x

[27] Percival SL, Vuotto C, Donelli G, Lipsky BA. Biofilms and wounds: an identification algorithm and potential treatment options. Adv. Wound Care (New Rochelle). 2015;4:389–397. doi:10.1089/wound.2014.0574

[28] Rhoads DD, Wolcott RD, Percival SL. Biofilms in wounds: management strategies. J. Wound Care. 2008;17:502–508. doi:10.12968/jowc.2008.17.11.31479

[29] Leaper D, Assadian O, Edmiston CE. Approach to chronic wound infections. Br. J. Dermatol. 2015;173:351–358. doi:10.1111/bjd.13677

[30] Leaper DJ, Schultz G, Carville K, Fletcher J, Swanson T, Drake R. Extending the TIME concept: what have we learned in the past 10 years? Int. Wound J. 2012;2:1–19. doi: 10.1111/j.1742-481X.2012.01097.x

[31] Sen CK, Gordillo GM, Roy S, Kirsner R, Lambert L, Hunt TK, Gottrup F, Gurtner GC, Longaker MT. Human skin wounds: a major and snowballing threat to public health and economy. Wound Rep. Reg. 2009;17:763–771. doi: 10.1111/j.1524-475X.2009.00543.x

[32] Dalton T, Dowd SE, Wolcott RD, Sun Y, Watters C, Griswold JA, Rumbaugh KP. An *in vivo* polymicrobial biofilm wound infection model to study interspecies interactions. PLoS One. 2011;6:e27317. doi:10.1371/journal.pone.0027317

[33] Clinton A, Carter T. Chronic wound biofilms: pathogenesis and potential therapies. Lab. Med. 2015;46:277–284. doi:10.1309/LMBNSWKUI4JPN7SO

[34] Gullo A, Volti GL, Ristagno G. New burns and trauma journal celebrating translational research. Burns Trauma 2013;1:47–50. doi:10.4103/2321-3868.118922

[35] Siddiqui AR, Bernstein JM. Chronic wound infection: facts and controversies. Clin. Dermatol. 2010;28:519–526. doi:10.1016/j.clindermatol.2010.03.009.

[36] Perencevich EN, Sands KE, Cosgrove SE, Guadagnoli E, Meara E, Platt R. Health and economic impact of surgical site infections diagnosed after hospital discharge. Emerg. Infect. Dis. 2003;9:196–203. doi:10.3201/eid0902.020232

[37] James GA, Swogger E, Wolcott R, Pulcini Ed, Secor P, Sestrich J, Costerton JW, Stewart PS. Biofilms in chronic wounds. Wound Repair Regen. 2008;16:37–44. doi:10.1111/j.1524-475X.2007.00321.x

[38] Daeschlein G. Antimicrobial and antiseptic strategies in wound management. Int. Wound J. 2013;10:9–14. doi:10.1111/iwj.12175

[39] Braunwarth H, Brill FHH. Antimicrobial efficacy of modern wound dressings: oligodynamic bactericidal versus hydrophobic adsorption effect. Wound Med. 2014;5:16–20. doi:10.1016/j.wndm.2014.04.003

[40] Percival SL, McCarty SM. Silver and alginates: role in wound healing and biofilm control. Adv. Wound Care (New Rochelle). 2015;4:407–414. doi:10.1016/j.wndm.2014.04.003

[41] Madhumathi K, Sudheesh Kumar PT, Abhilash S, Sreeja V, Tamura H, Manzoor K, Nair SV, Jayakumar R. Development of novel chitin/nanosilver composite scaffolds for wound dressing applications. J. Mater. Sci. Mater. Med. 2010;21:807–813. doi:10.1007/s10856-009-3877-z.

[42] Maiti S, Krishnan D, Barman G, Ghosh SK, Lah JK. Antimicrobial activities of silver nanoparticles synthesized from *Lycopersicon esculentum* extract. J. Anal. Sci. Technol. 2014;5:40. doi:10.1186/s40543-014-0040-3

[43] Seil JT, Webster TJ. Antimicrobial applications of nanotechnology: methods and literature. Int. J. Nanomedicine. 2012;7:2767–2781. doi:10.2147/IJN.S24805

[44] Yah CS, Simate GS. Nanoparticles as potential new generation broad spectrum antimicrobial agents. Daru 2015;23:43. doi:10.1186/s40199-015-0125-6

[45] Zhou EH, Watson C, Pizzo R, Cohen J, Dang Q, Ferreira de Barros PM, Park CY, Chen C, Brain JD, Butler JP, Ruberti JW, Fredberg JJ, Demokritou P. Assessing the impact of engineered nanoparticles on wound healing using a novel *in vitro* bioassay. Nanomedicine (Lond). 2014;9:2803–2815. doi:10.2217/nnm.14.40

[46] Rivero PJ, Urrutia A, Goicoechea J, Arregui FJ. Nanomaterials for functional textiles and fibers. Nanoscale Res. Lett. 2015;10:501. doi:10.1186/s11671-015-1195-6

[47] Chatterjee AK, Chakraborty R, Basu T. Mechanism of antibacterial activity of copper nanoparticles. Nanotechnology. 2014;25:135101. doi:10.1088/0957-4484/25/13/135101

[48] Lansdown AB, Mirastschijski U, Stubbs N, Scanlon E, Agren MS. Zinc in wound healing: theoretical, experimental, and clinical aspects. Wound Repair Regen. 2007;15:2–16. doi:10.1111/j.1524-475X.2006.00179.x

[49] Raguvaran R, Manuja A, Manuja BK. Zinc oxide nanoparticles: opportunities and challenges in veterinary sciences. Immunome Res. 2015;11:95. doi: 10.4172/1745-7580.1000095

[50] Apperlot G, Lipovsky A, Dror R, Perkas N, Nitzan Y, Lubart R, Gedanken A. Enhanced antibacterial activity of nanocrystalline ZnO due to increased ROS-mediated cell injury. Adv. Funct. Mater. 2009;19:842–852. doi:10.1002/adfm.200801081

[51] Salem W, Leitner DR, Zingl FG, 1, Schratter G, Prassl R, Goessler W, Reidl J, Schild S. Antibacterial activity of silver and zinc nanoparticles against Vibrio holera and enterotoxic *Escherichia coli*. Int. J. Med. Microbiol. 2015;305:85–95. doi:10.1016/j.ijmm.2014.11.005

[52] Raghupathi KR, Koodali RT, Manna AC. Size-dependent bacterial growth inhibition and mechanism of antibacterial activity of zinc oxide nanoparticles. Langmuir. 2011;27:4020–4028. doi:10.1021/la104825u

[53] Xie Y, He Y, Irwin PL, Jin T, Shi X. Antibacterial activity and mechanism of action of zinc oxide nanoparticles against Campylobacter jejuni. Appl. Environ. Microbiol. 2011;77:2325–2331. doi:10.1128/AEM.02149-10

[54] Reddy KM, Feris KV, Bell J, Wingett DG, Hanley C, Punnoose A. Selective toxicity of zinc oxide nanoparticles to prokaryotic and eukaryotic systems. Appl. Phys. Lett. 2007;90:213902-1–213902-3. doi:10.1063/1.2742324

[55] Ramyadevi J, Jeyasubramanian K, Marikani A, Rajakumar G, Rahuman A. Synthesis and antimicrobial activity of copper nanoparticles. Mater. Lett. 2012;71:114–111. doi: 10.1016/j.matlet.2011.12.055

[56] Ruparelia JP, Chatterjee AK, Duttagupta SP, Mukherji S. Strain specificity in antimicrobial activity of silver and copper nanoparticles. Acta Biomater. 2008;4:707–716. doi: 10.1016/j.actbio.2007.11.006

[57] Kornblatt AP, Nicoletti VG, Travaglia A. The neglected role of copper ions in wound healing. J. Inorg. Biochem. 2016;161:1-8. doi:10.1016/j.jinorgbio.2016.02.012

[58] Paladini F, Pollini M, Sannino A, Ambrosio L. Metal-based antibacterial substrates for biomedical applications. Biomacromolecules 2015;16:1873–1885. doi:10.1021/acs.biomac.5b00773

[59] Prabhu S, Poulose EK. Silver nanoparticles: mechanism of antimicrobial action, synthesis, medical applications, and toxicity effects. Int. Nano Lett. 2012;2:32. doi: 10.1186/2228-5326-2-32

[60] Morones JR, Elechiguerra JL, Camacho A, Holt K, Kouri JB, Ramirez JT, Yacaman MJ. The bactericidal effect of silver nanoparticles. Nanotechnology 2005;16:2346–2353. doi: 10.1088/0957-4484/16/10/059

[61] Li WR, Xie XB, Shi QS, Zeng HY, Ou-Yang YS, Chen YB. Antibacterial activity and mechanism of silver nanoparticles on *Escherichia coli*. Appl. Microbiol. Biotechnol. 2010;85:1115–1122. doi:10.1007/s00253-009-2159-5

[62] Feng QL, Wu J, Chen GQ, Cui FZ, Kim TN, Kim JO. A mechanistic study of the antibacterial effect of silver ions on *Escherichia coli* and *Staphylococcus aureus*. J. Biomed. Mater. Res. 2008;52:662–668. doi:10.1002/1097-4636(20001215)52:4<662::AID-JBM10>3.0.CO;2-3

[63] Sondi I, Salopek-Sondi B. Silver nanoparticles as antimicrobial agent: a case study on *E. coli* as a model for Gram-negative bacteria. J. Colloid Interface Sci. 2004;275:177–182. doi:10.1016/j.jcis.2004.02.012

[64] Marx DE, Barillo DJ. Silver in medicine: the basic science. Burns. 2014;40:S9–S18. doi: 10.1016/j.burns.2014.09.010

[65] Kim JS, Kuk E, Yu K, Kim JH, Park SJ, Lee HJ, Kim SH, Park YK, Park YH, Hwang CY, Kim YK, Lee YS, Jeong DH, Cho MH. Antimicrobial effects of silver nanoparticles. Nanomedicine 2007;3:95–101. doi:10.1016/j.nano.2006.12.001

[66] Gupta V, Kumar A. Nanosilver products – a review. Chem. Sci. Rev. Lett. 2014;3:717–727.

[67] Nam G, Rangasamy S, Purushothaman B, Song JM. The application of bactericidal silver nanoparticles in wound treatment. Nanomater. Nanotechnol. 2015,5:23. doi: 10.5772/60918

[68] Tian J, Wong KK., Ho CM, Lok CN, Yu WY, Che CM, Chiu JF, Tam PK. Topical delivery of silver nanoparticles promotes wound healing. Chem. Med. Chem. 2007;2:129–136. doi:10.1002/cmdc.200600171

[69] Deepachitra R, Pujitha Lakshmi R, Sivaranjani K, Helan Chandra J, Sastry TP. Nanoparticles embedded biomaterials in wound treatment: a review. J. Chem. Pharm. Sci. 2015;8:324–328.

[70] Velázquez-Velázquez JL, Santos-Flores A, Araujo-Meléndez J, Sánchez-Sánchez R, Velasquillo C, González C, Martínez-Castañon G, Martinez-Gutierrez F. Anti-biofilm and cytotoxicity activity of impregnated dressings with silver nanoparticles. Mater. Sci. Eng. C Mater. Biol. Appl. 2015;49:604–611. doi:10.1016/j.msec.2014.12.084

[71] Phillips PL, Yang Q, Davis S, Sampson EM, Azeke JI, Hamad A, Schultz GS. Antimicrobial dressing efficacy against mature *Pseudomonas aeruginosa* biofilm on porcine skin explants. Int. Wound J. 2015;12:469–483. doi:10.1111/iwj.12142

[72] Mei Dai, XiuLing Zheng, Xu Xu, XiangYe Kong, XingYi Li, Gang Guo, Feng Luo, Xia Zhao, Yu Quan Wei, and Zhiyong Qian. Chitosan-alginate sponge: preparation and application in curcumin delivery for dermal wound healing in rat. J. Biomed. Biotechnol. 2009;595126:8. doi:10.1155/2009/595126

[73] Kumar PT, Lakshmanan VK, Anilkumar TV, Ramya C, Reshmi P, Unnikrishnan AG, Nair SV, Jayakumar R. Flexible and microporous chitosan hydrogel/nano ZnO composite bandages for wound dressing: *in vitro* and *in vivo* evaluation. ACS Appl. Mater. Interfaces. 2012;4:2618–2629. doi:10.1021/am300292v

[74] Mohandas A, Kumar PTS, Raja B, Lakshmanan VK, Jayakumar R. Exploration of alginate hydrogel/nano zinc oxide composite bandages for infected wounds. Int. J. Nanomedicine. 2015;10:53–66. doi:10.2147/IJN.S79981

[75] Sudheesh Kumar P.T., Lakshmanan VK, Raj M, Biswas R, Hiroshi T, Nair SV, Jayakumar. Evaluation of wound healing potential of β-chitin hydrogel/nano zinc oxide composite bandage. R. Pharm. Res. 2013;30:523–537. doi:10.1007/s11095-012-0898-y

[76] Kumar PT, Lakshmanan VK, Biswas R, Nair SV, Jayakumar R. Synthesis and biological evaluation of chitin hydrogel/nano ZnO composite bandage as antibacterial wound dressing. J. Biomed. Nanotechnol. 2012;8:891–900. doi:10.1166/jbn.2012.1461

[77] Rakhmetova AA, Bogoslovskaya OA, Olkhovskaya IP, Zhigach AN, Ilyina AV, Varlamov VP, Gluschenko NN. Concomitant action of organic and inorganic nanoparticles in wound healing and antibacterial resistance: chitosan and copper nanoparticles in an ointment as an example. Nanotechnol. Russ. 2015;10:149–157. doi:10.1134/S1995078015010164

[78] Babushkina IV, Mamontova IA, Gladkova EV. Metal nanoparticles reduce bacterial contamination of experimental purulent wounds. Bull. Exp. Biol. Med. 2015;158:692–694. doi:10.1007/s10517-015-2837-5

[79] Klinkajon W, Supaphol P. Novel copper (II) alginate hydrogels and their potential for use as anti-bacterial wound dressings. Biomed. Mater. 2014;9:045008. doi: 10.1088/1748-6041/9/4/045008

[80] Akila S, Nanda A. *In-vivo* wound healing activity of silver nanoparticles: an investigation. Int. J. Sci. Res. 2014;3:1208–1212.

[81] Adhya A, Bain J, Ray O, Hazra A, Adhikari S, Dutta G, Ray S, Kumar Majumdar B. Healing of burn wounds by topical treatment: a randomized controlled comparison between silver sulfadiazine and nano-crystalline silver. J. Basic Clin. Pharm. 2014;6:29–34. doi:10.4103/0976-0105.145776

[82] Archana D, Singh BK, Dutta J, Dutta PK. PVP-nano silver oxide wound dressing: *in vitro* and *in vivo* evaluation. Int. J. Biol. Macromol. 2015;73:49–57 doi:10.1016/j.ijbiomac.2014.10.055

[83] Abboud EC, Legare TB, Settle JC, Boubekri AM, Barillo DJ, Marcet JE, Sanchez JE. Do silver-based wound dressings reduce pain? A prospective study and review of the literature. Burns. 2014;40:S40–S47. doi:10.1016/j.burns.2014.09.012

[84] Singh R, Singh D. Chitin membranes containing silver nanoparticles for wound dressing application. Int. Wound J. 2014;11:264–268. doi:10.1111/j.1742-481X.2012.01084.x

[85] Chaloupka K, Malam Y, Seifalian AM. Nanosilver as a new generation of nanoproduct in biomedical applications. Trends Biotechnol. 2010;28:580–588. doi:10.1016/j.tibtech.2010.07.006

[86] Chowdhury S, De M, Guha R, Batabyal S, Samanta I, Hazra SH, Ghosh TK, Konar A, Hazra S. Influence of silver nanoparticles on post-surgical wound healing following topical application. Eur. J. Nanomed. 2014;6:237–247. doi:10.1515/ejnm-2014-0030

[87] Rigo C, Ferroni L, Tocco I, Roman M, Munivrana I, Gardin C, Cairns WR, Vindigni V, Azzena B, Barbante C, Zavan B. Active silver nanoparticles for wound healing. Int. J. Mol. Sci. 2013;14:4817–4840. doi:10.1007/s10856-009-3877-z

[88] Oliveira RN, Rouzé R, Quilty B, Alves GG, Soares GD, Thiré RM, McGuinness GB. Mechanical properties and *in vitro* characterization of polyvinyl alcohol-nano-silver hydrogel wound dressings. Interface Focus. 2014;6:20130049. doi:10.1098/rsfs.2013.0049

[89] Nguyen TH, Kim YH, Song HY, Lee BT. Nano Ag loaded PVA nano-fibrous mats for skin applications. J. Biomed. Mater. Res. B Appl. Biomater. 2011;96:225–233. doi:10.1002/jbm.b.31756

[90] Singh R, Singh D. Radiation synthesis of PVP/alginate hydrogel containing nanosilver as wound dressing. J. Mater. Sci. Mater. Med. 2012;23:2649–2658. doi:10.1007/s10856-012-4730-3

[91] Lu S, Gao W, Gu HY. Construction, application and biosafety of silver nanocrystalline chitosan wound dressing. Burns. 2008;34:623–628. doi:10.1016/j.burns.2007.08.020

[92] Demling RH, Leslie De Santi MD. The rate of re-epithelialization across meshed skin grafts is increased with exposure to silver. Burns. 2002;28:264–266. doi:10.1016/S0305-4179(01)00119-X

[93] Kostenko V, Lyczak J, Turner K, Martinuzzi RJ. Impact of silver-containing wound dressings on bacterial biofilm viability and susceptibility to antibiotics during prolonged treatment. Antimicrob. Agents Chemother. 2010;54:5120–5131. doi:10.1128/AAC.00825-10

[94] Yang Y, Hu H. A review on antimicrobial silver absorbent wound dressings applied to exuding wounds. J. Microb. Biochem. Technol. 2015;7:228–233. doi:10.4172/1948-5948.1000212

[95] Percival SL, Slone W, Linton S, Okel T, Corum L, Thomas JG. The antimicrobial efficacy of a silver alginate dressing against a broad spectrum of clinically relevant wound isolates. Int. Wound J. 2011;8:237–243. doi:10.1111/j.1742-481X.2011.00774.x

[96] Slone W, Linton S, Okel T, Corum L, Thomas JG, Percival SL. The effect of pH on the antimicrobial efficiency of silver alginate on chronic wound isolates. J. Am. Col. Certif. Wound Spec. 2011;2:86–90. doi:10.1016/j.jcws.2011.01.001

[97] Seo SY, Lee GH, Lee SG, Jung SY, Lim JO, Choi JH. Alginate-based composite sponge containing silver nanoparticles synthesized *in situ*. Carbohydr. Polym. 2012;90:109–115. doi:10.1016/j.carbpol.2012.05.002.8

[98] Hooper SJ, Percival SL, Hill KE, Thomas DW, Hayes AJ, Williams DW. The visualisation and m peed of kill of wound isolates on a silver alginate dressing. Int. Wound J. 2012;9:633–642. doi:10.1111/j.1742-481X.2012.00927.x

[99] Wu J, Zheng Y, Song W, Luan J, Wen X, Wu Z, Chen X, Wang Q, Guo S. *In situ* synthesis of silver-nanoparticles/bacterial cellulose composites for slow-released antimicrobial wound dressing. Carbohydr. Polym. 2014;102:762–771. doi:10.1016/j.carbpol.2013.10.093

[100] Wu J, Zheng Y, Wen X, Lin Q, Chen X, Wu Z. Silver nanoparticle/bacterial cellulose gel membranes for antibacterial wound dressing: investigation *in vitro* and *in vivo*. Biomed. Mater. 2014;9(3):035005. doi:10.1088/1748-6041/9/3/035005

[101] Ye D, Zhong Z, Xu H, Chang C, Yang Z, Wang Y, Ye Q, Zhang L. Construction of cellulose/nanosilver sponge materials and their antibacterial activities for infected wounds healing. Cellulose 2016;23:749–763. doi:10.1007/s10570-015-0851-4

[102] Marie Arockianathan P, Sekar S, Sankar S, Kumaran B, Sastry TP. Evaluation of biocomposite films containing alginate and sago starch impregnated with silver nano particles. Carbohydr. Polym. 2012;90:717–724. doi:10.1016/j.carbpol.2012.06.003

[103] Shalumon KT, Anulekha KH, Nair SV, Nair SV, Chennazhi KP, Jayakumar R. Sodium alginate/poly(vinyl alcohol)/nano ZnO composite nanofibers for antibacterial wound dressings. Int. J. Biol. Macromol. 2011;49:247–254. doi:10.1016/j.ijbiomac.2011.04.005.

[104] Herron M, Agarwal A, Kierski PR, Calderon DF, Teixeira LB, Schurr MJ, Murphy CJ, Czuprynski CJ, McAnulty JF, Abbott NL. Reduction in wound bioburden using a silver-loaded dissolvable microfilm construct. Adv. Health Mater. 2014;3:916–928. doi:10.1002/adhm.201300537

[105] Abboud EC, Settle J, Legare TB, Marcet JE, Barillo DJ, Sanchez JE. Silver-based dressings for the reduction of surgical site infection: review of current experience and recommendation for future studies. Burns. 2014;40:S30–S39. doi:10.1016/j.burns.2014.09.011

[106] Pollini M, Paladini F, Licciulli A, Maffezzoli A, Sannino A, Nicolais L. Antibacterial natural leather for application in the public transport system. J. Coat. Technol. Res. 2013;10:239–245. doi:10.1007/s11998-012-9439-1

[107] De Simone S, Gallo AL, Paladini F, Sannino A, Pollini M. Development of silver nanocoatings on silk sutures as a novel approach against surgical infections. J. Mater. Sci. Mater. Med. 2014;25:2205–2214. doi:10.1007/s10856-014-5262-9

[108] Paladini F, Cooper IR, Pollini M. Development of antibacterial and antifungal silver-coated polyurethane foams as air filtration units for the prevention of respiratory diseases. J. Appl. Microbiol. 2014;116:710–717. doi:10.1111/jam.12402

[109] Paladini F, Sannino A, Pollini M. *In vivo* testing of silver treated fibers for the evaluation of skin irritation effect and hypoallergenicity. J. Biomed. Mater. Res. B Appl. Biomater. 2014;102:1031–1037. doi:10.1002/jbm.b.33085

[110] Paladini F, De Simone S, Sannino A, Pollini M. Antibacterial and antifungal dressings obtained by photochemical deposition of silver nanoparticles. J. Appl. Polym. Sci. 2014;131:40326.

[111] Paladini F, Picca RA, Sportelli MC, Cioffi N, Sannino A, Pollini M. Surface chemical and biological characterization of flax fabrics modified with silver nanoparticles for biomedical applications. Mater. Sci. Eng. C Mater. Biol. Appl. 2015;52:1–10. doi:10.1016/j.msec.2015.03.035

[112] Paladini F, Cooper IR, Pollini M. Development of antibacterial and antifungal silver-coated polyurethane foams as air filtration units for the prevention of respiratory diseases. J. Appl. Microbiol. 2014;116:710–717. doi:10.1111/jam.12402

[113] Paladini F, Meikle ST, Cooper IR, Lacey J, Perugini V, Santin M. Silver-doped self-assembling di-phenylalanine hydrogels as wound dressing biomaterials. Mater. Sci. Mater. Med. 2013;24:2461–2472. doi:10.1007/s10856-013-4986-2

[114] Harding K, Gottrup F, Jawień A, Mikosiński J, Twardowska-Saucha K, Kaczmarek S, Sopata M, Shearman C, Pieronne A, Kommala D. A prospective, multi-centre, randomised, open label, parallel, comparative study to evaluate effects of AQUACEL® Ag and Urgotul® Silver dressing on healing of chronic venous leg ulcers. Int. Wound J. 2012;9(3):285–294. doi:10.1111/j.1742-481X.2011.00881.x

[115] Silver S, Phung le T, Silver G. Silver as biocides in burn and wound dressings and bacterial resistance to silver compounds. J. Ind. Microbiol. Biotechnol. 2006;33(7):627–634. doi:10.1007/s10295-006-0139-7

[116] Said J, Walker M, Parsons D, Stapleton P, Beezer AE, Gaisford S. An *in vitro* test of the efficacy of an anti-biofilm wound dressing. Int. J. Pharm. 2014;474:177–181. doi:10.1016/j.ijpharm.2014.08.034

[117] Bidgoli SA, Mahdavi M, Rezayat SM, Korani M, Amani A, Ziarati P. Toxicity assessment of nanosilver wound dressing in Wistar rat. Acta Med. Iran. 2013;51:203–208.

[118] Konop M, Damps T, Misicka A, Rudnicka L. Certain aspects of silver and silver nanoparticles in wound care: a minireview. J. Nanomater. 2016;7614753:10. doi: 10.1155/2016/7614753

[119] Tocco I, Zavan B, Bassetto F, Vindigni V. Nanotechnology-based therapies for skin wound regeneration. J. Nanomater. 2012;714134:11. doi:10.1155/2012/714134

[120] Mordorski B, Rosen J, Friedman A. Nanotechnology as an innovative approach for accelerating wound healing in diabetes. Diabetes Manag. 2015;5:329–332. doi:10.2217/dmt.15.28

Section 4

Alternative Approaches for Tissue Regeneration

Chapter 21

Alternative Approaches to Wound Healing

Anuradha Majumdar and Prajakta Sangole

Additional information is available at the end of the chapter

http://dx.doi.org/10.5772/63636

Abstract

The history of wound healing across the globe abounds with usage of various herbs for treating simple cuts and bruises to serious burns. Wound healing is a complex and dynamic process and, moreover, depends a lot on the wound bearing person's immunity and mental status. Synthetic medicine may give rise to side effects of allergy and resistance with usually higher cost of treatment. Whereas the alternative and complementary medicine such as Ayurveda, Siddha, Unani, Chinese medicine, and ozone therapy can lessen these side effects considerably and offer treatment at lower costs, thus elevating the overall quality of life of the patient. In today's times the patient is more demanding and has the ability to partake in treatment decisions. It is then the moral responsibility of the scientists to apply modern up-to-date scientific acumen to provide evidenced-based concept to alternative therapies of wound healing to ensure that these practices are safe and efficacious.

Keywords: wound healing, alternative therapies, Ayurveda, Siddha, Unani, Traditional Chinese Medicine, ozone therapy

1. Introduction

Wound healing continues to pose a challenging clinical problem despite scientific developments in the field. A correct and efficient wound management is essential. Emphasis is required on new and alternative therapeutic approaches and development of technologies for acute and chronic wound management. A wound can be defined as a damage or a disruption to the normal anatomical structure and function [1]. This can range from a simple break in the epithelial integrity of the skin or it can be deeper, extending into subcutaneous tissue with damage to other structures such as tendons, muscles, vessels, nerves, parenchymal organs, and even bones [2]. Depending on the time of repair, wounds can be divided as acute, chronic, and complicated. Wound healing is a natural, complex, dynamic yet continuous process, and is initiated as any injury occurs and continues till the entire repair of the wound and tissue remodelling is complete. The process can be randomly divided into (i) coagulation and haemostasis, (ii) inflammation, (iii) proliferation, and (iv) wound remodelling with scar tissue formation. If the wound healing is interrupted by any infection, tissue hypoxia, edema, growth factor imbalance or nutritional, and metabolic status of the host, then the wound may take extended time for repair. Normal wound healing is a dynamic and complex process involving a series of coordinated events including bleeding, coagulation, initiation of an acute inflammatory response to the initial injury, regeneration, migration, and proliferation of connective tissue and parenchyma cells, as well as synthesis of extracellular matrix proteins, remodelling of new parenchyma, connective tissue, and collagen deposition [3–7]. Modern synthetic allopathy-based medicines have their share of limitations of allergy, resistance, cost, etc., which has prompted the scientists and wound care professionals to consider alternative approaches to wound healing and validating their use using modern technology. The perception toward alternative medicine such as Ayurveda, Siddha, Unani, and Chinese has changed. The World Health Organisation (WHO) defines traditional medicine as "the sum total of the knowledge, skills, ands practices based on the theories, beliefs, and experiences indigenous to different cultures, whether explicable or not, used in the maintenance of health as well as in the prevention, diagnosis, improvement or treatment of physical and mental illness" [8]. Each of the above-mentioned systems of medical practice offers a variety of medicines for wound management and has been traditionally practiced since ancient times in few parts of the world and is fast getting acceptance in rest of the globe. Ayurveda or Indian traditional and Chinese medicine have rich abundance of knowledge and have been well known as ethnopharmacological and folklore-based systems. Siddha also has origin in south of India, Tamilnadu, which aims in providing ultimate cure to both mind and body systems. "Food as medicine" is the principle behind Siddha treatment. Unani system of medicine has its origin in Iran and also has documented evidences of antimicrobial herbs possessing wound healing properties. Ozone therapy has been in use since World War I times and offers remarkable bactericidal action. The abovementioned alternative therapies offer an economical approach to wound healing. Besides this benefit, they have significant lesser side effects thus increasing patient compatibility as compared to modern medicine.

2. Alternative approaches in wound healing

2.1. Ayurvedic products

A rich heritage of knowledge on preventive and curative medicines is available in ancient scholastic work included in the Atharvaveda (an Indian religious book), Ayurveda (Indian traditional system of medicine), etc. Many Ayurvedic plants have a very important role in the process of healing of wounds (*vrana*). Plants are more potent healers because they promote the repair mechanisms in the natural way. Plant-based therapy not only accelerate healing process, moreover, also maintain the esthetics. More than 70% of wound healing Ayurveda-based pharma products are plant-based, 20% are mineral-based, and remaining contain animal

http://dx.doi.org/10.5772/63636

products as their base material. The plant-based materials are used as first aid—antiseptic coagulants and wound wash [9]. Different Ayurvedic preparations are made and used topically for healing of wounds. Ghee is used in many Ayurvedic traditional preparations and also finds use as an ointment base. It is rich source of essential fatty acids (EFAs), which regulate prostaglandin synthesis and hence induce wound healing. Cow ghee (*Goghrita*) specifically possesses regenerative properties promoting the growth of healthy cells and is clinically proven. *Bhasma* is a calcined preparation in which the gem or metal is converted into ash. *Grithas*, also called as *neyyu*, are medicated clarified butter. *Taila* or medicated oil is manufactured by steeping powdered medicinal substances, water, vegetable drugs in paste form and fragrance-producing materials such as cardamon, saffron, sandalwood, camphor. *Malam* (Cream) too is applied topically and has been documented in ancient ayurvedic texts for its helpfulness in wound healing. Some of the herbal drugs that are mentioned in Ayurvedic texts which have been specifically studied for their wound healing properties (*vranaropaka*) are mentioned below.

2.1.1. *Aloe vera*

A. vera finds a mention in Ayurvedic practice since centuries regarding its wound healing property. A study carried out by Yadav *et al.* [10] in 2012 provides the scientific rationale for the traditional use of *A. vera* gel for management of wound using wound excision model in experimental rats. The effect produced by *A. vera* gel with reference to wound contraction, wound closure, decrease in surface area of wound, tissue regeneration at the wound site, and histopathological characteristics were significant in treated rats. The effect of *A. vera* gel on biochemical studies revealed significant increase in collagen and decreased hexosamine content and malondialdehyde levels when compared with control. The authors concluded that *A. vera* gel is very effective on open wounds and a promising herbal drug. It also had a marked influence on the collagen level which is the precursor protein for wound healing mechanism. *A. vera* gel reportedly accelerated epithelialization, neovascularization, and increased wound contraction in the later stage of the wound healing process.

2.1.2. *Cleome rutidosperma DC.*

A study [11] justifies the use of folklore plant *C. rutidosperma* for the treatment of wounds. Petroleum ether, chloroform, methanol, and aqueous extracts of *C. rutidosperma* (Family: Capparidaceae) roots were evaluated for their wound healing activities in rats using excision and incision wound models, respectively. The effects of wound healing were assessed by the rate of wound closure, period of epithelialization, and wound breaking strength. Nitrofurazone (0.2% w/w) in simple ointment IP was used as reference standard for the activity comparison. The authors concluded that the animals treated with methanol and aqueous extracts of *C. rutidosperma* showed faster rate of wound healing compared with other extracts under study. The wound healing property of the roots can be attributed to the presence of flavonoids, triterpenoids, and tannins which possess the antimicrobial and astringent properties which seem to be responsible for wound contraction and increased rate of epithelialization.

2.1.3. *Kshatantak Malam*

It is a combination of *Acyranthes aspera, Allium cepa,* and *Cannabis sativa* also known as *Baharer nani* has been traditionally reported by Bengal School of Ayurvedic Physicians as external healer for open cuts, complicated wounds and burns but still a scientific document proving its quality was not available. Gangopadhyay *et al.* [12] reported its pharmacological evaluation and chemical standardization for its wound healing activity in rats. The test drug was applied topically on a 8 mm diameter full thickness punch in Wistar rats. Framycetin and povidone-iodine ointment were used as standard comparators. Parameters such as wound contraction size (mm^2), wound index, healing period (days), tensile strength (g), DNA (mg/g), RNA (mg/g), total protein (mg/g), hydroxyproline (mg/g), PAGE study, and histological analysis were carried out for analysing the effects of the malam. Out of the three constituents, *A. aspera* specifically possesses potent wound healing activity, *A. cepa* owns antimicrobial activity, and *C. sativa* is capable of tissue repair by virtue of its anti-inflammatory property.

2.1.4. *Katupila (Securinega leucopyrus) (Willd.)*

Another plant used since ancient times in Saurashtra region of India and Srilanka is known as *Katupila* in Srilanka and *Humari* in India. It is mentioned as one of the 60 measures for wound healing by *Acharya Sushruta* (Ancient spiritual Hindu teacher). *Katupila* leaves act as antiseptic, and the paste is capable of removing extraneous material from the wounds without the need of surgery [13].

2.1.5. *Ayurvedic polyherbal formulation*

Rawat and Gupta [14] reported wound healing activity of a prepared ayurvedic formulation containing *Jasad Bhasma, Gandhak, Tankankhar, and Ras Kapoor. J.* (*Yashad*) *Bhasma* is ash containing zinc. *Gandhak or Gandhaka Rasayan* is an ayurvedic mineral-based medicine, which contains detoxified sulfur processed with herbal juice as a main ingredient. *Gandhak Rasayan* is a great antibacterial, antiviral, and antimicrobial ayurvedic medicine. *Tankankhar* is borax applied topically for its analgesic property. Ras Kapoor are pills made out of camphor (*karpoora/ kapoor*), mercury compound (*Shuddha Hingula*), purified opium (*Papaver somniferum*), nutgrass (*Musta/ Cypeus rotundus*), Connessi seed (*Indrayava/ Holarrhena antidysenterica*), and Nutmeg (*Jatiphala/ Myristica fragrans*). The preparation was studied on excision and incision wound models in rats. The preparation exhibited remarkable wound healing in rats and the authors suggest further mechanism-based probing to prove the effectiveness of the constituents to be utilised in humans.

Few more folklore plants which were validated by means of preclinical wound healing studies are mentioned below in **Table 1**. Almost all the plants are shown to be wound healers by applying their extracts topically on wounds created by punches on rats. Their subsequent effect on wound healing models such as excision, incision, and dead space wound models in rats corroborate their wound healing properties. These plants ultimately are reported to stimulate wound contraction, increase hydroxyproline and eventually collagen content thus strengthening the wound area, increase the wound closure rate, reduce scar area, and epithelialization period. Few plants such as *A. cepa, Ageratum conyzoides*, and *Heliotropium indicum* are known to specifically heal the wounds by benefit of their antioxidant property. Dexamethasone is a potent anti-inflammatory glucocorticoid which is used in skin allografts but is known to delay wound healing. Plants such as *Ocimum sanctum, Gossypium herbaceum, Ficus hispida, Pyrus communis*, and *Tetrapleura tetraptera* have been specifically shown to promote dexamethasone suppressed wound healing tested in wound healing models (**Table 1**). *Alafia multiflora* is found to be one of the plants which contains retinoids and have shown marked interaction with steroids like dexamethasone and was reported to further delay the healing of dexamethasone-suppressed wounds. Thus, vitamin A even if known to hasten the process of wound healing is shown to interact with steroids and thus concomitant application should be avoided in dexamethasone suppressed wounds. Few plants such as *Echinacea* species, Vitamins such as A and E found in plants, Bromelain, and Grape seed extract have demonstrated few interactions with conventional therapies used for wound healing (**Table 1**).

No.	Name	Wound healing activity
Plants effective on acute wounds in rats		
1.	*Mimusops Elengi* (*Linn.*) (Sapotaceae)	The methanolic extract ointment of *M. elengi* in rats effectively stimulated wound contraction; increased tensile strength of incision and dead space wounds as compared to control group [15]
2.	*Carica papaya* (Caricaceae)	Contains a mixture of cysteine endopeptidases such as papain. Chympopapain A and B, papaya endopeptidase-II, papaya endopeptidase-IV, omega endopeptidase, chinitase, protease-inhibitors, and proteins. Papaya fruits possess wound healing properties; papaya latex was applied to the burn wound using hydrogel as a vehicle system [16]
3.	*Tephrosia purpurea* (*Linn.*) (Leguminosea)	Contains glycosides, rotenoids, isoflavones, flavones, chalcones, flavonoids and sterols. It is used in the treatment leprous wound and the juice is used for the eruption on skin [17]
4.	*Adhatoda vasica* (*Linn.*) (Acanthaceae)	Leaves and stems of the plant have been reported to contain an alkaloid mimosine, leaves also contain mucilage and root contains tannins. The methanolic, chloroform and Diethyl ether extract ointment (10% w/w) of *A. vasica* has significant wound healing activity. In both extract ointment, the methanolic extract ointment (10% w/w) showed significant effect when compare to standard drug and other two extract in excision wound model [18]
5.	*Piper betle* (Piperaceae)	In Indian folkloric medicine, betel leaf is popular as an antiseptic and is commonly applied on wounds and lesions for its healing effects. This particular property has paved way for further experimental studies, which have established pan extract to have antimicrobial and anti-leshmian properties. Fresh juice of betel leaves is also used in many Ayurvedic preparations [19]
6.	*Moringa oleifera* (*Linn.*) (Moringaceae)	It has anti-inflammatory, antibacterial and counter irritant action, which helps in wound healing. The aqueous extract was studied and it was found that there was

No.	Name	Wound healing activity
		significant increase in wound closure rate, skin-breaking strength, granuloma breaking strength, hydroxyproline content, granuloma dry weight and decrease in scar area was observed [20]
7.	*Eucalyptus globules* (Myrtaceae)	It is used for cuts, wounds and to boost the immune system [21]
8.	*Terminalia Chebula* (Combretaceae)	Traditionally, fruit pulp is used to stop bleeding. Recent studies showed that various aqueous and organic extracts increased cell proliferation and reduced free radical production thus promoting wound healing. Significant utility of the plant is in cases where ammonia accumulation is a limiting factor [22]
9.	*Aegel marmelos* (Bael) (Rutaceae)	Methanolic extract was found to heal wounds faster when tested in wound healing models in rats. *A. marmelos* treated wounds were reported to epithelialize faster and rate of wound contraction was higher as compared to control group of rats [23]
10.	*Alternanthera sessilis* (*Linn.*) (Amaranthaceae)	Consist of chemical constituents like α and β-spinosterols lupeal isolated from roots. The leaves are used for cuts and wounds. The wound healing property of *A. sessilis* (*Linn.*) attributed to sterols present in the plant [24]
11.	*Mussaenda frondosa.* (*Linn.*) (Rubiaceae)	The leaves extract was tested on wound healing models in rats. *M. frondosa* treated rats displayed Increased wound concentration and tensile strength, augmented hydroxyproline content along with antibacterial activity [25]
12.	*Aristolochia bracteata* (Aristolochiaceae) and *Cassia tora* (Leguminosae)	Wound contracting ability of the extracts was significantly greater than that of the control, which was comparable to that of the reference standard 0.02%w/w nitrofurazone ointment [26]
13.	*Mimosa pudica* (Mimosaceae)	Used in folklore medicine for arresting bleeding and in skin diseases. *M. pudica* has been reported to contain mimosine (an alkaloid), free amino acids, sitosterol, linoleic acid and oleic acid. The wound healing studies on roots indicated that phenols constituents/tannins play an important role in wound healing process. The result of excision wound model is indicating that significant increase in wound contraction compared with standard group, revealing that the extract has ability to induce cellular proliferation. The increase in tensile strength of wounded skin indicates the promotion of collagen fibers [27]
14.	*Anthocephalus Cadamba* (Rubiaceae)	The potent wound healing capacity was shown from the wound contraction and increased tensile strength has thus validated the ethno therapeutic claim [28]
15.	*Lantana camara* (*Linn.*) (Verbenaceae)	Showed considerable signs of dermal healing and significantly decrease mean wound healing time and reduced scarring at the wound enclosure [29]
16.	*Carapa guianensis* (Meliaceae)	The ethanolic leaf extract of *C. guianensis* showed increase in the rate of wound contraction, skin breaking strength, the rate of epithelialization [30]
17.	*Curcuma longa* (*Linn.*) (Zingiberaceae)	Curcumin has potent anti-inflammatory and analgesic activities. Volatile oil isolated from *C. longa* also exhibits antibacterial and potent anti-inflammatory activity. *C. longa* also contains protein, fats, vitamins (A, B, C, etc) all of which have an important role

No.	Name	Wound healing activity
		in would healing and regeneration. Turmeric has been used for treating the wounds in the rats. The presence of vitamin A and proteins in turmeric result in the early synthesis of collagen fibers by mimicking fibroblastic activity. Juice of the fresh rhizome is commonly applied to recent wounds, bruises and leech bites [31]
18.	*Tecomaria capensis* (Bignoniaceae)	*T. capensis* significantly stimulated wound contraction. The breaking strength of the treated incision wounds increased in *T. capensis* extract when treated groups compared with the control group [32]
19.	*Hyptis suaveolens* (*Linn.*) (Lamiaceae)	Aqueous, alcoholic and petroleum ether extracts were tested in rats in wound healing models. Petroleum ether extract was found to show enhanced wound healing activity compared to other extracts. Period of epithelialization, granulation strength, hydroxyproline content was found to be increased in petroleum ether extract as compared to other extracts. Histopathological study of this extract too revealed more collagen and macrophages as compared to other extracts [33]
20.	*Arnebia densiflora* (*Ledeb.*) (Boraginaceae)	Rats treated with *A. densiflora* showed rapid healing than the control group. Wound closure and collagen production were faster and healing occurred on the 14th day after wounding [34]
Plants possessing anti-oxidant property contributing to wound healing activity		
21.	*Allium cepa* (Liliaceae)	It contains kampferol, β-sitosterol, ferulic acid, myritic acid, prostaglandins. Flavonoids have been documented which is believed to be one of the most important components of wound healing. The enhanced wound healing in rats when *A. cepa* was administered orally may be due to free radical scavenging action and the antibacterial property of the phytoconstituents present in it [35]
22.	*Ageratum conyzoides* (Asteraceae)	The leaves are applied to the wounds act as septic and heel them quickly. Several Phytoconstituents like alkaloids and saponins are known to promote wound healing process due to their antioxidant anti-microbial activities. The wound healing property of *A. conyzoides* appears to be due to the presence of its active principles, which accelerate the healing process and confers breaking strength to the healed wound [36]
23.	*Heliotropium Indicum* (Boraginaceace)	Various extracts of *H. indicum* were tested in wound healing models in rats. The methanolic and aqueous extracts were shown to be working better than petroleum ether extract. Increase in the granulation tissue weight, hydroxyproline content, and increased activity of superoxide dismutase and catalase level was reported to be contributing factors for better wound healing of *H. indicum* as compared to 0.2% w/w nitrofurazone ointment [37]
Plants reported to improve dexamethasone suppressed wound healing		
24.	*Ocimum sanctum* (*Linn.*) (Labiaceae)	Ethanolic extract of *O. sanctum* significantly decreased the anti-healing effect of dexamethasone in all wound models like incision, excision and dead space wound model. It was reported that the plant has various actions like free radical scavenging effect, metal chelation and immune modulation [38]

No.	Name	Wound healing activity
25.	*Gossypium herbaceum* (*Linn.*) (Malvaceae)	Ethanol and ethyl ether fractions of *G. herbaceum* were tested in wound models to test the effect of the plant on diabetes and dexamethasone delayed wounds. The plant displayed significant increased wound contraction, breaking strength and decreased epithelization period. Hydroxyproline and collagen content was increased [39]
26.	*Ficus hispida* (*Linn.*) (Moraceae)	Ethanolic extract of roots of *F. hispida* was investigated in normal and dexamethasone depressed healing conditions, using incision, excision and dead space wound models in albino rats. Collagen and hydroxyproline content was increased thus proving the pro-healing effect of the plant [40]
27.	*Pyrus communis* (Rosaceae)	Ethanol and ethyl acetate extracts of *P. communis* were tested in dexamethasone delayed wound healing model in rats. The study reported that plant treated wounds displayed fast healing of infectious wound, in immunosuppressed and disease condition like diabetes [41]
28.	*Tetrapleura tetraptera* (Mimosaceae)	The stem bark aqueous extract was studied for effect on dexamethasone delayed wounds in excision and incision wound models in rats. The authors reported excellent potential of the plant related to epithelialization, contraction and tensile strength improvement [42]
Plant reported to display interaction with dexamethasone and further delay wound healing (drug–herb interaction)		
29.	*Alafia multiflora* (*Stapf.*) (*Apocynaceae*)	The study on *A. multiflora* highlights the drug-herb interaction. Aqueous extract of the plant was studied for its effect on normal and dexamethasone delayed wounds in rats utilizing excision and incision wound models. It showed beneficial effects in normal rats. But in dexamethasone delayed wounds, the plant extract further deteriorated the wound healing. This proved the known interaction between retinoids occurring in the plant and the steroid but also indicated at involvement of some other constituent contributing to the delayed wound healing [43]
Plants with interactions with conventional therapies and reported side effects		
30.	*Echinacea* species (*Echinacea purpurea, Echinacea pallida, Echinacea angustifolia*) (Asteraceae)	Risk of poor wound healing in chronic users [44]
31.	Vitamin A (Retinoic acid)	Interaction with steroids to further delay wound healing [45]
32.	Bromelain (Protein extract from pineapple, *Ananas sativus*)	Can improve wound healing but carries risk of bleeding. Recommended to stop its usage 2 weeks before surgery [46]
33.	Vitamin E	Can improve wound healing owing to its antioxidant property but carries risk of bleeding. Recommended to stop its usage 2 weeks before surgery [47]
34.	Grape seed extract	Possesses antioxidant activity owing to the presence of active proanthocyanidin content. Proanthocyanidin is a bioflavonoid that acts as a strong antioxidant, protecting DNA from harmful free radicals. Additionally, grape seed extract has been

No.	Name	Wound healing activity
		reported to reduce inflammation, stabilize collagen and elastin, act as a natural antihistamine, and protect and heal connective tissue. It seems safe overall with no studies pertaining to its interactions were found to be reported. Seems safe overall [48]

Table 1. Ayurvedic plants with reported wound healing activity.

2.2. Siddha medicines

Siddha is the traditional system of medicine practiced in Tamilnadu, South India, and Tamil speaking areas of the world. The Siddhars' (founders of Siddha medicine) used lots of herbs to treat cardiac and respiratory conditions, heal wounds, treat snake and scorpion bites, dreaded diseases like cancer, and documented them in the form of palm leaf manuscripts, stone, and copper scriptures, etc. The claim of the Siddha physicians is that the medicinal plants are commonly identifiable, easily available throughout the year, cost effective, and with lesser adverse effects [49]. The Siddha system of medicine aims at offering complete cure to mind and body. It follows the principle of "Food as medicine" [50]. The Siddhars have documented many oils (*Tailam*) and ointments (*Kalimbu*) effective in wound healing. There are few plants mentioned in Siddha system of traditional medicine which have been evaluated preclinically for their wound healing activity.

Few noteworthy studies using Siddha medicines are mentioned below.

2.2.1. Siddha polyherbal oils

Siddha medicine has used *Kayathirumeniennai, punguthailam, and mathanthailam* as polyherbal (medicated oils) since centuries, but recently, Sabarianandh *et al.* in 2014 made efforts to scientifically validate the use of these oils on experimentally induced burn wounds in Wistar rats. The study showed wound contraction was significantly decreased; epithelialization was increased as compared to the vehicle treated group. This was even confirmed by the histopathological analysis [51].

2.2.2. Heritage Sanjeevi

Pugalendhi *et al.* demonstrated the effect of Heritage *Sanjeevi* (a Siddha combination drug) on wound healing in Wistar rats. "Heritage *Sanjeevi*" is a medication made up of *Curcuma Aromatia, Psoralea Corylifolia, Vernonia Anthemintica* (*Willd.*), *Hydnicarpus Laurifolia, Elettaria Cadamomum*, coconut milk, mercury, sulphur, hydrogyrum schloride calomel, "Sulphie" of lead, copper sulphate, zinc sulphate, and camphor. The mixtures of these compounds were processed in the manner that all the inorganic material is detoxified using an ancient detoxin called *Pooneer*. The extracted oil is filtered and stored in glassware. It is used for external application only, and its shelf life is six years, and it has been claimed to have excellent healing property against burns, scalds, chemical burns, acid burns, and radiation burns. The medication was tested on Wistar rats by external application till the time the wound which was created using a punch was completely healed. The study results demonstrated significant reduction in the size of the wound. The authors claimed that wound healing can be credited to one or few constituents of the medication causing collagen production and thus helping in faster wound correction [52].

2.2.3. *Siddha Kalimbu*

Another study revealed the wound healing ability of a polyherbal Siddha formulation, *Siddha kalimbu* consisting of 10 gm each of *Ficus spp* (*Itthi*), *Adenanthera Pavonina* (*Manjeti*), sandalwood (*Santhanam*), jasmine (*malligai*), *Symplocos racemosa* (*Roxb.*) (*Vellilothram*), *Ficus hispida* (*Atthi*), *Alstonia scholaris* (*Satvin*), and dried roots of 12.5 gm of *Curcuma longa* (*Manjal*) when mixed with 60 ml of Eal oil (muscle relaxant drug), 10 ml neem oil (*Azadirachta indica*), 20 ml of coconut oil, and 10 ml *Millettia pinnata* (*Pungai*) oil. The formulation was tested on excision and incision wound models in rats, and it was reported that the Siddha treatment significantly healed the wound by synthesizing collagen and influencing the growth hormone. The topical application of the formulation increased the wound breaking strength, wound contraction, and period of epithelialization [53].

2.2.4. *Polyherbal formulation*

Krishnamoorty *et al.* in 2012 reported an *in vitro* study of a polyherbal formulation comprising of extracts of *Wrightia tinctoria*, *Aloe vera*, *Curcuma longa*, and *Terminalia chebula*. They studied the impact of the formulation on fibroblast cell migration and proliferation using scratch wound assay technique. Fibroblast cell migration and proliferation were studied employing cell migration assay. Carbomer-based gel with beeswax made for a novel delivery system and the formulation proved significantly effective in management of superficial wounds and first degree burns [54].

2.2.5. *Kungiliya vennai and Kalchunna thailam*

Vennai (*Butter*) *and thailam* (*Balm*) are mentioned and used in Siddha medicine as wound healing bases. *Kungiliya vennai* is herbal formulation containing *Shorea robusta*, *Sesamum indicum*, and *Cocos nucifera*. It is traditionally recommended by Siddha practitioners for wound healing. *Kalchunna thailam* finds a mention in Siddha medicine for wound healing and is a preparation of limestone and coconut oil mixed in equal proportions. In an excision wound model in Sprague Dawley rats, the *Kungiliya vennai and Kalchunna thailam* treated rats showed positive outcome in the wound healing process. The preparations were comparable with the standard 2% Mupirocin ointment. The authors reported *Kungiliya vennai* has additional property of regenerating adnexal structures such as hair follicles, sweat, and sebaceous glands [55].

Few more Siddha plants which were preclinically evaluated for wound healing activity are mentioned below (**Table 2**).

http://dx.doi.org/10.5772/63636

No.	Plant name	Wound healing activity
1.	Banyan tree (*Ficus benghalensis*)	Ethanolic and aqueous extracts of *F. benghalensis* were evaluated in excision and incision wound models. Both extracts exhibited significant wound-healing activity, which was proven by decrease in the period of epithelialization, an increase in the rate of wound contraction and skin-breaking strength. Proteoglycans and glucosaminoglycans have been shown to play important roles in wound healing [56]
2.	Common wireweed (*Sida acuta*)	Was studied respectively on two types of wound models in rats, (i) the excision and (ii) the incision wound model. Wound contracting ability of the *S. acuta* ointment (5% w/w) significantly greater than that of the control nitrofurazone ointment (0.2% w/w) which was employed as standard comparator drug [57]
3.	Barmuda grass (*Cynodon dactylon*)	Flavanoid fraction of *C. dactylon* in Swiss albino mice demonstarted the wound healing activity, when it was applied externally daily on excised wound area for 8 days [58]
4.	Country fig (*Ficus racemosa*)	Aqueous and ethanolic extract of roots of *F. racemosa* in Wistar albino rats showed significant increase in percentage closure by enhanced epithelialization. The effect can be linked to enhanced collagen synthesis. Results showed the herb hastened the wound healing process by decreasing the surface area of the wound [59]
5.	Purging nut (*Jatropha curcas*)	Bark extract showed significant wound healing activity in albino rats. It accelerated the healing process by increasing the skin breaking strength, wound contraction, dry granulation tissue weight, and hydroxyproline levels. Epithelization period was also significantly decreased [60]
6.	Maasikkai (*Quercus infectoria*)	Ethanol extract of the shade-dried leaves of was studied in rats and it showed a positive effect on wound healing, with a significant increase in the levels of the antioxidant enzymes, superoxide dismutase and catalase, in the granuloma tissue [61]
7.	Pomegranate (*Punica granatum*)	Ethanolic extract on Wistar rat showed significant the wound healing activity. It significantly increased the rate of wound contraction and collagen turnover [62]
8.	Red silk cotton (*Bombax malabaricum*)	Alcoholic Bark extract resulted in a significant decline in the wound in rats. When compared with standard drug, nitrofurazone, it was found superior in terms of wound contracting ability, wound closure time, and tensile strength [63]
9.	Rhus olina (*Lannea coromandelica*)	Ethanol and acetone extracts of barks were applied to male Wistar rats in the form of simple ointments exhibited wound healing activity in excision and incision methods. Framycetin sulphate was taken as standard control. It displayed potent wound healing activity in terms of significant wound contraction and increased tensile strength [64]
10.	Plantain tree (*Musa paradisiaca*)	The extract of *M. Paradisia*ca holds substantial wound healing activity in rat models [65]
11.	Kino tree (*Pterocarpus marsupium*)	The effect of heart wood extract of *P. marsupium* on wound healing has been studied in diabetic and normal animals. The effect has also been compared with standard (mupirocin ointment) application. The results show that application of heart wood extract significantly increased wound healing in both normal and diabetic animals [66]

Table 2. Siddha herbs with reported wound healing activity.

2.3. Unani medicines

Unani system of medicine has its origin in Iran and also has documented evidences of antimicrobial herbs possessing wound healing properties. Like Siddha, Unani system too has a mention of cow's ghee (*Roghan-e-gao*), *Shorea robusta*, etc. Following are examples of wound healing plants or medicines (*marham*) according to Unani system of medicine.

2.3.1. Iranian wound healing plants

Pirbalouti *et al.* reported the wound healing properties of five traditional Iranian plants on alloxan-induced diabetic wounds in rats. Wound area, epithelialization time, and histopathological characteristics were studied upon treatment with *Malva sylvestris, Punica granatum, Amygdalus communis, Arnebia euchroma, and Scrophularia deserti*. The results corroborated the traditional wound healing use of the above plants [67].

2.3.2. Marham-e-Ral

Similarly, a study described the wound healing effect of a Unani formulation *Marham-e-Ral* in rats. Ingredients of this formulation are *Shorea robusta Gaertn* (*Ral*), Camphor (*Kafoor*), Catechu (*Katha*), *Roghan-e-Gao*, and Beeswax. *Marham-e-Ral* was administered topically once a day till complete epithelialization occurred. Wound contraction and epithelialization were measured. Both excision and incision wound models were developed. Rate of wound contraction was significantly enhanced so was the epithelialization period. The plant extracts have revealed presence of flavonoids, triterpenoids, and tannins which are known to contribute to wound healing. They also possess astringent, antimicrobial and antiinflammatory effects. Based on their study, the authors claimed the prohealing stroke *Marham-e-Ral* possesses [68].

2.3.3. Aloe (Elva)

Aloe is one of the oldest plants documented across the globe and also features in Unani system of medicine where it is called as *'Elva'*. Oryan *et al.* [69] reported the detailed account of wound healing activity of *A. vera* in rats. They demonstrated that the wound healing was 50% faster with aqueous extract of *A. vera* as compared to silver sulfadiazine in case of open wounds.

2.3.4. Golnar-e-farsi

Punica granatum (*Linn.*), known as *Golnar-e-farsi* in Iran, popularly known as pomegranate flowers and *Achillea kellalensis* (*Bioss.*) and *Hausskn* a well known traditional herb used in tribal medicine of Iran is locally known as *Golberrenjas or Bumadaran-e-Sabzekoh* were studied scientifically by Pirbalouti *et al.* in 2010. The authors reported their significant wound healing properties in rat excision wound model owing to their increased wound contraction ability and collagen turnover [70].

2.3.5. *Shorea robusta*

Shorea robusta finds a mention in both Siddha and Unani systems of medicine. A study carried out by Wani *et al.* in 2011 reported the wound healing property of *S. robusta Gaertn. f.* in excisional and incisional wound models in rats. The ethanolic extract was found to accelerate wound contraction, increased tensile strength, and hydroxyproline content thus acting as a wound healer [71].

2.4. Chinese herbs

As are Ayurveda and Siddha to India and Unani to Iran, traditional Chinese system of medicine has been practiced for ages in China. Traditional Chinese Medicine (TCM) focuses on the concept of Yin and Yang which describes two opposing yet complementary aspects of any one phenomenon. Yin is associated with poor circulation and healing and stagnation, while Yang is related with being overheated and excess of scar tissue. Thus for optimum wound healing, an ideal balance needs to be struck between Yin and Yang. Raw Chinese formulas are created specific to each patient. A raw formula means simply that the herbs in the formula are in their natural state without modification. Traditionally, raw Chinese formulas are given in their organic form, cooked for several hours, and then ingested, but it tends to have an undesirable taste. However, with wound healing, a topical application is convenient, effective, and has no or less side effects. Herbs can be utilized in their natural state and with their maximum potency. Few of the examples of wound healer herbs of TCM are as follows:

1. Tam *et al.* [72] were the first to report a combination of *Radix astragali* and *Radix rehmanniae* in the ratio of 2:1 for the treatment of diabetic foot wounds. The herb combination showed its effectiveness in treating diabetic wound healing through the actions of tissue regeneration, angiogenesis and anti-inflammation.

2. *Angelica sinensis* (AS) called as *Dang-Gui* in Chinese, was analysed in detail by Hsiao *et al.* [73] using proteomics to demonstrate range of pharmacological effects associated with AS which will prove fruitful in developing it as a wound healing herb. The authors concluded that AS extract and its active component ferulic acid (FA) participate in the modulation of wound healing process associated with fibroblasts. FA specifically acts as a ROS scavenger. Additionally, FA is also able to trigger proteins like heme oxygenase-1 (HO-1), heat shock protein 70 (HSP70), Extracellular signal-regulated kinases (ERK ½), and Protein kinase B (Akt), which help cells to respond to environmental stress thus contributing to its enhanced wound healing ability.

3. Hou *et al.* [74] recently demonstrated the wound healing property of a four-herb Chinese medicine ANBP which is a pulverized mixture of four herbs including *Agrimonia eupatoria* (A), *Nelumbo nucifera Gaertn* (N), *Boswellia carteri* (B), and *Pollen Typhae Angustifoliae* (P) explored the effect of four-herb Chinese medicine ANBP. The herb was evaluated on the basis of wound healing and scar formation in rabbit ear hypertrophic scar models of full-thickness skin defect. Compared with the control group, local ANBP treatment not only significantly improved wound healing, but also reduced scar formation. The study results demonstrated that ANBP treatment along with reducing collagen synthesis, blocked

excessive deposition of collagen and also promoted collagen maturity, thus obstructing the formation of scar. The mechanism of the effect of ANBP on collagen expression is different in the early and late stages of wound healing, which is favourable for wound closure and scar contraction. Using proteomics approach, the authors suggested that ANBP promoted wound healing and condensed scarring by bidirectional regulation of the Transforming Growth Factor β (TGF- β)-/Smad-dependent pathway.

4. Chinese medicine book, Compendium of Materia Medica proclaims *Lucilia sericata* known as *'WuGuChong'* in Chinese for treating superficial purulent diseases like carbuncle. Zhang *et al.* reported that fatty acid extracts of *Lucilia sericata* can promote murine cutaneous wound healing by virtue of its remarkable angiogenic activity. Wound excision model in rats followed by Vascular Endothelial Growth factor (VEGF) expression analysis by western blotting, RT-PCR and immunohistochemistry strongly suggested the mechanism involved in wound healing property of the herb [75].

5. Chak *et al.* [76] demonstrated the effect of another Chinese medicine *Shiunko* consisting of sesame oil, *Lithospermi radix*, (*LR; Lithospermum erythrorhizon Sieb. et Zucc.*), *A. sinensis*, lard, and beeswax. The authors reported that *Shiunko*-treated fibroblasts induced range of biochemical events engaged in the wound healing process, including cell proliferation and anti-apoptosis, anti-oxidant activity, secretion of collagen, and cell mobility. It was also noted that Stathmin, a differentiation marker was greatly induced by *Shiunko*, which is a sign of good healing process. Proteomics suggested peroxiredoxin and glutathione S-transferase were involved in antioxidantion offered by *Shiunko*. Also, superoxide dismutase was enhanced after *Shiunko* treatment which again contributed to its wound healing property. TGF-β was upregulated on *Shiunko* treatment which happens to be upstream regulator of collagen expression and an indispensable factor for wound healing.

6. *Terminalia chebula* is mentioned in other systems of medicine like Ayurveda for its wound healing ability. Likewise, it was proven by Li *et al.* [77] that tannin extracts from immature *Terminalia chebula* fruits helps in cutaneous wound healing in rats. The immunohistochemical, transcriptional and translational levels of VEGF analysed in the study helped the authors conclude that the wound healing property was by the virtue of anti-angiogenic effects. Also, the proliferation of bacteria like *Staphylococcus aureaus* and *Klebsiella pneumonia* were inhibited by the extract thus conferring the much needed antibacterial effect beneficial for faster wound healing. Thus the study concluded that tannin extracts from immature fruits of *Terminalia chebula Fructus* (*Retz.*) stimulated cutaneous wound healing in rats.

2.5. Ozone therapy

Ozone therapy dates back to the year 1914 when it was used during World War I for the treatment of gas gangrene. Ozone has multiple therapeutic effects in wound healing due to the property of releasing nascent oxygen, which has been shown to have bactericidal capabilities and to stimulate antioxidant enzymes. There are few randomized clinical trials to verify the use of ozone therapy in the early stages of wound healing. To verify the same, Zhang *et al.* [78] recently carried out a study assessing the use of ozone therapy in the early stages of diabetic foot ulcer by estimating the expression of VEGF, TGF-β, and Platelet derived growth factor (PDGF). The authors claimed that the oxygen-ozone therapy increased the levels of all the above three endogenous growth factors which contributed to its enhanced wound healing ability. Similarly, Wainstain *et al.* [79] demonstarted that oxygen–ozone therapy along with conventional therapy for 24 weeks hastened the healing of diabetic foot ulcer. The theory that ozonated oil has wound healing property was investigated at our laboratory in an excision wound model using Sprague Dawley rats. The animals were divided into four groups, which were treated with sesame oil (vehicle), framycetin (standard), or two doses of ozonated sesame oil (peroxide values 500 and 700 mEq/1000 g, respectively). The formulations were topically applied on the excision wounds once daily for 11 consecutive days, and the animals were euthanized on the 12th day. Ozonated oil treated wounds had significantly higher tensile strength, collagen content, and superoxide dismutase activity than that of the vehicle treated wounds. Histopathological analysis of skin of the excised wound area treated with ozonated oil revealed better healing activity in comparison with the vehicle-treated wounds. Thus it was concluded that ozonated oil can be of potential remedial use for healing wounds [80]. Another animal study was carried out by Kim *et al.* [81] to evaluate the therapeutic effects of ozonated olive oil in guinea pigs in acute cutaneous wound healing model. Full thickness punch wound was created on the back of guinea pigs and ozonated olive oil treatment was compared with pure olive oil and no treatment control group. The immunohistopathological results demonstrated that topical application of ozonated olive oil increased the levels of VEGF, TGF-β, and PDGF thus accelerating acute cutaneous wound healing. A study conducted by Travagli *et al.* [82] reported a deleterious effect of ozone treatment on aged mice. The authors claimed that ozone therapy in 8-week mice enhanced wound healing, while when administered to 18-week mice, the full thickness excisional wound displayed delayed healing. This may also be attributed to reduced bacterial infection and/or increased O_2 tension by O_3 contact in wound area in younger population.

3. Clinical studies supporting the folklore use of alternative therapies

Scientists advocate more clinical studies to be conducted to provide robust proof-of-concept of folklore wound healing property of the herbs mentioned in alternative therapies. Few of the clinical studies carried out are documented subsequently.

3.1. Ayurveda-based clinical studies

3.1.1. Katupila study

A case study of diabetic wound of a 55-year-old female patient wherein *Katupila* paste [(*Securinega leucopyrus*) (*Willd.*)] was applied daily and after a month the wound was reported to have healed completely leaving a minimal scar. The healing properties of *Katupila* were attributed to its antimicrobial, antiseptic, and wormicidal qualities. Also it was shown to possess abundant quantities of flavonoids and tannins which offer the antioxidant effects [13].

3.1.2. Manjishthadi Gritha

A clinical study employing *Manjishthadi Gritha* was carried out by Baria *et al*. The *Gritha* was prepared using seven herbs namely, *Manjishtha* (*R. cordifolia Linn.*), *Daruharidra* (*B. aristata DC.*), *Mocharasa* (*Salmalia malabaricum*), *Dhatakipushpa* (*Woodfordia fruticosa* (*Linn.*) *Kurz.*), *madhuka* (*Madhuca indica J. F. Gmel*), *Lodhra* (*Symplocos racemosa Roxb.*) *and Rasanjana* (*Extractum berberis*). The *Gritha* was applied topically on wounds mostly from anorectal cases twice a day for 21 days. The observation period of 1 month recorded the results of the study. Out of 45 patients, 24 were treated with the *Gritha* and 21 with povidone iodine ointment. The *Gritha*-treated patients showed better wound healing, no left-over scar, no excess pigmentation, and absence of adverse effects. The authors reported *Manjishthadi Gritha* as an economical and effective wound healing combination [83].

3.1.3. Honey: A pilot study

Vijaya *et al.* [84] reported a pilot study using honey for healing the cutaneous wounds of 10 randomly selected patients of both sexes. Honey collected locally was applied daily for 20 days and the size of the wound was measured on day 7, 15, 20, and after complete wound healing. The authors concluded that honey was remarkable in healing the wounds and can be very effectively used as first aid dressing material. A case study [85] was reported employing honey for the cure of a chronic infected wound on the right lower limb of a 70-year-old female. Every morning the wound was cleaned with neem bark decoction, and Dabur® honey was applied on the wound. Along with the local application, following drugs were administered orally every 12 hours: *Glycerrhiza glabra* (*Linn.*), *Asparagus racemosus* (*Willd.*), *Tribulus terrestris*, *Tinispora cordifolia* (*Willd*). At the end of fifth week, the authors reported a complete healing of the wound leaving a minimal scar. Sushruta Samhita has mentioned *honey* (*madhu*) as a wound healer centuries ago. The above case study practically proved the effectiveness of honey. It is hyperosmolar so confers antibacterial effect. It has high viscosity so acts as physical barrier. Presence of enzyme catalase in honey gives it antioxidant properties. The four drugs given orally possess antioxidant, adaptogenic, and immunomodulatory activities. Clinical studies employing honey with bigger population although would yield more authentic conclusions.

3.2. Unani medicine-based study

3.2.1. Dragon's blood cream

Namjoyan *et al.* [86] reported a clinical study using Dragon's blood cream, a deep red resin obtained from four different sources, *Croton spp.*, *Dracaena spp.*, *Daemonorops spp.*, and *Pterocarpus spp.* 60 patients referred to remove their skin tags were included in this randomized clinical trial to receive either Dragon's blood cream or placebo cream. Wound measurement and process of healing was checked on 3rd, 5th, 7th, 10th, 14th, and 20th day of the trial. The patients receiving Dragon's blood cream showed significant wound healing. The phenolic compounds present in Dragon's blood cream reportedly contribute to its effective wound healing property.

3.3. Clinical study on ozone therapy

3.3.1. *Adjuvant ozone therapy*

Shah *et al.* [87] presented a case study of a 59-year-old female patient with an extensively infected wound and exposed tibia to about $^{4}/_{5}$th of its extent. Topical ozone therapy twice a day and ozone hemotherapy once a day along with daily dressings and parenteral antibiotics showed significant improvement in 15 days in the patient. After a follow-up of 20 months, the patient was able to walk with minimal disability. Ozone disintegrates into reactive oxygen species which further lead to increased growth factors contributing to faster wound healing. The study stated that oxidative injury is a possible side effect of ozone therapy but at therapeutic doses oxygen radicals are removed by the blood antioxidants and thus side effects are rare and only observed in overdose or compromised anti-oxidant system.

4. Conclusion

The folklore knowledge is abundant with mention of various herbs and medicines as wound healers across different civilizations and systems of medicines. Modern medicine is fast attempting to explore the ancestral data and test its effectiveness using current experimental methods. The focus is on analyzing the molecular basis of the effectiveness of the concerned plants. Proteomic and genomic-based evidences using robust markers blended with traditional knowledge can provide relevant answers and solutions for healing of wounds which affect the largest organ of human body. Although more randomized clinical trials are the need of the day to validate the ancient claims.

Author details

Anuradha Majumdar* and Prajakta Sangole

*Address all correspondence to: anuradha.majumdar@bcp.edu.in

Department of Pharmacology, Bombay College of Pharmacy, Kalina, Mumbai, India

References

[1] Robson MC, Steed DL and Franz MG. Wound healing: biologic features and approaches to maximize healing trajectories. Curr Probl Surg 2001; 38: 72–140. doi:10.1067/j.cpsurg.2008.10.004.

[2] Robson MC, Steed DL and Franz MG. The management of complex orthopaedic injuries. Surg Clin North Am 1996; 76: 879–903. doi:10.1016/S0039-6109(05)70486-2.

[3] Vanwijck R. Surgical biology of wound healing. Bull Mem Acad R Med Belg 2001; 115: 175–84. PMID: 11789398.

[4] Degreef H. How to heal a wound fast. Dermatol Clin 1998; 16 (2): 365-375. doi:10.1016/S0733-8635(05)70019-X.

[5] Attinger CE, Janis JE, Steinberg J, *et al.* Clinical approach to wounds: debridement and wound bed preparation including the use of dressings and wound-healing adjuvants. Plast Reconstr Surg 2006; 117(7 suppl): 72S–109S. doi:10.1097/01.prs.0000225470.42514.8f.

[6] Broughton G 2nd, Janis JE, Attinger CE, *et al.* Wound healing: an overview. Plast Reconstr Surg 2006; 117(7 suppl):1e–S–32e–S. doi:10.1097/01.prs.0000222562.60260.f9.

[7] Hunt TK, Hopf H, Hussain Z, *et al.* Physiology of wound healing. Adv Ski Wound Care 2000; 13: 6–11. PMID: 11110286.

[8] General Guidelines for Methodologies on Research and Evaluation of Traditional Medicine. WHO/EDM/TRM/2000.1: 1–71.

[9] Santhosh Aruna M, Shravanthi V, Jhansi Sri U, *et al.* An Overview of herbs possessing wound healing activity. Eur J Pharm Med Res 2015; 2(7): 329–332.

[10] Haritha Yadav K, Ravi Kumar J, Ilias Basha S, *et al* Wound healing activity of topical application of *aloe Vera* Gel in experimental animal models. Int J Pharma Bio Sci 2012; 3: 63–73.

[11] Mondal S, Dash GK and Bal SK. Anthelmintic activity of *Cleome rutidosperma DC.* roots. Indian Drugs 2009; 46: 47–49.

[12] Gangopadhyay KS, Khan M, Pandit S, *et al.* Pharmacological evaluation and chemical standardization of an ayurvedic formulation for wound healing activity. Int J Low Extrem Wounds 2014; 13: 41–49. doi:10.1177/1534734614520705.

[13] Dudhamal T, Gupta S, Mahanta V, *et al. Katupila Securinega leucopyrus* as a potential option for diabetic wound management. J Ayurveda Integr Med 2014; 5: 60. doi: 10.4103/0975-9476.128872.

[14] Rawat S and Gupta A. Development and study of wound healing activity of an ayurvedic formulation. Asian J Res Pharm Sci 2011; 1 : 26–28. ISSN: 2231-5659.

[15] Gupta N and Jain UK. Investigation of Wound Healing Activity of Methanolic Extract of Stem Bark of Mimusops Elengi Linn. Afr J Tradit Complement Altern Med. 2011; 8(2): 98–103.

[16] Azarkan M, El Moussaoui A, Van Wuytswinkel D, *et al.* Fractionation and purification of the enzymes stored in the latex of *Carica papaya*. J Chromatogr B Anal Technol Biomed Life Sci 2003; 790: 229–238. doi:10.1016/S1570-0232(03)00084-9.

[17] Deshpande SS, Shah GB and Parmar NS. Antiulcer activity of *Tephrosia purpurea* in rats. Ind J Pharmacol 2000; 35: 168–172.

[18] Subhashini S and Arunachalam K. Investigations on the phytochemical activities and wound healing properties of *Adhatoda vasica* leave in Swiss albino mice. Afr J Plant Sci 2011;5: 133–145.

[19] Verma A, Kumar N and Ranade SA. Genetic diversity amongst landraces of a dioecious vegetatively propagated plant, betelvine (*Piper betle L.*). J Biosci 2004; 29: 319–328. doi: 10.1007/BF02702614.

[20] Rathi BS, Bodhankar SL and Baheti AM. Evaluation of aqueous leaves extract of *Moringa oleifera Linn* for wound healing in albino rats. Indian J Exp Biol 2006; 44: 898–901.

[21] Hukkeri VT, Kardi RV, Akki KS, *et al.* Wound healing property of *Eucalyptus globulus* leaf extract. Indian Drugs 2002; 39: 481–483.

[22] Singh D, Singh D, Choi SM, *et al.* Effect of extracts of *Terminalia chebula* on Proliferation of Keratinocytes and Fibroblasts Cells: an Alternative Approach for Wound Healing. Evid Based Complement Alternat Med 2014; 2014: 1–13. doi:http://dx.doi.org/10.1155/2014/701656.

[23] Jaswanth A, Loganathan V, Manimaran S, *et al.* Wound healing activity of *Aegle marmelos*. Ind J Pharm Sci 2001;63: 41–44.

[24] Jalalpure S, Agrawal N, Patil M, *et al.* Antimicrobial and wound healing activities of leaves of *Alternanthera sessilis Linn*. Int J Green Pharm 2008; 2: 141. doi: 10.4103/0973-8258.42729.

[25] Patil SA, Joshi VG, Sutar PS, *et al.* Screening of alcoholic extract of *Mussaenda frondosa* leaf for wound-healing and antibacterial activities in albino rats. Pharmacologyonline 2010; 2: 761–773.

[26] Jayasutha A and Nithila SMJ. Evaluation of wound healing activity of Ethanolic extract of *Aristolochia bracteata* and *Cassia tora* on wistar Albino rats. Int J Pharmtech Res 2011; 3: 1547–1550.

[27] Pawaskar SM and Kale KU. Antibacterial activity of successive extracts of *Mimosa pudica*. Ind Drugs 2006; 43: 476–480.

[28] Sanjay PU, Kumar GS, Jayaveera KN, *et al.* Antimicrobial, wound healing and antioxidant activities of *Anthocephalus cadamba*. African J Tradit Complement Alternat Med 2007; 4: 481–487. doi:10.1089/ast.2006.0095.

[29] Nayak BS, Raju SS and Ramsubhag A. Investigation of wound healing activity of *Lantana camara L.* in Sprague Dawley rats using a burn wound model. Int J Appl Res Nat Prod 2008; 1: 15–19.

[30] Nayak BS, Kanhai J, Milne DM, *et al.* Experimental evaluation of ethanolic extract of *Carapa guianensis L.* leaf for its wound healing activity using three wound models. Evid Based Complement Alternat Med 2011; 2011. Article ID 419612: 1–6. doi:10.1093/ecam/nep160.

[31] Mehra KS, Mikuni I, Gupta U, *et al. Curcuma longa* (*Linn*) drops in corneal wound healing. Tokai J Exp Clin Med 1984; 9: 27–31.

[32] Saini N, Singhal M and Srivastava B. Evaluation of wound healing activity of *Tecomaria capensis* leaves. Chin J Nat Med 2012; 10(1 suppl): 138–141. doi:10.3724/SP.J.1009.2012.00138.

[33] Shenoy C, Patil MB, Kumar R., *et al.* Wound Healing Activity of *Hyptis suaveolens* (*L.*) *Poit* (Lamiaceae). Int J Pharm Tech Res 2009; 1: 737–744. ISSN: 0974-4304

[34] Kosger HH, Ozturk M, Sokmen A, *et al.* Wound healing effects of *Arnebia densiflora* root extracts on rat palatal mucosa. Eur J Dent 2009; 3: 96–99.

[35] Shenoy C, Patil MB, Kumar R, *et al.* Preliminary phytochemical investigation and wound healing activity of *Allium Cepa linn.* (Liliaceae). Int J Pharm Sci 2009; 2: 167–175.

[36] Jain S, Jain N, Tiwari A, *et al.* Simple evaluation of wound healing activity of polyherbal formulation of roots of *Ageratum conyzoides Linn.* Asian J Res Chem 2009; 2 (2): 135–138. ISSN: 0974–4169.

[37] Reddy JS, Rao PR and Reddy MS. Wound healing effects of *Heliotropium indicum, Plumbago zeylanicum* and *Acalypha indica* in rats. J Ethnopharmacol 2002; 79: 249–251. doi:10.1016/S0378-8741(01)00388-9.

[38] Udupa SL, Shetty S, Udupa AL, *et al.* Effect of *Ocimum sanctum Linn.* on normal and dexamathasone suppressed wound healing. Indian J Exp Biol 2006:49–54.

[39] Velmurugan C, Bhargava A, Vijaya Kumar S, *et al. Gossypium Herbaceum* hasten wound healing in dexamethasone delayed wound healing model in rats. Int J Phytopharm 2013; 4: 152–157.

[40] Murti K, Lambole V, Panchal M Effect of *Ficus hispida L.* on normal and dexamethasone suppressed wound healing. Brazilian J Pharm Sci 2011; 47: 855–860.

[41] Anitha KN, Reddy BS, Velmurugan C, *et al.* Pear fruit velocity of wound healing in dexamethasone delayed wound healing model in rats. Der Pharm Lett 2015; 7: 310–319.

[42] Tsala DE, Habtemariam S, Simplice FH, *et al.* Topically applied *Tetrapleura tetraptera* stem-bark extract promotes healing of excision and incision wounds in rats. J Intercult Ethnopharmacol 2014; 3: 63–67. doi:10.5455/jice.20140129034637.

[43] Tsala DE, Nga N, Joseph MN, *et al.* A dermal wound healing effect of water extract of the stem bark of *Alafia multiflora Stapf.* Phytopharmacology 2013; 4: 114–122.

[44] Barrett B. Medicinal properties of *Echinacea*: a critical review. Phytomedicine 2003; 10: 66–86.

[45] Wicke C, Halliday B, Allen D, *et al.* Effects of steroids and retinoids on wound healing. Arch Surg 2000; 135: 1265–1270. doi:10.1001/archsurg.135.11.1265.

[46] Maurer HR. Bromelain: biochemistry, pharmacology and medical use. Cell Mol Life Sci 2001; 58: 1234–1245.

[47] Miller ER, Pastor-Barriuso R, Dalal D, *et al.* Meta-analysis: high-dosage vitamin E supplementation may increase all-cause mortality. Ann Intern Med 2005; 142 (1): 37–46.

[48] Bagchi D, Bagchi M, Stohs SJ, *et al.* Free radicals and grape seed proanthocyanidin extract: importance in human health and disease prevention. Toxicology 2000; 148: 187–197. doi:S0300483X00002109 [pii].

[49] Merish S, Tamizhamuthu M and Thomas W. Styptic and wound healing properties of siddha medicinal plants – a review. Int J Pharm Bio Sci 2014; 5: 43–49.

[50] Thomas W, Merish S, Tamizhamuthu M. Review of *Alternanthera sessilis* with reference to traditional siddha medicine. Int J Pharmacogn Phytochem Res 2014; 6: 249–254.

[51] Sabarianandh JV, Uma VK, Fernandes DL, *et al.* Wound healing effect of three traditional medicated oils (*Kayathirumeniennai, Punguthailam* and *Mathanthailam*) on experimentally induced burn wounds in Wistar rats . World J Pharm Pharm Sci 2014; 3: 1307–1313.

[52] Pugalendhi V, Panicker TMR, Korath MP, *et al.* Effect of heritage sanjeevi (a siddha combination drug) on wound healing in Wistar rats. JIMSA 2010; 23: 233–234.

[53] Devi M, Kumar B. Evaluation of wound healing activity of polyherbal Siddha formulation. J Pharm Biomed Sci 2011; 5: 6–8.

[54] Krishnamoorthy JR, Sumitira S, Ranjith MS, *et al.* An in vitro study of wound healing effect of a poly-herbal formulations as evidenced by enhanced cell proliferation and cell migration. Egypt Dermatology Online J 2012; 8: 1–7.

[55] Bhat V, Amuthan A, Rosli BBM, *et al.* Effect of *Kungiliya vennai* and *Kalchunna thailam* on excision wound healing in albino Wistar rats. Int J Pharmacol Clin Sci 2015; 4: 52–57. doi:10.5530/ijpcs.4.3.4.

[56] Murti K, Kumar U, Panchal M. Healing promoting potentials of roots of *Ficus benghalensis L.* in albino rats. Asian Pac J Trop Med 2011; 4: 921–924. doi:10.1016/S1995-7645(11)60219-8.

[57] Akilandeswari S, Senthamarai R, Valarmathi R, *et al.* Wound healing activity of *Sida acuta* in rats. Int J Pharm Tech Res 2010; 2: 585–587. ISSN: 0974-4304.

[58] Saroja M, Santhi R and Annapoorani S. Wound healing activity of Flavanoid fraction of *Cynodon dactylon* in Swiss albino Mice. Int Res J Pharm 2012; 3 (2). 230–231.

[59] Murti K and Kumar U. Enhancement of wound healing with roots of *Ficus racemosa L.* in albino rats. Asian Pacific J Trop Med J Trop Med 2012: 276–280. doi:10.1016/S2221-1691(12)60022-7.

[60] Shetty S, Udupa SL, Udupa AL, *et al.* Wound healing activities of Bark Extract of *Jatropha curcas Linn* in albino rats. Saudi Med J 2006; 27: 1473–1476.

[61] Umachigi SP, Jayaveera KN, Ashok Kumar CK, *et al.* Studies on wound healing properties of *Quercus infectoria*. Trop J Pharm Res 2008; 7: 913–919.

[62] Pirbalouti AG, Azizi S, Koohpayeh A, Hamedi B. Wound healing activity of *Malva sylvestris* and *Punica granatum* in alloxan-induced diabetic rats. Acta Pol Pharm 2010; 67: 511–516. PMID: 20210088.

[63] Udaya chandrika P, Girija K, Lakshman K, *et al.* Evalution of wound healing activity of bark of *Bombax malabaricum*. Int J Bio Pharm Res 2010; 1: 50–55.

[64] Sathish R, Ahmed MH, Natarajan K, *et al.* Evaluation of wound healing and antimicrobial activity of *Lannea coromandelica* (*Houtt*) *Merr*. J Pharm Res 2010; 3: 1225–1228.

[65] Goel RK and Sairam K. Anti-ulcer drugs from indigenous sources with emphasis on *Musa sapientum, tamrabhasma, Asparagus racemosus* and *Zingiber officinale*. Indian J Pharmacol 2002; 34: 100–110.

[66] Gupta M, Soni R, Singhal A, *et al.* Evaluation of wound healing potential of *Pterocarpus marsupium* heart wood extract in normal and diabetic rats. Chronicles Young Sci 2012; 3 (1): 42–47. doi:10.4103/2229-5186.94313.

[67] Pirbalouti AG, Azizi S, Koohpayeh A. Healing potential of Iranian traditional medicinal plants on burn wounds in alloxan-induced diabetic rats. Brazilian J Pharmacogn 2012; 22: 397–403. doi:10.1590/S0102-695X2011005000183.

[68] Mokhtar MA, Ahmad MA, Nizami Q, *et al.* Wound healing effect of a unani formulation *Marham-e-Ral*. Int J Adv Pharm Med Bioallied Sci 2014; 2 (1): 20–24.

[69] Oryan A, Naeini AT, Nikahval B, *et al.* Effect of aqueous extract of *Aloe vera* on experimental cutaneous wound healing in rat. Vet Arch 2010; 80: 509–522. ISSN: 0372-5480.

[70] Pirbalouti AG, Koohpayeh A and Karimi I. The wound healing activity of flower extracts of *Punica granatum* and *Achillea kellalensis* in Wistar rats. Acta Pol Pharm Ñ Drug Res 2010; 67: 107–110.

[71] Wani T, Chandrashekara H and Kumar D. Wound healing activity of ethanolic extract of *Shorea robusta Gaertn. f.* resin. Indian J Exp Biol 2012; 50: 277–281. PMID: 22611916

[72] Tam JCW, Lau KM, Liu CL, *et al.* The in vivo and in vitro diabetic wound healing effects of a 2-herb formula and its mechanisms of action. J Ethnopharmacol 2011; 134: 831–838. doi:10.1016/j.jep.2011.01.032.

[73] Hsiao CY, Hung CY, Tsai TH, *et al.* A study of the wound healing mechanism of a Traditional Chinese Medicine, *Angelica sinensis*, using a proteomic approach. Evid Based Complement Alternat Med 2012; 2012. doi:10.1155/2012/467531.

[74] Qian H, Wen-Jun H, Hao-Jie H, *et al.* The four-herb chinese medicine ANBP enhances wound healing and inhibits scar formation via bidirectional regulation of transformation growth factor pathway. PLoS One 2014; 9: 1–15. doi:10.1371/journal.pone.0112274.

[75] Zhang Z, Wang S, Diao Y, *et al.* Fatty acid extracts from *Lucilia sericata* larvae promote murine cutaneous wound healing by angiogenic activity. Lipids Health Dis 2010; 9. doi: 10.1186/1476-511X-9-24.

[76] Chak K-F, Hsiao C-Y and Chen T-Y. A study of the effect of shiunko, a traditional Chinese herbal medicine, on fibroblasts and its implication on wound healing processes. Adv Wound Care 2013; 2: 448–455. doi:10.1089/wound.2012.0368.

[77] Li K, Diao Y, Zhang H, *et al.* Tannin extracts from immature fruits of *Terminalia chebula Fructus Retz*. promote cutaneous wound healing in rats. BMC Complement Alternat Med 2011; 11: 86. doi:10.1186/1472-6882-11-86.

[78] Zhang J, Guan M, Xie C, *et al.* Increased growth factors play a role in wound healing promoted by noninvasive oxygen-ozone therapy in diabetic patients with foot ulcers. Oxid Med Cell Longev 2014; 2014, Article ID 273475: 1–8. doi:10.1155/2014/273475.

[79] Wainstain J, Feldbrin Z, Boaz M, *et al.* Efficacy of ozone-oxygen therapy for the treatment of diabetic foot ulcers. Diabetes Technol Ther 2011; 13: 1255–1260. doi: 10.1089/dia.2011.0018.

[80] Pai SA, Gagangras SA, Kulkarni SS, *et al.* Potential of ozonated sesame oil to augment wound healing in rats. Ind J Pharm Sci 2014; 76: 87–92. PMID: 24799744.

[81] Kim HS, Noh SU, Han YW, *et al.* Therapeutic effects of topical application of ozone on acute cutaneous wound healing. J Korean Med Sci 2009; 24:368–374. doi:10.3346/jkms.2009.24.3.368.

[82] Travagli V, Zanardi I, Valacchi G, *et al.* Ozone and ozonated oils in skin diseases: a review. Mediators Inflamm 2010; 2010. doi:10.1155/2010/610418.

[83] Baria J, Gupta SK and Bhuyan C. Clinical study of *Manjishthadi Ghrita* in *vrana ropana*. Ayu 2011;32:95–9. doi:10.4103/0974-8520.85738.

[84] Vijaya KK and Nishteswar K. Wound healing activity of honey: a pilot study. Ayu 2012; 33: 374–347. doi:10.4103/0974-8520.108827.

[85] Dudhamal TS, Gupta SK and Bhuvan C. Role of honey (madhu) in management of wounds (*Dushta vrana*). Int J Ayur Res 2010; 1: 271–273. doi:10.4103/0974-7788.76793.

[86] Namjoyan F, Kiashi F, Beigom Moosavi Z, *et al*. Efficacy of Dragon's blood cream on wound healing: a randomized, double-blind, placebo-controlled clinical trial. J Tradit Chinese Med Sci 2014. doi:10.1016/j.jtcme.2014.11.029.

[87] Shah P, Shyam AK and Shah S. Adjuvant combined ozone therapy for extensive wound over tibia. Indian J Orthop 2011; 45: 376–379.

Chapter 22

Medicinal Plants and Natural Products with Demonstrated Wound Healing Properties

Christian Agyare, Emelia Oppong Bekoe,
Yaw Duah Boakye, Susanna Oteng Dapaah,
Theresa Appiah and Samuel Oppong Bekoe

Additional information is available at the end of the chapter

http://dx.doi.org/10.5772/63574

Abstract

This section reviews the current literature on medicinal plants including extracts, fractions, isolated compounds and natural products that have been demonstrated to have wound healing properties. Various electronic databases such as PubMed, Science Direct, SciFinder and Google Scholar were employed to search for plants, natural plant constituents and natural products that have been scientifically demonstrated to have wound healing activity using *in vivo* and *in vitro* wound models. Parameters used in the evaluation of an agent with wound healing properties include rate of wound contraction, tensile strength, antioxidant and antimicrobial activities, hydroxyproline content assay and histological investigations including re-epithelization, collagen synthesis, granulation, proliferation and differentiation of fibroblasts and keratinocytes in excision and incision wound model studies. Eighty-five medicinal plants belonging to 45 families, phytoconstituents including phenolics, oils and other substances including honey were identified as potential wound healing agents or possess wound healing properties using various wound healing models.

Keywords: wounds, wound healing, medicinal plants, natural products, incision, excision

1. Introduction

Wounds are physical injuries that result in an opening or break of the skin that causes disturbance in the normal skin anatomy and function. They result in the loss of continuity of epithelium with or without the loss of underlying connective tissue [1, 2]. Wounds that are most difficult to heal include delayed acute wounds and chronic wounds. Current estimates indicate that nearly 6 million people suffer from chronic wounds worldwide [3, 4]. Foot and leg ulcer is a common disorder, and approximately 1% of the European population suffers from such chronic and recurrent ulceration [3, 5]. Non-healing or chronic wounds result in enormous health care expenditures, with the total cost estimated at more than $3 billion *per* year [3, 4]. Wounds such as injuries, cuts, pressure, diabetic, burns, gastric and duodenal ulcers continue to have severe impact on the cost of health care to patients as well as their families, dependents and health care institutions globally with increasing aging population.

Over the last decades, the search for newer and potent agents from nature (plants, marine environment, fungi and other microorganisms) to manage chronic wounds especially, in patients with underlying metabolic disorders has increased immensely. This is mainly due to the high risk of loss of function, loss of mobility, amputations and huge financial cost as well as death in some cases associated with chronic wounds [6, 7]. The situation is also compounded by the increase in the number of non-communicable diseases such as diabetes and ulcers and longer life expectancy in most developed countries where the prevalence and impact of chronic wounds are on the increase [8].

Most chronic wounds are ulcers that are associated with ischemia, diabetes mellitus, venous stasis disease, or pressure. Between 70% and 80% of people living in the developing countries especially in Africa and Asia depend on herbal medicine for their health needs including wounds, infectious and metabolic diseases [5]. For some time now, there have been increased use of herbal and natural products for the management and treatment of various disease conditions among people in the developed countries including the United States, Europe and Japan.

With respect to the use of medicinal plants and natural products for the treatment of various diseases including metabolic and infectious diseases, specific diagnoses using various modern tools and equipment are not normally made but the treatment is based on the signs and symptoms of the diseases with which these products have been used for over a long period of time with successful treatment outcomes.

This section highlights the importance of medicinal plants and natural products as a major source of wound healing agents with the potential to be developed into phytotherapeutic agents to treat and/or manage wounds and their associated complications. This will also provide a starting point for future studies aimed at isolation, purification, and characterization of bioactive compounds present in these plants as well as exploring the underlying pharmacological mechanisms of action and potential niche market of these medicinal plants and natural products.

2. Properties of a good wound healing agent from herbal or natural product

Wound healing agents are agents that can stimulate fibroblast proliferation, induce keratinocytes proliferation and differentiation, increase collagen formation, exhibit antimicrobial, antioxidant and anti-inflammatory properties. In most cases, for an agent from medicinal plants or natural product to be classified as a good wound healing agent, it should possess two or more of the above properties [9, 10].

3. *In vivo* models for assessing wound healing activity

In vivo models include both artificial and tissue models. Artificial models include subcutaneous chamber/sponges and subcutaneous tubes. Tissue models such as excision wounds, incision wounds, superficial wounds, dead space and burn wounds are usually used to determine the degree of re-epithelialization, collagenation, neovascularization and tensile or breaking strength of wounds [11–13]. Models such as rabbit ear chamber, the hamster cheek pouch, the rabbit corneal pocket and the chick chorioallantoic membrane can also be employed to investigate the extent of re-epithelialization, neovascularization and dermal reconstitution [14].

4. *In vitro* models for assessing wound healing activity

In vitro models are generally simple, rapid and involve minimal ethical consideration compared to whole animal work and allow insight into the biochemical and physiological processes induced by the test agent. Many pharmacological agents at different concentrations can be evaluated concurrently without intrinsic heterogenecity associated with *in vivo* models [14]. As regenerative skin is characterized by connective as well as epithelial tissues, both cell types, dermal fibroblasts as well as human fibroblasts (either primary cells or cell lines), should be used for complete assessment of wound healing activity. *In vitro* models are relevant in study of cell-cell and cell-matrix interaction to mimic cell migration during wound healing. *In vitro* models can employ single cell systems, three dimensional systems, multicellular systems or organ cultures in assessing the wound healing properties of wound healing agents or compounds [14, 15].

5. Methods used for pinpointing herbal materials and natural products with wound healing property

Electronic databases such as PubMed, Scifinder® and Google Scholar were used to search medicinal plants that have been evaluated for wound healing. All filtered articles were appraised to determine whether they contain any validated *in vitro* or *in vivo* wound model. Primary search results were independently screened by two investigators. Included articles were reviewed concerning plant botanical names, part of plants used in the respective study and type of plant extracts, active constituents or compounds and wound models used (*in vivo* or *in vitro*) or standardized clinical trials with clearly demonstrated wound healing activity in the models used. Consideration was given to the significant differences between test group and control group with respect to wound contraction, wound tensile strength, period of epithelialization, neovascularization, collagenation, keratinization and fibrosis. In case of clinical studies, the respective design, number of patients, interventions, duration of treatment, and data related to the efficacy and tolerability of the patients to treatment were also monitored.

6. Medicinal plants used in wound care

6.1. Acanthaceae

Justicia flava (Forssk.) Vahl has widespread uses in tropical Africa. It is used in traditional medicine for the treatment of cough, paralysis, fever, epilepsy, convulsion and spasm, and skin infections and disorders. The roots are also used for diarrhea and dysentery [16, 17]. The methanol leaf extract of *J. flava* (7.5% w/w) has been found to reduce wound size significantly ($p < 0.01$) as compared to the untreated wounds in rats excision wound model. The extract also significantly ($p < 0.01$) increased the tensile strength of wounds compared to the untreated wounds. Wound tissues form animals treated with the test extract showed improved angiogenesis, collagenation, and re-epithelialization compared to the untreated wound tissue [16].

Adhatoda vasica L., commonly known as Chue Mue, grows in India. Leaves and stems of the plant have been reported to contain an alkaloid mimosine. Leaves also contain mucilage and root contains tannins. The methanol, chloroform and diethyl ether extract ointment (10% w/w) of *A. vasica* showed significant effect when compared to standard drug in excision wound model [18].

6.2. Amaranthaceae

Achyranthes aspera L., locally known as "Telenge or ambulale," is one of the traditionally used plants in the indigenous health care delivery system for the treatment of various kinds of wounds especially in Ethiopia and India. The leaves of *A. aspera* (2.5%, 5% and 10% w/w) simple ointment when applied topically have been shown to significantly ($p < 0.05$) enhance the rate of wound contraction, breaking strength and epithelization in excision wound model compared to the control. Histological evaluation of *A. aspera*-treated wound tissues revealed well organized epidermal layer, increased number of fibrocytes, improved neovascularization and epithelialization compared to the control group [19]. Barua et al. [20] further reported that 5% ointment of methanol leaf extract of *A. aspera* significantly ($p < 0.05$) increased the wound contraction rate, hydroproline and protein production, vitamin C content as well as elevates antioxidant enzymes such as superoxide dismutase and catalase levels in burn wound bed compared to control. The study via gelatin zymography also revealed an increased expression of matrix metalloproteinases (MMP-2 and 9) and improved granulation tissues, collagen and fibroblast deposition in wound bed of *A. aspera*-treated animals compared to control group in subsequent histological examinations.

Alternanthera sessilis (L.) R. Br. ex DC is a tropical plant which is traditionally used for the treatment of ulcers and cuts and wounds, fevers, ophthalmia, gonorrhea, pruritis, burning sensations, diarrhea, skin diseases, dyspepsia, hemorrhoids, liver and spleen diseases [21]. The oral application of chloroform extract from the leaves of *A. sessilis* at a dose of 200 mg/kg body weight significantly reduced wound area ($p < 0.005$) and increased re-epithelialization ($p < 0.0001$) compared to the untreated wound tissues. Furthermore, in excision wound model, scar area after complete epithelialization ($p < 0.0008$) with increased wound breaking strength ($p < 0.0001$) compared with the untreated wounds in incision wound model [22]. Antibacterial property of the leaves and aerial parts of *A. sessilis* has been reported by [23] and antibacterial activity is an ideal property of good wound healing agent [9].

Pupalia lappacea (L.) Juss is an annual or perennial herb found widespread in the tropics and subtropical regions in Africa and it is used in folklore medicine for treatment of boils, chronic wounds and skin infections [10, 24]. Histological studies of wound tissues treated with extracts revealed appreciable collagenation, re-epithelialization, granular tissue formation and angiogenesis for wounds treated with 2% and 10% (v/w) of ethanol leaf extract creams as well as 1% chloroform extract creams to untreated control wound tissues. The ethanol and chloroform extracts also exhibited high rate of wound closure [25]. However, Udegbunam et al. [26] also reported that higher concentrations (10% and 20% (w/v) ointment of methanol leaf extract of *P. lappacea*) significantly ($p < 0.05$) accelerated wound healing, thereby the 20% ointment having the highest percentage wound contraction and rate of epithelialization. The extract also exhibited antimicrobial activity with MIC of 3.0–9.0 mg/mL and MBC of 7–10 mg/mL against *Pseudomonas aeruginosa, Staphylococcus aureus* and *Bacillus subtilis.*

6.3. Anacardiaceae

Buchanania lanzan Spreng, commonly known as char, achar and chironji, is an evergreen tree commonly found in the dry deciduous tropical forests of India and it is used to treat cough, constipation, skin disorders and stomach disorders [27]. Topical application of methanol root extract of *B. lanzan* (10% (w/w) ointment) significantly ($p < 0.05$) increased the tensile strength in the incision wound model. *B. lanzan* also showed significant wound healing activity in excision wound model [28]. However, a study conducted by Chitra et al. [29] showed that the methanol fruit extract of *B. lanzan* did not significantly ($p > 0.05$) promote wound healing when compared to the control in excision, incision and dead space wound models.

Lannea welwitschii (Hiern.) Engl. is found growing in deciduous and secondary forests of Africa from Cote d'Ivoire to Cameroon and extending to Uganda and Angola. Decoction of the leaves is used traditionally for the treatment of diarrhea, dysentery, swellings, gout, gingivitis, topical infections, and wounds [10]. Methanol leaf extract of *L. welwitschii* (7.5%, w/w) significantly ($p < 0.05$) reduced wound size as compared to the untreated in excision wound model in rats. The extract also significantly ($p < 0.01$) increased the tensile strength, improved angiogenesis, collagenation, and re-epithelialization of wounds compared to the untreated wounds [16].

6.4. Apiaceae

Centella asiatica (L.) Urban is a tropical plant native to Southeast Asian countries such as India, Sri Lanka, China, Indonesia, and Malaysia as well as South Africa and Madagascar [30]. It is used for treatment of burns and postoperative hypertrophic scars [31, 32]. Asiaticoside, isolated from *C. asiatica,* has been studied in normal as well as delayed-type wound healing in guinea pigs. Topical applications of 0.2% (v/w) asiaticoside on wounds induced a 56% increase in hydroxyproline, 57% increment in tensile strength, increased collagen formation and improved re-epithelialization. Also in streptozotocin-diabetic rats, where wound healing is typically delayed, topical application of 0.4% (v/w) asiaticoside over punch wounds increased hydroxyproline content, tensile strength, collagen content and epithelialization thereby facilitating the healing. Asiaticoside was also found to be active by the oral route at a dose of 1 mg/kg in the guinea pig punch wound model. It promoted angiogenesis in the chick chorioallantoic membrane model at 40 μg/disk concentration [33]. Triterpene compounds such as asiatic acid, madecassic acid and madecassoside are the principal components of *C. asiatica,* responsible for wound healing. The action has been demonstrated both for the extracts as well as for the triterpene *in vitro* and *in vivo* studies [31, 32].

Cuminum cyminum L. is one of the oldest cultivated medicinal food herbs in Africa, Asia and Europe and seeds have been commonly used for culinary and flavoring purposes and folklore therapy since antiquity in various countries [34–36]. Alcoholic extract of the seeds and its petroleum ether fraction showed better re-epithelialization ($p < 0.001$), therefore promoted wound healing compared to the untreated wounds [37].

6.5. Apocyanaceae

Catharanthus roseus L. is native to the Caribbean Basin, Madagascar and has been found growing in tropical Africa. The fresh juice from the flowers of *C. roseus* made into a tea has been used by Ayurvedic physicians in India to treat skin infections, dermatitis, eczema and acne. Ethanol flower extract of *C. roseus* significantly ($p < 0.001$) increased the wound breaking strength in the incision wound model compared to controls. The extract-treated wounds were found to epithelialize faster, and wound contraction was significantly ($p < 0.001$) increased in comparison to control wounds and hydroxyproline content in a dead space wound model increased significantly ($p < 0.05$) [38].

Strophanthus hispidus DC. is found all over Africa including savannah forests in Ghana, Senegal, Sudan, Congo DR, Uganda, and Tanzania. It is used for the treatment of syphilis ulcers, bony syphilis, and guinea worm sores and wounds [39]. The influence of the leaf and root extracts of *S. hispidus* on rate of wound closure was investigated using the excision wound model. The extract (7.5%, w/w) showed significantly ($p < 0.05$) improved wound contraction compared to the untreated wounds. Extract-treated wound tissues with showed improved collagenation, re-epithelialization and rapid granulation formation compared with untreated wound tissues [40].

Wrightia tinctoria R. Br., commonly known as Indrajauis, is a small deciduous tree distributed in Asia and some tropical countries in Africa such as Ghana, Nigeria and Cameroun. It is used traditionally to treat various skin diseases and wounds [41–43]. *In vivo* investigations revealed that ethanol stem bark extract of *W. tinctoria* exhibited significant wound healing activity. The extract improved breaking strength ($p < 0.01$) increased the percentage wound closure and decreased epithelialization time ($p < 0.001$) compared to the control. It also significantly increased ($p < 0.001$) hydroxyproline content of ten-day-old granuloma of extract-treated animals compared to control animals in dead space wound model. The pro-healing action seems to be due to the increased synthesis of collagen and its cross-linking as well as better alignment and maturation [44].

Saba florida (Benth.) is widely distributed in tropical Africa in countries such as Senegal, Nigeria, Cameroon, Sudan and Tanzania. It is used to treat rheumatism, diarrhea, gonorrhea and as antidote against food poisoning as well as snake bites [45]. Alcohol extract of *S. florida* when administered topically (10%, w/w) and orally (100–400 mg/kg body weight) significantly stimulate wound healing in excision and incision wound models [46].

6.6. Asclepiadaceae

Calotropis gigantea R. Br. is a perennial under-shrub found chiefly in wastelands throughout India, and in some African countries such as Angola, Gabon, DR Congo, Kenya, Sudan, Tanzania and Mozambique. The whole plant is used for treatment of skin diseases, boils and sores. *C. gigantea* is also used in some parts of India for wound healing in combination with other plants [47–49]. The whole plant extract increased the percentage of wound contraction, scar area and decreased re-epithelialization time. Breaking strength of extract-treated wounds and hydroxyproline content increased compared to untreated [50].

Calotropis procera W. T. Aiton is a well-known plant in the Ayurvedic system of medicine. *C. procera* originated from the Afro-Asian monsoonal regions. It spreads on an arc expanding from north western Africa including Mauritania, Senegal, through the Arabian Peninsula and Middle-East to the Indian subcontinent. It was introduced to subtropical America, the Mascarene Islands, drier parts of Australia and probably Southeast Asia [51]. The latex of *C. procera* (1%, w/v) significantly facilitated the wound healing process by increasing collagen, DNA and protein synthesis and epithelialization leading to a marked reduction in wound area compared to the control [52].

6.7. Asteraceae

Achillea biebersteinii Afan is a perennial herb which is used in folkloric medicine in Turkey to treat abdominal pain, wounds and stomachache. N-hexane aerial parts extract of *A. biebersteinii* showed marked increase in wound contraction rate and tensile strength in excision and incision wound models, respectively. However ointment incorporated with 1% chloroform, ethyl acetate and methanol extract showed no significant influence on the wound healing process in both excision and incision wound models [53].

Ageratum conyzoides L. has long been known in herbal medicine as a remedy for various ailments in Africa [54], Asia, and South America [55, 56]. It is used by the Fipa in South Africa and central Africa for the treatment of fresh wounds and burns [57]. The wound healing activities of petroleum ether, chloroform, methanol and aqueous extracts of *A. conyzoides* were evaluated using the excision, incision and dead space wound models. Methanol and aqueous leaf extracts of *A. conyzoides* showed faster rate of wound healing compared to other extracts [58].

Chromolaena odorata L. is a perennial shrub that is native in Africa [59, 60]. Extracts from the leaves of *C. odorata* have been shown to be beneficial for treatment of wounds. The crude ethanol extract of the plant had been demonstrated to be a powerful antioxidant in protecting fibroblasts and keratinocytes *in vitro*. Phenolic acids including protocatechuic, p-hydroxybenzoic, p-coumaric, ferulic and vanillic acids and complex mixtures of lipophilic flavonoid aglycones (flavanones, flavonols, flavones and chalcones) were antioxidants found to protect cultured skin cells against oxidative damage in colorimetric and lactate dehydrogenase release assay [61].

Centaurea iberica Trev. ex Spreng also called Iberian star thistle is native to the Mediterranean region, southern Europe and northern Africa. Several *Centaurea* species are used in Turkish folk medicine to alleviate pain and inflammatory symptoms in rheumatoid arthritis, high fever, headache and wounds. Particularly, the aerial parts have found to improve wound healing. Histopathological evaluation of both ointment of aqueous and methanol extracts treated and untreated wound tissues from rats supported the healing process with remarkable increase in the proliferation of fibroblasts, differentiation of keratinocytes, re-epithilization and remodeling [62].

Sphaeranthus indicus L. is distributed throughout Africa, India, Sri Lanka and Australia. It is an important medicinal plant used for the treatment of styptic gastric disorders, skin diseases, anthelmintic, glandular swelling, and nervous depression. The decoction and powdered material of the plant are used for the treatment of bronchitis, asthma, leucoderma, jaundice, piles and scabies [63–65]. Extract of the aerial parts of *S. indicus* significantly enhanced the rate of wound contraction and the period of epithelialization comparable to neomycin in pigs [66].

Tridax procumbens L. is commonly known as 'coat buttons' among English folks. The plant is native to tropical America and naturalized in tropical Africa, Asia, Australia and India. The influence of whole plant extract and aqueous extract of *T. procumbens* on lysyl oxidase activity, protein and nucleic acid contents as well as the tensile strength which are relevant to wound healing resulted in significant ($p < 0.01$) increment in the above parameters in albino rat treated with whole plant aqueous extract and aqueous extract fractions compared to the untreated in dead space wound healing model. Butanol and petroleum ether fractions treated wound tissues showed a decrease in all these parameters except tensile strength. In these two groups, the hexosamine levels were increased ($p < 0.001$). Whole plant extract were more active as compared to the other extracts in dead space wound model [67]. Yaduvanshi et al. [68] reported that, excision wounds treated with extract of the juice of *T. procumbens* (1 mg/g) and VEGF (1 μg/mL) exhibited a significant ($p < 0.05$) increase of 38.81% and 47%, respectively in collagen biosynthesis compared to the vehicle-treated wounds. Histological investigations also showed increased infiltration of inflammatory cells, fibroblast proliferation and re-epithelialization with moderate vascularity in dermal wound tissues treated with extract of the juice of *T. procumbens*. However, dermal wounds treated with extract of the juice of *T. procumbens* at a dose of 4 mg/g induced inflammation, edematous tissue and decreased vascularity. Ethanolic and aqueous leaf extract *T. procumbens* significantly ($p < 0.05$) increase in wound tensile strength. In the excision model, biochemical markers such as hydroxyproline, collagen and hexosamine increased significantly ($p < 0.05$) compared to the untreated control group [69].

Calendula officinalis L., also known as pot marigold or garden marigold, is a common garden plant which is native to Southern Europe and Egypt. Traditionally it is used to treat various skin disorders such as burns and wounds, eczema, psoriasis and variety of skin infections. It can also be used to treat seizures, haemorrhoids and lungs, mouth and throat infections [70]. The effects of oral application of *C. officinalis* flower ethanol extract at dose of 20 and 100 mg/kg body weight have been reported to significantly ($p < 0.01$) promote wound closure and re-epithelialization compared to the control group in excision wound model. In addition, there was significant ($p < 0.05$) increases in hydroxyproline and hexosamine content in the 100 mg/kg extract-treated wounds compared with the untreated animals [71].

6.8. Bignoniaceae

Kigelia africana (Lam.) Benth. is found widespread across tropical Africa including Ghana, Sierra Leone, Gambia, Sudan and Nigeria and also found growing in wet savannah and near river bodies where it occurs in abundance [72]. It is used to treat skin ailments including fungal infections, boils, psoriasis and eczema, leprosy, syphilis, and cancer. The roots, wood and leaves have been found to contain kigelinone, vernolic acid, kigelin, iridoids, luteolin, and 6-hydroxyluteolin [73]. The iridoids have antibacterial property [74]. The methanol stem bark extract of *K. africana* (7.5%, w/w aqueous cream) in rat excision wound model showed significant ($p < 0.05$) wound contraction on day 7 with 72% of wound closure compared to the untreated control group. Wound tissues treated with the extracts showed improved collagenation, re-epitheliazition and rapid granulation formation compared to untreated wound tissues [40].

Spathodea campanulata P. Beauv. is used in folkloric medicine in Ghana and several African countries to treat various forms of wounds [9, 10, 75]. Excision wounds treated with 20% (w/w) *S. campanulata* cream and Cicatrin® cream showed a rapid and comparable decrease ($p < 0.05$) in wound size in rats. In uninfected wounds, both 20% (w/w) *S. campanulata* cream and Cicatrin® cream application resulted in 95% wound closure seen on day 20, and a complete closure seen on day 24. In infected wounds, both 20% (w/w) *S. campanulata* cream and Cicatrin® cream administration led to approximately 91% wound closure on day 24 and a complete wound contraction on day 28 [76].

Tecoma capensis Thumb. Lindl, commonly called Cape honeysuckle, is a shrub which is native of South Africa. The leaf extract of *T. capensis* (5% and 10%, w/w ointment) have been reported to exert significant increase rate wound closure and wound breaking strength in excision and incision wound models, respectively. Again, oral administration of 200 and 400 mg/kg leaf extract significantly increased granuloma breaking strength and hydroxyproline contents in dead space wound model [77].

6.9. Boraginaceae

Heliotropium indicum L. has a pantropical African distribution, but is probably native of tropical America and it is widespread throughout Africa. It is used as an analgesic (rheumatism), diuretic and for treatment of skin problems including yaws, urticaria, scabies, ulcers, eczema, impetigo and wounds [17, 78, 79]. *H. indicum* extracts (petroleum ether, chloroform, methanol and aqueous) promoted wound healing activity. The highest activity was observed with the methanol fraction. Significant increase in the granulation tissue weight, increased hydroxyproline content, and increased activity of superoxide dismutase and catalase level with the animals treated with methanol extract in dead space wound model further augmented the wound healing potential of *H. Indicum* [80].

6.10. Cactaceae

Opuntia ficus-indica (L.), commonly known as cactus or prickly pear, is a tropical and subtropical plant that grows in arid and semi-arid climates with a geographical distribution encompassing Mexico, Latin America, South Africa and Mediterranean countries [81, 82]. It has been used in folklore medicine for the treatment of diseases including inhibition of stomach ulceration [83]. The methanol stems extract of *O. ficus-indica* and its hexane, ethyl acetate, *n*-butanol and aqueous fractions were evaluated for their wound healing activity in rats. The extract and less polar fractions showed significant ($p < 0.05$) wound healing effects compared to the untreated wounds [84]. The wound-healing potential of two lyophilized polysaccharide extracts obtained from *O. ficus-indica* (L.) cladodes applied on large full-thickness wounds in the rat have been reported. When topically applied for 6 days, polysaccharides with a molecular weight >10(4) Da accelerated the re-epithelialization and remodeling phases, also by affecting cell-matrix interactions and by modulating laminin deposition. However, the wound-healing activity is high with polysaccharides with a MW ranging between 10(4) and 10(6) Da than for those with molecular weight >10(6) Da [85].

6.11. Caricaceae

Carica papaya L. is commonly known as pawpaw. The edible part of *C. papaya* is widely used all over the world and is cultivated in most tropical countries. The leaves are used traditionally as a dressing component for wounds [86]. The aqueous leaf extract of *C. papaya* (5% and 10%, w/v extract in vaseline and solcoseryl jelly) accelerated wound healing compared to the wounds treated with blank vaseline [87]. In streptozotocin-induced diabetic rats using excision and dead space wound models, the aqueous extract exhibited 77% reduction in the wound area compared to the controls. The wet and dry granulation tissue weight and hydroxyproline content increased significantly when compared to controls [88]. Carbopol gel containing 1.0% and 2.5% (w/w) of dried papaya latex have been found to accelerate wound closure, increase hydroxyproline content and stimulate epithelialization compared to the control in burn wound model [89].

6.12. Cecropiaceae

Myrianthus arboreus P. Beauv is a dioecious shrub or tree which grows up to 20 m tall. It is found growing in forest zones of tropical Africa including Ghana, Sierra Leone, Sudan, Ethiopia, southern part of DR Congo, Tanzania and Angola. Extracts of the leaves and leafy shoots of *M. arboreus* are used in the treatment of dysentery, diarrhea, wounds, boils, dysmenorrhea and incipient hernia and vomiting. The study revealed that 5% (w/w) methanol leaf extracts of *M. aboreus* cream has potent wound healing capacity with better wound closure ($p < 0.05$) on day 1 and day 9 ($p < 0.001$) compared with untreated wounds in excision wound model. Histological investigations showed enhanced wound tissue proliferation, fibrosis and re-epithelialization compared with the untreated wound tissues [90].

6.13. Combretaceae

Terminalia arjuna (Roxb. Ex DC) Wight and Arn. is native to India and Sri Lanka but it has been planted and naturalized in many African countries. In Mauritius, it is traditionally used in the management of dysentery and rheumatism. The effect of topical application of fractions (fractions I, II and III) obtained from a hydro-alcoholic extract of the stem bark were assessed on the healing of rat dermal wounds. The fractions significantly increased the tensile strength of the incision wounds and degree of re-epithelialization of excision wounds compared to control animals ($p < 0.05$). However, topical treatment with fraction I, consisting mainly of tannins, was found to demonstrate a comparatively high increase in the tensile strength of incision wounds and exhibited the fastest rate of epithelialization and increased hexosamine content [91].

Combretum mucronatum Schum. & Thonn. grows in west Africa in countries such as Ghana Senegal, DR Congo and Gabon. The leaves are traditionally used for treatment of wounds and skin infections. Aqueous leaf extract of *C. mucronatum* has been shown to stimulate viability of human keratinocytes and dermal fibroblasts. The extract stimulated cellular differentiation of primary keratinocytes significantly at 1 and 10 μg/mL. An isolate, procyanidin B2 from *C. mucronatum* at 1 and 10 μM was shown to be responsible for the induction of this cellular differentiation, while epicatechin and procyanidins B5, C1 and D1 also isolated from the extract were inactive [92].

6.14. Crassulaceae

Bryophyllum pinnatum Lam. is a perennial herb that grows in the tropical, subtropical and temperate regions of the world. The plant is well known as an agent for wound healing in folkloric medicine in most part of Asia especially in India. Petroleum ether, alcohol and aqueous leaf extract of *B. pinnatum* at an oral dose of 400 mg/kg showed significant ($p < 0.001$) increase in the breaking strength of incision wound as compared to control group. In the dead space wound healing, granuloma breaking strength and hydroxyproline content of granulation tissue increased significantly ($p < 0.001$) compared to control group. The aqueous extract of *B. pinnatum* also showed significant ($p < 0.001$) increase in wound contraction and formation of scars compared to the control in excision wound model [93].

6.15. Curcubitaceae

Momordica charantia L. also known as bitter gourd or bitter lemon is found in tropical regions including west Africa and it is used in the management of wounds, peptic ulcer, fever, piles and skin infections and parasitic infections [86, 94]. In excision wound model, the methanol leaf extract of *M. charantia* showed significant ($p < 0.05$) wound closure and histological investigation of the wound tissues revealed high fibrosis and collagenation compared to the untreated wound tissues in rats [94].

6.16. Cyperaceae

Cyperus rotundus L. is indigenous to India, but now it is found in tropical, subtropical and temperate regions from Asia, Africa and South America [95]. *C. rotundus* is used in folkloric medicine for the treatment of dyspepsia, fever, pruritis, wounds and pains [64, 96]. An alcoholic extract of tuber parts of *C. rotundus* ointments showed an increase in wound contracting ability, tensile strength and a decrease in wound closure time [97].

6.17. Euphorbiacea

Phyllanthus muellerianus (Kuntze) Exell. is found growing in most tropical region including Africa and Asia and it is used for the treatment of boils, wounds, stomach sores, menstrual disorders, fevers and other skin eruptions. Geraniin is the major phytochemical constituents in the leaves of *P. Mullerianus* [98]. In the excision wound healing, aqueous extract (PLE) of *P. muellerianus* (0.25%, 0.5% and 1%, w/w) and geraniin (0.1%, 0.2% and 0.4%, w/w) significantly ($p < 0.001$) reduced wound area, increased hydroxyproline content and tensile strength compared to the untreated wounds. Histological studies of wound tissues showed high number of fibroblasts and increased collagenation in PLE and geraniin-treated wound tissues. Immunohistochemical investigations revealed high levels of TGF-β_1 in PLE (0.25%, 0.5% and 1%, w/w) and geraniin-treated (0.1%, 0.2% and 0.4%, w/w) wound tissues compared to the untreated wound tissues. Protein band analysis of coomassie stained SDS-PAGE showed significantly ($p < 0.001$) high levels of TGF-β_1 in both PLE (0.25%, 0.5% and 1%, w/w) and geraniin-treated (0.1%, 0.2% and 0.4% ,w/w) wound tissues compared to the untreated wound tissues. SOD activity increased significantly ($p < 0.001$) in both PLE (0.25%, 0.5% and 1%, w/w) and geraniin-treated (0.1%, 0.2% and 0.4%, w/w) wound tissues compared to the untreated wound tissues. SOD, CAT and APx activity increased significantly ($p < 0.01$) in both PLE (0.25%, 0.5% and 1% ,w/w) and geraniin-treated (0.1%, 0.2% and 0.4%, w/w) wound tissues compared to the untreated tissues. However, MPO activity decreased significantly ($p < 0.01$) in PLE (0.25%, 0.5% and 1%, w/w) and 0.2% and 0.4% (w/w) geraniin-treated wound tissues compared to the untreated wound tissues [99]. Hydrophilic extracts from *P. muellerianus* and especially the major isolate, geraniin, exhibited stimulating activity on dermal fibroblasts and keratinocytes, leading to increased cell proliferation, barrier formation and formation of extracellular matrix proteins [98].

Alchornea cordifolia (Schum. &Thonn.) Muell. Arg. is an evergreen dioecious shrub which grows in the eastern part of Senegal to Kenya and Tanzania and throughout Central Africa to Angola.

The poultice of the leaves is used for the treatment of wounds. The leaves and root bark of *A. cordifolia* are externally applied to treat leprosy and as antidote to snake venom [10, 86]. Aqueous leaf extracts of *A. cordifolia* cream (10%, w/w) in an excision wound model, exhibited potent wound healing capacity with better wound closure ($p < 0.05$) at day 1 and day 9 ($p < 0.001$) compared with untreated wounds. Histological investigations showed enhanced wound tissue proliferation, fibrosis and re-epithelialization compared with the untreated wound tissues [90].

Jatropha curcas L. also called physic nut is a perennial poisonous shrub originated from Central America but has spread to other tropical and subtropical countries and mainly grows in Asia and Africa. The plant has been employed in the management of many ailments including ulcer and sores in some parts of Africa [99, 100]. The leaf and stem bark extracts of *J. curcas* have been found to accelerate the healing process by increasing the skin breaking strength, granulation tissue breaking strength, wound contraction, dry granulation tissue weight and hydroxyproline levels. A marked decrease in epithelialization period was also observed. The histological examination of granulation tissue also showed the presence of more collagen, which has organized to form bundles indicative of advance wound healing [101].

Arabinogalactan protein (JC) from *J. curcas* seed endosperm (mean molecular weight 140 kDa) was isolated by cold water extraction and characterized concerning sugar and amino acid composition. At 10 and 100 μg/mL JC stimulated mitochondrial activity (MTT assay) of HaCaT keratinocytes and dermal fibroblasts and the ATP status of primary keratinocytes. JC did not influence the cellular proliferation, while primary keratinocytes were triggered into differentiation status. Investigations on a potential mode of action of JC were performed on complex organotypic skin equivalents. JC induced HGF, KGF and TGF-β expression, with TGF-β being the main inductor for the differentiation-inducing effect of JC. Also the expression of GM-CSF was stimulated strongly by JC. This *in vitro* activity profile indicated JC to be a potent inductor of cellular differentiation via stimulation of growth hormones and TGF-β-induced cell signaling [102].

Mallotus oppositifolius (Geiseler) Müll. Arg. is found growing in tropical African region regions including Ghana and Nigeria. A leaf or stem bark infusion is applied to cuts and sores as haemostatic and used to treat burns, skin eruptions and rashes [78, 86, 103]. Methanol leaf extract of *M. oppositifolius* showed significant ($p < 0.05$) wound closure, fibrosis and collagenation in excision wound model [94].

Phyllanthus emblica L. also known as *Emblica officinalis* is a native plant from Asia. It is used in folkloric medicine as a wound healing agent either in single formulation or in combination with other medicinal plants. Topical application of ethanol fruit extract (200 μL) of *P. emblica* increases cellular proliferation and cross-linking of collagen at the wound site, which is evidenced by an increase in the activity of extracellular signal-regulated kinase 1/2, along with an increase in DNA, type III collagen, acid-soluble collagen, aldehyde content, shrinkage temperature and tensile strength. Higher levels of tissue ascorbic acid, alpha-tocopherol, reduced glutathione, superoxide dismutase, catalase and glutathione peroxidase support the fact that *P. emblica* promotes antioxidant activity at the wound site in excision wound model [104]. Again, aqueous extract of the fruit of *P. emblica* (0.1 μg/mL) in scratch assay using human umbilical vein endothelial cells (HUVEC) was shown to promote endothelial cell function and wound healing by significantly ($p < 0.05$) promoting NO production, endothelial wound closure, endothelial sprouting, and VEGF mRNA expression which provides further evidence to support the traditional use of *P. emblica* as a wound healing agent [105].

6.18. Fabaceae

Mimosa pudica L. originated in tropical Central and South America and naturalized throughout the tropics including Africa. Its wound healing properties were studied in three different wound models in rats (excision, incision and estimation of biochemical parameter) using both aqueous and methanol root bark extract. Treatment of wounds with ointment containing 2% (w/w) of methanol and aqueous extract exhibited significant ($p < 0.001$) wound healing activity by increasing rate of wound contraction, tensile strength and hydroxyproline content compared to the control. The period for re-epithelialization was reduced compared to the control [106].

Indigofera enneaphylla L. is an under-shrub widely grown throughout India. The plant is used traditionally to treat scurvy, stomach disorders, pain, skin infections and wounds. showed that Ethanol extract of the whole plant extract of *I. enneaphylla* (0.5% and 1%, w/w ointments) significantly increased ($p < 0.001$) rate of wound contraction on day 18 post wounding in excision wound model when compared to the control group. In the incision wound model, both doses of extract also exhibited significant ($p < 0.001$) increase in tensile strength [107].

Tephrosia purpurea L. is an herb which grows in the tropical regions. It is traditionally used in the treatment of bronchitis, boils, bleeding piles, pimples, roots and seeds are used as insecticidal, vermifuge, leprous wound and the juice is used for the eruption on skin. It has found to contain glycosides, rotenoids, isoflavones, flavones, chalcones, flavonoids and sterols. Ethanol aerial parts extract of *T. purpurea* formulated into a 5% (w/w) simple ointment stimulated ($p < 0.05$) wound contraction, tensile strength, hydroxyproline content, protein level in excision, incision and dead space wound models. Histological examination of the wound tissue showed significant ($p < 0.05$) increase in fibroblast cells, collagen fibers and blood vessels formation [104].

6.19. Fagaceae

Quercus infectoria Olivier is a small tree found in Greece, Asia and Iran. The galls of *Q. infectoria* are used traditionally to treat inflammatory diseases including toothache and gingivitis. The wound healing activity of ethanol extract of the galls of *Q. infectoria* was investigated using the incision, dead space and excision wound models in rats. The study revealed a (400 and 800 mg/kg body weight) significantly ($p < 0.05$) increase in tensile strength in extract-treated wound tissues compared to the control group in the incision wound model. In the dead-space wound model the extract significantly ($p < 0.05$) increased dry granuloma weight, granuloma breaking strength and hydroxyproline content compared to the control group. *Q. infectoria* was also identified to significantly ($p < 0.05$) promote wound contraction rate as well as increase levels of superoxide dismutase and catalase activity in wound bed compared to the control in the excision wound model [108].

6.20. Flacourtiaceae

Hydnorcarpus wightiana Blume is widely distributed in India and its neighboring countries. The oil referred to as "chaulmoogra" which is extracted from *H. wightiana* and other species is well known for its anti-leprosy activity. The oil at a dose of 45 mg/kg is also reported to significantly ($p < 0.01$) enhance wound healing by increasing breaking strength and collagen and hydroxyproline contents of wounds compared to the control in incision and dead space wound models, respectively. *H. wightiana* oil administered orally significantly ($p < 0.001$) promoted epithelialization, but not wound contraction rate in excision wound model [109, 110].

6.21. Gentianaceae

Anthocleista nobilis G. Don is used in local medicine in Ghana and other parts of West Africa for curing fever, stomach ache, diarrhea, gonorrhea and also as poultice for sores [72, 111]. Methanol extract of *A. nobilis* at concentration of 33.3% (w/w) significantly ($p < 0.02$) enhanced wound closure and hydroxyproline production compared to the control in the excision wound model in rats. In the incision wound model, the extract significantly increased tensile strength of *A. nobilis* treated-wounds compared to the control. However, the methanol extract of *A. nobilis* had no significant effect on the proliferation of human dermal fibroblast at concentrations as high 50 μg/mL. Doses over 50 μg/mL showed cytotoxic effects on the human dermal fibroblasts [112].

6.22. Ginkgoaceae

Ginkgo biloba L. also known as maiden hair tree is believed to be native of China. The plant has been used in folkloric medicine for its therapeutic purposes especially in mental sicknesses. Bairy and Rao [113] reported that intraperitoneal administration of the 50 mg/kg dried leaf extract of *G. biloba* significantly ($p < 0.01$) promoted the breaking strength and hydroxyproline content of granulation tissue in dead space wounds in rats. However, in excision wounds while it did not affect the wound contraction but epithelization period was significantly ($p < 0.01$) shortened compared to the control.

6.23. Hypericaceae

Hypericum patulum Thumb. is a perennial plant distributed in Southern Africa, Asia and North America. It is used traditionally to treat dog bites and bee sting [114]. Methanol leaf extract of *H. patulum* in the form of an ointment (5% and 10%, w/w) enhanced wound contraction rate, re-epithelialization, tissue granulation and increased tensile strength in rats compared with the control group [115].

Hypericum perforatum L., commonly called St John Worts, Klamath weed, tipton weed, goat weed, and enola weed, is a perennial flowering herb native to Europe, but has spread to temperate locations in Asia, Africa, Australia, Europe and North and South America [116]. Olive oil extracted from the aerial parts of *H. perforatum* is a popular folk remedy for the treatment of wounds in Europe. Aerial parts of *H. perforatum* have been found to possess remarkable wound healing activities. Flavonoids including hyperoside, isoquercitrin, rutin and (–)-epicatechin, and naphthoquinones especially hypericins were found as the active components of *H. perforatum* [117]. The total extract of *H. perforatum* in *in vivo* experimental wound models of linear incision, circular excision and thermal burn showed that topical treatment improve wound contraction rate and period of re-epithelialization [118]. A plant-derived wound dressing containing a mixture of hypericum oil and neem oil (*Azadirachta indica* A. Juss.) in scalp wounds with exposed bone [119] and pediatric burn wounds [120] promoted healing in rats by enhancing granulation tissues formation and re-epithelialization.

6.24. Lamiaceae

Occimum sanctum L. occurs naturally in tropical America, Africa and Asia. It is used traditionally in the treatment of diverse ailments like infections and skin diseases [121]. The wound healing parameters were evaluated by using incision, excision and dead space wound models in rats. The alcoholic (400 and 800 mg/kg) and aqueous (400 and 800 mg/kg) extracts of *O. sanctum* significantly ($p < 0.05$) increased wound contraction rate, wound breaking strength, hydroxyproline, hexuronic acid, hexosamines, superoxide dismutase, catalase and reduced glutathione levels. Lipid peroxidation was significantly ($p < 0.05$) reduced when compared with the control group [101]. Goel et al. [122] also reported that 10% *O. sanctum* aqueous leaf extract in petroleum jelly increased rate of wound contraction and re-epithelialization compared to the control in excision model of wound repair in Wistar albino rats.

Occimum gratissimum L. is an aromatic plant found in tropical Africa including Ghana, Nigeria and Kenya among others. The leaves are rubbed between the palms and sniffed as a treatment for blocked nostrils [115]. Leaf extract of *O. gratissimum* promote wound healing by significant wound contraction ($p < 0.05$) on day 10 in extract-treated rats group compared with the control group. Histology of the healed scar showed non-significant ($p > 0.05$) decrease in the mean fibroblast count for the experimental group compared to the control group [123, 124].

Hoslundia opposita Vahl. is used in ethnomedicine to treat sore throats, colds, sores, veneral diseases, herpes and other skin diseases [125], malaria, microbial infections, epilepsy, fever and inflammation [126, 127]. Methanol leaf extract of H. *opposita* at concentration of 33.3% (w/w) significantly ($p < 0.01$) increased wound contraction and hydroxyproline content compared to the control in the excision wound model in rats. In the incision wound model, the extract significantly improved tensile strength of wounds compared to the control. The extract had no significant effect on the growth of human dermal fibroblast up to concentrations of 50 μg/ml and higher concentrations exhibited toxic effects [112].

Hyptis suaveolens (Poit), commonly called bush tea, is a native to tropical America, but it is also widespread in tropical Africa, Asia and Australia. *H. suaveolens* is used in traditional medicine for treatment of various diseases including wounds, skin infections etc. Ethanol leaf extract of *H. suaveolens* (400 and 800 mg/kg body weight) increased skin breaking strength, granuloma breaking strength, wound contraction, hydroxyproline content and dry granuloma weight and decreased the re-epithelialization period in rats. A supportive study made on granuloma tissue to estimate the levels of catalase and superoxide dismutase recorded a significant ($p < 0.05$) increase in the level of these antioxidant enzymes which resulted enhanced collagenation [128]. Shenoy et al. [129] also showed the effect of petroleum ether, alcohol, and aqueous leaf extracts of *H. suaveolens* on excision, incision and dead space wound models using Wistar albino rats. All three extracts at a dose of 500 mg/kg enhanced wound healing by accelerating wound closure and period for re-epithelialization compared to the control. Tensile strength, dry weight granulation tissue, breaking strength of granulation tissue and hydroxyproline content were also increased compared to the control.

Leucas hirta is found in East Africa and India [130, 131]. Decoctions of dry and fresh herbs of *L. hirta* are used for skin diseases and as gargle for the treatment of thrush, respectively. Roots are also used for snake bites [132]. A leaf poultice is used on swelling and boils. The latex of *L. hirta* is applied on lower eyelids to cure eye sores. The wound healing effect of aqueous and methanol leaf extracts of *L. hirta* at a dose of 35 mg/kg was evaluated in excision, incision and dead space wound models in rats. The methanol and aqueous leaf extracts were found to possess significant wound healing activity which was evidenced by decrease in the period of re-epithelialization, increase in the rate of wound contraction, skin breaking strength, granulation tissue dry weight, hydroxyproline content and breaking strength of granulation tissue. Histological study of the granulation tissue showed increased collagenation when compared to the respective control group of animals [133].

6.25. Liliaceae

Allium cepa L. is a biennial herbaceuos plant with edible bulb. It is commonly known as onion. Since ancient times, it has been used traditionally for the treatment of different diseases including various types of wounds, skin problems etc. It contains kampferol, β-sitosterol, ferulic acid, myritic acid, prostaglandins [134]. Shenoy et al. [129] reported that alcohol extract exhibits significant ($p < 0.05$) wound contraction rate, improved tensile strength and increased wound breaking strength, dry weight granuloma and hydroxyproline content compared to the control in excision, incision and dead space wound models in rats.

6.26. Lythraceae

Lawsonia inermis L. is widely distributed throughout Africa. It also occurs in the Middle East. Ethanol leaf extract of *L. inermis* (200 mg/kg/day) demonstrated high rate of wound contraction ($p < 0.001$), a decrease in the period of epithelialization ($p < 0.001$), high skin breaking strength ($p < 0.001$), a significant increase in the granulation tissue weight ($p < 0.001$) and hydroxyproline content ($p < 0.05$). The extract-treated rats showed 71% reduction in the wound area when compared with controls which was 58%. Enhanced wound contraction, increased skin breaking strength, hydroxyproline and histological findings suggest the use of *L. inermis* in the management of wounds in humans may be justified [135].

Punica granatum L., commonly called pomegranate, originated from Iran. It is widely distributed in Mediterranean, Europe, Africa and Asia. Leaf extract of *P. granatum* possess wound healing activity at concentrations of 2.5% and 5% (w/w) in rats. The amount of hydroxyproline increased by twofold in the group treated with 5.0% gel. The extract was found to contain gallic acid and catechin as major compounds [136].

6.27. Malvaceae

Hibiscus rosa sinensis L. is native in the tropics and subtropics [137]. It has been used traditionally for the treatment of a variety of diseases as well as to promote wound healing. Ethanol leaf extract (120 mg/kg/day) exhibited an 86% reduction in the wound area compared with controls, which exhibited a 75% reduction in rats. The extract-treated animals showed a significant epithelialization ($p < 0.002$) and had significantly ($p < 0.002$) higher skin-breaking strength than controls. The dry and wet weight of granulation tissue and hydroxyproline content also increased significantly when compared with controls [138]. Bhaskar and Nithya [139] also reported the influence of ethanol flower extract of *H. rosa sinensis* (5% and 10%, w/w) on wound healing in Wistar albino rats using excision, incision and dead space wound model. The extract increased cellular proliferation and collagen synthesis at the wound site, as evidenced by increase in DNA, total protein and total collagen content of granulation tissues. The extract significantly ($p < 0.001$) promoted wound healing which was indicated by improved rates of epithelialization and wound contraction as well as increased wound tensile strength and wet and dry granulation tissue weights compared to the control.

Thespesia populnea (L.) Soland Ex. Corr, also known as Indian Tulip tree, is found growing from West Bengal to South India. It is used locally to treat skin ailments like scabies, psoriasis, wounds and ulcers. Shivakumar et al. [140] reported that ointments containing 5% (w/w) of petroleum ether, alcohol and aqueous leaf extracts *of T. populnea* promote wound contraction and wound breaking strength significantly ($p < 0.01$) when compared to the control groups in excision and incision wound models in rats, respectively.

6.28. Meliaceae

Carapa guianensis Aublet is found in Guiana and Africa. The leaves of *C. guianensis* are used to treat ulcers, skin parasites and skin problems. The ethanol leaf extract of *C. guianensis* exhibited significant reduction ($p < 0.01$) in the wound area when compared to controls with significant decrease in the epithelialization period. Skin breaking strength ($p < 0.001$), wet ($p < 0.002$) and dry ($p < 0.02$) granulation tissue and hydroxyproline content ($p < 0.03$) were significantly higher in extract-treated animals. The increased rate of wound contraction, skin breaking strength and hydroxyproline content may support application of *C. guianensis* for treatment of wounds [141].

Azadirachta indica A. Juss (Neem tree) is a native of Asia but has now naturalized in West Africa. In excision wound model in rats, aqueous leaf extract of *A. indica* significantly increased ($p < 0.05$) the rate of wound closure of extract-treated group compared to control group [142]. Methanol leaf extract (5%, w/w ointment) of *A. indica* has also been reported to significantly ($p < 0.05$) promote the wound healing activity in both excision and incision wound models in rats [20]. Pandey et al. [143] reported that *A. indica* oil increases wound tensile strength and wound closure rate in animals using incision and excision wound models, respectively.

6.29. Moraceae

Ficus religiosa L., which is commonly known as bo tree, Pepal tree, Bodhi tree, peepul or sacred fig, is abundantly distributed throughout India, Southeast Asia, Southwest China and the Himalayan foothills. *F. religiosa* is reported to have wound healing, anti-inflammatory, analgesic, antioxidant (lipid peroxidation) properties. Application of simple ointment containing hydro-alcohol leaf extract of *F. reliogiosa* (5% and 10%, w/w) significantly promoted wound contraction rate, epithelization and wound breaking strength in excision and incision wound models, respectively, when compared to the control [144].

6.30. Moringaceae

Moringa oleifera Lam. is commonly known as drumstick and is widely distributed in India, Arabia and cultivated in tropical Africa, tropical America, Sri Lanka, India, Mexico and Malaysia [145]. The whole plant is used in the treatment of psychosis, eye diseases and fever and also as an aphrodisiac. Its leaf poultice is used in the management of wounds [146]. Qualitative phytochemical investigation confirmed the presence of phytosterols, glycosides, tannins, and amino acids in the various leaf extracts of *M. oleifera* whereas its seed extracts showed the presence of phytosterols, glycosides, phenolic compounds, carbohydrates and amino acids. The ethanol and ethyl acetate extracts of the seeds showed significant antipyretic activity in rats, whereas ethyl acetate leaf extract exhibited significant wound healing activity (10%, w/w ointment) on excision, incision and dead space (granuloma) wound models in rats [142].

6.31. Musaceae

Musa sapientum L. originated from native south-western Pacific home and spread to India and to the Islands of the Pacific, then to the West Coast of Africa [147]. It has an ulcer healing activity [148]. Aqueous and methanol extracts (100 mg/kg) have been found to increase wound breaking strength and levels of hydroxyproline, hexuronic acid, hexosamine, superoxide dismutase, reduced glutathione in the granulation tissue and decreased percentage of wound area, scar area and lipid peroxidation when compared with the control group in rats. The wound healing effect of *M. sapientum* may be due to its antioxidant effect and on various wound healing biochemical parameters [149].

6.32. Myrsinaceae

Embelia ribes Burm. is found in the hilly parts of India and grows in southern China, Indonesia and East Africa [150]. Traditionally the seeds are employed as a remedy for toothache, headache and snakebite. The seeds are mainly used for maintaining healthy skin and to support the digestive function [64]. It is also effective in the treatment of fever, abdominal disorders, lung diseases, constipation, fungus infections, mouth ulcer, sore throat, pneumonia, heart disease and obesity [150]. Ethanol leaf extract of *E. ribes* and its isolated quinone compound, embelin, were screened for wound healing activity in rats. In embelin-treated group (4 mg/mL in a 0.2%, w/v sodium alginate gel), re-epithelialization of the incision wound was faster with a high rate of wound contraction. The tensile strength of the incision wound was significantly increased in embelin-treated group than the ethanol extract. In dead space wound model also the weight of the granulation was increased indicating increase in collagenation. The histological examination of the granulation tissue of embelin-treated group showed increased cross-linking of collagen fibers and absence of monocytes [151].

6.33. Oleaceae

Jasminum auriculatum Vahl. is a small, evergreen, climbing shrub widely distributed in Eastern Asia including India, Nepal and Sri Lanka. The leaves are normally used to treat mouth ulcers. Mittal et al. [152] reported that ointment base incorporated with 16% (w/w) of ethanol leaf extract of *J. auriculatum* significantly ($p < 0.05$) decreased the period of re-epithelialization in excision wound model. In the incision wound model, there was significant increase in wound breaking strength and collagen content. Histological examination of wound tissues revealed increased fibroblast proliferation, collagen deposition and neovascularization.

Jasminum grandiflorum L. is an evergreen or deciduous shrub found in East tropical Africa countries including Sudan, Eritrea, Ethiopia, Somalia, Uganda, Kenya, Rwanda as well as in Asia. Traditionally it is used as an aphrodiasic, expectorant, painkiller and also to treat skin diseases including mouth ulcers and skin eruptions. Topical application of ointment *J. grandifolium* leaf extract (2% and 4%, w/w) on excision wounds in rats accelerated the healing process. Tissue growth and collagen synthesis were significantly ($p < 0.05$) higher which was determined by total hydroxyproline, hexosamine, protein and DNA content. The rate of wound healing was faster as determined by wound contraction, tensile strength and other histopathological changes. In addition, the 4% extract-treated wounds showed enhanced ($p < 0.05$) the activity of superoxide dismutase (SOD) and catalase (CAT) with high GSH content and low lipid peroxidation products in wound tissue compared to the control [153].

6.34. Papaveraceae

Argemone mexicana L. is a prickly, glabrous, branching annual herb with yellow juice and showy yellow flowers found in West Indies and Mexico. Traditionally, the plant is used as diuretic, purgative, painkiller, laxative and treatment for skin diseases, wounds and poisons [154]. In excision and incision wound models in rats, methanol, aqueous and chloroform leaf extracts of *A. mexicana* (10%, w/w) ointment significantly ($p < 0.05$) enhanced wound closure, re-epithelialization and breaking strength in wound bed compared to the control group. Histological studies of the extract-treated wound tissues revealed improved collagen deposition and fibroblast proliferation with reduced macrophage infiltration and edema. The methanol extract-treated animals showed significant ($p < 0.01$) increase in dry weight of granulation tissue and hydroxyproline content in dead space wound model. Superoxide dismutase and catalase level in the granulation tissue were significantly increased in methanol extract-treated rats ($p < 0.01$) when compared to the control in dead space wound model. The methanol extract also significantly ($p < 0.05$) improved wound healing in bacterial (*Pseudomonas aeruginosa* and *Staphylococcus aureus*) infected wounds [80].

6.35. Pedaliaceae

Sesamum indicum L. is used in native medicine in Africa and Asia for a variety of diseases. Mucilaginous leaves or leaf sap are used to treat fever, as a remedy for cough and sore eyes, dysentery and gonorrhea. In eastern and southern Africa, the leaves are used for the treatment of ulcers. The seeds of *S. indicum* are used traditionally for the treatment of various kinds of wounds. Seeds and oil treatment (2.5% and 5%, w/w) exhibited significant ($p < 0.05$) decrease in the period of epithelialization and wound contraction, and increased the breaking strength of rat wound tissues compared to the control. Also, the seeds and oil treatment (250 and 500 mg/kg; *po*) in dead space wound model produced a significant increase in the breaking strength, dry weight and hydroxyproline content of the granulation tissue which suggest that the extract and its oil possess wound healing property [155].

6.36. Piperaceae

Piper betel L. is extensively grown in India, Srilanka, Malaysia, Indonesia, Philippines and East African countries [156]. Ointment of white soft paraffin containing 1% of dried residue of aqueous extract of *P. betel* has been reported to possess wound healing activity [157].

6.37. Potulacaceae

Portulaca oleracea L. is a cosmopolitan weed occurring especially in warm areas; it occurs throughout tropical Africa. It is eaten in many African countries including Côte d'Ivoire, Benin, Cameroon, Kenya, Uganda, Angola, South Africa, Sudan and Egypt. It is used for the treatment of ulcers, eczema and dermatitis [158, 159]. Fresh homogenized crude aerial parts of *P. oleracea* accelerated the wound healing process in mice by decreasing the surface area of the wound and increased the tensile strength. The highest rate of contraction was found at dose of 50 mg, followed by 25 mg [160].

6.38. Phyllanthaceae

Bridelia ferruginea Benth. is a common savannah species. Ethnomedicines prepared from the bark, leaves and fruits are used for the treatment of bruises, boils, burns, wounds and skin disease [79]. Ethanol stem bark extract of *B. ferruginea* on wound contraction and epithelization in rats significantly enhanced wound contraction and epithelialization [161] (Udegbunam et al., 2011) and the extract (1–30 μg/mL) has been reported to influence the proliferation of dermal fibroblasts significantly ($p < 0.05$) compared to the untreated cells [162].

6.39. Rubiaceae

Morinda citrifolia L. is one of the most important traditional Polynesian medicinal plants. The primary indigenous use of this plant appears to be of the leaves, as a topical treatment for wound healing. The ethanol leaf extract (150 mg/kg/day, *p.o*) was used to evaluate the wound healing activity in rats, using excision and dead space wound models. The extract exhibited

71% reduction in the wound area when compared with controls which exhibited 57%. The granulation tissue weight and hydroxyproline content in the dead space wounds were also increased significantly in extract-treated animals compared with controls ($p < 0.002$). Enhanced wound contraction, decreased epithelialization time, increased hydroxyproline content and histological characteristics may indicate that noni leaf extract may be beneficial in wound healing [163].

Pentas lanceolata Pentas Benth. originated from East Africa and is commonly called the "Red Egyptian star". The ethanol flowers extract of *P. lanceolata* given by oral route to rats at a dose of 150 mg/kg per day for 10 days was evaluated on its effect on wound healing, using excision wound model. There was significant ($p < 0.05$) increment in granulation tissue weight, tensile strength, hydroxyproline and glycosaminoglycan content. There was marked increment in the wound contraction in extract treated group as compared to that of controls and these effects may be due to increased collagen deposition as well as better alignment and maturation [164].

Rubia cordifolia L. is popular all over the world for its medicinal uses in skin diseases like eczema, dermatitis and skin ulcers. *R. cordifolia* has an extremely large area of distribution, ranging from Africa to tropical Asia, China, Japan and Australia. In Africa, it is found from Sudan and Ethiopia to South Africa. Hydrogel of the alcoholic extract has been found to improve wound contracting ability, wound closure, decrease in surface area of wound, tissue regeneration at the wound site significantly ($p < 0.01$) in treated mice [165].

6.40. Rutaceae

Aegle marmelos L., commonly called Bael in Hindu, is a perennial plant indigenous to dry forests on hills and plains of India, Pakistan, Bangladesh, Sri Lanka, Myanmar, Nepal, Vietnam, Laos, Cambodia and Thailand. The fruits and leaves are used to treat pain, fever, inflammation, respiratory disorders, cardiac disorders, dysentery and diarrhea in folk and Ayuverdic medicine. Jaswanth et al. [166] reported the wound healing effect of methanol root extract of *A. marmelos* (5% and 10%, w/w in simple ointment base) using excision and incision wound models in rats. The extract-treated wounds showed significant ($p < 0.01$) increase in wound contracting ability, reduced wound closure time and increase in the tensile strength compared to the control in excision and incision wound models, respectively. Gautam et al. [167] also reported that rats treated with 200 mg/kg *A. marmelos* ethanol leaf extract significantly ($p < 0.05$) increase wound breaking strength and improved ($p < 0.05$) wound contraction rate in *A. marmelos*-treated wounds compared to the control in excision wound model. This was also supported by histological examination of excised wounds which revealed increased granulation tissues formation and reduced inflammatory cell infiltration in 200 mg/kg treated wound tissues compared to the control. Granulation tissues showed increased ($p < 0.001$) collagen content compared to the control group. Catalase, superoxide dismutase and gluthathionine levels were markedly elevated, whereas lipid peroxidation, myeloperoxidation and nitric oxide levels were markedly ($p < 0.05$) lower in *A. marmelos*-treated wounds compared to the control group.

6.41. Sapotaceae

Mimusops elengi L. is native to India, Sri Lanka, the Andaman Islands, Myanmar and Indo-China, but is commonly planted as an ornamental tree throughout tropical countries including Ghana, Tanzania, Mozambique, Réunion Island and Mauritius. In Asia, the leaves are used medicinally to treat headache, toothache, wounds and sore eyes, and are smoked to cure infections of the nose and mouth. A decoction of the bark mixed with the flowers has been used for treatment of fever, diarrhea, inflammation of the gums, toothache, gonorrhea and wounds. The flowers have been used for the management of diarrhea [161, 168, 169]. Methanol bark extract of *M. elengi* (5%, w/w) exhibited significant ($p < 0.05$) influence on the rate of wound closure, tensile strength and dry granuloma weight. Histological investigation of the wound tissues revealed similar effects consistent with its *in vivo* wound healing properties [170].

6.42. Solanaceae

Datura metel L. is found growing in most tropical countries in Africa and it is used for the treatment of haemorrhoids, boils, sores and skin diseases [171, 172]. The ethanol leaf extract increased cellular proliferation and collagen synthesis at the wound site, as evidenced by increase in synthesis of DNA, total protein and total collagen content of granulation tissues. The extract-treated wounds were found to heal much faster with improved rates of epithelialization and wound contraction and these observations were confirmed by histological examinations of the wound tissues. The leaf extract of *D. metel* significantly ($p < 0.001$) increased the wound breaking strength compared to the controls. Wet and dry granulation tissue weights increased significantly ($p < 0.001$). There was a significant increase in wound closure rate, tensile strength, dry granuloma weight, wet granuloma weight and a decrease in epithelialization period in *D. metel* extract treated group when compared to control and commercial drug treated groups [173].

Solanum xanthocarpum Schrad and Wendl is known as Indian night shade or yellow berried night shade plant. It is more commonly used for the management of diseases like bronchial asthma, cough, worms etc. The fruits facilitate the seminal ejaculation, alleviate worms, itching, and fever and reduce fats [86]. Ethanol leaf extract of *S. xanthocarpum* significantly ($p < 0.01$) improved wound healing via increased re-epithelialization, tensile strength and hydroxyproline content which may be due to the presence of secondary metabolites such as alkaloids, glycosides, saponins, carbohydrates, tannins, phenolic compounds, proteins and fats [174].

6.43. Vitaceae

Cissus quadrangularis L. is a perennial climber popularly known as "Hadjod" in India and is widely distributed in the tropics. Traditionally, it is used to treat gastritis, bone fractures, skin infections, constipations, eye diseases, piles, anemia, asthma, irregular menstruation, burns and wounds. Treatment of wounds with ointment containing 2% (w/w) methanol extract and 2% w/w aqueous extract of *C. quadragularis* significantly ($p < 0.001$) enhanced wound closure and breaking strength compared to the control group in excision and incision wound models, respectively in rats [175].

6.44. Verbenaceae

Clerodendron splendens G. Don is a climbing shrub, mostly found growing on cultivated lands between food crops in Ghana and other West African countries. The plant is used in ethnomedicine in Ghana for the treatment of vaginal thrush, bruises, wounds and various skin infections [72]. The methanol aerial parts extract of *C. splendens* improved wound closure and hydroxyproline biosynthesis compared to the control group in the excision wound model in rats. The extract also increased the tensile strength of wounds compared to the control group [176].

Lantana camara L. occurs widely in the Asia-Pacific region, Australia, New Zealand, Central and South America, West Indies and Africa. It is used in herbal medicine for the treatment of skin itches, wounds, leprosy and scabies [177]. Treatment of the wounds in animals with leaf extract of *L. camara* enhanced the rate of wound contraction, synthesis of collagen and decreased mean wound healing time [138].

6.45. Zingiberaceae

Curcuma aromatica Salisb. is a medicinal plant cultivated most extensively in India, Bangladesh, China, Thailand, Cambodia, Malaysia, Indonesia, and Philippines. It has been grown in most tropical regions in Africa, America, and Pacific Ocean Islands. Rhizomes of *C. aromatica* are used as a stomachic, carminative and emmenagogue remedies for skin diseases [178] and also for snakebites [179] (Chopra et al., 1941). Report by Santhanam and Nagarajan [157] has shown that ointment of white soft paraffin containing 1% of powdered *C. aromatic* rhizome promotes wound contraction and epithelialization. Kumar et al. [137] also reported that ethanol dried rhizome of *C. aromatica* extract significantly ($p < 0.001$) improved wound contraction in rat excision wound model.

Curcuma longa L., commonly known as tumeric, is a rhizomatous perennial herb native to India. In traditional medicine, it is used to treat skin ailments, wound, worm infestation and as blood purifier. *C. longa* contains three major curcuminoids, namely, curcumin, demethoxycurcumin, and bis-demethoxycurcumin [180]. *C. longa* possesses antibacterial, anti-inflammatory, anti-arthritic, anti-hepatotoxic (liver protective) and anti-allergic properties. Topical application (5% and 10%, w/w simple ointment) of ethanol rhizome extract of *C. longa* promotes significantly ($p < 0.01$) enhanced wound contraction, increased hydroxproline and tensile strength of wounds in excision and incision wound models in rats and rabbits. Histological studies also showed increased collagen, fibroblasts and blood vessels formation [181, 182]. Sidhu et al. [183] reported via immunohistochemical investigations that *C. longa*-treated wounds show highly localized transforming growth factor-β1 in wound bed compared with untreated wounds. There was an increment in the mRNA transcripts of transforming growth factor-β1 and fibronectin in curcumin-treated wounds.

Curcuma purpurascens Blume. is commonly known as "Temu tis" and "Koneng tinggang" in Indonesia. The rhizome of this plant has been reported to have extensive traditional uses in rural communities against different skin ailments and dermatological disorders, especially wounds and burns. Macroscopic evaluation of wounds showed conspicuous elevation in wound contraction ($p < 0.05$) after topical administration of hexane extract of the rhizome of *C. purpurascens* (100 and 200 mg/kg body weight) to wounded rats. Histological analysis revealed enhanced collagen content and fibroblast proliferation and scanty inflammatory cells in the granulation tissues of *C. purpurascens*-treated wounds compared to the control. At the molecular level, *C. purpurascens* facilitated wound-healing process by down-regulating Bax and up-regulating Hsp70 protein at the wound site. In addition, the plant enhanced catalase, glutathione peroxidase, superoxide dismutase activity and reduced malondialdehyde levels in wound tissues compared to the control group [184].

6.46. Zygophyllaceae

Balanites aegyptiaca (L.) Diel is widely distributed in tropical regions of Africa. The plant is used in folk medicine for treatment of circumcision wounds, worm infestation, abdominal and chest pains, and as an abortifacient and contraceptive [177, 185]. Methanol extract of *B. aegyptiaca* at concentration of 33.3% (w/w) significantly ($p < 0.001$) improved wound closure, tensile strength and hydroxyproline production compared to the control in the excision wound model in rats [112].

7. Phenolic compounds with wound healing properties

Though many crude plant extracts have been scientifically demonstrated to have wound healing activities, enriched fractions and isolated compounds from some of these plants have also been shown to possess specific promising wound healing properties. The commonly known effects of the active constituents of plant extracts towards wound healing are known to be through blood clotting, antimicrobial, antioxidant, mitogenic activities and also enhancing the expression of vascular endothelial growth factor thereby improving angiogenesis and blood flow as the tissue repair process advances [179, 186–188]. In chronic wounds, agents inducing differentiation of keratinocytes play an important role.

Plant polyphenols are among the most abundant phytochemicals present in the human diet, and they range from simple molecules such as phenolic acids to highly polymerized compounds, such as condensed tannins [189]. Several plants extracts used in wound healing contain phenolics in the form of procyanidins, flavonoids and phenolic acids [187] as their active ingredients. Tannins and procyanidins are known to actively facilitate wound healing [190].

Resveratrol is a natural polyphenol found predominantly in the skin of red grapes that has been studied extensively for its potential health benefits [191]. Resveratrol is a popular nutritional supplement and ingredient in over-the-counter skin care products. In humans, resveratrol was shown to protect against sun damage to the skin, enhance moisture and elasticity, reduce wrinkle depth and intensity of age spots, and protected keratinocytes from nitrous oxide-induced death [191, 192]. Its positive effect on keratinocytes has beneficial effect on wound healing. Resveratrol administration significantly increased the tensile strength of the abdominal fascia, and increased the hydroxyproline 1 levels *in vivo*. The acute inflammation scores, collagen deposition scores and the neovascularization scores on postoperative days 7 and 14 were found to be significantly higher in the resveratrol treatment group. The amount of granulation tissue and the fibroblast maturation scores were found to be significantly higher on postoperative day 14 in the treatment group when compared to the control group [193].

7.1. Tannins

Tannins are natural polyphenols and in many cases the active constituents in plants in which they are found. Tannins have a wide range of pharmacological activities including antimicrobial, wound healing, antioxidant and anti-inflammatory activities. The physical and chemical properties of tannins suggest that they may act by virtue of their complexation, astringent, antioxidant and radical scavenging activities, and their ability to form complex with proteins [194].

7.2. Ellagitannins

Ellagitannins, namely geraniin and furosin isolated from *Phyllanthus muellerianus*, were demonstrated to stimulate cellular activity, differentiation and collagen synthesis of human skin keratinocytes and dermal fibroblasts. Geraniin and furosin increased the cellular energy status of human skin cells (dermal fibroblasts NHDF, HaCaT keratinocytes) and triggered the cells towards higher proliferation rates. Furosin and geraniin stimulated the biosynthesis of collagen from normal human dermal fibroblasts. Geraniin also significantly stimulated the differentiation in normal human epidermal keratinocytes while furosin had a minor influence on the expression of involucrin and cytokeratins K1 and K10. The study proved that geraniin exhibit stimulating activity on dermal fibroblasts and keratinocytes, leading to increased cell proliferation, barrier formation and formation of extracellular matrix proteins [98].

7.3. Flavanols and proanthocyanidins

Flavanols are a sub-family of flavonoids which are present in plants as aglycones, as oligomers, or esterified with gallic acid and the most common oligomers of procyanidins present in edible plants are derived from epicatechin [189].

Flavanols and procyanidins are chemically able to prevent oxidation, and their administration has been associated with a decrease in oxidative stress markers in humans with improve blood supply to the wounded area to accelerate wound healing. They have been shown to exert a wide range of biological activities including wound healing property. The known biological activities of proanthocyanidins include antioxidant activity, anti-inflammatory activity, antimicrobial activities and wound healing activities [92, 189, 195].

A redox-active grape seed proanthocyanidin extract has been shown to up regulate oxidant and tumor necrosis factor-α inducible VEGF expression in human keratinocytes. Furthermore this grape seed proanthocyanidin extract was shown to accelerate wound contraction and closure *in vivo*, to enhance deposition of connective tissue and to improve histological architecture [186].

Wound healing property of *Camellia sinensis,* also known as green tea, has been linked to the presence of proanthocyanidins which are mainly made up of epicatechin, epigallocatechin, epicatechin-3-gallate and epigallocatechin-3-gallate and these induce differentiation of epidermal keratinocytes and also accelerate epithelial neoformation during wound healing [196].

Similarly, a fraction of the methanol extract of *Persea americana* Mill. seeds, containing high amounts of procyanidins B1 and B2 as well as an A-type trimer, was shown to stimulate proliferation of normal primary keratinocytes and fibroblasts cells but on another hand inhibited the proliferation of HaCaT-keratinocytes [197].

A study conducted on a proanthocyanidins rich fraction from *Hamamelis verginiana* showed that this fraction strongly increased the proliferation of skin cells. This effect was attributed to the tannin fraction, consisting of hydrolysable and condensed tannins, which account to 12% of Hamamelis bark [198].

A study of the wound healing activities of the hydrolyzable tannins from the hydro-alcoholic stem bark extract of *Poincianella pluviosa* enhanced the proliferation of human keratinocytes and dermal fibroblasts, which suggests that epidermal barrier formation can be accelerated by the use of *P. pluviosa* [199]. Treatment of keratinocytes with apple procyanidins has been shown to inhibit apoptosis and promote cell proliferation, migration and survival, necessary for revascularization and re-epithelialization of the wound. *In vivo* studies have shown that apple procyanidins (also known as procyanidins B1, B2 and C1) not only stimulate angiogenesis but also cause epithelial cells to grow mimicking keratinocyte re-epithelialization [200].

Epicatechin also blocks radiation-induced apoptosis via down-regulation Jun N-terminal kinase and p-38 in the HaCaT cells [201]. Epicatechin and procyanidins dimers are known to inhibit NADPH-oxidase and the subsequent superoxide production by directly binding to the enzyme or regulating calcium influx, or potentially inhibiting the binding of ligands that trigger NADPH-oxidase activation to their receptors (e.g. TNF-α). These functions are means by which epicatechin may provide cytoprotection to the cell. Both epicatechin and the respective procyanidin dimers can interact with the DNA-binding site of the nuclear factor kappa B (NF-κB) proteins, preventing the interaction of NF-κB with κB sites in gene promoters, thus inhibiting gene transcription [189]. The reduced NF-κB activation results in the suppression of inflammatory cytokines [200].

Procyanidins are known to induce the differentiation of keratinocytes. It has been reported that epigallocatechin-3-gallate induces differentiation of human epidermal keratinocytes [202]. In comparison to epigallocatechin-3-gallate, procyanidin B2 is more inductive to differentiation at lower concentrations [92].

Procyanidin B2 is also known to have beneficial effects in pathologies with pro-inflammatory components by inhibiting NF-κB-driven gene expression, including various cytokines and anti-apoptotic prote [203, 204]. It has been reported that several selective protein kinase C inhibitors, including procyanidin B-2, promote hair epithelial cell growth [205]. This presupposes that procyanidin B2 could be useful for aesthetic purposes during wound healing by stimulating the regrowth of skin appendages in the wounded area.

Procyanidin C1 inhibits nitric oxide production and the release of pro-inflammatory cytokines (IL-6 and TNF-α). Additionally, the potent anti-inflammatory effect of procyanidin C1 occurs through inhibition of mitogen-activated protein kinase and NF-κB signaling pathways. These two factors play a major role in controlling inflammation in the wounds [206]. In wound healing, procyanidin C1 activity presents a novel and effective means of inflammation control. Procyanidin dimers and trimers extracted from grape seeds are also known to exhibit higher growth-promoting activity than the monomer on hair epithelial cells *in vivo* [207].

7.4. Flavonoids

Flavonoids are a chemically defined group of polyphenols that have a basic structure of two aromatic rings (A and B) linked through three carbons that usually form an oxygenated heterocycle (C ring). The chemical characteristics of the C ring define the various subgroups of flavonoids by providing different arrangements of hydroxy, methoxy, and glycosidic groups, and the bonding with other monomers [208].

An important effect of flavonoids is the scavenging of oxygen-derived free radicals, reduction of liquid peroxidation, anti-inflammatory and wound healing activities. A drug that inhibits lipid peroxidation is believed to increase the viability and strength of collagen fibers and prevents cell damage by promoting DNA synthesis Flavonoids prevent or delay the onset of cell necrosis and also improve vascularity to the wounded area [179].

Several flavonoids, including quercetin, result in a reduction in ischemia-reperfusion injury through the activity of constitutive nitric-oxide synthase which is important in maintaining the dilation of blood vessels [209]. Quercetin, in particular, inhibits both cyclooxygenase and lipoxygenase activities, thus diminishing the formation of their inflammatory metabolites [210, 211].

Certain flavonoids, notably diosmin and hesperidin, have been used routinely in Europe for many years to treat varicose veins, hemorrhoids, and the edema that accompanies chronic venous insufficiency. These flavonoids have now been employed in the treatment of wounds. Purified micronized flavonoid fraction, comprising 90% diosmin and 10% hesperidin, is basically used as a phelebotonic and vasculoprotector agent. It also has anti-inflammatory and anti-edematous actions. In a clinical study, groups with infected wounds that were orally and topically treatment, accelerated wound healing when compared to the untreated control group. This was confirmed with surface area measurements and histopathological evaluation. This study showed that oral or topical administration of micronized flavonoid fraction in infected wounds is beneficial [212].

A flavonoid rich fraction of *Martynia annua* L. has also been shown to induce mature collagen fibers and promote fibroblasts with improved angiogenesis in an *in vivo* model [213]. Isovitexin and vitexin are the major flavonoid constituents of *Jatropha multifida* L. which is used commonly for the treatment of infected wounds and skin [214].

Flavonoids from *Vernonia arborea* and *Pentas lanceolata* have been reported to promote wound healing by their astringent and antimicrobial properties, which seems to be responsible for wound contraction and increased rate of epithelialization [215].

Martynia annua L. is a plant that has tannins, phenols, flavonoids, carbohydrates and anthocyanins as its constituents [216]. A flavonoid rich fraction and luteolin isolated from *M. annua* was shown to improve wound healing in streptozotocin induced diabetic rats. The results showed that, percent wound contraction were significantly greater for the flavonoid rich fraction and luteolin-treated groups. Presence of matured collagen fibers and fibroblast with better angiogenesis were observed histopathologically in these groups [213].

8. Fats and oils with wound healing properties

Several unsaturated fatty acids such as oleic, linoleic, eicosapentanoic and arachidonic acids are among the natural ligands for perosisome proliferative activator receptors (PPAR) which are involved in wound healing. These PPAR are nuclear hormone receptors and are up regulated in keratinocytes after injury and have been found to be important regulators of re-epithelialization [217, 218]. Also ω-3 polyunsaturated fatty acids (PUFA) eicosapentaenoic acid (EPA) and docosahexaenoic acid (DHA) affect the synthesis and activity of proinflammatory cytokines which to a large extent initiate the inflammatory stage of wound healing [219, 220]. It can therefore be said that the presence of these fatty acids in plant extracts and other compounds could contribute to the survival and differentiation of keratinocytes through the activation of PPAR. Also they may promote the recovery of the epidermal barrier, skin homeostasis and anti-inflammatory activity to the skin during the wound healing process.

8.1. Eucalyptus oil (Dinkum oil)

This oil is obtained by steam distillation of fresh leaves of *Eucalyptus globules* which belongs to the family Myrtaceae. It is indigenous to Australia and Tasmania. It is cultivated in United States, Spain, Portugal and India. It contains eucalyptol, pinene, camphene, phellandrene, citronellal and geranyl acetates. In skin care, it is used to treat burns, blisters, herpes, cuts, wounds, skin infections and insect bites [221].

8.2. Aroeira (*Schinus terebinthifoliu*) oil

The aroeira tree (*Schinus terebinthifolius* Raddi.) belongs to the family Anacardiaceae and it is popularly known as Brazilian pepper, Florida Holly, rose pepper and Christmas berry. It is used to treat wounds and ulcers of skin and mucous membranes, against infections of the respiratory system, digestive system, genito-urinary tract, hemoptysis and metrorrhagia [222]. The essential oil of *S. terebinthifoliu* is obtained by hydro-distillation of crushed fresh leaves. Aroeira oil is reported to accelerate the healing process of wounds by significantly ($p < 0.01$) increasing contraction of oil-treated wounds in rats [223].

8.3. Virgin coconut oil

Cocos nucifera L. (Arecaceae), commonly known as coconut, is a palm, which thrives within the tropical zone. Its fresh kernel is consumed by people all over the world. Oil of *C. nucifera* which is extracted from the dried inner flesh of coconut [224] predominantly contains medium chain triglycerides, with 86.5% saturated fatty acids, 5.8% monounsaturated fatty acids, and 1.8% polyunsaturated fatty acids. Virgin coconut oil is also known to have antibacterial and antifungal properties [225, 226]. Excised wounds treated with virgin coconut oil healed much faster, as indicated by a decreased time of complete epithelization and increased in pepsin-soluble collagen, as well as an increase in fibroblast proliferation and neovascularization [227]. Also in burn wounds, there was improvement in wound contraction and decreased period of epithelialization when treated with coconut oil [224].

8.4. *Vitis vinifera* (grape) oil

Oil extracted from the seeds of grapes *Vitis vinifera* (Family Vitaceae) has been found to exhibit wound healing activity. In the excision wound model, grape oil-treated animals had increased wound area contraction and hydroxyproline content. Also histological analysis of the grape oil-treated wound tissue showed increased well organized collagen band [228].

8.5. *Vaccinium macrocarpon* (cranberry) oil

Vaccinium macrocarpon (family Ericaceae) is an evergreen creeping shrub native to North America [229]. Excision wounds on animals treated with cranberry oil showed faster rates of wound area contraction with higher hydroxyproline content. The cranberry oil-treated wound tissue had well organized bands of collagen [228].

8.6. *Melaleuca alternifolia* (Tea tree) oil

The essential oil derived from steam distillation of the leaves and terminal branches of *Melaleuca alternifolia* (family Myrtaceae) commonly known as tea tree [230], is composed of a mixture of monoterpenes, 1-terpinen-4-ol, cineole and other hydrocarbons. Tea tree oil possesses antimicrobial, anti-inflammatory and analgesic properties [231]. Tea tree oil has been reported to aid in healing of bacterial infected wounds, including diabetic wounds, characterized by reduced healing time, rapid reduction in inflammation, pain and wound odor [232, 233].

8.7. *Vitellaria paradoxa* (Shea tree) oil

Vitellaria paradoxa (family Sapotaceae) commonly known as shea butter is an indigenous species of Sub-Saharan African [234]. The nuts and seeds are a very rich source of fats and oils, from which shea butter is derived. Shea butter is known to accelerate healing after circumcision [235]. The healing effect of shea butter may be attributed to the presence of allantoin, since it is a substance known to stimulate the growth of healthy tissues in ulcerous wounds [236].

8.8. Virgin fatty oil of *Pistacia lentiscus*

Pistacia lentiscus L. (Anacardiaceae) is a dioecious sclerophyllous evergreen species widely distributed along the Mediterranean basin. The essential oil of *P. lentiscus* obtained by hydro-distillation of leaves, fruits or trunk exudates called mastic gum [229] contains 73% unsaturated fatty acids (oleic and linoleic) and 25.8% saturated fatty acids (palmitic and stearic) and has been proven to exhibit antimicrobial, antioxidant, anti-inflammatory and antiatherogenic activities [237, 238]. The virgin fatty oil of *P. lentiscus* exhibited wound healing property in burn wound model in rabbits. *P. lentiscus* oil treated wounds showed higher wound contraction and faster time of healing as compared to the untreated wounds. *P. lentiscus* virgin fatty oil promoted significantly ($p < 0.05$) wound contraction and reduces epithelization period in rabbit model [239].

9. Miscellaneous substances

9.1. Wound healing properties of honey

Honey is a collection of nectar processed by honey bees [240]. It is rich in nutrients and defined substances such as glucose, fructose, sucrose, minerals, vitamins, antioxidants, amino acids and many other products, which may be responsible for its numerous therapeutic roles and potency [241]. Its therapeutic properties include antimicrobial activity which may be attributed to its osmotic effect, a naturally low pH, and the production of hydrogen peroxide [242, 243]. Honey attacks antibiotic-resistant strains of bacteria and prevents bacterial growth even when wounds are heavily infected [244]. Again, honey has been reported to exhibit antioxidant activity [245, 246]. In wound care, honey has been used extensively as wound healing agent for almost all kinds of wounds. It has been assessed for the treatment of venous leg ulcers, burns, chronic leg ulcers, pressure ulcers, as well as diabetic wound [247], with scarless healing in cavity wounds, less edema, fewer polymorphonuclear and mononuclear cell infiltrations, less necrosis, better wound contraction, improved epithelialization, lower glycosaminoglycan and proteoglycan concentrations, increased granulation tissue formation and tissue growth, collagen synthesis and development of new blood vessels in the bed of wounds [241].

10. Conclusion

Most of these medicinal plants and natural products traditionally used for the treatment and management of these various types of wounds had their wound healing properties, including wound contraction, tensile strength, antioxidant and antimicrobial activities, hydroxyproline content assay and histological investigations namely re-epithelization, collagen synthesis, granulation, proliferation and differentiation of fibroblasts and keratinocytes, assessed and evaluated through *in vitro* and *in vivo* model studies. Hence there is a need to subject these products to both primary and advanced clinical studies with specific types of wounds to ascertain or confirm the reported wound healing properties. These trials must be done after safety profiles of these products have been determined.

Author details

Christian Agyare[1*], Emelia Oppong Bekoe[2], Yaw Duah Boakye[1], Susanna Oteng Dapaah[1], Theresa Appiah[1] and Samuel Oppong Bekoe[3]

*Address all correspondence to: cagyare.pharm@knust.edu.gh; chrisagyare@yahoo.com

1 Department of Pharmaceutics, Faculty of Pharmacy and Pharmaceutical Sciences, Kwame Nkrumah University of Science and Technology, Kumasi, Ghana

2 Department of Pharmaceutics and Pharmaceutical Microbiology, School of Pharmacy, University of Ghana, Legon, Accra, Ghana

3 Department of Pharmaceutical Chemistry, Faculty of Pharmacy and Pharmaceutical Sciences, Kwame Nkrumah University of Science and Technology, Kumasi, Ghana

References

[1] Ramzi SC, Vinay K, Stanley R. Pathologic Basis of Diseases, 5th ed., WB Saunders Company, Philadelphia; 1994. p. 86.

[2] Strodtbeck F. Physiology of wound healing. Newborn Infant Nurs Rev. 2001; 1: 43–45.

[3] Mathieu D, Linke JC, Wattel F. Non-healing wounds. In: Handbook on hyperbaric medicine, Mathieu DE (ed). Netherlands: Springer; 2006; p. 812.

[4] Menke NB, Ward KR, Witten TM, Bonchev DG, Diegelmann RF. Impaired wound healing. Clin Dermatol. 2007; 25: 19–25.

[5] Nelzen O, Bergqvist D, Lindhagen A. The prevalence of chronic lower-limb ulceration has been underestimated: results of a validated population questionnaire. Br J Surg. 1996; 83: 255–258.

[6] Baranoski S, Ayello EA. Wound dressings: an evolving art and science. Adv Skin Wound Care. 2012; 25: 87–92.

[7] Benbow M. Debridement: wound bed preparation. J Community Nurs. 2011; 25: 18–23.

[8] MacDonald J. Global initiative for wounds and lymphedema. J Lymphedema. 2009; 4: 92–95.

[9] Houghton PJ, Hylands PJ, Mensah AY, Hensel A, Deters A. *In vitro* tests and ethnopharmacological investigations: wound healing as an example. J Ethnopharmacol. 2005; 100: 100–107.

[10] Agyare C, Asase A, Lechtenberg M, Niehues M, Deters A, Hensel A. An ethnopharmacological survey and *in vitro* confirmation of ethnopharmacological use of medicinal

plants used for wound healing in Bosomtwi-Atwima-Kwanwoma area, Ghana. J Ethnopharmacol. 2009; 125: 393–403.

[11] Davidson JM. Animal models for wound repair. Archives Derm Res. 1998; 290: 1–11.

[12] Dorsett-Martin WA, Wysocki AB. Rat models of skin wound healing. In: Source Book of Models for Biomedical Research, Humana Press; 2008. p. 778.

[13] Gal P, Kilik R, Mokry M, Vidinsky B, Vasilenko T, Mozes S, Lenhardt L. Simple method of open skin wound healing model in corticosteroid-treated and diabetic rats: standardization of semi-quantitative and quantitative histological assessments. Vet Med. 2008; 53: 652–659.

[14] Gottrup F, Argen MS, Karlsmark T. Models for use in wound healing research: a survey focusing on *in vitro* and *in vivo* adult soft tissue. Wound Repair Regen. 2000; 8: 83–96.

[15] Tarnuzzer RW, Schultz GS. Biochemical analysis of acute and chronic wound environments. Wound Repair Regen. 1996; 4: 321–325.

[16] Agyare C, Bempah SB, Boakye YD, Ayande PG, Adarkwa-Yiadom M, Mensah KB. Evaluation of antimicrobial and wound healing potential of *Justicia flava* and *Lannea welwitschii*. Evid Based Complement Altern. 2013. Article ID 632927, 10 pp.

[17] Burkill HM. 1985. The Useful Plants of Tropical West Africa. Royal Kew Botanical Gardens K, London, UK; 1985; pp. 293–295.

[18] Shubhashini S, Kantha DA. Investigations on the phytochemica activities and wound healing properties of *Adhatoda vasica* leave in Swiss albino mice. Afr J Plant Sci.2011; 5(2): 133–145.

[19] Fikru A ME, Eguale T, Debella A, Mekonnen GA. Evaluation of *in vivo* wound healing activity of methanol extract of *Achyranthes aspera* L. J Ethnopharmacol. 2012; 143: 469–474.

[20] Barua CC, Talakdar A, Barua AG, Chakraborty A, Sarma RK, Bora RS. Evaluation of the wound healing activity of methanolic extract of *Azadirachta Indica* (Neem) and *Tinospora cordifolia* (Guduchi) in rats. Pharmacologyonline. 2010; 1: 70–77.

[21] Hossain AI, Faisal M, Rahman S, Jahan R, Rahmatullah M. A preliminary evaluation of antihyperglycemic and analgesic activity of *Alternanthera sessilis* aerial parts. BMC Complement Altern Med. 2014; 14: 169.

[22] Jalalpure SS, Arawal N, Patil MB, Chimkode R, Tripathi A. Antimicrobial and wound healing activities of leaves of *Alternanthera sessilis* Linn. Int J Green Pharm. 2008; 2: 141–144.

[23] Ullah MO, Haque M, Urmi KF, Zulfiker AH, Anita ES, Begum M, Hamid K, Uddin SJ. Anti-bacterial activity and brine shrimp lethality bioassay of methanolic extracts of

fourteen different edible vege's from Bangladesh. Asian Pac J Trop Biomed. 2013; 3: 1–7.

[24] Neeharika V, Fatima H, Reddy BM. Evaluation of antinociceptive and antipyretic effect of Pupalia lappacea Juss. Int Curr Pharm J. 2013; 2: 23–28.

[25] Apenteng JA, Agyare C, Adu F, Ayande PG, Boakye YD. Evaluation of wound healing potential of different leaf extracts of *Pupalia lappacea*. Afr J Pharm Pharmacol. 2014; 8: 1039–1048.

[26] Udegbunam SO, Udegunam RI, Muogbo CC, Ayamwu MV, Nwaehugor CO.Wound healing and antibacterial properties of methanolic extract of *Pupulia lappacea* Juss in rats. BMC Complement Altern Med. 2014; 14: 157.

[27] Siddiqui MZ, Chowhury, Prasad N, Thomas M. Buchanania lanzan: a species of enormous potentials. World J Pharm Sci. 2014; 2: 374–379.

[28] Pattnaik A, Sarkar R, Sharma A, Yadav KK, Kumar A, Roy P, Sen T. Pharmacological studies on Buchanania lanzan Spreng.-A focus on wound healing with particular reference to anti-biofilm properties. Asian Pac J Trop Biomed. 2013; 3: 967–974.

[29] Chitra V, Dharabu PP, Pavan KK, Alla NR. Wound healing activity of alcoholic extract of *Buchanania lanzan* in Albino rats. Int J ChemTech Res. 2009; 1: 1026–1031.

[30] Jamil SS, Nizami Q, Salam M. Centella asiatica (Linn.) Urban: a review. Nat Prod Radiance. 2007; 6: 158–170.

[31] Bylka W, Znajdek-Awiżeń P, Studzińska-Sroka E, Brzezińska M. *Centella asiatica* in cosmetology. Postepy Dermatol Alergol. 2013; 30: 46–49.

[32] Bylka W, Znajdek-Awiżeń P, Studzińska-Sroka E, Dańczak-Pazdrowska A, Brzezińska M. Centella asiatica in dermatology: an overview. Phytother Res. 2014; 28: 1117–1124.

[33] Shukla A, Rasik AM, Jain GK, Shankar R, Kulshrestha DK, Dhawan BN. *In vitro* and *in vivo* wound healing activity of asiaticoside isolated from *Centella asiatica*. J Ethnopharmacol. 1999; 65: 1–11.

[34] Rechinger KH. Flora Iranica, Apiaceae. Academische Druck-U-Verganstalt. Graz: Austria. 1981; 162: 140–142.

[35] Mozaffarian V. A Dictionary of Iranian Plant Names. Tehran: Farhang Moaser Publisher; 1996. p. 739.

[36] Gohari AR, Saeidnia SA. Review on Phytochemistry of *Cuminum cyminum* seeds and its standards from field to market. Pharmacognosy J. 2011; 3: 1–5.

[37] Patil DN KA, Shahapurkar AA, Hatappakki BC. Natural cumin seeds for wound healing activity in albino rats. Int J Biol Chem. 2009; 3: 148–152.

[38] Nayak BS, Pinto-Pereira ML. Catharanthus roseus flower extract has wound-healing activity in Sprague Dawley rats. BMC Compliment Altern Med. 2006; 6: 41–39.

[39] Krasner DL RG, Sibbald RG. Chronic wound care: A Clinical source book for health professionals, HMP Communications, Malvern, Ala, USA, 4th ed.; 1990.

[40] Agyare C, Dwobeng AS, Agyepong N, Boakye YD, Mensah KB, Ayande PG, Adarkwa-Yiadom M. Antimicrobial, antioxidant, and wound healing properties of *Kigelia africana* (Lam.) Beneth. and *Strophanthus hispidus* DC. Adv Pharmacol Sci. 2013. Article ID 692613, 10 pp.

[41] Singh VP, Sharma SK, Kare VS. Medicinal plants from Ujjain District Madhya Pradesh, Indian Drugs. 1980; 17: 7–12.

[42] Shah GL, Gopal GV. Ethnomedical notes from the tribal inhabitants of the north Gujarat (India). J Ecotoxicol Bot. 1988; 6: 193–221.

[43] Joshi MC, Patel MB, Mehta PJ. Some folk medicines of Dangs, Gujarat State. Bull Med Ethnobot Res. 1980; 1: 8–24.

[44] Veerapur VP, Palkar MB, Srinivasa H, Kumar MS, Patra S, Rao PGM, Srinivasan KK. The effect of ethanol extract of *Wrightia tinctoria* bark on wound healing in rats. J Nat Prod. 2004; 4: 155–159.

[45] Omale J, Ubimago UOTG. In-vitro anthelmintic activity of *Saba florida* (Benth) extracts against Nigerian adult earth worm (*Terrestris lumbricoides*). Am J Phytomed Clin Ther. 2014; 2(6), 758–766.

[46] Omale J, Victoria IA. Excision and incision wound healing potential of *Saba florida* (Benth) leaf extract in *Rattus novergicus*. Int J Pharm Biomed Res. 2010; 1: 101–107.

[47] Ahmed KKM, Rana AC, Dixit VK. *Calotropis* species (Ascelpediaceae) – A comprehensive review. Pharmacog Mag. 2005; 1: 48–52.

[48] Chitme HR, GhobadiR, Chandra M, Kaushik S. Studies on anti-diarrhoeal activity of *Calotropis gigantea* R. Br. in experimental animals. J Pharm Pharm. Sci. 2004; 7: 70–75.

[49] Argal A, Pathak AK. Antidiarrhoeal activity of *Calotropis gigantea* flowers. Indian J Nat Prod. 2005; 21: 42–44.

[50] Deshmukh PT, Fernandes J, Atul A, Toppo E. Wound healing activity of *Calotropis gigan*tea root bark in rats. J Ethnopharmacol. 2009; 125; 178–181.

[51] Parsons WT, Cuthbertson EG. Noxious weeds of Australia. CSIRO Publishing; 2001. 712.

[52] Rasik MA, Raghubir R, Gupta A, Shukla A, Dubey MP, Srivastava S, Jain HK, Kulshrestha KD. Healing potential of *Calotropis procera* on dermal wounds in guinea pigs. J Ethnopharmacol. 1999; 68: 261–266.

[53] Akkol EK, Koca U, Pesin I, Yilmazer D. Evaluation of the wound healing potential of *Achillea biebersteinii* Afan.(Asteraceae) by *in vivo* excision and incision models. Evid-Based Complement Altern Med. 2011. Article ID 474026, 7 pp., 2011.

[54] Almagboul AZ, Farroq AA, Tyagi BR. Antimicrobial properties of certain Sudanese plants used in folk medicine: screening for antibacterial activity part 2. Fitoterapia. 1985; 56: 103–109.

[55] Ekundayo OS, Sharma S, Rao EV. Essential oils of *Ageratum conyzoides*. Linn Planta Med. 1987; 54: 55–57.

[56] Borthakur N, Baruah AKS. Search for precocenes in *Ageratum conyzoides* L. of Northeast India. J India Chem Soc. 1987; 64: 580–581.

[57] Watt JM, Breyer-Brandwijk MG. The medicinal and poisonous plants of South and Eastern Africa.197–8. 2nd Edn. London. E&S Livingstone Ltd., London, UK; 1962. 1457.

[58] Oladejo OW, Imosemi IO, Osuagwu FC, Oluwadara OO, Aiku A, Adewoyin O, Ekpo OE, Oyedele OO, Akang EEU. Enhancement of cutaneous wound healing by methanolic extracts of *Ageratum conyzoides* in the Wistar rat. Afr J Biomed Res. 2003; 6: 27–31.

[59] De Rouw DEA. The fallow period as weed-break in shifting cultivation (tropical wet forests). Agric Ecosys Environ. 1995; 54: 31–43.

[60] Olaoye SOA. *Chromolaena odorata* in the tropics and its control in Nigeria. In: Moody K. (Ed.) Weed control in tropical crops. Volume II. Weed Science Society of the Los Banos, Philippines, 1986, pp. 279–293.

[61] Phan T, Wang Lee, See P, Grayer JR, Chan S, Lee ST. Phenolic compounds of *Chromolaena odorata* protect cultured skin cells from oxidative damage: implication for cutaneous wound healing. Biol Pharm Bull. 2001; 24: 1373–1379.

[62] Koca U, Suntar PI, Keles H, Yesilada E, Akkol EK. *In vivo* anti-inflammatory and wound healing activities of *Centaurea iberica* Trev. ex Spreng. J Ethnopharmacol. 2009; 126: 551–556.

[63] Nadkarni AK. Indian Materia Medica. Popular Prakashan Private Limited. Bombay: 3rd ed; 2007. 1163.

[64] Chopra RN, Nayar SL., Chopra IC. Glossary of Indian Medicinal Plants, Publications and Information Directorate, CSIR, New Delhi; 1956. 88–89.

[65] Kirtikar KR, Basu BD. Dehra Dun: International Book Distributors. Indian Medicinal Plants; 1999; 1347.

[66] Sadaf F, Saleem R, Ahmed M, Ahmad SI. Healing potential of cream containing extract of *Sphaeranthus indicus* on dermal wounds in guinea pigs. J Ethnopharmacol. 2006, 107: 161–163.

[67] Udupa AL, Kulkarni DR, Udupa SL. Effect of *Tridax Procumbens* on wound healing. Pharm Biol. 1995; 33: 37–40.

[68] Yaduvanshi B, Mathur R, Mathur SR, Velpandian T. Evaluation of wound healing potential of topical formulation of leaf juice of *Tridax procumbens* L. in mice. Indian J Pharm Sci. 2011; 73: 303–306.

[69] Yogesh PT, Biswaddeep D, Tania P, Deeali YT, Kishori GA, Pradeep BP. Evaluation of wound healing potential of aqueous and ethanolic extracts of *Tridax procubens* Linn. in Wistar Rat. Asian J Pharm Clin Res. 2012; 5: 4, 141–145.

[70] Leach MJ. Calendula officinalis and wound healing: A Systematic review. Wounds. 2008; 20: 236–243.

[71] Preethi KC, Kuttan R. Wound healing activity of flower extract of *Calendula offlcinalis*. J Basic Clin Physiol Pharmacol. 2009; 20: 73–80.

[72] Irvine FR. Woody Plants of Ghana. Oxford University Press, Oxford, UK 1961. 868.

[73] Houghton PJ. Tesausage tree (*Kigelia pinnata*): Ethnobotany and recent scientific work. S Afr J Bot. 2002; 68: 14–20.

[74] Picerno P AG, Marzocco S, Meloni M, Sanogo R, Aquino RP. Anti-inflammatory activity of verminoside from *Kigelia africana* and evaluation of cutaneous irritation in cell cultures and reconstituted human epidermis. J Nat Prod. 2005; 68: 1610–1614.

[75] Mensah AY, Fleischer TC, Adu F, Agyare C, Ameade AE. Antimicrobial and antioxidant properties of two Ghanaian plants used traditionally for wound healing. J Pharm Pharmacol. 2003; 55: S-4.

[76] Ofori-Kwakye K KA, Bayor MT. Wound healing potential of methanol extract of *Spathodea campanulata* stem bark formulated into a topical preparation. Afr J Trad Complement Altern Med. 2011; 8: 218–223.

[77] Saini NK SM, Srivastava B. Evaluation of wound healing activity of *Tecomaria capensis* leaves. Chin J Nat Med. 2012; 10: 138–141.

[78] Iwu MM. Handbook of African medicinal plants. CRC Press BR, Florida, United States; 1993. p. 464.

[79] Sofowora A. Medicinal plants and traditional medicines in Africa. New York CJ, Wiley & Sons, UK; 1993. p. 320.

[80] Dash GK, Murthy PN. Evaluation of *Argemone mexicana* L. leaves for wound healing activity. J Nat Prod Plant Res. 2011; 1: 46–56.

[81] Butera D, Tosoriere L, Di Gaudio F, Bongiorno A, Allegra M, Pintaudi AM, Kohen R, Livrea M. A. Antioxidant activities of sicilian prickly pear (*Opuntia ficus indica*) fruit extracts and reducing properties of its betalains: Betanin and indicaxanthin. J Agric Food Chem. 2002; 50: 6895–6901.

[82] Hassan F, El-RazekA, Hassan AA. Nutritional value and hypoglycemic effect of prickly cactus pear (*Opuntia Ficus-Indica*) fruit juice in alloxan-induced diabetic rats. Aust J Basic Appl Sci. 2012; 5: 356–377.

[83] Galati EM, Mondello MR, Giufferida D, Dugo G, Miceli N, Pergolizzi S, Taviano MF. Chemical characterization and biological effects of Sicilian *Opuntia ficus indica* (L.) Mill. Fruit juice: antioxidant and antiulcerogenic activity. J Agric Food Chem. 2003; 51: 4903–4908.

[84] Park EH, Chun MJ. Wound healing activity of *Opuntia ficus-indica*. J Ethnopharmacol. 2001; 72: 165–167.

[85] Trombetta D, Puglia C, Perri D, Licata A, Pergolizzi S, Lauriano ER, Bonina FP. Effect of polysaccharides from *Opuntia ficus-indica* (L.) cladodes on the healing of dermal wounds in the rat. Phytomedicine. 2006; 13: 352–358.

[86] Burkill HM. The Useful Plants of West Tropical Africa ne, vol 3:11, Royal Kew Botanical Gardens, Kew, London, UK; 1995. 868p.

[87] Mahmood AA, Sidik K, Salmah I. Wound healing activity of *Carica papaya* L. aqueous leaf extract in rats. Int J Mol Med Adv Sci. 2005; 1: 398–401.

[88] Nayak BS, Pereira LP, Maharaj D. Wound healing activity of *Carica papaya* L. in experimentally induced diabetic rats. Indian J Exp Biol. 2007; 45: 739.

[89] Gurung S, Škalko-Basnet N. Wound healing properties of *Carica papaya* latex: in vivo evaluation in mice burn model. J Ethnopharmacol. 2009; 121: 338–341.

[90] Agyare C, Ansah AO, Ossei PPS, Apenteng JA, Boakye YD. Wound healing and anti-infective properties of *Myrianthus arboreus* and *Alchornea cordifolia*. Med Chem. 2014; 4: 533–539.

[91] Chaudhari M, Mengi S. Evaluation of phytoconstituents of *Terminalia arjuna* for wound healing activity in rats. Phytother Res. 2006; 20: 799–805.

[92] Kisseih E, Lechtenber M, Petereit F, Sendker J, Brandt S, Agyare C, Hensel A. Phytochemical characterization and in vitro wound healing activity of leaf extracts from *Combretum mucronatum* Schum. & Thonn.: Oligomeric procyanidins as strong inductors of cellular differentiation. J Ethnopharmacol. 2015; 174: 628–636.

[93] Khan M, Patil PA, Shobha JC. Influence of *Bryophyllum pinnatum* (Lim.) leaf extract on wound healing in albino rats. J Nat Remedies. 2004; 4: 41–46.

[94] Agyare C, Amuah E, Adarkwa-Yiadom M, Osei-Asante S, Ossei SPP. Medicinal plants used for the treatment of wounds and skin infections: assessment of wound healing and antimicrobial properties of *Mallotus oppositifolius* and *Momordica charantia*. Int J Phytomedicine. 2014; 6: 50–58.

[95] Gordon-Gray KD. Cyperaceae in Natal. National Botanical Institute P, South Africa; 1995. p. 218.

[96] Chopra RN, Chopra IC, Varma BS. Glossary of Indian Medicinal Plants, CSIR, New Delhi; 1969. p. 119.

[97] Puratchikody A, Devi CN, Nagalakshmi G. Wound healing activity of *Cyperus rotundus* Linn Indian J Pharm Sci. 2006; 68: 97–101.

[98] Agyare C, Lechntenberg M, Deters A, Petereit F, Hensel A. Ellagitannins from Phyllanthus muellerianus (Kuntze) Exell.: Geraniin and furosin stimulate cellular activity, differentiation and collagen synthesis of human skin keratinocytes and dermal fibroblasts. Phytomedicine. 2011; 18: 617–624.

[99] Gonasekera MM, Gunawardan VK, Mohammed SG, Balasubramania S. Pregnancy terminating effects of *Jatropha curcas* in rats. J Ethnopharmacol. 1995; 47: 117–123.

[100] Igoli JO, Ogaji D. Tor-Anyim TA, Igoli NP.Traditional Medicine practice among the Igede people of Nigeria. Afr J Trad Compliment Altern Med. 2005; 2: 134–152.

[101] Shetty S, Udupa L. Evaluation of antioxidant and wound healing effects of alcoholic and aqueous extract of *Ocimum sanctum* Linn in rats. Evid-Based Complement Altern Med. 2008; 5: 95–101.

[102] Zippel J, Wells T, Hensel A. Arabinogalactan protein from Jatropha curcas L. seeds as TGFβ1-mediated inductor of keratinocyte in vitro differentiation and stimulation of GM-CSF, HGF, KGF and in organotypic skin equivalents. Fitoterapia. 2010; 81: 772–778.

[103] Kabran FA, Maciuk A, Okpekon TA, Leblanc K, Seon-Meniel B, Bories C, Champy P, Djakouré L A, Figadère B. Phytochemical and biological analysis of *Mallotus oppositifolius* (Euphorbiaceae). Planta Med. 2012; 78: 1381.

[104] Lodhi S, Pawar RS, Jain AP, Singhai AK. Wound healing potential of *Tephrosia purpurea* (Linn.) Pers. in rats. J Ethnopharmacol. 2006; 108: 204–210.

[105] Chularojmontri L, Suwatronnakorn M, Wattanapitayakul SK. *Phyllanthus emblica* L. enhances human umbilical vein endothelial wound healing and sprouting. Evid-Based Complement Altern Med. 2013. Article ID 720728, 9 pp., 2013.

[106] Kokane DD, More YR, Kale BM, Nehete NM, Mehendale CP, Gadgol HC. Evaluation of wound healing activity of root of *Mimosa pudica*. J Ethnopharmacol. 2009; 124: 311–315.

[107] Sivagamy M, Jeganathan, Manavalan R, Senthamarai R. Wound healing activity of *Indigofera enneaphylla* Linn. Int J Adv Pharm Chem Biol. 2012; 1: 211–214.

[108] Umachigi SP, Jayaveera KN, Kumar CA, Kumar GS¸ Kumar DK. Studies on wound healing properties of *Quercus infectoria*. Trop J Pharm Res. 2008; 7: 913–919.

[109] Oommen ST, Rao M, Raju CVN. Effect of oil of Hydnocarpus on wound healing1. Int J Lepr Other Mycobact Dis. 1999; 67: 154.

[110] Oommen ST. The effect of oil of hydnocarpus on excision wounds. Int J Lepr Other Mycobact Dis. 2000; 68: 69–70.

[111] Dokosi OB. Herbs of Ghana. Ghana Universities Press; 1998. p. 765.

[112] Annan K, Dickson R. Evaluation of wound healing actions of *Hoslundia opposita* Vahl, *Anthocleista nobilis* G. Don. and *Balanites aegyptiaca* L. J Sci Tech (Ghana), 2008; 28(2): 26–35.

[113] Bairy KL, Rao CM. Wound healing profiles of *Ginkgo biloba*. J Nat Remedies. 2001; 1: 25–27.

[114] Baruah A, Sarma D, Saud J, Singh RS. In vitro regeneration of *Hypericum patulum* Thunb.-A medicinal plant. Indian J Experiment Biol. 2001; 39: 947–949.

[115] Mukherjee KP, Verpoorte R, Suresh B. Evaluation of *in-vivo* wound healing activity of *Hypericum patulum* (Family: Hypericaceae) leaf extract on different wound model in rats. J Ethnopharmacol. 2000; 70: 315–321.

[116] Gleason HA, Cronquist A. Manual of Vascular Plants of Northeastern United States and Adjacent Canada. 2nd ed. Bronx, NY: The New York Botanical Garden; 1991. 810.

[117] Süntar IP, Akkol EK, Yılmazer D, Baykal T, Kırmızıbekmez H, Alper M, Yeşilada E. Investigations on the in vivo wound healing potential of *Hypericum perforatum* L. J Ethnopharmacol. 2010; 127: 468–477.

[118] Prisăcaru AI, Andritoiu CV, Andriescu C, Hăvârneanu EC, Popa M, Motoc AGM, Sava A. Evaluation of the wound-healing effect of a novel *Hypericum perforatum* ointment in skin injury. Rom J Morphol Embryol. 2013; 54: 1053–1059.

[119] Laeuchli S, Vannotti S, Hafner J, Hunziker T, French L. A Plant-derived wound therapeutic for cost-effective treatment of post-surgical scalp wounds with exposed one. Res Complement Med. 2014; 21: 88–93.

[120] Mainetti S, Carnevali F. An experience with pediatric burn wounds treated with a plant-derived wound therapeutic. J Wound Care. 2013; 22: 681–689.

[121] Godhwani S, Godhwani JL, Vyas DS. *Ocimum sanctum* – a preliminary study evaluating its immunoregulatory profile in albino rats. J Ethnopharmacol. 1988; 24: 193–198.

[122] Goel A, Kumar S, Singh DK, Bhatia AK. Wound healing potential of *Ocimum sanctum* Linn. with induction of tumor necrosis factor-alpha. Indian J. Exp. Biol. 2010; 48: 402–406.

[123] Osuagwu FC, Oladepo OW, Imosemi IO, Adewoyin BA, Adewoyin OO, Ekpe OE, Olumadara OO. Wound healing activities of methanolic extracts of *Ocimum gratissum* leaf in Wistar rats – a preliminary study. Afr J Med Sci. 2004; 33: 23–26.

[124] Chah KF, Eze CA, Emuelosi CE, Esimone CO. Antibacterial and wound healing properties of methanolic extracts of some Nigerian medicinal plants. J Ethnopharmacol. 2006; 104: 164–167.

[125] Abbiw DK. Useful plants of Ghana: West African uses of wild and cultivated plants. Intermediate Technology Publications and The Royal Botanic Gardens; Kew, UK 1990. p. 337.

[126] Olajide OA, Oladiran OO, Awo SO, Makinde JM. Pharmacological evaluation of *Hoslundia opposita*. Phytother. Res. 1998; 12: 364–366.

[127] Moshi MJ, Kagashe GA, Mwambo ZH. Plants used to treat epilepsy in Tanzanian tradition. J Ethnopharmacol. 2005; 97: 327–336.

[128] Shirwaikar A, Shenoy R, Udupa AL, Udupa SL, Shetty S. Wound healing property of ethanolic extract of leaves of *Hyptis suaveolens* with supportive role of antioxidant enzymes. Indian J Exp Biol. 2003; 41: 238–241.

[129] Shenoy C, Patil MB, Kumar R, Patil S. Preliminary phytochemical investigation and wound healing activity of *Allium cepa* Linn. (Liliaceae). Int J Pharm Pharm Sci. 2009; 2: 167–175.

[130] Mukerjee SK. *A revision of the Labiatae of the Indian Empire* (Doctoral dissertation), University of Edinburgh.

[131] Ryding O. Phylogeny of the Leucas Group (Lamiaceae). Syst Botany. 1998; 23: 235–247.

[132] Williamson EM. Major herbs of Ayurveda L, Churchill Livingstone, UK; 2002. p. 361.

[133] Manjunatha BK, Vidya SM, Krishna V, Mankani KL. Wound healing activity of *Leucas hirta*. Indian J Pharm Sci. 2006; 68: 380–384.

[134] Dahanukar SA, Kulkarni RA, Rege NN. Pharmacology of medicinal plants and natural products. Indian J Pharmacol. 2000; 32: S81–S118.

[135] Nayak BS, Isitor G, Davis EM, Pillai GK. The evidence based wound healing activity of *Lawsonia inermis* Linn. Phytother Res. 2007; 21(9): 827–831.

[136] Chidambara MKN, Vittal KR, Jyothi MV, Uma DM. Study on wound healing activity of *Punica granatum* peel. J Med Food. 2004; 7: 256–259.

[137] Kumar A, Singh A. Review on Hibiscus Rosa sinensis. Int J Res Pharm Biomed Sci., 2012; 3: 534–538.

[138] Nayak BS, Raju SS, Eversley M, Ramsubhag A. Evaluation of wound healing activity of *Lantana camara* L. – a preclinical study. Phytother Res. 2009; 23: 241–245.

[139] Bhaskar A, Nithya V. Evaluation of the wound-healing activity of *Hibiscus rosa sinensis* L. (Malvaceae) in Wistar albino rats. Indian J Pharmacol. 2012; 44: 694–698.

[140] Shivakumar H, Prakash T, Rao RN, Swamy BJ, Nagappa AN. Wound healing activity of the leaves of *Thespesia populnea*. J Nat Remedies. 2007; 7: 120–124.

[141] Nayak SB KJ, Milne MD, Pinto-Pereira L, Swanston HW. Extract of *Carapa guianensis* L. Leaf for its wound healing activity using three wound models. Evid-Based Complement Altern Med. 2011, Article ID 419612, 6 pp.

[142] Hukkeri VI, Nagathan CV, Karadi RV, Patil BS. Antipyretic and wound healing activities of *Moringa oleifera* Lam. in rats. Indian J Pharm Sci. 2006; 68:124–126.

[143] Pandey IP, Ahmed SF, Chhimwal S, Pandey S. Chemical composition and wound healing activity of volatile oil of leaves of *Azadirachta indica* A. Juss. Adv Pure Appl Chem. 2012; 1: 62–66.

[144] Roy K, Shivakumar, Sarkar S. Wound healing potential of leaf extracts of *Ficus religiosa* on Wistar albino strain rats. Int J Pharm Tech Res, 2009; 1: 506–508.

[145] Kirtikar KR, Basu BD. In; Indian Medicinal Plants, 1st edn. Vol. III, International Book Publishers, Dehradun; 1980; 676.

[146] Chopra RN. In: Indigenous Drugs of India, 2nd edn., Vol. I. Academic Publishers, Kolkata; 1993; 792.

[147] Rahman MM. Bangladesh: (IUCN) International Union for Conservation of Nature. Invasive plants of Sundarbans. Interim report under SBCP Project; 2003. p.132.

[148] Goel RK KSA-udfisweoMs, Tamrab hasma, *Asparagus racemosus* and *Zingiber officinale*. Indian J Pharmacol. 2002; 34: 100–110.

[149] Agarwal PK, Singh A, Gaurav K, Goel S, Khanna HD, Goel RK. Evaluation of wound healing activity of extracts of plantain banana (*Musa sapientum* var. *paradisiaca*) in rats. Indian J Exp Biol. 2009; 47:32–34.

[150] Lal B, Mishra N. Importance of *Embelia ribes*: An update. Int J Pharm Sci Res. 2013; 4: 3823–3838.

[151] Kumara SHM, Krishna V, Shankarmurthy K, Abdul RB, Mankani KL, Mahadevan KM, Harish BG, Raja NH. Wound healing activity of embelin isolated from the ethanol extract of leaves of *Embelia ribes* Burm. J Ethnopharmacol. 2007; 109: 529–534.

[152] Mittal A, Satish SS, Anima P. Evaluation of wound healing, antioxidant and antimicrobial efficacy of *Jasminum auriculatum* Vahl. leaves. Avicenna J Phytomed. 2015: 1–11.

[153] Chaturvedi AP, Kumar M, Tripathi YB. Efficacy of *Jasminum grandiflorum* L. leaf extract on dermal wound healing in rats. Int Wound J. 2013; 10: 675–682.

[154] Rajvaidhya S, Nagori BP, Singh GK, Dubey BK, Desai P, Jain S. A review on *Argemone mexicana* Linn.-an Indian medicinal plant. Int J Pharm Sci Res. 2012; 3: 2494–2504.

[155] Kiran K, Asad M. Wound healing activity of *Sesamum indicum* L. seed and oil in rats. Ind. J Exp Bio. 2008; 46: 777–782.

[156] Parmer VS JS, Bisht KS. Phytochemistry of genus *Piper*, Phytochemistry. 1997; 46: 597–673.

[157] Santhanam G, Nagarajan S. Wound healing activity of *Curcuma aromatica* and *Piper betle*. Fitoterapia. 1990; 61: 458–459.

[158] Rubatzky VE, Yamaguchi M. World vegetables: principles, production and nutritive values. 2nd edn. Chapman & Hall, New York, United States; 1997. p. 843.

[159] P Phillips SM. Portulacaceae. In: Beentje, H.J. (Ed). Flora of Tropical East Africa. A.A. Balkema, Rotterdam, Netherlands; 2002; p. 40.

[160] Rashed NA, Afifi UF, Disi AM. Simple evaluation of the wound healing activity of a crude extract of *Portulaca oleracea* L. (growing in Jordan) in *Mus musculus* JVI-1. J Ethnopharmacol. 2003; 88:131–136.

[161] Pennington TD. The genera of Sapotaceae. Royal Botanic Gardens K, Richmond, United Kingdom and the New York Botanical Garden, New York, United States; 1991. p. 307.

[162] Adetutu A, Morgan WA, Corcoran O. Ethnopharmacological survey and *in vitro* evaluation of wound-healing plants used in South-western Nigerian. J Ethnopharmacol. 2011; 137: 50–56.

[163] Nayak BS, Sandiford S, Maxwell A. Evaluation of the wound-healing activity of ethanolic extract of *Morinda citrifolia* L. Leaf. Evid-Based Complement Altern Med. 2009; 6: 351–356.

[164] Nayak SB, Vinuta B, Geetha B, Sudha B. Experimental evaluation of *Pentas lanceolata* flowers for wound healing activity in rats. Fitoterapia. 2005; 76: 671–675.

[165] Karodi, Jadhav M, Rub R, Bafna A. Evaluation of the wound healing activity of a crude extract of *Rubia cordifolia* L. (Indian madder) in mice. Int J Appl Res Nat Prod. 2009; 2: 12–18.

[166] Jaswanth A, Sathya S, Ramu S, Puratchikody A, Ruckmani K. Effect of root extract of *Aegle marmelos* on dermal wound healing in rats. Anc Sci life. 2001; 20: 111.

[167] Gautam MK, Purohit V, Agarwal M, Singh A, Goel RK. In vivo healing potential of *Aegle marmelos* in excision, incision, and dead space wound models. Sci World J. 2014. Article ID 740107, 9 pp.

[168] Lemmens RHMJ. *Mimusops elengi* L. In: Louppe D, Oteng-Amoako, A. A., Brink, M. (Editors). Prota 7(1): Timbers/Bois d'œuvre 1 [CD-Rom]. PROTA, Wageningen, Netherlands; 2005.

[169] Shah PJ, Gandhi MS, Shah MB, Goswami SS, Santani D. Study of *Mimusops elengi* bark in experimental gastric ulcers. J Ethnopharmacol. 2003; 89: 305–311.

[170] Gupta N, Jain UK. Investigation of wound healing activity of methanolic extract of stem bark of *Mimusops elengi* Linn. Afr J Tradit Complement Altern Med. 2011; 8: 98–103.

[171] Ratsch C. The Encyclopedia of Psychoactive Plants: Ethnopharmacology and its Applications. Rochester: Park Street Press 1998: p. 944.

[172] Avery AG. "Historical Review." In Blakeslee – the Genus Datura, New York: Ronald Press; 1959: 3–15.

[173] Nithya V. Evaluation of the wound healing activity of Datura metel L. in Wistar albino rats. Inventi Rapid: Ethnopharmacol. 2011; 4.

[174] Dewangan H BM, Jaiswal V, Verma VK. Potential wound healing activity of the ethanolic extract of *Solanum xanthocarpum* Schrad and Wendl leaves. Pak J Pharm Sci. 2012; 25: 189–194.

[175] Bharti M, Bias M, Singhasiya A. Evaluation of wound healing activity of *Cissus quadrangularis*. World J Pharm Pharm Sci. 2014; 3: 822–834.

[176] Gbedema SY, Kisseih E, Adu F, Annan K, Woode E. Wound healing properties and kill kinetics of *Clerodendron splendens* G. Don, a Ghanaian wound healing plant. Pharmacog Res. 2001; 2:63–68.

[177] Liu HW, Nakanishi K. The structure of balanitins; potent molluscicides isolated from *Balanites aegyptiaca*. Tetrahedron. 1982; 38:513–519.

[178] Kojima H, Yanai T, Toyota A. Essential oil constituents from Japanese and Indian *Curcuma aromatica* rhizomes. Planta Med. 1998; 64: 380–381.

[179] Arun MSS, Anima P. Herbal boon for wounds. Int J Pharmacy Pharm Sci. 2013; 5, 1–12.

[180] Bhagavathula N, Warner RL, DaSilva M, McClintock SD, Barron A, Aslam MN, Varani J. A combination of curcumin and ginger extract improves abrasion wound healing in corticosteroid-impaired hairless rat skin. Wound Repair and Regen. 2009; 17: 360–366.

[181] Pawar RS, Toppo FA, Mandloi AS, Shaikh S. Exploring the role of curcumin containing ethanolic extract obtained from *Curcuma longa* (rhizomes) against retardation of wound healing process by aspirin. Indian J Pharmacol. 2015; 47:160–166.

[182] Kundu S, Biswas TK, Das P, Kumar S, De DK. Turmeric (*Curcuma longa*) rhizome paste and honey show similar wound healing potential: a preclinical study in rabbits. The Int J Lower Extre Wounds. 2005; 4: 205–213.

[183] Sidhu GS, Singh AK, Thaloor D, Banaudha KK, Patnaik GK, Srimal RC, Maheshwari RK. Enhancement of wound healing by curcumin in animals. Wound Repair Regen. 1998; 6: 167–177.

[184] Rouhollahi E, Moghadamtousi SZ, Hajiaghaalipour F, Zahedifard M, Tayeby F, Awang K, Mohamed Z. *Curcuma purpurascens* Bi. rhizome accelerates rat excisional wound healing: involvement of hsp70/Bax proteins, antioxidant defense, and angiogenesis activity. Drug Des Dev Ther. 2015; 9: 5805–5813.

[185] Kamel MS, Ontani K, Kurokawa T, Assaf HM, El-Shannawany MA. Studies on *Balanites aegyptiaca* fruits, an antidiabetic Egyptian folk medicine. Phytochemistry. 1991; 31: 3565–3569.

[186] Khanna S, Venojarvi M, Roy S, Sharma N, Trikha P, Bagchi D, Bagchi M, Sen CK. Dermal wound healing properties of redox-active grape seed proanthocyanidins. Free Rad Biol Med 2002; 33: 1089–1096.

[187] Ghosh P, Gaba A. Phyto-extracts in Wound healing. J Pharm Sci. 2013; 16: 760–820.

[188] Thakur R, Jain N, Pathak R, Sandhu SS. Practices in wound healing studies of plants. Evid-Based Complement Alternat Med. 2011; 17. Article ID 438056.

[189] Fraga CG, Oteiza PI. Dietary flavonoids: role of (−)-epicatechin and related procyanidins in cell signaling. Free Rad Biol Med 2011; 51: 813–823.

[190] Fakhim SA, Babaei H, Nia AK, Ashrafi J. Wound healing effect of topical grape seed extract (*Vitis Vinifera*) on rat palatal mucosa. Int J Curr Res Aca Rev. 2015; 3(6):477–489.

[191] Shirley D, McHale C, Gomez G. Resveratrol preferentially inhibits IgE-dependent PGD2 biosynthesis but enhances TNF production from human skin mast cells. Bioch Bioph Acta 2016; 1860: 678–685

[192] Novelle MG, Wahl D, Diéguez C, Bernier M, de Cabo R. Resveratrol supplementation: Patel, H. H., and Insel, P. A. Lipid rafts and caveolae and their role in compartmentation of redox signaling. Antioxidant and Redox Signaling 2009; 11: 1357–1372.

[193] Yaman I DH, Kara C, Kamer E, Diniz G, Ortac R, Sayin O. Effects of resveratrol on incisional wound healing in rats. Surg Today. 2013; 43(12): 1433–1438.

[194] Haslam, E. Natural polyphenols (vegetable tannins) as drugs: possible modes of action. J Nat Prod. 1996; 59: 205–215.

[195] Aerts RJ, Barry TN and McNabb WC. (Polyphenols and agriculture: beneficial effects of proanthocyanidins in forages. Agric Ecosys Environ. 1999; 75: 1–12.

[196] Neves ALA, Komesu MC, Di Matteo, MA. Effects of green tea use on wound healing. Int J Morphol. 2010; 28: 905–910.

[197] Ramos-Jerz MDR, Villanueva S, Jerz G, Winterhalter P, Deters AM. *Persea americana* Mill. Seed: Fractionation, characterization, and effects on human keratinocytes and fibroblasts. Evid-Based Complement Alternat Med. 2013; 2013: 391247.

[198] Deters A, Dauer A, Schnetz E, Fartasch M, Hensel, A. High molecular compounds (polysaccharides and proanthocyanidins) from *Hamamelis virginiana* bark: Influence on human skin keratinocyte proliferation and differentiation and influence on irritated skin. Phytochemistry. 2001; 58: 949–958.

[199] Bueno FG, Panizzon GP, Souza EV, Mello DL, Lechtenberg M, Petereit F, João Carlos J, de Mello P, Hensel A. Hydrolyzable tannins from hydroalcoholic extract from *Poincianella pluviosa* stem bark and its wound-healing properties: phytochemical investiga-

tions and influence on in vitro cell physiology of human keratinocytes and dermal fibroblasts. Fitoterapia. 2014; 99: 252–260.

[200] McKelvey K, Xue M, Whitmont K, Shen K, Cooper A, Jackson C. Potential anti-inflammatory treatments for chronic wounds. Wound Pract Res. 2012; 20: 86–89.

[201] Shin YS, Shin HA, Kang SU, Kim JH, Oh YT, Park KH, Kim CH. Effect of epicatechin against radiation-induced oral mucositis: *In vitro* and *in vivo* study. PLoS ONE 2013; 8: e69151.

[202] Balasubramanian S, Efimova T, Eckert RL. Green tea polyphenol stimulates Ras, MEKK1, MEK3 and p38 cascade to increase activator protein 1 factor-dependent involucrin gene expression in normal human keratinocytes. J Biol Chem. 2002; 277: 1828–1836.

[203] Mackenzie GG, Adamo AM, Decker NP, Oteiza PI. Dimeric procyanidin B2 inhibits constitutively active NF-kappa B in Hodgkin's lymphoma cells independently of the presence of Ikappa B mutations. Biochem Pharmacol. 2008; 75: 1461–1471.

[204] Mackenzie GG, Delfino JM, Keen CL, Fraga CG, Oteiza PI. Dimeric procyanidins are inhibitors of NF-kappa B-DNA binding. J Biol Chem. 2002; 277: 1828–1836.

[205] Kamimura A, Takahashi T. Procyanidn B-2 extracted from apples, promotes hair growth: a laboratory study. Brit J Dermatol. 2002; 146: 41–51.

[206] Byun EB, Sung NY, Byun EH, Song DS, Kim JK, Park JH, Song BS, Park SH, Lee JW, Byun MW and Kim JH. The procyanidin trimer C1 inhibits LPS-induced MAPK and NF-κB signaling through TLR4 in macrophages. Int J Immunopharmacol. 2013; 15: 450–456.

[207] Takahashi T, Kamiya T, Hasegawa A, Yokoo Y. Procyanidin oligomers selectively and intensively promote proliferation of mouse hair epithelial cells *in vitro* and activate hair follicle growth *in vivo*. J Invest Dermatol. 1999; 112: 310–316.

[208] Crozier A, Jaganath IB, Clifford MN., Deters A, Dauer A, Schnetz E, Fartasch M, Hensel, A. High molecular compounds (polysaccharides and proanthocyanidins) from *Hamamelis virginiana* bark: influence on human skin keratinocyte proliferation and differentiation and influence on irritated skin. Phytochemistry. 2001; 58: 949–958.

[209] Nijveldt RJ, van Nood E, van Hoorn DE, Boelens PG, van Norren K, van Leeuwen PA. Flavonoids: a review of probable mechanisms of action and potential applications. Am J Clin Nutr. 2001; 74 (4): 418–425.

[210] Robak J, Gryglewski RJ. Bioactivity of flavonoids. Pol J Pharmacol 1996; 48: 555.

[211] Ferrandiz ML, Nair AG, Alcaraz MJ. Inhibition of sheep platelet arachidonate metabolism by flavonoids from Spanish and Indian medicinal herbs. Pharmazie 1990; 45: 206–208.

[212] Hasanoglu A, Ara C, Ozen S, Kali K, Senol M, Ertas E. Efficacy of micronized flavonoid fraction in healing of clean and infected wounds. Int J Angiol. 2001; 10(1): 41–44.

[213] Lodhi S, Singhai KK. Wound healing effect of flavonoid rich fraction and luteolin isolated from *Martynia annua* Linn. on streptozotocin induced diabetic rats. Asian Pac J Trop Med. 2013; 6: 253–259.

[214] Hirota BCK, Miyazaki CMS, Mercali CA, Verdan MC, Kalegari M, Gemin C, Lordello AL, Miguel MD, Miguel OG. C-glycosyl flavones and a comparative study of the antioxidant, hemolytic and toxic potential of *Jatropha multifida* leaves and bark. Int J Phytomedicine 2012; 4: 1–5.

[215] Ambigas S, Narayanan R, Gowri D, Sukumar D, Madhavan S. Evaluation of wound healing activity of flavonoids from *Ipomea carnea* Jacq. Ancient Sci Life 2007; 26: 45–51.

[216] Mali PC, Ansari AS, Chaturvedi M. Antifertility effect of chronically administered *Martynia annua* root extract on male rats. J Ethnopharmacol. 2002; 82(3): 61–67.

[217] Goldstein JT, Dobrzyn A, Clagett-Dame M, Pike JW, DeLuca HF. Isolation and characterization of unsaturated fatty acids as natural ligands for the retinoid-X receptor. Arch Biochem Biophys. 2003; 420(1): 185–193.

[218] Michalik L, Wahli W. Peroxisome proliferator-activated receptors (PPARs) in skin health, repair and disease. Biochim Biophys Acta (BBA)-Mol Cell Biol Lipids. 2007; 1771 (8): 991–998.

[219] Efron PA, Moldawer LL. Cytokines and wound healing: the role of cytokine and anticytokine therapy in the repair response. J Burn Care Res. 2004; 25(2): 149–160.

[220] Calder PC. n–3 Polyunsaturated fatty acids and inflammation: from molecular biology to the clinic. Lipids. 2003; 38(4): 343–352.

[221] Hukkeri VI, Karadi R V, Akki KS, et al. Wound healing property of Eucalyptus globulus L. leaf extract'. Indian Drugs. 2002; 39(9): 481–483.

[222] Medal JC, Vitorino MD, Habeck DH, Gillmore JL, Pedrosa JH, De Sousa LP. Host specificity of *Heteroperreyia hubrichi* Malaise (Hymenoptera: Pergidae), a potential biological control agent of Brazilian peppertree (*Schinus terebinthifolius* Raddi). Biol Control. 1999; 14(1): 60–65.

[223] Estevão LRM, Mendonca FDS, Baratella-Evêncio L, et al. Effects of aroeira (*Schinus terebinthifoliu* Raddi) oil on cutaneous wound healing in rats. Acta Cir Bras. 2013; 28(3): 202–209.

[224] Srivastava P, Durgaprasad S. Burn wound healing property of *Cocos nucifera*: an appraisal. Indian J Pharmacol. 2008; 40(4): 144–146.

[225] Bergsson G, Arnfinnsson J, Steingrimsson Ó, Thormar H. Killing of Gram-positive cocci by fatty acids and monoglycerides. Note Apmis. 2001; 109 (10): 670–678.

[226] Chadeganipour M, Haims A. Antifungal activities of pelargonic and capric acid on *Microsporum gypseum*. Mycoses. 2001; 44(3–4):109–112.

[227] Nevin KG, Rajamohan T. Effect of topical application of virgin coconut oil on skin components and antioxidant status during dermal wound healing in young rats. Skin Pharmacol Physiol. 2010; 23(6): 290–297.

[228] Shivananda NB, Dan Ramdatg D, Marshall JR, Isitor G, Xue S, Shi J. Wound-healing properties of the oils of *Vitis vinifera* and *Vaccinium macrocarpon*. Phyther Res. 2011; 25(8): 1201–1208.

[229] Castola V, Bighelli A, Casanova J. Intraspecific chemical variability of the essential oil of *Pistacia lentiscus* L. from Corsica. Biochem Syst Ecol. 2000; 28(1): 79–88.

[230] Carson CF, Riley T V. Antimicrobial activity of the essential oil of *Melaleuca alternifolia*. Lett Appl Microbiol. 1993; 16(2): 49–55.

[231] Carson CF HK, Riley TV. *Melaleuca alternifolia* (tea tree) oil: a review of antimicrobial and other medicinal properties. Clin Microbiol Rev. 2006; 19(1): 50–62.

[232] Halcón L, Milkus K. *Staphylococcus aureus* and wounds: a review of tea tree oil as a promising antimicrobial. Am J Infect Control. 2004; 32(7): 402–408.

[233] Edmondson M, Newall N, Carville K, Smith J, Riley T V, Carson CF. Uncontrolled, open-label, pilot study of tea tree (*Melaleuca alternifolia*) oil solution in the decolonisation of methicillin-resistant *Staphylococcus aureus* positive wounds and its influence on wound healing. Int Wound J. 2011; 8 (4): 375–384.

[234] Carette C, Malotaux M, van Leeuwen M, Tolkamp M. Shea nut and butter in Ghana: opportunities and constraints for local processing. Rep Proj Oppor Shea Nuts North Ghana. 2009. pp. 1–88.

[235] Goreja WG. Shea Butter: The Nourishing Properties of Africa's Best-Kept Natural Beauty Secret. TNC International Inc; Stone Mountain, Georgia 2004.

[236] Wallace-Bruce S, Appleton H. Shea Butter Extraction in Ghana. Intermediate Technology Publications Ltd (ITP); London, UK 1995.

[237] Benhammou N, Bekkara FA, Panovska TK. Antioxidant and antimicrobial activities of the *Pistacia lentiscus* and *Pistacia atlantica* extracts. Afri J Pharm Pharmacol. 2008; 2(2): 22–28.

[238] Dedoussis GVZ, Kaliora AC, Psarras S, et al. Antiatherogenic effect of *Pistacia lentiscus* via GSH restoration and downregulation of CD36 mRNA expression. Atherosclerosis. 2004; 174(2): 293–303.

[239] Djerrou J, Maameri Z, Hamdo-Pacha Y, et al. Effect of virgin fatty oil of Pistacia lentiscus on experimental burn wound's healing in rabbits. Afri J Trad Complement Altern Med. 2010; 7(3): 258–263.

[240] El-Soud A, Helmy N. Honey between traditional uses and recent medicine. Maced J Med Sci. 2012; 5(2): 205–214.

[241] Al-Waili N SK, Al-Ghamdi AA. Honey for wound healing, ulcers, and burns; data supporting its use in clinical practice. Sci World J. 2011; 11: 766–787.

[242] Bang LM, Buntting C, Molan P. The effect of dilution on the rate of hydrogen peroxide production in honey and its implications for wound healing. J Altern Complement Med. 2003; 9(2): 267–273.

[243] Subrahmanyam M, Sahapure AG, Nagane NS, Bhagwat VR, Ganu J V. Effects of topical application of honey on burn wound healing. Ann Burns Fire Disasters. 2001; 14(3): 143–145.

[244] Maeda Y, Loughrey A, Earle JAP, et al. Antibacterial activity of honey against community-associated methicillin-resistant *Staphylococcus aureus* (CA-MRSA). Complement Ther Clin Pract. 2008; 14(2): 77–82.

[245] Islam A, Khalil I, Islam N, et al. Physicochemical and antioxidant properties of Bangladeshi honeys stored for more than one year. BMC Complement Altern Med. 2012; 12(1): 1.

[246] Al-Mamary M, Al-Meeri A, Al-Habori M. Antioxidant activities and total phenolics of different types of honey. Nutr Res. 2002; 22(9): 1041–1047.

[247] Alam F, Islam MA, Gan SH, Khalil MI. Honey: a potential therapeutic agent for managing diabetic wounds. Evid-Based Complement Altern Med. 2014; 2014: 16